Low-Cost Approaches to Promote Physical and Mental Health

Low-Cost Approaches to Promote Physical and Mental Health

Theory, Research, and Practice

Edited by

Luciano L'Abate
Professor Emeritus of Psychology
Georgia State University
Atlanta, Georgia

Springer

Luciano L'Abate
Georgia State University
2079 Deborah Drive
Atlanta, GA 30345-3917
Email: llabate3@bellsouth.net

Library of Congress Control Number: 2001012345

ISBN-10: 0-387-36898-1 (Hardbound)
ISBN-13: 978-0-387-36898-6 (Hardbound)
e-ISBN-10: 0-387-36899-X
e-ISBN-13: 978-0-387-36899-3

Printed on acid-free paper.

10 9 8 7 6 5 4 3 2 1

springer.com

This book is dedicated to my beloved grandchildren,
Alessandra and Ian Sterling L'Abate,
so as they grow up
they can use some of the approaches in this book
and to Dennis D. Embry, Ph.D.,
who started the ball rolling with his vaccine metaphor.

Preface

The purpose of this book is to cover the wide range of prescriptive approaches that have been found to produce noticeable and known physical, behavioral and psychological benefits with a minimum of cost and maximal mass-administration. Being possibly self-initiated and self-administrated activities, or interventions administered by others, face-to-face (f2f) contacts and talk are kept to a minimum. After learning how to use a particular activity, participants can go on their own without further contact with whoever is administering the approaches. In most cases, short written instructions may suffice.

In editing this book, to keep its focus clear and specific, there was no interest in including or overlapping with prevention-oriented approaches (Albee & Gullotta, 1997; Baum & Singer, 2001; Bloom, 1996; Camic & Knight, 1998; Dalton, Elias, & Wandersman, 2001; Gullotta & Bloom, 2003; Kessler, Goldston, & Joffe, 1992). Consequently, no prolonged and costly approaches were included, such as training in social, or psycho-educational skills, assertiveness training, or anger management. Also not included were prolonged face-to-face talk-based interactions between participants and professionals, like traditional primary, secondary, and tertiary prevention approaches, such as psychotherapy, or crisis activity. The aim was to create a new tier of promotional approaches in their own right. If these approaches are contained within what has been called primary universal prevention, so much the better.

The classification of prescriptive approaches, as defined by the Table of Contents, is completely new and cannot and will not be found anywhere else in the psychological literature, as far as this editor knows. This book is a "first" in many respects. To support this contention, one needs to compare its contents with those of other authoritative sources. For instance, its closest competitors can be found in Jason and Glenwick (2002), Bloom (1996), Norcross et al. (2000), and Gullotta & Bloom (2003). In Jason and Glenwick's book, for instance, except for a chapter about promoting mental health in later life, all chapters deal with primary and secondary prevention. It does not cover specific approaches the way we do here: Approaches covered in this volume are physical survival and mental health enjoyment as dependent variables. All the chapters in Jason and Glenwick's work are based on programs and research relying on prolonged interactions and complex methods to prevent physical and mental illness. Furthermore, none of the approaches covered in the present book are anywhere to be found in that book. Hence, the overlap between these two volumes is minimal. To make this point clear, readers will not need a research grant to implement any of the approaches covered in the present book unless they are interested in evaluating whether a particular approach works or not.

In stark contrast with programs reviewed in Jason and Glenwick, the present book contains a different set of easy-to-administer, simple-to-implement, and sufficiently concrete approaches to represent standard operating procedures repeatable from one participant to another, or from one intermediary to another, either at no cost, low cost, or cost effectively. Most of the approaches reviewed in the present book fall within the province of being administered by sub professional, para professional, or semi-professional intermediaries, by mail or through the Internet. These approaches do not address the complex outcomes of earlier preventive work, such as delinquency, homicide, child abuse, and the effects of racism, among many others. The same conclusion about complexity and length leveled about programs covered by Jason and Glenwick's book could be repeated about standard health psychology texts (Camic & Knight, 1998; Sarafino, 1994).

Bloom's (1996) contents also could be compared with this book. He *did cover* nutrition (5 pages), lifelong exercise (5 pages), and social support, mutual assistance, and self-help groups (6 pages altogether). This book devotes one chapter for each topic, bringing them up-to-date with recent research and practice.

The only overlap between the contents of this book and another text could be found in Norcross et al.'s (2000) guide. The guide covers self-help books, audio- and video-tapes, films, as well as Internet resources available for help, autobiographies and support groups. This is why we have kept self-help books, audio- and video-tapes, and films out of this volume. However, various structures of writing (Section IV this volume) including self-help workbooks, were not contained in Norcross et al. The research to demonstrate the usefulness of many resources reviewed in this "authoritative guide" is limited, questionable, and not very encouraging. We hope to do a better job in two overlapping areas, autobiographies (Chapter 12 this volume) and support groups (Chapter 23 this volume).

Another distinction between prescriptive approaches, as defined here, and traditional primary preventive approaches, as commonly practiced (Gullotta & Bloom, 2003), must be made. Traditionally, preventive approaches have been intended to *avoid* negative behaviors, as found, for instance, among high-risk populations, addicts, abusers, and criminals. To use Jason and Glenwick's (2002) work as a representative example of such primary prevention practices, 10 of their 15 chapters were related to preventing physical and sexual abuse; school failure; delinquency and antisocial behavior; depression in youth; alcohol, tobacco, and other substance abuse; HIV and AIDS; chronic health problems; marital disorder; and racism and sexism. Even chapters devoted to promoting effective parenting practices, mental health in later life, and healthy communities through community development presented rather complex programs that at first blush appear difficult to replicate unless a research grant is obtained.

Another example of a competing source can be found in Gullotta and Bloom's (2003) encyclopedic work on primary prevention and health promotion. In this work, preventive and promotional approaches seem to overlap without any clear delineation and differentiation between promotion and prevention. Even one chapter devoted exclusively to a brief history and analysis of "health promotion" (Bingenheimer, Repetto, Zimmerman, & Kelly, 2003), or another chapter on theories of prevention and promotion (Silverman, 2003) included physical diseases and their prevention. Furthermore, most contents of the whole work included few positive conditions to promote prevention, such as: academic success, five chapters devoted to creativity across the entire life span, environmental health, strengthening families, health promotion in older adulthood, identity promotion in adolescence, marital enhancement and satisfaction, five chapters on nutrition over the entire life cycle, four chapters on parenting over the life cycle, perceived personal control, physical fitness, four chapters on religion and spirituality over the life cycle, resilience, self-esteem, social competency in adolescence, and three chapters on social and emotional learning in early childhood, childhood, and adolescence, and sports. These chapters composed about one third of the topics reviewed.

The major difference between Gullotta and Bloom's (2003) work and the present classification lies in their considering topics by the nature of the behaviors to be prevented, while the classification presented in the present work is by replicable methods to promote physical and mental health in functional populations. Very few, if any, methods to promote physical and mental health were included in Gullotta and Bloom (2003). Hence, the aims of the present classification are different from those found in the prevention literature, including Gullotta and Bloom, among others. The latter, encyclopedic treatise, covers any possible condition known to date. However, it differs from this book in several ways:

1. Their encyclopedia fails to distinguish between primary prevention and health promotion, and lumps them together as if they were synonymous. There is no clear line of demarcation between promotion and prevention, as achieved in this book.
2. Their encyclopedia is organized around topics to be prevented, rather than methods, and lumps together positive as well as negative conditions. For instance, creativity, religion and spirituality,

among other positive topics, are included without distinction with the bulk of the book that deals with negative topics, like abuse, criminality, etc.

3. By dealing with topics to be prevented, their encyclopedia fails to stress the importance of no-cost or low-cost methods to promote physical and mental health. As already noted, positive and negative topics are lumped together without distinguishing, as we do, between primary prevention versus health promotion. For instance, it is difficult, if not impossible to know which methods of prevention have been used, if any. Admittedly, we do separate between Part I, Physical, and Part II, Mental Health, strictly to break down the two parts. We know full well that a demarcating line between the physical and mental is artificial and no longer sustainable, conceptually as well as empirically.
4. In their encyclopedia, no attention is given to costs, in spite of having a whole chapter on cost-effectiveness analysis. Traditional lengthy and complex prevention approaches are included that are difficult, if not impossible to replicate without external funding. Indeed, there is a whole chapter devoted to financing primary prevention and health promotion, definitely very important and relevant topics for prevention but not for promotion.
5. In their book, one chapter devoted entirely to health promotion covers diseases that have been effectively reduced by a variety of physical means, like medication, exercise and diet. Hence, the distinction was not made between promotion to approach and augment health and prevention to avoid and decrease risks of disease.

Hence, there is little if any overlap between the contents of the present book and the monumental encyclopedia by Gullotta and Bloom (2003) that represents a milestone in the progress of prevention of mental illness.

In sum, as far as prevention goes, all the approaches reviewed in selected sources are based on *prolonged rather than short-lived*, low-cost approaches. Many programs used in most prevention or community programs covered in those references will not be replicated. They cost too much. For instance, many promising and interesting preventive programs covered in these references have not been replicated, as far as this writer knows. Most preventive programs receive support from research grants and from the federal government. Consequently these and other preventive programs found in the edited books cited above are limited to researchers who qualify for external funds. If funds are limited, these programs do not occur. None of the approaches we cover here need grant money. They can be implemented with very little monetary investment if any.

Furthermore, many texts cited here and elsewhere in the present book are no longer up-to-date with the conclusions of the New Freedom Commission on Mental Health (2003) or the recommendations of the Surgeon General of the United States by the Department of Health and Human Welfare (U.S. Public Health Service Office of the Surgeon General, 1999) about mental health and prevention. Both reports either ignore prevention altogether or leave it to future efforts, let alone promotion. Most, if not all, approaches covered in this volume require a minimum of external support.

Intended Audiences

The intended, primary audience for this book includes professionals, teachers and researchers who subscribe to a public health rather than to a private health ideology. Even in the latter case, these approaches might convince professionals in clinical practices to prescribe as many approaches reviewed here to couple with face-to-face talk-based approaches. These approaches can be administered by practically anybody, volunteers, graduate students, practitioners, and researchers in the mental health helping professions (clinical psychology, psychiatry, social work, marriage and family therapy, school counseling). Professionals in prevention, psychotherapy, and rehabilitation, as well as graduate students and professionals in related disciplines, such as nutrition, sports, physical education, and leisure time activities, could conceivably profit by using the approaches reviewed in this book.

The Need for Theory to Account for Practice

Contributors to each chapter of this book were allowed complete freedom to link their specific approaches to whatever conceptual or theoretical framework or model best suited that activity. What about a theoretical framework that would account for the field of health promotion as contained in this book?

As noted above, while prescriptive approaches are directed toward the *approach* of positive low-cost activities to increase physical and mental health, most preventive efforts are directed toward the reduction and *avoidance* of mental illness. This important distinction finds its theoretical basis in Higgins' (1998) seminal distinction that leads to further theoretical expansions, especially in the area of motivation (Elliot & Church, 1997; Elliot & Covington, 2001; Impett, Peplau, & Gable, 2005). A dimension based mostly on *distance*, and defined by extremes in approach-avoidance, therefore, forms the basis for communal/expressive relationships based on closeness (love, care, concern, and compassion) covered in some ways in Section V of this book. By the same token, another dimension, based on *control*, and defined by extremes in discharge-delay, forms the basis for agentic/instrumental relationships covered in some ways in Section VI of this volume, involving bargaining, problem-solving, and negotiation (L'Abate, 2005). This distinction finds its physiological counterparts in Gray's (1987) distinction between appetitive activation and aversive inhibition (Gable, Reis, & Elliot, 2000). Chapter 1 expands on this distinction while this distinction is expanded at a biological level elsewhere (L'Abate, 2006).

Above and beyond theoretical distinctions, the notion of prescriptive approaches used in this book is in line with approaches based on positive psychology. Indeed, this notion finds its validation in positive psychology. For instance, self-help exercises, administered through the Internet and lasting a few minutes a day for one week, produced effects lasting up to six months in two out of five exercises. Writing about three good things that happened in one day and using signature strengths of character each day, showed that these exercises indeed performed as vaccines, that is, they were: (1) easily self-administered, (2) economical to administer to a large mass of participants, and (3) produced significant effects that lasted for some time (Seligman, Steen, Park, & Peterson, 2005).

Organization of the Book

The first section serves as an historical introduction with a chapter devoted to distinguishing promotion from prevention approaches (Chapter 1, L'Abate). Even though there is a very thin line between physical and mental health, for purposes of classification, the first part of this book focuses on approaches that are primarily related to physical health, such as nutrition and physical activities. In the first section nutritional approaches cover diets and weight control (David Katz et al., Chapter 3) and the current obesity epidemic (Chapter 4, Finke and Huston). Omega-3 fatty acids require a Chapter 4 of their own because of the amount of research devoted to their benefits (Umhau and Dauphinais).

In Chapter 5 Edward Giovannucci covers the vitamins, minerals and supplements most beneficial to most consumers. Along the same lines, in Chapter 6, Sharin Akhondzadeh explores how simple, inexpensive herbal medicines help in treating psychiatric and neurological disorders. At this point the reader may ask why this chapter was included since it involves "treatment of diseases" rather than promotion of health. This editor feels justified in including this chapter for the very simple reason that "herbal medicines" are available to practically everybody without a medical prescription. Consequently, they follow within the rubric of "low-cost prescriptive approaches."

Section III covers secondary approaches related to motoric, nonverbal vaccines. In Chapter 7, Calogero and Pedrotty discuss their original distinction between "mindless" and "mindful" exercise, a very important distinction that they follow up with very clear guidelines. In Chapter 8, Angele McGrady covers relaxation, meditation, and related techniques, like mindlessness, imagery, and acceptance. In Chapter 9, Dianne Dulicai and Schelly Hill cover expressive movements, as seen in dancing. In Chapter 10, Joan S. Anderson covers pleasant, pleasurable, and positive activities in relation to their health benefits.

The second part covers approaches that impact more directly on mental health. Section IV includes secondary approaches based strictly on writing. In Chapter 11, Minna Levine and Ronald Calvanio review what in the past might have been called journaling and diaries but which now implies recording of personal information as an activity and as electronic health support. In Chapter 12, Duccio Demetrio and Chiara Borgonovi cover autobiographical methodology that involves more than just requiring participants to simply "Write your autobiography." It takes more than this instruction to write an autobiography. In Chapter 13, Ewa Kacewicz, Richard Slatcher, and James W. Pennebaker et al. cover what has now become known as the "Pennebaker paradigm" formerly known also as "Expressive Writing." In Chapter 14, Luciano L'Abate and Demian Goldstein review application of workbooks to promote mental health and life-long learning. They confront the paradox that in outpatient therapy, workbooks seem to prolong the number of sessions while in a hospital, workbooks seem to reduce the number of days spent there. In Chapter 15, Myron Pulier, Tim Mount, Joe McMenamin, and Marlene Mahue review the revolutionary effects that computers and the Internet already have had and will have on our lives.

Section V includes secondary relational approaches, where an interaction between two or more human beings is involved. In Chapter 16, Ruth Feldman reviews parent-infant skin-to-skin contact as a contributor to physical, cognitive, social, and emotional growth. In Chapter 17, Nancy Aaron Jones and Krystal Mize review the research evidence from normative and at-risk groups about how tactile stimulation and massage positively affect development. In the same vein, in Chapter 18, Andrew K. Gulledge, Michael Hill, Zephon Lister, and Carolyn Sallion review how close, nonsexual physical contact, like affection, leads directly to mental and physical benefits. In Chapter 19, Chad Cross and Gerald Weeks survey whether sex, sexuality and sensuality show any demonstrable physical and mental benefits, while in Chapter 20 Anita Vangelisti and Gary Beck demonstrate the benefits of intimacy and the costs of avoiding it, especially when intimacy is defined as the sharing of joys and hurts. In Chapter 21, Lindsey Root and Michael McCullough review low-cost approaches to promote forgiveness and its connection to physiological concomitants. Closely allied but still separate from forgiveness lies the difficult area of spirituality covered in Chapter 22 by Leonard Sperry, Louis Hoffman, Richard H. Cox, and Betty Ervin Cox. In Chapter 23 by Patricia M. Sias with Heidi Bartoo survey how friendships and social support show direct links to physical and mental health.

Section VI consists of tertiary approaches that involve the presence of more than two individuals. In Chapter 24, Luciano L'Abate reviews the widespread use of animal companions and their effects on mental and physical health. In Chapter 25 David Ryback and Laura Sweeney survey applications of emotional intelligence in the classroom and the workplace.

In the final Section VI and conclusive Chapter 26, Cornelius Hogan shows with direct applications how prescriptive approaches do promote physical health with serious implications for policy, promotional, epidemiological, and public health ideologies and approaches.

Luciano L'Abate
April 30, 2006

References

Albee, G. W., & Gullotta, T. P. (Eds.). (1997). *Primary prevention works*. Thousand Oaks, CA: Sage.

Baum, A., & Singer, J. (Eds.). (2001). *Book of health psychology*. Mahwah, NJ: LEA.

Bingenheimer, J. B., Repetto, P. B., Zimmerman, M. A., & Kelly, J. G. (2003). A brief history and analysis of health promotion. In T. Gullotta, & M. Bloom (Eds.), *Encyclopedia of primary prevention and health promotion* (pp. 23–26). New York: Kluwer Academic.

Bloom, M. (1996). *Primary prevention practices*. Thousand Oaks, CA: Sage.

Camic, P., & Knight, S. (Eds.). (1998). *Clinical handbook of health psychology*. Seattle, WA: Hogrefe & Huber.

Dalton, J. H., Elias, M. J., & Wandersman, A. (2001). *Community psychology: Linking individuals with communities*. Belmont, CA: Wadsworth/Thompson Learning.

Elliot, A. J., & Church, M. A. (1997). A hierarchical model of approach and avoidance achievement motivation. *Journal of Personality and Social Psychology, 72*, 218–232.

Elliot, A. J., & Covington, M. V. (2001). Approach and avoidance motivation. *Educational Psychology, 13*, 73–92.

Gable, S. L., Reis, S. T., & Elliot, A. J. (2000). Behavioral activation and inhibition in everyday life. *Journal of Personality and Social Psychology, 78*, 1135–1149.

Gray, J. (1987). *The psychology of fear and stress*. New York: Cambridge University Press.

Gullotta, T. P., & Bloom, M. (Eds.). (2003). *Encyclopedia of primary prevention and health promotion*. New York: Kluwer Academic.

Higgins, E. T. (1998). Promotion and prevention: Regulatory focus of a motivational principle. *Advances in Experimental Social Psychology, 30*, 1–46.

Impett, E. A., Peplau, L. A., & Gable, S. L. (2005). Approach and avoidance sexual motives: Implications for personal and interpersonal well-being. *Personal Relationships, 12*, 465–482.

Jason, L. A., & Glenwick, D. S. (2002). Introduction: An overview of preventive and ecological perspectives. In L. A. Jason, & D. S. Glenwick (Eds.), *Innovative strategies for promoting health and mental health across the life span* (pp. 3–16). New York: Springer.

Kessler, M., Goldston, S. E., & Joffe (Eds.). (1992). *The present and future of prevention: In honor of George W. Albee*. Newbury Park, CA: Sage.

L'Abate, L. (2005). *Personality in intimate relationships: Socialization and psychopathology*. New York: Springer.

L'Abate, L. (2006). Toward a relational theory for psychiatric classification. *American Journal of Family Therapy*, 34, 1–15.

New Freedom Commission on Mental Health (2003). *Achieving the promise: Transforming mental healthcare in America: Executive summary*. Rockville, MD: DHHS Publication No. SMA-03-3831.

Norcross, J. C., Santrock, J. W., Campbell, L. F., Smith, T. P., Sommer, R., & Zuckerman, E. L. (2000). *Authoritative guide to self-help resources in mental health*. New York: Guilford.

Sarafino, F. P. (1994). *Health psychology: Biosocial approaches*. New York: Wiley.

Seligman, M. E. P., Steen, T. A., Park, N., & Peterson, C. (2005). Positive psychology progress: Empirical validation of approaches. *American Psychologist, 60*, 410–421.

Silverman, M. M. (2003). Theories of primary prevention and health promotion. In T. Gullotta, & M. Bloom (Eds.), *Encyclopedia of primary prevention and health promotion* (pp. 27–41). New York: Kluwer Academic.

United States Public Health Service Office of the Surgeon General (1999). *Mental health: A report of the Surgeon General*. Rockville, MD: Department of Health and Human Services.

Acknowledgements

I am grateful to Susan Milmoe, formerly with Lawrence Erlbaum Associates (LEA), who accepted the initial proposal with enthusiasm and support. Her successor at LEA, Steven Ritter (now with Routledge Publications), was equal to the task of supporting me throughout the gestation of the whole volume. He was very helpful in paying special attention to the introductory chapter and keeping me focused on what needed to be done throughout a whole year. Grazie mille, Steve (he speaks Italian!).

I am very grateful to my long-time friend and editor, Sharon Panulla, Executive Editor at Springer, and to Janice Stern, Health and Behavior Editor, for their quick and enthusiastic acceptance of this volume and for helping me with a difficult first chapter. I am also indebted to Natacha Menar, who offered her editing assistance, above and beyond what is expected from her position.

Last but not least, I am grateful to the collaborators of this volume. They seemed to understand from the outset what I was trying to accomplish and responded to my editorial requests with speed and graciousness. It was a distinct pleasure and honor to work with such a distinguished group of collaborators. I am very proud of their contribution and to have them as my colleagues.

Contents

List of Contributors

* denotes lead authorship

Shahin Akhondzadeh, Ph.D., Professor of Clinical Neuropharmacology, Psychiatric Research Center, Roozbeth Hospital, Tehran University of Medical Sciences, South Kargar Street, Tehran 13185, Iran. Address Correspondence to: No: 29, 39th Street, Gisha Street, Tehran 14479, Iran, s.akhond@neda.net

Joan S. Anderson, Ph.D., Independent Practice, Apt. C, 1714 Nantucket Drive, Houston, TX 77057-2977, JSidney@aol.com

Heidi Bartoo, M.A., Doctoral candidate, Department of Communication, University of Vermont, hbartoo:uvm.edu

Gary Beck, M.A., Department of Communication Studies, 1 University Station, A110 University of Texas at Austin, Austin, TX 78712-1105, garyb@utexas.edu

Chiara Borgonovi, Ph.D. in philosophy and Ph.D. candidate and instructor in pedagogical sciences, University of Milano-Bicocca, chiara.borgonovi@unimib.it

* Rachel Calogero, M.A., Post-doctoral student in Social Psychology, Part-Time Teacher, University of Kent at Canterbury, UK; Address: 64 London Road, Canterbury, Kent, UK, CT2 8Jzi, rmcalogero@hotmail.com

Ronald Calvanio, Ph.D., SymTrend, Inc., 89 Bay State Rd., Belmont, MA 02478-0002, see Minna Levine

Betty Ervin Cox, Ph.D., Dean of Students, Colorado School of Professional Psychology 555 E. Pikes Peak Ave, #108, Colorado Springs, CO 80922, ervin-cox@cospp.edu

Richard H. Cox, Ph.D., M.D., D.Min, Provost, Colorado School of Professional Psychology; 555 E. Pikes Peak Ave, #108; Colorado Springs, CO 80922, cox@cospp.edu

* Chad. L. Cross, Ph.D., N.C.C., Associate Professor of Biostatistics Director, Program in Epidemiology & Biostatistics, School of Public Health, University of Nevada, Las Vegas 4505 Maryland Parkway, M/S 3063; Las Vegas, NV 89154-3063, Chad.Cross@ccmail.nevada.edu

Karl M. Dauphinais, M.D., Yale Primary Care Internal Medicine, Chase Outpatient Center, 140 Grandview Ave, Waterbury, CT; Home Address: 78 Cove St #1; New Haven, CT 06512, kdauphinais@yahoo.com

* Duccio Demetrio, Ph.D., Professor of Philosophy of Education, University of Milano-Bicocca, Piazza Ateneo Nuovo, 1, Milano 20149, Italy; Founder of Free University of Autobiography, Anghiari (Arezzo, Italy), duccio.demetrio@unimib.it

Dianne Dulicai, Ph.D., A.D.T.R., Founder and Senior Consultant, Hahnemann-Drexel Dance/Movement Therapy Program, Drexel University; 7700 Willowbrook Rd. Fairfax Station, VA 22039, dianne.dulicai@cox.net

Ruth Feldman, Ph.D., Department of Psychology and Gonda Brain Sciences Center, Bar-Ilan University, Ramat-Gan, Israel 52900, feldman@biu.ac.il

* Michael S. Finke, Ph.D., Assistant Professor, Department of Consumer and Family Economics, 239 Stanley Hall, University of Missouri, Columbia, MO 65211, FinkeM@Missouri.edu

Edward Giovannucci, M.D., Ph.D., Harvard University School of Public Health, 665 Huntington Avenue, Boston, MA 02115l, edward.giocannucci@channing.harvard.edu

Demian F. Goldstein, Licensed Psychologist, JUNKAL 1221, 6th, Buenos Aires 1062, Argentina, cognitas@fibertel.com.ar

* Andrew K. Gulledge, M.S., 117 Corsica Dr., Newport Beach, CA 92660, akgulledge@hotmail.com, Andrew@CaliforniaMarriages.org

Ellen Schelly Hill, A.D.T.R., M.M.T., N.C.C., L.P.C.; Director, Dance/movement Therapy Section, Hahnemann-Drexel Creative Arts Therapy Department; work address: Hahnemann-Drexel University, Creative Arts Therapy Department, M.S. 501; College of Nursing and Health Professions; 245 N. 15th Street, Philadelphia, PA 19102, es42@drexel.edu

Michael Hill, M.A., Oklahoma State University, 3242 208th St. EastFaribault, MN 55021, michaeltthill@yahoo.com

Louis Hoffman, Ph.D.; Acting Dean of Faculty; Core Faculty, Colorado School of Professional Psychology; 555 E. Pikes Peak Ave, #108, Colorado Springs, CO 80922, hoffman@cospp.edu

Cornelius Hogan, Sr. Fellow, Center for the Study of Social Policy, Washington, DC. Home Office Address; 324 Gouyeau Rd., Plainfield, VT 05665, chogan@conhogan.com

Sandra J. Huston, Ph.D., Assistant Professor, Consumer and Family Economics, University of Missouri-Columbia, Columbia, MO, Sandra.huston@ttu.edu

* Nancy Aaron Jones, Ph.D., Infant Behavior and Development Center, Florida Atlantic University; 5353 Parkside Drive, Jupiter, FL 33458, njones@fau.edu

Ewa Kacewicz, B.A., Department of Psychology, University of Texas at Austin, Austin, TX 78712, see James Pennebaker

* David L. Katz, M.D., M.P.H., F.A.C.P.M., F.A.C.P., Associate Clinical Professor of Epidemiology & Public Health, Director, Prevention Research Center Yale University School of Medicine, Griffin Hospital, 130 Division Street, Derby, CT 06418, katzdl@pol.net

* Luciano L'Abate, Ph.D., Professor Emeritus of Psychology, Georgia State University. Address correspondence to: 2079 Deborah Drive, Atlanta, GA 30345-3917, llabate3@bellsouth.net

* Minna Levine, Ph. D., SymTrend, Inc., 89 Bay State Rd., Belmont, MA 02478-0002, mlevine@symtrend.com

Zephon Lister, M.A., M.S., Loma Linda University, 7848 Wisteria Ct. Highland, CA 92346, buddyz00@hotmail.com

Marlene M. Maheu, Ph.D., 6987 Ridge Manor Ave., San Diego, CA 92120-3146, drmm@cox.net

Michael E. McCullough, Ph.D., Department of Psychology, University of Miami, P.O. Box 248185, Office: 437 Flipse Building, Coral Gables, FL 33124-2070, mikem@miami.edu

Angele McGrady, Ph.D., M.Ed., LPCC, Professor, Department of Psychiatry, Director, Complementary Medicine Center, Medical College of Ohio, 3120 Glendale Ave. Toledo, Ohio 43614, amcgrady@meduohio.edu

Joseph P. McMenamin, J.D., McGuire Woods, LLP, One James Center, 901 E Cary St. Richmond, VA 23219-4030, jmcmenamin@mcguirewoods.com

Krystal D. Mize, B. A., Florida Atlantic University, 5353 Parkside Drive, Jupiter, FL 33458, see Nancy Jones

Timothy G. Mount, 6207 Caminito Andreta, San Diego, CA 92111, tmount@cox.net

Meghan O'Connell, M.P.H., Senior Research Associate, Yale-Griffin Prevention Research Center, Griffin Hospital, 130 Division Street, Derby, CT 06418, meghan.oconnell@yalegriffinprc.org

Kelly Pedrotty, M.S., Delaware County Intermediate Unit, The Refrew Center, Philadelphia, PA. Address: 124 Wood St., Conshohocken, PA 19428, kpedrotty@dciu.org

* James W. Pennebaker, Ph.D., Professor and Chair, Psychology Department, University of Texas, Austin, TX 78712, pennebaker@psy.utexas.edu

* Myron L. Pulier, M.D., Clinical Associate Professor of Psychiatry, UMDNJ-NJ Medical School 800 W End Ave #13E, New York, NY 10025-5467, pulierml@umdnj.edu

* Lindsey M. Root, Graduate Assistant, Department of Psychology, University of Miami, P.O. Box 248185, Coral Gables, FL 33124-2070, see Michael McCullough

* David Ryback, Ph.D., President, EQAssociates, 1534 N. Decatur Rd., Atlanta, GA, 30324, Eqassoc@aol.com

Carolyn Sallion, M.F.T.T., M.P.H., R.N., Loma Linda University, PO Box 432; Loma Linda, CA 92354, see Andrew K. Gulledge

* Patricia M. Sias, Ph.D., Professor, Edward R. Morrow School of Communication, Washington State University, Pullman, WA 99164-2520, psias@wsu.edu

Richard B. Slatcher, M.A., Department of Psychology, University of Texas at Austin, Austin, TX 78712, see James Pennebaker

* Len Sperry, M.D., Ph.D., Professor and Coordinator of Doctoral Program in Counseling, Florida Atlantic University; and Clinical Professor of Psychiatry, Medical College of Wisconsin; 777 Glades Road, Boca Raton, FL 33431, Lsperry@fau.edu

Laura Sweeney, Ed.D., 1018 Autumn Trace, Monroe, GA 30656, laurainmonroe@aol.com

* John C. Umhau, M.D., M.P.H., Senior Clinical Investigator, Laboratory of Clinical Studies, National Institutes of Health, National Institute on Alcohol Abuse and Alcoholism; 10 Center Drive, Building 10-CRC, Hatfield Center, Room 1-5330, MSC 1108; Bethesda, MD, 20892-1108, johnu@lcs.niaaa.nih.gov

* Anita L. Vangelisti, Ph.D., Department of Communication Studies, 1 University Station, A1105; University of Texas at Austin, Austin, TX 78712-1105, a.vangelisti@utexas.edu

Gerald R. Weeks, Ph.D., Professor & Chair, Department of Counseling, University of Nevada at Las Vegas, 4505 Maryland Parkway, Box 453045; Las Vegas, NV 89154-3045, gweeks@univ.nevada.edu

Ming-Chin Yeh, Ph.D., Assistant Professor, Nutrition and Food Science Track Program in Urban Public Health, Hunter College, City University of New York, 425 East 25th Street, New York, NY 10010, myeh@hunter.cuny.edu

Section I

Introduction

The introductory chapter in this section will review the field of health promotion as clearly distinguished from sickness prevention. Up to now, health promotion has been the Cinderella of prevention, not receiving what prevention has received with the lion share of academic research, federal support, and research grants. This neglect was due to the inadequate definition of the field of health promotion and especially mental health promotion. If a field is not defined or ill-defined by its own approaches, how can it be defined?

This chapter will argue for health promotion constituting a tier of approaches well defined by their low cost included in this book. By creating a new tier of its own, the health promotion approaches included here will allow health promoters, sickness preventers, psychotherapists, and primary health professionals to expand their repertoires according to a successive sieves approach to healthcare, suggested years ago (L'Abate, 1990). Depending on the level of functionality, this approach begins with the least expensive sieve progressing to more expensive sieves, going from promotion first, then to prevention, and from prevention to treatment. Hence, the contents of this book constitute a dream come true, a dream started more than a quarter of a century ago.

Reference

L'Abate, L. (1990). *Building family competence: Primary and secondary prevention strategies*. Newbury Park, CA: Sage.

1

Low-Cost Approaches to Promote Physical and Mental Health

Luciano L'Abate

The purpose of this edited work is to present and review low-cost or cost-effective, large scale, mass-oriented approaches to promote physical and mental health. These approaches can be implemented with a minimum of bureaucratic obstacles or research grants. Hence, this book means to advance the importance of self-administered, economical, and long-lasting, evidence-based prescriptive approaches that have been demonstrated to promote physical and mental health. These approaches include all three modes of communication: talk, motor or nonverbal (including nutrition), and writing (L'Abate, 1990, 1997, 1999).

The purpose of this chapter is to introduce the notion of "prescriptive, promotional approaches" for low-cost or cost-effective approaches included in this book. Prescriptive means some type of instruction, as short as a sentence and as long as a recipe in a cookbook, given through any channel of communication. The purpose of each prescription is to indicate how and how much the interventional approaches should be used, their dosage, frequency, rate, and duration or possible side-effects, if any. With some approaches these instructions are not even necessary, as in support-self-help groups, for instance.

Prescriptive, promotional approaches mean simple, concrete, easily replicable activities or operations that can be self-initiated and self-administered, or interventions administered to large populations with minimum costs and maximum benefits. By the same token, approaches included in this volume intend to make people more refractory to physical and mental illnesses by making them more resilient and less liable to become physically or mentally "sick". Therefore, "promotional" and "prescriptive" will be used interchangeably.

The major conceptual and practical distinction between prescriptive approaches that promote physical and mental health lies in their being different from traditional preventive approaches. The former stress *approach* toward positive habits and behaviors from the outset. The latter try to help people avoid or give up already existing negative habits and behaviors. Prescriptive approaches lie in the promotion and strengthening of physical and mental health in the general population. Prevention attempts to decrease or even eliminate the effects of negative behaviors in targeted populations. Primary prevention wants to *avoid* destructive and hurtful behaviors from augmenting and spreading even further in at-risk populations (Gullotta & Bloom, 2003).

Hence, prescriptive approaches constitute a tier of their own in stressing physical and mental health promotion, earlier and even before primary, secondary, or tertiary prevention, even though terms like promotion and prevention are used interchangeably in basic textbooks (Gullotta & Bloom, 2003) or lead articles (Weisz, Sandler, Durlak, & Anton, 2005). Therefore, one way to define and differentiate approaches to promote physical and mental health from preventive approaches is to apply the notion of prescriptive promotions. Health promotion is a completely different tier of approaches usually included in primary, secondary, and tertiary prevention, as discussed in the Preface of this volume. The purpose of approaches included in this work is definitely focused on *promotion of health* rather than on *prevention of disease*. These promotional, prescriptive approaches, of course, can be inserted, incorporated, and added into primary, secondary, and tertiary prevention, including psychotherapeutic and medical interventions to obtain synergistic outcomes.

An important issue, relating to the simplicity, concreteness, and ease of administration of promotional approaches relates to their replicability. This advantage speaks to the core of preventive programs reviewed in most references cited in the Preface and elsewhere in this chapter. In addition to their relying on external funding for implementation, because of their complexity and prolonged, f2f verbal contacts between participants and professionals, many preventive approaches thus far implemented have failed to demonstrate integrity (Dane & Schneider, 1998). Integrity means that their complexity makes it difficult to rely on treatment protocols that are replicable from one setting to another. Promotional approaches, on the other hand, are easily replicable with low-cost, or minimum cost and few, if any side-effects. Indeed, there may be many side-benefits. For instance, improved physical health may improve mental health. By the same token, improvements in mental health may lead toward greater attention to physical health. If costs are involved, they occur at the beginning of the learned activity, rather than throughout its prolongation.

A difference between promotional approaches and traditional preventive approaches may lie in when the intervention occurs. Ideally, these approaches should be administered *before* behaviors deteriorate. Traditional preventive approaches sometimes occur either during or after negative, identified and targeted behaviors have already deteriorated. Whether this distinction holds up conceptually and empirically remains to be seen. Nonetheless, this distinction may help toward a supplementary classification and expansion of primary prevention to a separate tier of prescriptive, promotional approaches.

Excluded from this definition is any form of intervention i.e., prolonged, expensive, that requires f2f contact and talk between participants and professionals (L'Abate, in press). F2f talk still remains the major if not the only medium of communication and healing, not only in psychotherapy, but even in preventive practices (Albee & Gullotta, 1997; De Maria, 2003; Gullotta & Bloom, 2003). Approaches with a protracted exchange of money over time are also excluded, including money supplied by participants themselves or by supporting agencies, like third party payments, managed care, insurance companies, and external support. In addition to costs and difficulties in replicability, traditional preventive approaches that tend to avoid negative self-other habits or behaviors are also excluded, such as protracted psycho-educational and social skills training programs (L'Abate & Milan, 1985).

Consequently, psychotherapy is excluded, as well as its offshoots such as bibliotherapy, for instance, where confounds between effects of self-help books and personal contact with a therapist have not yet been disentangled (Gregory, Schwer-Canning, Lee, & Wise, 2004). Even though these approaches might have demonstrable and demonstrated benefits, they are centered around prolonged relationships between participants and professionals, based on exchange of money. Consequently, they are expensive, and inaccessible to large sections of our populations. Furthermore, they are designed to avoid dysfunctionalities rather than approach and promote functionalities.

Additionally, psychotherapies are difficult to replicate and vary from one therapist to another, making their preventive application difficult if not impossible. This exclusion in no way means to eliminate prolonged f2f talk-based contacts between participants and professionals, any more than it would eliminate medical approaches or even medications from being administered. All three approaches, medical, preventive, and psychotherapeutic, when needed, can and should work together synergistically with promotional approaches to improve physical and mental health in as many people as possible.

One important aspect of prescriptive approaches relates to their being used voluntarily, while preventive and therapeutic approaches require some degree of immediate need, not necessarily shared by promotional activities. The latter are based on a long-term view of results, like mortality, while preventive and therapeutic interventions, can only assess short-term effects, at the most after six months or at best one year. Prescriptive approaches, on the other hand, because of their simplicity, concreteness, and ease of administration, can be administered by nonprofessional laypersons and subprofessionals, not by professionals. These approaches should last a lifetime.

The greater the functionality the greater is the need for promotional self-initiated and self-administered activities or activities administered by a hierarchy of personnel at various levels of education, including laypersons (see Table 1.1). The greater the dysfunctionality the greater is the need for semi- and full-fledged professional interventions. In health promotion, professionals could fulfill advisory, supervisory, supportive, and research roles according to a hierarchical structure found in the realities of business, commerce, medicine, law, and industry (see Table 1.2). Doctorate-level professionals alone will not be sufficient to deal with the sheer numbers and functions needed to implement promotional and preventive approaches necessary for the immense numbers of people in need of help, as discussed below. A hierarchical structure of personnel is necessary (L'Abate, 1990, 2002; Table 1.2) if we ever hope to make a dent in the growing physical and mental health problems that are besetting our nation, as indicated by the New Freedom Commission on Mental Health (2003) and earlier by the Surgeon General's Report on Mental Health (United States Public Health Service, 1999).

Consequently, the purpose of this book is to gather, under one cover evidence necessary to support the existence and growth of the field of physical and mental health promotion to justify its existence. By the same token, the notion of health promotion in public health requires that completely different

Table 1.1. Criteria to differentiate and discriminate among preventive approaches.*

Criteria	Types of Approaches Primary Proactive Pretherapeutic	Secondary Para-active Paratherapeutic	Tertiary Reactive Therapeutic
1. Risk	Low to minimal	High: in need but not critical	Very high: critical
2. Reversibility	High: 100% to 33%	Medium 33% to 66%	Low to very low 66% to 0%.
3. Probability of breakdown	Low but potential	Medium but probable	High and real
4. Population	Nonclinical and not diagnosable	Preclinical and diagnosable	Clinical: critical and diagnosed
5. Ability to learn	High	Medium	Low
6. Goals	Increase competence and resistance to breakdown	Decrease stress and chance of crisis	Restore to minimal functioning
7. Type of involvement	Voluntary: Many choices	Obligatory: Decrease in choices	Mandatory: No other choices available
8. Recommendation	"Could benefit by it." "It would be nice."	"You need it before, it's too late" "Recommend strongly that you do it."	"It is necessary." "Nothing else will work." "Other choices would be more expensive (i.e. hospitalization, incarceration)."
9. Cost	Low	Medium	High
10. Effectiveness	High (?)	Questionable yet to be found	Relatively low
11. Personnel	Lay volunteers and pre-paraprofessionals	Middle-level professionals	Professionals
12. Types of interventions	General, learning, strengthening, enrichment	More specific to behavior, programmed materials	Specialized therapies
13. Degree of structure	High	Medium	Low
14. Degree of specificity	General and topical	Individualized	Specific to the symptom

Source: From L'Abate (1990). Reprinted with permission.

specialized professionals might be needed (L'Abate, 2005c). Promotional approaches require a whole hierarchy of professionals, semi-professionals, volunteer paraprofessionals, and laypersonnel working at a distance from participants through various media, including computers and the Internet among others, as discussed later in this chapter (see Chapter 15 in this volume).

What growing physical and mental problems are besetting our nation? We will need to look at them squarely in the face without denying their severity and their widespread presence.

Facing the Present Reality

There are at least four disparate areas that make up the reality of pervasive social disorders we are presently facing. They need all the possible

Table 1.2. Toward a hierarchy of mental health personnel.

Educational level	Skills and responsibilities
Board diplomate	Directorship and major responsibility for leadership. Support and supervision of doctorate level professionals. Research and personnel management skills. Knowledge of skills requited at various educational levels.
Doctorate	Crisis intervention. Decision making to discriminate among promotional, preventive, and psychotherapeutic interventions. Treatment plans based on conclusions from evaluation (history, objective tests, diagnosis). Supervision and support of master-level personnel. Quality control, maintenance of ethical, professional, and scientific standards.
Master or equivalent degree	Responsibility to oversee, support, and encourage volunteers and paraprofessional personnel in promotional and preventive. Direct face-to-face, talk based interventions.
Bachelor or equivalent degree	Administration of promotional and preventive activities, including administration and feedback of homework assignments. Technical skills.
High school diploma	Administration and scoring of standard test and clerical responsibilities.

Source: Adapted from L'Abate (2002, p. 230).

promotional, preventive, therapeutic, medical, community, and epidemiological approaches that we can muster. They are mental disorders, addictions, criminalities, and poverties, disabilities, and disenfranchisements.

Mental Disorders

To make sure that this reality is free of interpretation and possible distortions, it is presented *verbatim* from its original sources. These sources are in the public domain (National Institute of Mental Health, 2001). In the USA, mental disorders are diagnosed based on the Diagnostic and Statistical Manual of Mental Disorders, fourth edition (DSM-IV). Mental disorders are common in the United States and internationally (U.S. Bureau of Census, 2004). An estimated 22.1% of Americans ages 18 and older – about 1 in 5 adults – suffer from a diagnosable mental disorder in a given year. When applied to the 1998 US Census residential population estimate, this figure translates to 44.3 million people. In addition, 4 of the 10 *leading causes of disability* in the US and other developed countries are mental disorders – major depression, bipolar disorder, schizophrenia, and obsessive-compulsive disorder. Many people suffer from more than one mental disorder at a given time

Depressive Disorders

Depressive disorders encompass major depressive disorder, dysthymic disorder, and bipolar disorder. Bipolar disorder is included because people with this illness have depressive episodes as well as manic episodes. Approximately 18.8 million American adults, or about 9.5% of the US population age 18 and older in a given year, (http://www.nimh.nih.gov/publicat/numbers.cfm#1) have a depressive disorder. Nearly twice as many women (12.0%) as men (6.6%) are effected by a depressive disorder each year. These figures translate to 12.4 million women and 6.4 million men in the US Depressive disorders may be appearing earlier in life in people born in recent decades compared to the past. Depressive disorders often co-occur with anxiety disorders and substance abuse.

Major Depressive Disorder

Major depressive disorder is the leading cause of disability in the US and established market economies worldwide. Major depressive disorder effects approximately 9.9 million American adults, or about 5.0% of the US population age 18 and older in a given year. Nearly twice as many women (6.5%) as men (3.3%) suffer from major depressive disorder each year. These figures translate to 6.7 million women and 3.2 million men. While major depressive disorder can develop at any age, the average age at onset is the mid twenties.

Dysthymic Disorder

Symptoms of dysthymic disorder (chronic, mild depression) must persist for at least 2 years in adults (1 year in children) to meet criteria for the diagnosis. Dysthymic disorder effects approximately 5.4% of the US population age 18 and older during their *lifetime*. This figure translates to about 10.9 million American adults (http://www.nimh.nih.gov/publicat/numbers.cfm#5). About 40% of adults with dysthymic disorder also meet criteria for major depressive disorder or bipolar disorder in a given year. Dysthymic disorder often begins in childhood, adolescence, or early adulthood.

Bipolar Disorder

Bipolar disorder effects approximately 2.3 million American adults, or about 1.2% of the US population age 18 and older in a given year (http://www.nimh.nih.gov/publicat/numbers.cfm#1). Men and women are equally likely to develop bipolar disorder (http://www.nimh.nih.gov/publicat/numbers.cfm#5). The average age at onset for a first manic episode is the early twenties.

Suicide

In 2000, 29,350 people died by suicide in the US More than 90% of people who kill themselves have a diagnosable mental disorder, commonly a depressive disorder or a substance abuse disorder. The highest suicide rates in the US are found in white men over age 85. In 2000, suicide was the third leading cause of death among 15–24 year olds. Four times as many men as women die by suicide; however, women attempt suicide two to three times as often as men.

Schizophrenia

Approximately 2.2 million American adults, or about 1.1% of the population age 18 and older in a given year (http://www.nimh.nih.gov/publicat/numbers.cfm#1), have schizophrenia. Schizophrenia effects men and women with equal frequency. Schizophrenia often first appears in men in their late teens or early twenties. Women are generally effected in their twenties or early thirties.

Anxiety Disorders

Anxiety disorders include panic disorder, obsessive-compulsive disorder, posttraumatic stress disorder, generalized anxiety disorder, and phobias (social phobia, agoraphobia, and specific phobia). Approximately 19.1 million American adults ages 18–54, or about 13.3% of people in this age group in a given year, have an anxiety disorder. Anxiety disorders frequently cooccur with depressive disorders, eating disorders, or substance abuse. Many people have more than one anxiety disorder. Women are more likely than men to have an anxiety disorder. Approximately twice as many women as men suffer from panic disorder, posttraumatic stress disorder, generalized anxiety disorder, agoraphobia, and specific phobia, though about equal numbers of women and men have obsessive-compulsive disorder and social phobia.

Panic Disorder

Approximately 2.4 million American adults ages 18–54, or about 1.7% of people in this age group in a given year, have panic disorder. Panic disorder typically develops in late adolescence or early adulthood. About one in three people with panic disorder develop agoraphobia, a condition in which they become afraid of being in any place or situation where escape might be difficult or help unavailable in the event of a panic attack.

Obsessive-Compulsive Disorder (OCD)

Approximately 3.3 million American adults ages 18–54, or about 2.3% of people in this age group in a given year, have OCD. The first symptoms of OCD often begin during childhood or adolescence.

Posttraumatic Stress Disorder (PTSD)

Approximately 5.2 million American adults ages 18–54, or about 3.6% of people in this age group in a given year, have PTSD. PTSD can develop at any age, including childhood. About 30% of Vietnam veterans experienced PTSD at some point after the war (http://www.nimh.nih.gov/publicat/numbers.cfm#17). The disorder also frequently occurs after violent personal assaults such as rape, mugging, or domestic violence; terrorism; natural or human-caused disasters; and accidents.

Generalized Anxiety Disorder (GAD)

Approximately 4.0 million American adults ages 18–54, or about 2.8% of people in this age group in a given year, have GAD. GAD can begin across the life cycle, though the risk is highest between childhood and middle age.

Social Phobia

Approximately 5.3 million American adults ages 18–54, or about 3.7% of people in this age group in a given year, have social phobia. Social phobia typically begins in childhood or adolescence.

Agoraphobia and Specific Phobias

Agoraphobia involves intense fear and avoidance of any place or situation where escape might be difficult or help unavailable in the event of developing sudden panic-like symptoms. In a given year, approximately 3.2

million American adults ages 18–54, or about 2.2% of people in this age group, have agoraphobia. Specific phobias involve marked and persistent fear and avoidance of a specific object or situation. Approximately 6.3 million American adults ages 18–54, or about 4.4% of people in this age group in a given year, have some type of specific phobia.

Other Disorders

Under this category are included eating, attention deficit/hyperactivity, autism, and Alzheimer disorders.

Eating Disorders: The three main types of eating disorders are anorexia nervosa, bulimia nervosa, and binge-eating disorder. Females are much more likely than males to develop an eating disorder. Only an estimated 5–15% of people with anorexia or bulimia and an estimated 35% of those with binge-eating disorder (http://www.nimh.nih.gov/publicat/numbers.cfm#19) are male. In their lifetime, an estimated 0.5–3.7% of females suffer from anorexia and an estimated 1.1–4.2% suffer from bulimia. Community surveys have estimated that between 2% and 5% of Americans experience a binge-eating disorder in a 6-month period. The mortality rate among people with anorexia has been estimated at 0.56% per year, or approximately 5.6% per decade, which is about 12 times higher than the annual death rate due to all causes of death among females ages 15–24 in the general population.

Attention Deficit Hyperactivity Disorder (ADHD): ADHD, one of the most common mental disorders in children and adolescents, effects an estimated 4.1% of youths ages 9–17 in a 6-month period. About two to three times more boys than girls are effected. ADHD usually becomes evident in preschool or early elementary years. The disorder frequently persists into adolescence and occasionally into adulthood.

Autism: Autism effects an estimated 1–2 per 1,000 people. Autism and related disorders (also called autism spectrum disorders or pervasive developmental disorders) develop in childhood and generally are apparent by age 3. Autism is about four times more common in boys than girls. Girls with the disorder, however, tend to have more severe symptoms and greater cognitive impairment. Within this *category*, one needs to consider also Asperger's disorders, which are still not clearly identified in the general population.

Alzheimer's Disease: Alzheimer's disease, the most common cause of dementia among people age 65 and older, effects an estimated 4 million Americans. As more and more Americans live longer, the number effected by Alzheimer's disease will continue to grow unless a cure or effective prevention is discovered. The duration of illness, from onset of symptoms to death, averages 8–10 years.

Addictive Disorders

This report presents the first information from the 2004 National Survey on Drug Use and Health (NSDUH), an annual survey of the civilian, noninstitutionalized population of the United States aged 12 years old or older. Prior to

2002, the survey was called the National Household Survey on Drug Abuse (NHSDA). This initial report on 2004 data presents national estimates of rates of use, numbers of users, and other measures related to illicit drugs, alcohol, and tobacco products.

Illicit Drug Use

In 2004, 19.1 million Americans, or 7.9% of the population aged 12 or older, were current illicit drug users. Current drug use means use of an illicit drug during the month prior to the survey interview. The rate of illicit drug use among persons aged 12 or older in 2004 was similar to the rates in 2002 and 2003 (8.3% and 8.2%). Among youths aged 12–17, the rate declined between 2002 and 2004 (11.6% in 2002, 11.2% in 2003, and 10.6% in 2004). Marijuana was the most commonly used illicit drug in 2004, with a rate of 6.1% (14.6 million current users). There were 2.0 million current cocaine users, 467,000 of whom used crack. Hallucinogens were used by 929,000 persons, and there were an estimated 166,000 heroin users. All of these estimates are similar to estimates for 2003. Between 2002 and 2004, past month marijuana use declined for male youths aged 12–17 (9.1% in 2002, 8.6% in 2003, and 8.1% in 2004), but it remained level for female youths (7.2%, 7.2%, and 7.1%, respectively) during the same time span. The number of current users of Ecstasy decreased between 2002 and 2003, from 676,000 to 470,000, but the number did not change between 2003 and 2004 (450,000). In 2004, 6.0 million persons were current users of psychotherapeutic drugs taken nonmedically (2.5%). These include 4.4 million who used pain relievers, 1.6 million who used tranquilizers, 1.2 million who used stimulants, and 0.3 million who used sedatives. These estimates are all similar to the corresponding estimates for 2003. There were significant increases in the lifetime prevalence of use from 2003 to 2004 in several categories of pain relievers among people aged 18–25. Specific pain relievers with statistically significant increases in lifetime use were Vicodin, Lortab, or Lorcet (from 15.0% to 16.5%); Percocet, Percodan, or Tylox (from 7.8% to 8.7%); hydrocodone products (from 16.3% to 17.4%); OxyContin (from 3.6% to 4.3%); and oxycodone products (from 8.9% to 10.1%). Among youths aged 12–17, rates of current illicit drug use varied significantly by major racial/ethnic groups in 2004. The rate was highest among American Indian or Alaska Native youths (26.0%). Rates were 12.2% for youths reporting two or more races, 11.1% for white youths, 10.2% for Hispanic youths, 9.3% for black youths, and 6.0% for Asian youths. In 2004, 19.2% of unemployed adults aged 18 or older were current illicit drug users compared with 8.0% of those employed full-time and 10.3% of those employed part-time. However, of the 16.4 million illicit drug users aged 18 or older in 2004, 12.3 million (75.2%) were employed either full- or part-time.

Alcohol Use

In 2004, 121 million Americans aged 12 or older were current drinkers of alcohol (50.3%). Fifty five million (22.8%) participated in binge drinking, defined as five or more drinks on at least one occasion in the 30 days prior to the survey. 16.7 million (6.9%) were heavy drinkers, defined as binge drinking on 5 or more days in the past month. These numbers are all similar to the corresponding estimates for 2002 and 2003. The highest prevalence of binge and heavy drinking in 2004 was for young adults aged 18–25 (41.2%

and 15.1%, respectively). The peak rate of both measures occurred at age 21 (48.2% and 19.2%, respectively). The rate of underage drinking remained the same in 2004 as in 2002 and 2003. About 10.8 million persons aged 12–20 reported drinking alcohol in the month prior to the survey interview in 2004 (28.7% of this age group). Of these, nearly 7.4 million (19.6%) were binge drinkers, and 2.4 million (6.3%) were heavy drinkers.

Among persons aged 12–20 in 2004, past month alcohol use rates were 16.4% among Asians, 19.1% among blacks, 24.3% among American Indians or Alaska Natives, 26.4% among those reporting two or more races, 26.6% among Hispanics, and 32.6% among whites. Among pregnant women aged 15–44, 11.2% reported past month alcohol use and 4.5% reported past month binge drinking, based on combined 2003 and 2004 data. 32.5 million persons aged 12 or older in 2004 (13.5%) drove under the influence of alcohol at least once in the 12 months prior to the interview. This was similar to the rate in 2003. Young adults aged 18–22 enrolled full-time in college were more likely than their peers not enrolled full-time to use alcohol, binge drink, and drink heavily in 2004 (this category includes part-time college students and persons not enrolled in college). Binge and heavy use rates for college students were 43.4% and 18.6%, respectively, compared with 39.4% and 13.5%, respectively, for other persons aged 18–22.

Tobacco Use

In 2004, 70.3 million Americans were current users of a tobacco product. This is 29.2% of the population aged 12 or older. 59.9 million (24.9%) smoked cigarettes, 13.7 million (5.7%) smoked cigars, 7.2 million (3.0%) used smokeless tobacco, and 1.8 million (0.8%) smoked tobacco in pipes. The rate of tobacco use declined between 2002 and 2004, from 30.4% to 29.2%, primarily due to a decline in cigarette use from 26.0% to 24.9%. The rate of cigar use remained steady, but smokeless tobacco use dropped from 3.3% to 3.0%. Young adults aged 18–25 continued to have the highest rate of past month cigarette use (39.5%). The rate did not change significantly between 2002 and 2004. The rate of cigarette use among youths aged 12–17 declined from 13.0% in 2002 to 11.9% in 2004. A higher proportion of males than females aged 12 or older smoked cigarettes in 2004 (27.7% vs. 22.3%). Among youths aged 12–17, however, girls (12.5%) were more likely than boys (11.3%) to smoke. Based on 2003 and 2004 data combined, 18.0% of pregnant women aged 15–44 smoked cigarettes in the past month compared with 30.0% of women in that age group who were not pregnant. However, among those aged 15–17, this pattern did not hold. The rate of cigarette smoking among pregnant women aged 15–17 was 26.0% compared with 19.6% among nonpregnant women of that age (not a statistically significant difference). In completely rural nonmetropolitan counties, current cigarette use among persons aged 12 or older declined from 31.8% in 2002 to 22.8% in 2004. Among the 93.4 million persons who ever had smoked cigarettes daily in their lifetime, nearly half (46.2%) had stopped smoking in 2004; i.e., they did not smoke at all in the past 30 days. The remaining 53.8% were still current smokers.

Initiation of Substance Use (Incidence)

Based on a new approach to estimating incidence, the 2004 NSDUH shows that the illicit drug category with the largest number of new users was nonmedical use of pain relievers. Within the past 12 months, 2.4 million persons used pain relievers nonmedically for the first time. The average age at first use among these new initiates was 23.3 years. In 2004, 2.1 million persons had used marijuana for the first time within the past 12 months. This estimate was not significantly different from the number in 2003 (2.0 million). The average age at first use among the 2.1 million recent marijuana initiates was 18.0 years. Most (63.8%) of the recent initiates were younger than age 18 when they first used. In 2004, 4.4 million persons had used alcohol for the first time within the past 12 months. The number of alcohol initiates increased from 3.9 million in 2002 and 4.1 million in 2003. Most (86.9%) of the 4.4 million recent alcohol initiates in 2004 were younger than age 21 at the time of initiation. The number of persons who smoked cigarettes for the first time within the past 12 months was 2.1 million in 2004, not significantly different from the estimates in 2002 (1.9 million) or 2003 (2.0 million). About two thirds of new smokers in 2004 were under the age of 18 when they first smoked cigarettes (67.8%).

Youth Prevention-Related Measures

The percentage of youths aged 12–17 indicating that smoking marijuana once a month was a great risk increased from 32.4% in 2002 to 34.9% in 2003, but did not change between 2003 and 2004 (35.0%). There were declines between 2003 and 2004 in the percentages of youths perceiving a great risk in using cocaine and heroin. Perceived risk of cigarette use increased between 2003 and 2004, but there was no change in the perceived risk of having four or five drinks of alcohol nearly every day or having five or more drinks once or twice a week. The percentage of youths reporting that it would be easy to obtain marijuana declined between 2002 and 2003, from 55.0% to 53.6%, and again between 2003 and 2004, to 52.2%. The percentage of youths reporting that LSD would be easy to obtain also decreased between 2002 and 2004, from 19.4% to 16.9%, as did the perceived availability of heroin (15.8% to 14.0%). Most youths (89.8%) reported that their parents would strongly disapprove of their trying marijuana or hashish once or twice. Among these youths, only 5.1% had used marijuana in the past month. However, among youths who perceived that their parents would only somewhat disapprove or neither approve nor disapprove of their trying marijuana, 30.0% used marijuana.

Substance Dependence, Abuse, and Treatment

In 2004, 22.5 million Americans aged 12 or older were classified with past year substance dependence or abuse (9.4% of the population), about the same number as in 2002 and 2003. Of these, 3.4 million were classified with dependence on or abuse of both alcohol and illicit drugs, 3.9 million were dependent on or abused illicit drugs but not alcohol, and 15.2 million were dependent on or abused alcohol but not illicit drugs. In 2004, 19.9% of unemployed adults aged 18 or older were classified with dependence or abuse, while 10.5% of full-time employed adults and 11.9% of part-time employed adults were classified as such. However, most adults with substance dependence or abuse were employed either full- or part-time. Of the 20.3 million adults classified with dependence or abuse, 15.7 million (77.6%) were employed. In 2004, 3.8 million people aged 12 or older (1.6% of the population) received treatment in the past 12 months for a drug or alcohol use problem. Of these, 2.3 million received treatment at a specialty facility for substance use treatment, including 1.7 million at a rehabilitation facility as an outpatient, 947,000 at a rehabilitation facility as an inpatient, 775,000 at a hospital as an inpatient, and 982,000 at a mental health center as an outpatient.

Nonspecialty treatment locations were self-help groups (2.1 million persons), private doctor's offices (490,000 persons), emergency rooms (453,000 persons), and prisons or jails (310,000 persons). (Note that the estimates of treatment by location include persons reporting more than one location.) Persons dependent on or abusing a substance in the past 12 months, or who received specialty treatment for a substance use problem within the past 12 months, are classified as needing treatment. In 2004, the number of persons aged 12 or older needing treatment for an alcohol or illicit drug use problem was 23.48 million (9.8%). Of these, 2.33 million received treatment at a specialty facility in the past year. Thus, 21.15 million people needed but did not receive treatment at a specialty facility in 2004. The number needing but not receiving treatment did not change significantly from 2002 to 2004. *6.6 million people needed but did not receive treatment for an illicit drug use problem in 2004* (italics mine). Of these, 598,000 (9.0%) felt they needed treatment. This number increased from 362,000 in 2002 and from 426,000 in 2003. *Of the 598,000 persons who felt they needed treatment in 2004, 194,000 (32.4%) reported that they made an effort but were unable to get treatment, and 404,000 (67.6%) reported making no effort to get treatment* (italics mine). The topic of treatment will be revisited at the end of this chapter.

Crime and Criminalities

The US Federal Bureau of Investigation (Department of Justice, 2003) released the following statistics on crimes for the year 2002. During that year there were 11,877.00 violent crimes that included murder and nonnegligent manslaughter, forcible rape, robbery, and aggravated assault. There were 10,451.000 property crimes that included burglary, larceny-theft, and motor vehicle theft. There were significant differences among crimes in large metropolitan areas and smaller cities versus rural areas, where crimes were less frequent. These figures support an estimate of approximating more than two million inmates in federal and state prisons (Department of Justice, 2003). What can be done to prevent crimes and rehabilitate those who commit them? How can one use words to treat individuals who rely mostly on physical actions to commit crimes?

Poverties, Disabilities, and Disenfranchisements

Perhaps, this category is different from the three previous ones. However, "For decades of research have delineated the need for improved psychotherapeutic opportunities for poor participants" (Smith, 2005, p. 687). Smith accused psychotherapists of remaining "contradictory" in regard to what has been done for the poor. She suggested that: "...unexamined classist assumptions" (p. 687) remain at the base of this neglect. Even though this suggestion may be valid, another possibility may be just as valid, and i.e., traditional talk-based, face-to-face (f2f), psychotherapy may be an inappropriate medium of communication with the poor, the handicapped, the shut-in, and other marginalized and disenfranchised populations. Perhaps combinations of nutritional (Section II this volume), nonverbal (Section III this volume), writing (Section IV this volume), and relational (Section V this volume) approaches may be more appropriate areas to explore when dealing with poverty and other debilitating conditions. Furthermore, the poor also bear the added burden of more frequent mental disorders, addictions, and criminalities. Consequently, a single approach, like talk-based, f2f psychotherapy would be insufficient and probably ineffective, if not inappropriate, when there are other more immediate needs that must be addressed. Additionally, what about seniors, military, and missionary families, who in some ways are disenfranchised? Many live close to poverty levels. How are we going to reach all these populations? We need to consider low-cost, evidence-based, mass-oriented approaches that will reach these populations in more effective ways than traditional f2f talk-based psychotherapy or even prevention (Veroff, Kulka, & Douvan, 1981).

If those statistics are not enough, what is happening within the wider context of the workplace? Productivity losses related to personal and family health problems cost US employers $1,685 per employee per year or about $226 billion annually (Caminiti, 2005, p. S2). Healthcare costs are projected to keep soaring in the US with no public policy solution in sight. The money spent on healthcare is projected to grow 7% or more annually over the next ten years, taking up nearly a fifth of our nation's GDP (Caminiti, 2005, p. S14).

What can be concluded from these general, stark and discouraging statistics? One is bound to conclude that, at any given time, with overlaps among the four completely different types of dysfunctionality, mental illnesses, addictions, criminalities, poverties, and other debilitating conditions, conservatively at least 20–30% of the total population may be dysfunctional, or at least not functioning at appropriate or desirable levels (Dew & Bromet, 1993). Even the lowest percentage of 20% means that at least 58–60 million people need some kind of help. If one considers that, at best, there may be approximately half a million mental health professionals in the US, this number is never going to be sufficient to reach all the troubled people in need of help. We need to find more cost-effective and innovative ways to meet the mental health needs we are presently facing. Hence the purpose of this book.

Given the statistics given above, what percentage of these populations is helped or will be helped by existing f2f talk-based prevention and psychotherapy? Even using groups and families, as suggested by the New Freedom Commission on Mental Health (2003), f2f talk-based prevention and psychotherapy models, aren't and won't reduce those statistics. L'Abate (1999, in press) has even argued that the talk-based f2f model, if it is to help all those in need of help, is inefficient, relatively ineffective, expensive, and in need of serious modifications. What about preventive approaches? Unless supported by research grants, many preventive approaches are not sufficiently effective or long-lasting to make a dent in specific populations that need those services. What other approaches can we use? We cannot understand the nature of prescriptive approaches unless we understand its preceding historical context within prevention. Let's see what has happened to prevention in the past and, perhaps, learn from it to promote health promotion in the present and the future.

Learning from the Past: A Few Historical Highlights

In this section the historical background of preventive approaches will be briefly reviewed because past health promotion efforts, if any thus far, were imbedded in them. For a thorough summary of the historical antecedents of prevention the interested reader may want to consult Mrazek and Haggerty (1994). We need to learn from this history to understand how promotion, as a more recent development, is different conceptually and practically from prevention. The preventive psychology movement owes its roots to a variety of sources and strands. Within this movement one needs to add the more recent health promotion movement.

Early Beginnings

Only during the second half of the last century, did prevention become viable in the US. Caplan (1964) was the first to indicate the need for prevention in psychiatry. Albee, with his milestone report (1959) on mental health personnel needs (Kessler, Goldston, & Joffe, 1992), was one of the first to stress the need for prevention in psychology. Accordingly, he started the Vermont Conference on Prevention that spawned a variety of research projects and kept alive the importance of prevention. During the Carter administration years (1977–1980) and especially through the efforts of Roselynn Carter, offices of prevention were introduced at the federal and state levels (Klein & Goldston, 1977). During that period, quite a few publications formed the bases for community psychology (Bloom, 1975; Iscoe, Bloom, & Spielberger, 1977). Another seminal work by the Joint Commission on Mental Illness and Health (1961) formed the basis for preventive efforts.

Among the many roots for preventing efforts, one cannot omit the results of (a) the Headstart program at the preschool level, (b) the influence of Sesame Street on TV at the toddler level, and (c) the community mental health movement (Rappaport, 1992). These efforts were coupled with the success of preventive programs in dentistry (fluoride), medicine (heart disease), and HIV/AIDS (Baum & Posluszny, 1999; Camic & Knight, 1998; Reppucci, Woolard, & Fried, 1999; Schneiderman, Antoni, Saab, & Ironson, 2001). These successes promoted the development and existence of the specialty area of health psychology, which overlapped with community and prevention psychology (Baum & Singer, 2001; Edelstein & Michelson, 1986; Felner, Jason, Moritsugu, & Farber, 1983; Sarafino, 1994).

An often ignored but crucial milestone in the inevitable evolution from psychotherapy toward prevention lies in Margaret Rioch's research (1970) which showed how briefly trained housewives might obtain comparable results as professionally trained psychotherapists. This research raised so many outcries from professional organizations that it failed to receive further support from the National Institutes of Mental Health. Yet, it remains an important step in what was to become the paraprofessional revolution in mental health (Guerney, 1969).

The Psycho-Educational Social Skills Training Movement

The last quarter of a century, starting in the mid 1960s and evolving in the 1970s, witnessed the growth of what has been called the Psycho-Educational

Social Skills Training (PE-SST) movement. This approach consists of a variety of structured programs, with a definite topic that defines how the clientele might profit by the program, usually with a predetermined number of sessions and costs. Although this movement purports to be preventive, the proof of prevention is very difficult to substantiate (De Maria, 2003; L'Abate, 1980, 1981, 1986, 1990; Phillips, 1985). It takes decades to demonstrate that any program designed to be preventive has produced its desired, long-term, positive effects. At best, its immediate effects, usually following termination of a program, have been evaluated, while, as far as this writer knows, there are very few studies of long-term effects for any preventive approach (L'Abate & Milan, 1985). An exception may lie in Cusinato's (2004) follow-up study of couples trained in Treviso's Family Center (Italy). Ten years after entering a Catholic marriage preparation course, modeled in part after Olson's PREPARE-ENRICH program, only 2% of 10,000 couples were divorced. These results compared well with an Italian national divorce rate of at least 20–30%.

A variety of sources sparked the PE-SST movement, as exemplified earlier (in the late 1930s) by the now commercially available Dale Carnegie training programs. Earlier (1965), this movement was started by the Marriage Encounter Movement (Father Calvo) and its many offshoots in various religious denominations (Berger & Hannah, 1999; Levant, 1986). During the same year (1970), two major publications spawned further developments of this movement (a) the successful Assertiveness Training (Alberti & Emmons, 1970) and its offshoots, (b) Parent Effectiveness Training (Gordon, 1970) and its offshoots. Later, (c) Goldstein's (1973) Structured Therapy for juveniles, (d) The Divorce Mediation Movement, as another structured approach, and, finally (e) the Couple and Family Enrichment Movement (L'Abate & Weinstein, 1987) were the bases for growth in preventive, social skills training programs for targeted conditions (assertiveness, parenting, etc.), or targeted populations (children, adolescents, adults) with a specific disorder (aggression, phobias, etc.).

All these various strands indicated that many approaches in mental health do not need to be administered by professionals. Properly trained, responsible, responsive, and caring semi- or subprofessionals, and even unpaid, part-time volunteers, could perform many of the functions that were previously thought to be the restricted province of professionals with doctorates.

The Nonprofessional Revolution

This movement was sparked in part by Ellsworth (1968) showing how crucial psychiatric aides were in the rehabilitation and recovery of schizophrenic participants. It was followed by Grosser, Henry, and Kelly's (1969) expansions to other clinical conditions, and by Guerney's (1969) demonstration of how parents and teachers could be used in the therapy of children.

Being at the frontline of approaches to deal with psychopathology and its etiology, subprofessionals are the very people who spearhead a pyramidal structure necessary to deal successfully with the prevention of serious mental disorders (Sobey, 1970). Behind them should exist a ladder of professionals available to intervene in cases of crisis. In addition to demystifying the halo of professionals, this movement has helped to demonstrate that professional qualifications alone are not enough, and that personal qualities, sometimes lacking in professionals, might be more important than formal degrees (L'Abate, 1983, 1987a, 2001).

The Self-Help Revolution

Starting with Alcoholics Anonymous in the mid 1930s of the last century and proliferating to other self-help groups, let alone alcoholics, the self-help movement is tantamount to a revolution in mental health. An effect size of 0.76 for self-help approaches at posttreatment and of 0.53 at follow-up (Gould & Clum, 1993) indicates how much self-help can help improve physical and mental health (Kelly, 2003). The major issue still lies in its evaluation. Who will benefit by self-help? Who will benefit by which approach? Who will need prescriptive approaches, prevention, psychotherapy, or medication? Who will need a combination all of different approaches?

The Evolution of Family Life Education

A related but independent resource in the evolution of subprofessional influence was education, the field of family life (L'Abate, 1987b). From a didactically passive, classroom stance with little if any research, this approach began to develop more active and interactive stances. It was hampered, however, by the lack of evaluation and research, and by the unavailability of a delivery system, except the classroom with students not yet married. Nonetheless, it became the basis for knowledge about couple and marital relationships that were otherwise not considered by the initially monadic social skills training movements. Family life education was further influenced by the social skills and family enrichment movements to become more assertive and interactive rather than limiting itself to abstract book learning, as it originally started out doing (Arcus, Schvaneveldt, & Moss, 1993).

The Construct of Competence

Theoretically, the prevention movement was helped by the pioneer work of Leslie Phillips and Ed Zigler (Phillips, 1968) about deficits in the social skills of schizophrenics, as incorporated in E. Lakin Phillips' work (1978). Underlying all of the above approaches, usually most of them a-theoretical, lies the positive construct of *competence*, in contrast with the negative view of illness followed in prevention, psychiatry, and psychotherapy. This construct became a rallying point for the prevention movement. Based on White's seminal suggestion (1959) of competence as a motivational concept, this construct sparked a whole series of papers, chapters, and books on the same concept (Marlowe & Weinberg, 1985; Sternberg & Kolligian, 1990), among many others (Elliot & Dweck, 2005).

More recently, L'Abate's theory of relational competence in intimate relationships (L'Abate, 1994, 2005a, 2006a; L'Abate & Baggett, 1997; L'Abate & De Giacomo, 2003; L'Abate & Menar, 2006), however, went one step further in specifying in greater detail two major sets of competencies necessary for survival in life: the ability to love (communal/expressive) and the ability to negotiate (agentic/instrumental) (Bakan, 1968). This distinction is present in differentiating Sections II, III, and IV from Section V in this book.

Furthermore, the selfhood model of this relational theory, how importance is attributed and expressed to self or to intimate others through four personality propensities, predicts about: (1) 25% of the population being severely dysfunctional, where self and intimate others are denied importance, (2) 50% being borderline in functionality, where either self or intimate others are denied importance, and (3) only 25% being fully functioning, when importance is expressed positively toward both self and intimate others. When one compares the statistics given at the beginning of this chapter, and the predictions given by this model, one can see that the model is not too far off from the stark reality of those statistics. It fares well with results given from studies, among them (Dew & Bromet, 1993), and the famous Midtown Manhattan Study (Srole et al., 1962) which found that only 20% of the population was fully functional.

Why Promotion? A Brief Rationale for Promotion

If promotion is defined as the administration of prescriptive approaches, here is a list of reasons for using them earlier than expensive preventive or even more expensive crisis-based interventions, such as psychotherapy and even hospitalization. In the past, the standard dictum for prevention was "An ounce of prevention is worth a pound of cure." This dictum can be changed once we define health promotion as a specialty area preceding prevention. Consequently, here is how that dictum is (re)used.

1. *Promotion is cheaper than prevention*: "An ounce of promotion is worth one pound of prevention and a ton of cure," because it can rely on itself and, if and when necessary, a hierarchy of nonprofessional laypersons, subprofessionals, semi-professionals, and professionals to get the job done. By themselves doctorate level professionals can't deal with all the physical, social, and mental ills present in our country, as documented above. Even an orthopedist needs a physical therapist to restore an operated limb. Dentists use assistants to clean teeth. Lawyers use paralegals to deal with routine matters. Architects and engineers need technicians and laborers to build skyscrapers. Only in mental health have we tried to help troubled people through f2f talk and, when talk fails, medication or hospitalization No training, or promotional approaches are included, except perhaps rehabilitation during hospitalization.
2. *Promotion can reach more people per unit of professional time* than prevention or psychotherapy, especially if audio-video tapes, films, TV, and online computers are used (Norcross et al., 2000). This point implies that most prevention approaches need administration at a distance between administrators and participants, who will use writing as a major medium of communication rather than f2f talk (Section IV this volume).
3. *Promotion allows to recruit more volunteer laypersons and paraprofessionals to help.* The ease, simplicity, and concreteness of approaches reviewed in this book makes them ideal for administration at various levels of personal, technical, and semi-professional competence.
4. *Promotion yields a wider number of less expensive options than prevention*, crisis-intervention, psychotherapy, medication, or more

expensive approaches (hospital, jail). The range of approaches reviewed in this book is such that no longer does one need to consider "nothing," i.e., no intervention, versus prevention, psychotherapy, or medication, or worst, hospitalization or even incarceration. Promoting health even before preventing and before "curing" illnesses is always the more rational and sensible way to deal with many physical and mental problems.

5. *There are never going to be enough professionals to deal with the many social ills confronting our society*, as illustrated above. Overall statistics given at the outset of this chapter concerning the extent of dysfunctionalities in the US, may already be outdated. Full-fledged professionals will not be sufficient to stem the growth of physical and mental disorders.
6. *Once promotional approaches are added to prevention, they can be subdivided into various levels*: (a) *promotion for everybody*, (b) primary prevention for *selected* populations, as in social, psycho-educational skill training approaches, (c) secondary for *specific* populations, i.e., adult children of alcoholics, and (d) tertiary, as in crisis intervention and psychotherapy for clinical intervention with clinically or psychiatrically "sick" populations (L'Abate, 1990), as detailed in Table 1.1.

The original differentiation among primary, secondary, and tertiary, prevention (L'Abate, 1990, p. 31; 1994, p. 221) used 14 criteria to discriminate among *pro-active "at risk"* (primary), *paraactive "in need"* (secondary), and *reactive "in crisis"* (tertiary) prevention approaches. This information is introduced here to allow even further discrimination between promotional, prescriptive and preventive approaches. Prescriptive approaches, therefore, qualify as one earlier and universal aspect of primary prevention, even though one would not want to confuse promotion with prevention, as has been done by various authors (see Preface this volume). L'Abate's (1990) criteria were reproduced practically *verbatim* by Mrazek and Haggerty (1994), without attribution. The original contribution made by those authors consisted of calling primary prevention "universal," secondary prevention "targeted," and tertiary prevention "necessary," terms that, in one way or another, were already contained in the original presentation, as shown in Table 1.1.

A similar model was presented by Weisz et al. (2005). They enlarged on L'Abate's (1990) model, and Mrazek and Haggerty's (1994) reproduction of that model, by proposing a circular ring composed of various wedges, starting with a separate wedge for health promotion and positive development. Wedges increased according to the level of dysfunctionality from prevention to treatment and ending to inpatient hospitalization and other treatment settings. Even though promotion was the first wedge in their model, these authors failed to differentiate promotion from prevention any further than considering promotion as part of universal prevention, without any further specification. Here is where the notion of promotional, prescriptive approaches contained in this book help us to differentiate health promotion from prevention. The inclusion of *prescriptive approaches* may further enlarge the field of primary prevention by suggesting one earlier, independent promotion tier, perhaps earlier than the three major tiers of primary prevention approaches shown in Table 1.1.

Conceptual and Practical Issues in Health Promotion

Five conceptual and practical issues, in some ways deriving from the background given above, need to be introduced before going any further into promoting promotion: (a) promotion before prevention, (b) health promotion and prevention, (c) the concept of structure in promotional interventions, (d) toward a sieves or stepped approach to health promotion and disease prevention, and (e) definitional issues that include a progression of criteria from approaches classification to traditional preventive approaches.

Promotion before Prevention

The statistics given at the beginning of this chapter plus the recent summary of the President's New Freedom Commission on Mental Health (2003) found that existing mental health treatments in the US are seriously inadequate. Traditional approaches based on f2f talk and personal contact between participants and professionals are unable to deal with existing and growing mental health needs that beset ours as well as other nations. While past traditional approaches focused mainly on individuals, families and groups instead will be the focus of future mental health approaches. The many recommendations of this Commission repeated those of the Surgeon General (1999). In addition to costs, fragmentation, and proliferation of inadequate approaches, both reports either ignored or were pessimistic about the future of prevention. Both reports acknowledged that prevention was so handicapped by so many barriers (political, economic, societal, professional), to be considered unobtainable at the present time. Unfortunately, both reports were written as if prevention were separate and independent from psychotherapy and rehabilitation in mental health, let alone promotion (De Maria, 2003).

Furthermore, both reports ignored that, in the future, health promotion, preventive and psychotherapeutic approaches will need to rely on a hierarchy of professionals, semi-professionals, paraprofessionals, and laypersons working with willing participants at a distance, using computers, mail, and the Internet. Without all communication media, it will be practically impossible to reach all the people in stress and distress who need and want help. The traditional paradigm of f2f talk is giving way, albeit slowly, to distance writing, with participants responding in writing to written homework assignments through computers and the Internet (see Section V this volume; Kazantzis, Deane, Ronan, & L'Abate, 2005; Kazantzis & L'Abate, 2007).

Health Promotion and Disease Prevention

The inadequacy of long-term effects for preventive needs consideration if progress is to be made in the field of health promotion. Past prevention advocates (Lofquist, 1983; National Mental Health Association, 1986; Pransky, 1991; Roberts & Peterson, 1984), for example, proclaimed emphatically that "An ounce of prevention is worth a pound of cure," including in their arguments its cost-effectiveness. From the physical-medical field (diet, exercise, fluoride, etc.), we have learned that most prevention approaches do work, suggesting that, in the long run, indeed: "Prevention does pay." Preventive approaches in mental health, however, as argued by one of its most severe critics and skeptics in this field, have failed to show definite dollar benefits (Russell, 1986). One needs to be aware of these criticisms, to consider fully information about pros and cons of preventive efforts, before embarking on an out-and-out advocacy of promotional approaches (L'Abate, 1986).

More to the point, we need to be mindful that, since there are no classifications and job descriptions in state merit systems for "preventers," let alone "health promoters," the melancholy and negative conclusion at this point, is the opposite, and i.e., "Illness prevention does not pay." Or, if this conclusion is too negative: "We need to demonstrate that preventive approaches do show substantially positive long-term effects to be included in state merit systems."

As far as we know thus far, there are no paid positions below policy levels for health promoters and disease preventers as yet available at state and federal levels. Furthermore, very few state laws determining mental health practices contain the term "health promotion" or even "disease prevention." Very few health promoters or prevention-oriented practitioners in full-time private practice can make a living from it, with the exception of a few stars who might "make it" in the marketplace of workshops and presentations. Most preventers work in academic positions that allow and encourage them to apply for research grants. Third parties, managed care and health insurance companies do not pay for disease prevention, let alone health promotion, hence, the need for external sources to fund primary and secondary prevention. Prescriptive approaches, on the other hand, are so inexpensive that very little external support is needed.

In addition to the academic community, one needs to look at federal and state bureaucracies for the creation of promotional opportunities in state merit systems with parallel job descriptions. The creation of offices of prevention, both at federal and state levels, under the leadership of Mrs. Roselynn Carter, boded well for positive beginnings. These beginnings may require legislative fiat to create new job descriptions detailing and prescribing the responsibilities of "preventers" (Heller, 1996; Munoz, Mrazek & Haggerty, 1996; Reiss & Price, 1996). By the same token, advocacy at political, national levels may be necessary to inform policy makers of the need for approaches to promote physical and mental health services, as discussed in Chapter 26 in this volume.

Albee (1984, 1996) served as a corrective force in this area, stressing more balanced and more realistic approaches than what appear *prima facie* as solely research-oriented efforts on the part of the federal government. If we were to find that health promotion is more cost-effective than prevention and psychotherapy, then promotion-related approaches may become substitutes for prevention and therapy in a good number of people who need some type of intervention. In conclusion, the question is: "We all want physical and mental health promotion and disease prevention, but how are we going to obtain both, and who is going to pay for them?"

The fields of promotion, prevention, and psychotherapy act separately from each other, as if they were three separate tracks without any ties between to link them. The list of promotion approaches found in this book, for instance, does not include prevention or psychotherapy. Prevention treatises in community and health psychology do not contain psychotherapeutic approaches (Bloom, 1996; Camic & Knight, 2000; Dalton, Elias, & Wandersman, 2001; Jason & Glenwick, 2002). Psychotherapy treatises do not contain preventive approaches, let alone promotional ones (De Maria, 2003). This separation hurts those very people who could use an integration of all three approaches in ideologies and in methods of intervention (L'Abate, 2005b).

The Concept of Structure to Promote Physical and Mental Health

The concept of competence promotion, mentioned earlier, needs to be included within the context of structure. If we conceive of promotion as Green and Kreuter (1999) did, promotion would consist of a planned combination of educational, regulatory, and community efforts to promote physical and mental health. For a thorough background on the history of health promotion, interested readers are referred to the relevant chapter by Bingenheimer, Repetto, Zimmerman and Kelly (2001). These approaches follow or claim to follow a structure, consisting of reproducible and replicable operations. For instance, promotional practices are based on written instructions, or recipes, that indicate the structure of how, when, and where a particular approach should be used.

Structure is not only defined by the number of sessions but also by content and cost. In psycho-educational skill training programs, for instance, prospective participants know beforehand (a) the cost of the program, if any, (b) the number of sessions needed, and (c) the content of topic(s) to be covered, such as assertiveness, parental effectiveness, couple relationships, etc. Since these programs are usually administered to groups rather than to individuals, less professional time is required to administer them. The time of semi-professionals and paraprofessional volunteers, who would run these groups, perhaps under the support and direction of a professional, is less costly then the time of professionals. In contrast to preventive approaches, prescriptive approaches should not require more than one, or at the most, two to three sessions to train participants in the particular area in which they want to become involved. In some cases, like self-help groups, entering into a group and talking is all that is necessary.

The important issue of evaluation and identification needs to be expanded if the fields of health promotional and preventive mental health are to advance and progress (L'Abate, 1990). However, one factor that differentiates promotion from prevention lies in the former being a volunteer activity, while in prevention participants are solicited to participate. Unless we can discriminate and identify levels of functionality among participants, the whole health promotion and disease prevention enterprise will be considered futile by policy makers and critics. Such identification may not be needed in administering compatible prescriptive approaches because participation is voluntary.

An additional feature of prescriptive approaches is validation. It is much easier (cheaper, more feasible) to validate the usefulness of low-cost promotional approaches because of their structured nature. A clear structure is easier to validate than a structure i.e., complex, unclear, minimal, or "non-structured." Most therapeutic approaches, for instance, because of their very unstructured nature, are extremely difficult to validate empirically through replication. This statement does not deny that preventive and therapeutic approaches have been validated; rather, it asserts that structured approaches are easier (cheaper, more feasible, etc.) to replicate and validate than unstructured ones.

In addition to people in crisis, who may need immediate, unstructured (open-ended as far as number of sessions is concerned and open to content) therapeutic help, there are also many more people who could use promotional, structured approaches, as indicated in greater detail in this volume as well as in past reviews of the prevention literature (see Preface this volume).

Prevalence and Treatment of Mental Health Problems

As already presented earlier in this chapter and reframed here to stress the importance of low-cost approaches, there were 35.1 million (14.7%) persons aged 12 or older who had at least one major depressive episode (MDE) in their lifetime. Of these, 19.3 million persons (8.1% of the population) had an MDE in the past 12 months, including 2.2 million youths aged 12–17 and 17.1 million adults aged 18 or older. That past year prevalence of MDE was highest for persons aged 18–25 (10.1%) and lowest for those aged 26 or older (7.6%). The rate among youths aged 12–17 was 9.0%. Females were more likely than males to have MDE in the past year (10.6% vs. 5.5%). Persons with past year MDE were more likely than those without MDE to have used an illicit drug in the past year (28.8% vs. 13.8%). Similarly, substance dependence or abuse was more prevalent among persons with MDE than among those without MDE (22.0% vs. 8.6%, respectively). Among persons aged 12 or older with past year MDE, 62.3% received treatment (i.e., saw or talked to a medical doctor or other professional or used prescription medication) for depression within the past 12 months. While MDE estimates describe persons with a specific mental disorder, the survey also produces estimates of serious psychological distress (SPD), which describe persons with a high level of distress due to any type of mental problem. In 2004, there were 21.4 million adults aged 18 or older with SPD. This represents 9.9% of all adults, a rate that increased since 2002 when it was 8.3%. SPD was highly correlated with substance dependence or abuse. Among adults with SPD in 2004, 21.3% (4.6 million) were dependent on or abused alcohol or illicit drugs, while the rate among adults without SPD was 7.9%. Among the 21.4 million adults with SPD in 2004, 10.3 million, or 48.1%, received treatment for a mental health problem in the past year. Among the 4.6 million adults with SPD and a substance use disorder in 2004, 47.5% (about 2.2 million) received treatment for mental health problems, and 11.0% (503,000) received specialty substance use treatment. Only 6.0% (274,000) received both types of treatment. In 2004, 27.5 million adults (12.8%) received treatment for mental health problems in the past year. This estimate is similar to the estimates in 2002 and 2003. The most prevalent type of treatment for mental health problems among adults in 2004 was prescription medication (10.5% of the population), followed by outpatient treatment (7.1%). 1.9 million adults (0.9%) received inpatient care for mental health problems at some time within the past 12 months. In 2004, 5.7 million youths aged 12–17 (22.5%) received treatment or counseling for emotional or behavior problems in the year prior to the interview. This is higher than the estimates for 2002 (19.3%) and 2003 (20.6%). Clearly, we do need a variety of cost-effective approaches to reach populations that are difficult to reach and to retain in any type of intervention.

Progression in the Classification of Prescriptive Approaches

The classification of promotional approaches contained in this book, as well as in the continuum of preventive and psychotherapeutic approaches (Table 1.1) follows a progression along five major dimensions: costs, complexity, temporality, specificity, and internality-externality. The three prevention tiers (Table 1.1), for instance, could be classified according to criteria used to include and classify approaches: costs, easy and simplicity of administration, concreteness, replicability, and degree of involvement required of participants. For instance, costs may be one criterion for classification of promotional approaches, with universal approach being the cheapest (Section II), followed by primary nonverbal (Section III), secondary writing (Section IV), tertiary relational (Section V), and quartic, multi- relational (Section VI), and ending with community-wide approaches. The latter community approaches are not included in this book, because they require a section of their own, with more information and space than this book can provide. *Preventive* programs requiring lengthier and more complex manuals, guidelines, and more prolonged relationships over a period of time, will be, by necessity, more costly and constitute a fifth, separate tier of their own.

A sixth tier might include skills training programs for specific conditions for targeted populations, adult children of alcoholics, for instance, with a specified number of sessions, with each session dedicated to a specific topic (De Maria, 2003; L'Abate & Milan, 1985). They would constitute an area of secondary prevention, shared, among others, by writing and self-help workbooks (Section V this volume), because of their targeted nature for specific conditions.

Costs

One reason many people in need of help fail to receive treatment lies in costs of physical and mental health approaches that are not covered for people without insurance. Hence, costs are a crucial factor in people receiving or not receiving needed physical and mental health help (Chamberlin, 2004). Stress on no-cost, low-cost, and cost-effectiveness for prescriptive approaches adds a dimension that might have been ignored by therapeutic approaches, and, in spite of claims to the contrary, by traditional preventive approaches, since the latter may need research grants to survive.

Complexity

The classification of approaches used here (see Table of Contents) follows a progressive sequence, from simple nutritional to more complex nonverbal, and even more complex relational and multi-relational ones, with the most complex being community-wide approaches, not contained here. The increase in complexity limits progressively the populations that can profit by a specific approaches. The more complex the approach, the more limited is the population it can be administered to, with costs increasing accordingly (Lombard, Haddock, Talcott, & Reynes, 1998). Nonetheless, as considered in Section VI (Chapter 26 this volume), it is possible to access large populations at minimal costs when promotional policies are involved.

Temporality

The issue of complexity is also related to temporality. Some approaches show immediate results while others have delayed effects. Exercise, for instance, may have an immediate effect as well as a delayed effect, while diet, vitamins, and supplements may have more delayed effects. Some effects may be immediately felt and visible, as in state-wide promotional approaches (Chapter 26 this volume), while the effects of other approaches may be more difficult to experience and to report on.

Specificity

The more complex a approaches is the more specific it will become in being used by more selected and specific groups of participants. Primary nutritional approaches, for instance, are the simplest in this classification and more generally universal. However, writing requires skills that may limit the populations it can be administered to. By the same token, dancing and expressive movements may be followed by illiterate people who can coordinate a tune with body movements. Some people, normal otherwise, may not have the ability or be inclined to coordinate music with body movements. People do not need to read or write to dance or to talk.

Internality

For a approach like food, for instance, internality means the approach is completely in the hands of participants, self-initiated and self-administered, as in the case of simple, universal approaches, like nutrition. More complex approaches, on the other hand, may depend on some training, some supervision and follow-up by external agents or by lay or volunteer workers. However, once the approaches is implemented, it can go its course without any further instructions.

Toward a Sieves or Stepped Approach to Health Promotion and Disease Prevention

Unfortunately, the scheme cited above does not indicate how concretely we can differentiate among levels of individual, dyadic, and multi-relational functioning. We need such a discrimination if we want to match participants with a specific promotion or prevention track (Mitchell, Stevenson, & Florin, 1996). In the past, a "sieves or hurdles model," was suggested, going from the least expensive (primary) to the most expensive (tertiary) intervention (L'Abate, 1990). If participants "fail" to profit by primary prevention, then secondary prevention strategies would be added. If these strategies fail, then tertiary prevention, crisis-oriented strategies would be used. The issue here consists of finding objective, intersubjective criteria that would distinguish according to levels of functionality from the very outset of offering any type of intervention. The technology to achieve such differentiation is available but it is not yet widely used.

In addition to the myriad of promotional technologies now available, as evidenced by the number of chapters in this book, the following model is suggested, using cost and length of treatment as major criteria:

1. Functional participants, self-selected and willing to participate, need no evaluation or scoring low on objective test batteries to measure individual

functioning and potential for future conflict, would receive just one or at most two prescriptive approaches, before primary and/or secondary prevention program. If one fails to gain from approaches at this level, one would need to "progress" to a more expensive sieve.
2. Semi-functional participants, scoring in the middle range on objective test batteries to measure individual or relational functioning, and with a specific issue or problem in the referral, would receive a preventive program directed toward the topic or issue needed or asked for by participants (McFarlane, 1991).
3. Semi-functional participants, already identified, who do not benefit from a preventive program, may benefit from brief, crisis-oriented psychotherapy with or without written homework assignments, as presented in Section IV, including online journaling (Chapter 11 this volume), autobiographies (Chapter 12 this volume), expressive writing (Chapter 13 this volume), and self-help, mental health workbooks (Chapter 14 this volume).
4. Dysfunctional participants, scoring high on test batteries to assess individual, dyadic, or family functioning, would receive crisis intervention plus specific, psycho-educational, social skills training programs. Depending on the nature of the referring question, long-term psychotherapy, i.e., *tertiary* or "*indicated*" prevention, would include none, some, or all of the techniques used in primary and secondary prevention plus medication when indicated.

Indeed, as the Seligman's (1996) Consumer's Report indicates, in spite of its many flaws and criticisms (Strupp, 1996; VandenBos, 1996), individuals who have been involved in prolonged therapeutic relationships are those who also report the greatest benefits. This conclusion is supported by Norcross' (2004) recent review. However, Norcross reported that "Most of the available studies (76%) found a significant, inverse relation between level of impairment and treatment outcome (p. 22)." This conclusion supports the suggestion that the greater the degree and type of dysfunctionality, the greater is the need for more than one approach to deal with it. Clearly, future research should concentrate on comparing structured versus unstructured approaches using the same number of sessions, with or without homework assignments (Kazantzis et al., 2005; Kazantzis & L'Abate, 2007; Tompkins, 2004).

The Urgent Need to Train Health Promoters

The field of physical and mental health promotion cannot be launched effectively until a properly trained and credentialed profession is created (L'Abate, 1983, 1987a). One effect that managed care may have on the profession of psychotherapy will be to force many psychotherapists to expand to new and diverse populations. These populations could consist of those who, for whatever reason, are in need or at risk and who could use promotional and primary and secondary preventive approaches rather than crisis intervention or psychotherapy (tertiary prevention). This means that unless colleges and universities begin efforts in the direction of creating new and specific course work and curricula in health promotion and prevention, no new, separately innovative profession can be created (L'Abate, 2005c). To wit, Perry, Albee, Bloom, and Gullotta (1996) argued that "Increasingly undergraduates and graduate students as well as mid-career professionals are deciding to pursue careers focused on the primary prevention of mental disorders and the promotion of mental health." These authors suggested various "...training and career options available to prospective students." Among these options these authors presented "a compendium of prevention resources [that] is not readily available" (p. 357). Among the disciplines that may offer training in prevention are: public health, community psychology, social work, counseling, and education. As laudably useful as this thesis may be for individuals contemplating such a career, one would need to substantiate the point that the majority of students and professionals are seeking careers in primary prevention. No data were offered to support such a position. It would be wonderful for physical and mental health promotion if such an increase were indeed present and substantiated. Yet, at the present time, this thesis seems more of an intangible wish than an established fact.

This conclusion, therefore, indicates the need for a completely new and different profession, and i.e., a profession or specialization of "promoters/ preventers" who will specialize in mastering such approaches (L'Abate, 1983, 1987a). These approaches could reach people who may not need crisis-oriented therapy but who are in need or at risk for possible breakdown, and who could profit and benefit by structured, promotional activities or interventions included in this book. Trainers for these populations could be part of an online curriculum that would require completely novel sets of skills not shared by traditional mental health professions, since these structured techniques are not part of most psychotherapeutic approaches (L'Abate, 2005a, 2005b, 2005c).

The field of promotional and preventive programs is an extremely wide one. It is vast enough to require specialization at the graduate level and able to meet most of the needs of functional and semi-functional people. Low-cost approaches promoting physical and mental health, therefore, have the potential to provide those very skills that are not available anywhere else but that are necessary to become effective persons, partners, and parents.

Differentiating Among Skills for Promotion and Prevention

Once the field of promotion is differentiated from preventive approaches, this scheme suggests a hierarchical structure in promotion involving differentiating between minimal skills, versus technical, versus professional skills. Unless such a differentiation finds a rationale, it will be impossible to create a much-needed hierarchal pyramid of skills and competencies in promotion, prevention, and psychotherapy, namely: clerical, technical, semi-professional, and professional. Even volunteer laypersons who want to be involved in some helpful activity will need to possess minimal technical skills but show also personal qualifications of responsible and responsive concern, caring, compassion, and intellectual capacities.

In pre-post intervention evaluation, the range of skills covered may vary from simply clerical, like filing or answering phone calls, to technical. The latter would consist of the administration and scoring of objective, group-oriented instruments. Subprofessionals could administer many structured programs. Professional skills, on the other hand, would consist of interpreting test results and reporting them with diagnostic conclusions and treatment implications. On the axes of Time versus Knowledge (L'Abate, 1994), technical skills take more time but require less education, knowledge, and training. Professional skills may take less time but require more education and more knowledge. To wit, it takes about an hour to administer an intelligence test and about half an hour to score it. But it may take a few minutes for a professional to interpret and report what the scores mean.

Technical skills may consist of administration of structured programs or materials, like enrichment, and keeping in touch with volunteers, clerical personnel, participants, and with supervising or consulting professionals. Professional skills may be needed for crisis intervention and symptom reduction with decision making about the type of course of treatment needed, with support and supervision of technical personnel. Educationally, volunteers and paraprofessionals need to show responsible and caring characteristics. They need motivation to help others but do not have the necessary education and expertise. A high school diploma may be needed for clerical skills, while some college may be needed for administration and scoring of standard test batteries, and administration of structured programs. Middle-level professionals will need a masters degree for direct services in secondary and tertiary prevention according to training and level of interests and experience. Professionals may need a doctorate or equivalent education for direction, research, support, supervision, and direction of treatment with crisis intervention (L'Abate, 2001, 2002).

If it is valid to conclude that for every participant (individuals, couples, or families) that is in therapy there are at least ten other potential participants who could use some other form of educative, promotional, or preventive intervention, then only a hierarchical personnel structure will be able to deal with so many participants. Some nonprofessional promoters/preventers, for instance, may not possess professional skills but may possess sufficient human skills (Carl Rogers' warmth, empathy, and unconditional positive regard) to receive restricted training and supervision from a more knowledgeable professional in one specific, structured prevention program rather than in a wide range of programs or unstructured techniques.

The fields of health promotion and disease prevention are so large that only few professionals can master them. Semi-professionals and paraprofessionals may master a much smaller number of approaches. Nonprofessional volunteers, for instance, may master just one approach. If indeed there are many more participants in need of alternative promotional and preventive approaches than there are professionals available for them, the challenge of the future will lie in training a vast hierarchy of health promoters and disease preventers who will take pride in identifying themselves as such, without seeing themselves as second-class therapists.

Looking at the Future

If we have learned anything from the past, we need to look at various issues implicit in the future of health promotion. These issues involve motivation, dissemination, implications for practice, and what will happen in the future?

Issues of Motivation

Motivation is and will remain a major issue in the delivery of approaches in general. It also is and will remain a major issue in the delivery of selected approaches to special populations in particular. Very likely, motivation will be determined by (a) the specific nature of the approaches, with primary, universal, nutritional approaches being used without any prodding except hunger, (b) specific needs of participants who select which secondary or tertiary approaches they like and want to enjoy life, (c) education and societal pressures to assure a better quality of life, and (d) societal and cultural changes that will in part determine the motivation of needy populations.

This motivation inside individuals will be increased or decrease according to the (a) involvement of mass media in distributing information about the usefulness of these approaches, (b) involvement of mental health organizations in making these approaches part of their training programs and of educational requirements for professional advancement, (c) resistance to change in mental health professionals who may see promotional approaches as a potential threat to their livelihood, (d) involvement of governmental agencies in requiring the use of approaches as part of an adoption of approaches as standard operating procedures required of most professionals (Chapter 26 this volume), and (e) influence of managed care companies in requiring the use of approaches as reimbursable payments for services.

Issues of Dissemination

It is an open question whether the Federal Government should be involved except for disseminating information or in a more direct ways as in the past, supporting directly preventive approaches. Clearly, some efforts at dissemination through the media as well as through professional organization will be necessary (Crits-Christoph, 1996; Gotham, 2004; Kettlewell, 2004; Southam-Gerow, 2004; Winett et al., 1995).

More recently, the introduction of new technology, like virtual reality and the Internet have made the whole enterprise of mental health promotion, prevention, and treatment available to more people than it has been possible heretofore (Chapter 16 this volume; Gullotta & Bloom, 2003; L'Abate, 2005c).

Implications for Practice

It is questionable whether the mental health profession is willing and able to change outdated and expensive preventive and clinical practices in favor of modern technology and cost-effective approaches (L'Abate, 1997, 1999, 2003). Change for mental health professionals, if it is to occur, will include the judicious use of all three media of communication – nonverbal, spoken, and written – including Virtual Reality (North, North, & Cogle, 1996) and greater reliance on technological advances found on TV, videos, pagers/beepers, phones, and computers (De Maria, 2003; Kalichman, 1996; L'Abate & Odell, 1995).

To further the mission of approaches administration to as many willing participants, there is no doubt that this practice of promotion needs to be solidly based on theory as well as on research. It would help the cause of promotion, prevention, and psychotherapy if both theory and research went hand-in-hand with each other (L'Abate, 1990, 1994, 1997, 2005a; L'Abate & De Giacomo, 2003).

The Need for Theory to Underlie Research

Smith (1999) decried the lack of theory to underlay most preventive and psychotherapeutic practices. The advent of empirically based approaches has taken first place to theoretical considerations. Theoretical views are not even considered as secondary. These considerations are actually not even brought forth in the relevant literature on empirically-based interventions. For instance, many relational approaches (Section V this volume) are based on close physical contact to strengthen attachment bonds, would fall within the realm of communal/expressive skills. Secondary and tertiary relational skills (Sections IV and VI this volume) would fall within the agentic/instrumental realm (L'Abate, 2005a).

Consequently, without an underlying theory, research about promotional, preventive, and psycho-therapeutic practices are bound to proliferate aimlessly, without a comprehensive umbrella that will allow them to integrate and even expand on the basis of empirical evidence guided by theory rather than by the whims and will of investigators.

The Need for Research to Underlie Practice

The present and long overdue emphasis on empirically supported approaches is welcome, provided it does not become a hindrance to creativity and productivity. Consequently, prescriptive approaches for physical and mental health need to be not only theory-derived, they must also be empirically-based (Weisz et al., 2005). Otherwise, theory without research evidence is a useless pursuit, while research without an underlying theoretical framework would lead to another Tower of Babel, with a great many research projects completely unrelated to each other and without an overarching theoretical framework (L'Abate, 2004c).

Theory-derived, Empirically-based Practice

The administration of some, but not all approaches, involves some learning and comfort on how to work at a distance from participants, with a minimum of f2f contacts and talk, with reliance on homework assignments, and phones, mail, fax, computers and Internet. As indicated above, progressive sieves or stepped sieves going *from the least expensive to the most expensive hurdle* (L'Abate, 1990), i.e., from universal approaches, without professional supervision, not requiring f2f contact and talk, to more expensive f2f talk with professional, i.e., "Take this general promotional approach and call me in the morning." If that does not work, let's try this nonverbal approaches, "If that does not work let's try, etc."

Here is where the five dimensions of progressions in costs, complexity, temporality, specificity, and internality mentioned earlier, come into their practical applications. Interventions with approaches then would follow a rational progression from least expensive approaches first, as in nutrition, to secondary nonverbal and writing approaches, second, and relational approaches, third. One could go as far as to make seeing and talking with a professional f2f contingent on participants' successful completion of homework assignments for some approaches. Instead of evaluating solely through talk, the level of motivation to change in participants could be evaluated through actual completion of assigned tasks, as practiced by Gould (2001) for years with thousands of participants. Professional f2f talk, i.e., crisis intervention or psychotherapy, would be used fourth in this progression, with medication, fifth, and, being most expensive, hospitalization sixth. What is the best way to demonstrate whether people want to change? The answer lies in giving participants different options to demonstrate their motivation by actual doing rather than by just talking.

What Will Happen in the Future?

A very likely prediction that is certain to happen relates to the transformation that promotion will undergo as a natural consequence in the inevitable process of greater differentiation and specialization. As systems survive, they tend to become institutionalized and absorbed into the mainstream. Hence, as part of this differentiation a greater and greater fragmentation of parts will occur. There will be greater differentiation of promotional activities, as considered elsewhere (L'Abate, 2004c).

Distance Approaches

By the same token, the future will see greater reliance on distance writing approaches (Section IV this volume), whether as written homework assignments or as computer assisted training (Bloom, 1992; Esterling et al., 1999; Gould, 2001; Williams, Boles, & Johnson, 1995). The cost-effective nature of these approaches, away from f2f contact with a professional, but under the guidance of a professional (via mail, phone, and E-mail), will facilitate access to populations that heretofore would have been impossible to reach. The essence of a public versus private health approach is indeed reliance on mass-oriented and cost-effective approaches rather than individualized ones.

Adding Promotion to Existing Preventive and Psychotherapeutic Practices

A greater integration of preventive programs with therapeutic practices will allow a hierarchical organization to come into effect. For instance, as illustrated by Kochalka, Buzas, L'Abate, McHenry, and Gibson (1987), it was possible to use paraprofessionals to administer enrichment programs to families after they had terminated crisis-oriented psychotherapy. Hence, *a reversed sieves model* could be operational here. Instead of going from the least expensive to the most expensive approach, as suggested earlier, participants (individuals, couples, and families) in crisis would be seen initially by a professional for time-limited crisis-intervention. Once the crisis is decreased, it would be followed by health promoting approaches in the hands of paraprofessional personnel supervised by professionals, or preventive, psycho-educational skill training programs (De Maria, 2003).

Greater Use of Homework Assignments

There is not denying that the use of homework assignments, whether in writing or verbally, is bound to increase (Kazantzis et al., 2005; Kazantzis & L'Abate, 2007; L'Abate, 2004a, b; Tompkins, 2004). Even though homework is supposed to shorten therapy, it will be crucial to find out which kind of homework will shorten psychotherapy and which will not. For instance, L'Abate, L'Abate, and Maino (2005) found that written homework assignments, i.e., workbooks, significantly lengthened the number of therapy sessions for individuals, couples, and families. Contrary to L'Abate's (1992, 2001, 2002) repeated claims of cost-effectiveness, these results would suggest that, at least written homework assignments, rather than any other kind of homework, may produce greater involvement and investment in participants. On the other hand, Goldstein, as reported in Chapter 15 (this volume), found that a problem-solving workbook cut in half the length of hospital stays in women with personality disorders. If that is the case, then further testing and evidence will be necessary to find which part of the outcome in promotion, prevention, and psychotherapy is due to f2f effects, which is due to homework assignments in general, and which is due to what kind of homework, for instance, administered in writing versus administered orally.

Comparative Testing

Comparative testing of promotional approaches together with parallel testing comparing the effectiveness of preventive or therapeutic approaches will be necessary if not vital. For instance, comparative testing of validated versus nonvalidated promotions will allow comparative testing of promotion versus prevention versus validated therapies according to cost-effectiveness and length (Beutler, 2004; Hays, Follette, Dawes, & Grady, 1995). By the same token, once comparative testing of manualized versus free-floating psychotherapy takes place, eventually, comparison of validated versus nonvalidated psychotherapeutic approaches will serve as backdrop for comparative testing between and among promotional and preventive approaches. As Tompkins (2004) commented on this issue: "...current manuals offer therapists...little guidance on how to implement therapy homework, even though we know that their ability to effectively assign and review homework can influence whether the participants improve or not" (p. ix).

The future is ready and ripe for prescriptive approaches as well as for preventive programs (structured, manualized, or validated, with or without homework assignments) for groups of individuals, couples, and families. However, each specialty area will need to prove itself in the arena of comparative cost-effectiveness. Once cost-effectiveness has been demonstrated (in either direction!), it will be easier to convince insurance companies, managed care organizations, and politicians that promotion and disease prevention indeed do pay. We will need to prepare a new profession of health promoters and disease preventers who will know all the pros and cons of both promotional and preventive programs (L'Abate, 2005c). None of the above, however, will take place unless comparative cost-effectiveness testing occurs in promotional and preventive programs themselves.

Conclusion

The purpose of this chapter is to introduce and to expand on the need for low-cost and cost-effective health promotion approaches that are called "prescriptive promotions." These approaches are easy to self-initiate and self-administer, or easy to be administered by others. They are simple to implement and relatively concrete to be available to a wide range of populations, those who might not need professional help as well as those who do need professional help. Most promotional approaches have shown noticeable or known benefits on physical and mental health. The introduction of these approaches has a broad implication on how mental health services in prevention and psychotherapy will be delivered in this coming century. A hierarchical structure of approaches administrators would include unpaid lay volunteers, paid semi- or subprofessionals, and supervising and advisory full-fledged professionals. Whether these changes will occur and be implemented depends on many factors that involve scientific disciplines, professional organizations, the Federal Government, private foundations, and the dissemination of information about prescriptive approaches above and beyond guild and proprietary interests.

References

Albee, G. W. (1959). *Mental health manpower trends*. New York: Basic Books.

Albee, G. W. (1984). Prologue: A model for classifying prevention programs. In J. M. Joffe, G. W. Albee, & L. D. Kelly (Eds.), *Readings in primary prevention of psychopathology* (pp. ix-xviii). Hanover, VT: University Press of New England.

Albee, G. W. (1996). Revolutions and counterrevolutions in prevention. *American Psychologist, 51*, 1130–1133.

Albee, G. W., & Gullotta, T. P. (Eds.). (1997). *Primary prevention works*. Thousand Oaks, CA: Sage.

Alberti, R. E., & Emmons, M. L. (1970). *Your perfect right: A guide to assertive behavior*. San Louis Obispo, CA: Impact.

Arcus, M. E., Schvaneveldt, J. D., & Moss, J. J. (Eds.). (1993). *Book of family life education: The practice of family life education*. Newbury Park, CA: Sage.

Bakan, D. (1968). *Disease, pain, and sacrifice: Toward a psychology of suffering*. Boston, MA: Beacon Press.

Baum, A., & Posluszny, D. M. (1999). Health psychology: Mapping biobehavioral contributions to health and illness. *Annual Review of Psychology, 50*, 137–163.

Baum, A., & Singer, J. (Eds.). (2001). *Book of health psychology*. Mahwah, NJ: Earlbaum.

Berger, R., & Hannah, M. T. (Eds.). (1999). *Preventive approaches in couples therapy*. Philadelphia, PA: Brunner/Mazel.

Bingenheimer, J. B., Repetto, P. B., Zimmerman, M. A., & Kelly, J. G. (2001). A brief history and analysis of health promotion. In T. Gullotta & M. Bloom (Eds.), *Encyclopedia of primary prevention and health promotion* (pp. 23–26). New York: Kluwer Academic.

Bloom, B. L. (1975). *Community mental health: A general introduction*. Monterey, CA: Brooks/Cole.

Bloom, B. L. (1992). Computer-assisted psychological intervention: A review and commentary. *Clinical Psychology Review, 12*, 169–197.

Bloom, M. (1996). *Primary prevention practices*. Thousand Oaks, CA: Sage.

Bureau of Census (2004). *Statistical Abstract of the U.S., 2004–05*. Washington, DC.

Camic, P., & Knight, S. (Eds.). (1998). *Clinical book of health psychology*. Seattle, WA: Hogrefe & Huber.

Caminiti, S. (2005). A better RX for what ails us. *Fortune, 152*, S1–S16.
Caplan, G. (1964). *Principles of preventive psychiatry*. New York: Basic Books.
Chamberlin, J. (2004). Survey says: More Americans are seeking mental health treatment. *Monitor on Psychology, 35*, 17.
Crits-Christoph, P. (1996). The dissemination of efficacious psychological treatments. *Clinical Psychology: Science and Practice, 3*, 260–263.
Cusinato, M. (2004). Marriage preparation and maintenance. In L. L'Abate (Ed.), *Using workbooks in mental health: Resources in prevention, psychotherapy and rehabiliation for clinicians and researchers* (pp. 217–245). Binghamton, NY. Haworth.
Dalton, J. H., Elias, M. J., & Wandersman, A. (2001). *Community psychology: Linking individuals with communities*. Belmont, CA: Wadsworth/Thompson Learning
Dane, A. V., & Schneider, B. H. (1998). Program integrity in primar and early secondary prevention: Are implementation effects out of control? *Clinical Psychology Review, 18*, 23–45.
De Maria, R. (2003). Psycho-education and enrichment: Clinical considerations for couple and family therapy. In L. Sexton, G. Weeks, & M. Robbins (Eds.), *Book of family therapy* (pp. 411–430). New York: Brunner-Routledge.
Department of Justice (2003). United States Federal Bureau of Investigation (Released October, 2003). *Crimes and crime rates, 2002*. <http://www.fbi.gov/wcr/02cins/htm> Washington, DC.
Dew, M. A., & Bromet, E. J. (1993). Epidemiology. In A. S. Bellack, & M. Hersen (Eds.), *Psycho-pathology in adulthood* (pp. 21–40). Boston, MA: Allyn & Bacon.
Edelstein, B. A., & Michelson, L. (Eds.). (1986). *Book of prevention*. New York: Plenum Press.
Elliot, A. J., & Dweck, C. S. (Eds.). (2005). *Book of competence and motivation*. New York: Guilford.
Ellsworth, R. B. (1968). *Nonprofessionals in psychiatric rehabilitation: The psychiatric aide and the schizophrenic patient*. New York: Appleton-Century-Crofts.
Esterling, B. A., L'Abate, L., Murray, E., & Pennebaker, J. M. (1999). Empirical foundation for writing in prevention and psychotherapy. *Clinical Psychology Review, 19*, 79–96.
Felner, R. D., Jason, L. A., Moritsugu, J. N., & Farber, S. S. (Eds.). (1983). *Preventive psychology: Theory, research, and practice*. New York: Pergamon Press.
Goldstein, A. P. (1973). *Structured learning therapy: Toward a psychotherapy for the poor*. New York: Academic Press.
Gordon, T. (1970). *Parental effectiveness training*. New York: Wyden Books.
Gotham, H. J. (2004). Diffusion of mental health and substance abuse treatments: Development, dissemination, and implementation. *Clinical Psychology: Science and Practice, 11*, 160–176.
Gould, R. L. (2001). A feedback-driven computer program for outpatient training. In L. L'Abate (Ed.), *Distance writing and computer-assisted interventions in psychiatry and mental health* (pp. 43–111). Westport, CT: Ablex.
Gould, R. A., & Clum, G. A. (1993). A meta-analysis of self-help treatment approaches. *Clinical Psychology Review, 13*, 169–186.
Green, E. C., & Kreuter, M. W. (1999). *Health promotion planning: An educational and ecological approach*. Mountain View, CA: Mayfield.
Gregory. R. J., Schwer-Canning, S., Lee, T. W., & Wise, J. C. (2004). Cognitive bibliotherapy for depression: A meta-analysis. *Professional Psychology: Research & Practice, 35*, 275–280.
Grosser, C., Henry, W. E., & Kelly, J. G. (1969). *Nonprofessionals in he human services*. San Francisco, CA: Jossey-Bass.
Guerney, B. L., Jr. (Ed.). (1969). *Psychotherapeutic agents: New roles for nonprofessionals, parents, and teachers*. New York: Holt, Rinehart & Winston.
Gullotta, T. P., & Bloom, B. L. (Eds.). (2003). *Encyclopedia of primary prevention and health promotion*, New York:Kluwer Academic.

Hays, S. C., Follette, V. M., Dawes, R. M. & Grady, K. E. (Eds.). (1995). *Scientific standards of psychological practice: Issues and recommendations*. Reno, NV: Context Press.

Heller, K. (1996). Coming of age of prevention science. *American Psychologist, 51*, 1123–1127.

Iscoe, I., Bloom, B. L., & Spielberger, C. D. (1977). *Community psychology in transition*. New York: Halstead Press.

Jason, L. A., & Glenwick, D. S. (Eds.). (2002) *Innovative strategies for promoting health and mental health across the life span*. New York: Springer.

Joint Commission on Mental Illness and Health. (1961). *Action for mental health*. New York: Basic Books.

Kalichman, S. C. (1996). HIV-AIDS prevention videotapes: A review of empirical findings. *The Journal of Primary Prevention, 17*, 259–279.

Kazantzis, N., Deane, F. P., Ronan, K. R., & L'Abate, L. (Eds.). (2005). *Homework assignments in cognitive-behavioral therapy*. New York: Brunner/Routledge.

Kazantzis, N., & L'Abate, L. (Eds.). (2007). *Handbook of homework assignments in psychotherapy: Theory, research, and prevention*. New York: Springer-Science.

Kelly, J. F. (2003). Self-help for substance-use disorders: History, effectiveness, knowledge gaps, and research opportunities. *Clinical Psychology Review, 23*, 639–664.

Kessler, M., Goldston, S. E., & Joffe, J. M. (Eds.). (1992). *The present and future of prevention: In honor of George W. Albee*. Newbury Park, CA: Sage.

Kettlewell, P. W. (2004). Development, dissemination, and implementation of evidence-based treatments: Commentary. *Clinical Psychology: Science and Practice, 11*, 190–195.

Klein, D. C., & Goldston, S. E. (Eds.). (1977). *Primary prevention: An idea whose time has come*. DHEW Publication No.77–447. Washington, DC: Government Printing Office.

Kochalka, J., Buzas, H., L'Abate, L., McHenry, S., & Gibson, E. (1987). Structured enrichment: Training and implementation with paraprofessionals. In L. L'Abate (Ed.), *Family psychology II: Theory, therapy, enrichment, and training* (pp. 279–287). Lanham, MD: University Press of America.

L'Abate, L. (1980). Toward a theory and technology for social skills training: Suggestions for curriculum development. *Academic Psychology Bulletin, 2*, 207–228.

L'Abate, L. (1981). Skill training programs for couples and families. In A. S. Gurman, & D. P. Kniskern (Eds.), *Book of family therapy* (pp. 631–661). New York: Brunner/Mazel.

L'Abate, L. (1983). Prevention as a profession: Toward a new conceptual frame of reference. In D. R. Mace (Ed.), *Prevention in family services: Approaches to family wellness* (pp. 49–62). Beverly Hills, CA: Sage.

L'Abate, L. (1986). Prevention of marital and family problems. In R. A. Edelstein, & L. Michelson (Eds.), *Book of prevention* (pp. 177–193). New York: Plenum.

L'Abate, L. (1987a). A graduate curriculum in preventive psychology. In L. L'Abate (Ed.), *Family psychology II: Theory, therapy, enrichment, and training* (pp. 257–266). Lanham, MD: University Press of America.

L'Abate, L. (1987b). The evolution of family life education: A historical perspective. In L. L'Abate (Ed.), *Family psychology II: Theory, therapy, enrichment, and training* (pp. 181–194). Lanham, MD: University Press of America.

L'Abate, L. (1990). *Building family competence: Primary and secondary prevention strategies*. Newbury Park, CA: Sage.

L'Abate, L. (1992). *Programmed writing: A self-administered approach for interventions with individuals, couples and families*. Pacific Grove, CA: Brooks/Colc.

L'Abate, L. (1994). *A theory of personality development*. New York: Wiley.

L'Abate, L. (1997). The paradox of change: Better them than us! In R. S. Sauber (Ed.), *Managed mental health care: Major diagnostic and treatment approaches* (pp. 40–66). Bristol, PA: Brunner/Mazel.

L'Abate, L. (1999). Taking the bull by the horns: Beyond talk in psychological interventions. *The Family Journal: Therapy and Counseling for Couples and Families, 7*, 206–220.

L'Abate, L. (Ed.). (2001). *Distance writing and computer-assisted approaches in psychiatry and mental heath*. Westport, CT: Ablex.

L'Abate, L. (2002). *Beyond psychotherapy: Programmed writing and structured computer-assisted interventions*. Westport, CT: Ablex.

L'Abate, L. (2003). *Family psychology III: Theory building, theory testing, and psychological interventions*. Lanham, MD: University Press of America.

L'Abate, L. (2004a). *A guide to self-help workbooks for clinicians and researchers*. Binghamton, NY: Haworth.

L'Abate, L. (Ed.). (2004b). *Using workbooks in mental health: Resources in prevention, psychotherapy, and rehabilitation for clinicians and researchers*. Binghamton, NY: Haworth.

L'Abate, L. (2005a). *Personality in intimate relationships: Socialization and psychopathology*. New York: Springer-Science.

L'Abate, L. (in press). What I really believe about family psychotherapy. (Journal of Family Psychotherapy.).

L'Abate, L. (2005c). *A proposed graduate curriculum for structured online mental heath interventions*. (unpublished manuscript).

L'Abate, L. (2006a). Toward a relational theory for psychiatric classification. *American Journal of Family Therapy, 34*, 1–15.

L'Abate, L., & Baggett, M. S. (1997). *The self in the family: A classification of personality, criminality, and psychopathology*. New York: Wiley.

L'Abate, L., & De Giacomo, P. (2003). *Intimate relationships and how to improve them: Integrating theoretical models with preventive and psychotherapeutic applications*. Westport, CT: Praeger.

L'Abate, L., L'Abate, B. L., & Maino, E. (2005). Reviewing 25 years of clinical practice: Written homework assignments and length of therapy. *American Journal of Family Therapy, 33*, 19–31.

L'Abate, L. & Menar, N. (2006). *A theory of personality socialization in intimate relationships*. Manuscript submitted for publication.

L'Abate, L., & Milan, M. (Eds.). (1985). *Handbook of social skills training*. New York: Wiley.

L'Abate, L., & Odell, M. (1995). Enlarging practices and roles of family clinicians. In M. Harway (Ed.), *Treating the changing family: Handling normative and unusual events* (pp. 321–339). New York: Wiley.

L'Abate, L., & Weinstein, S. E. (1987). *Structured enrichment programs for couples and families*. New York: Brunner/Mazel.

Levant, R. F. (Ed.). (1986). *Psychoeducational approaches to family therapy and counseling*. New York: Springer.

Lofquist, W. A. (1983). *Discovering the meaning of prevention*. Tucson, AZ: AYD Publications.

Lombard, D., Haddock, C. K., Talcott, G. W., & Reynes, R. (1998). Cost-effectiveness analysis: A primer for psychologists. *Applied & Preventive Psychology, 7*, 101–108.

Marlowe, H. A., Jr., & Weinberg, R. B. (1985). *Competence development: Theory and practice in special populations*. Springfield, IL: Thomas.

McFarlane, W. R. (1991). Family psychoeducational treatment. In A. S. Gurman, & D. P. Kniskern (Eds.), *Book of family therapy: Volume II* (pp. 363–395). New York: Brunner/Mazel.

Mitchell, R. E., Stevenson, J. F., & Florin, P. (1996). A typology of prevention activities: Applications to community coalitions. *The Journal of Primary Prevention, 16*, 413–436.
Mrazek, P. J., & Haggerty, R. J. (Eds.). (1994). *Reducing risks for mental disorders: Frontiers for preventive intervention research.* Washington, DC: National Academy Press.
Munoz, R. F., Mrazek, P. J., & Haggerty, R. J. (1996). Institute of Medicine report on prevention of mental disorders. *American Psychologist, 51*, 1116–1122.
National Institute of Mental Health (2001). *The Numbers Count: Mental Disorders in America: A summary of statistics describing the prevalence of mental disorders in America.* Rockville, MD: Department of Health and Human Services.
National Mental Health Association Commission on the Prevention of Mental-Emotional Disabilities (1986). *The prevention of mental-emotional disorders: Report and resource papers.* Alexandra, VI: National Mental Health Association.
New Freedom Commission on Mental Health (2003). *Achieving the promise: Transforming mental healthcare in America: Executive summary.* Rockville, MD: DHHS Publication No. SMA-03-3831.
Norcross, J. C. (2004). Empirically supported therapy relationships. *The Clinical Psychologist, 57*, 19–24.
Norcross, J. C., Santrock, J. W., Campbell, L. F., Smith, T. P., Sommer, R., & Zuckerman, E. L. (2000). *Authoritative guide to self-help resources in mental health.* New York, NY: Guildford.
North, M. M., North, S. M., & Cogle, J. R. (1996). *Virtual reality therapy: An innovative paradigm.* Colorado Springs, CO: IPI Press.
Perry, M. J., Albee, G. W., Bloom, M., & Gullotta, T. P. (1996). Training and career paths in primary prevention. *Journal of Primary Prevention, 16*, 357–371.
Phillips, E. L. (1978). *The social skills basis of psychopathology: Alternative to abnormal psychology.* New York: Grune & Stratton.
Phillips, E. L. (1985). Social skills: History and prospect. In L. L'Abate, & M. Milan (Eds.), *Handbook of social skills training and research* (pp. 3–21). New York: Wiley.
Phillips, L. (1968). *Human adaptation and its failures.* New York: Academic Press.
Pransky, J. (1991). *Prevention: The critical need.* Springfield, MO: Burrell Foundation.
Rappaport, J. (1992). The death and resurrection of the community mental health movement. In M. Kessler, S. E. Goldston, & M. Joffe (Eds.), *The present and future of prevention: In honor of George W. Albee* (pp. 78–98). Newbury Park, CA: Sage.
Reiss, D., & Price, R. H. (1996). National research agenda for prevention research. *American Psychologist, 51*, 1109–1113.
Reppucci, N. D., Woolard, J. L., & Fried, C. S. (1999). Social, community, and preventive interventions. *Annual Review of Psychology, 50*, 387–418.
Rioch, M. (1970). Should psychotherapists do therapy? *Professional Psychology, 2*, 139–142.
Roberts, M. C., & Peterson, L. (1984). *Prevention of problems in childhood: Psychological research and applications.* New York: Wiley-Interscience.
Russell, L. B. (1986). *Is prevention better than cure*? Washington, D. C.: The Brookings Institution.
Sarafino, F. P. (1994). *Health psychology: Biosocial interventions.* New York: Wiley.
Schneiderman, N., Antoni, M. H., Saab, P. G., & Ironson, G. (2001) Health psychology: Psychological and biobehavioral aspects of chronic disease management. *Annual Review of Psychology, 52*, 555–580.
Seligman, M. E. P. (1996). Good news for psychotherapy: The Consumer Report study. *The Georgia Psychologist*, Winter, 42–45.
Smith, D. A. (1999). The end of theoretical orientations? *Applied & Preventive Psychology*, 8, 269–280.

Smith, L. (2005). Psychotherapy, classism, and the poor: Conspicuous by their absence. *American Psychologist, 60*, 687–696.

Sobey, F. (1970). *The nonprofessional revolution in mental heath*. New York: Columbia University Press.

Southam-Gerow, M. A. (2004). Some reasons that mental health treatments are not technologies: Toward treatment development and adaptation outside labs. *Clinical Psychology: Science and Practice, 11*, 186–189.

Srole, L., Langner, T. S., Michael, S. T., Kirkpatrick, P., et al. (1962). *Mental health in the metropolis: The Midtown Manhattan study*. New York: Harper & Row.

Sternberg, R. J., & Kolligian, J. Jr. (Eds). (1990). *Competence considered*. New Haven, CT: Yale University Press.

Strupp, H. H. (1996). The tripartite model and the Consumer Reports study. *American Psychologist, 51*, 1017–1024.

Tompkins, M. A. (2004). *Using homework in psychotherapy: Strategies, guidelines, and forms*. New York: Guilford.

United States Public Health Service Office of the Surgeon General (1999). *Mental health: A report of the Surgeon General*. Rockville, MD: Department of Health and Human Services.

VandenBos, G. R. (1996). Outcome assessment of psychotherapy. *American Psychologist, 51*, 1005–1006.

Veroff, J., Kulka, R. A., & Douvan, E. (1981). *Mental health in America*. New York: Basic Books.

Weisz, J, R., Sandler, I. N., Durlak, J. A., & Anton, B. S. (2005). Promoting and protecting youth mental health through evidence-based prevention and treatment. *American Psychologist, 60*, 628–648.

White, R. W. (1959). Motivation reconsidered: The concept of competence. *Psychological Review, 66*, 297–333.

Williams, R. B., Boles, M., & Johnson, R. E. (1995). Patient use of a computer for prevention in primary care practice. *Patient Education and Counseling, 25*, 283–292.

Winett, R. A., Anderson, E. S., Desiderato, L. L., Solomon, L. J., et al. (1995). Enhancing social diffusion theory as a basis for prevention specificity, and internality come into the foreground of practice intervention: A conceptual and strategic framework. *Applied & Preventive Psychology, 4*, 233–245.

Section II

Primary Interventions: Nutritional Approaches

Americans are literally obsessed with foods, diets, vitamins, minerals, supplements, and herbs. What a generation ago was considered, in some circles, derisively, as "alternative medicine," and not part of the mainstream, it is now the mainstream. The costs of such products, above and beyond the cost of needed foods, runs in the billions. Many, if not most American households, are bombarded by books, pamphlets, flyers, advertisements, and newsletters proclaiming miracle cures and important breakthroughs in the fight against illnesses, obesity, diabetes, high blood pressure, and other physical and mental diseases, real or imagined. Popular literature is replete with books that advocate using alternative ways to prevent illness and promote wellness, especially by eating certain foods (Carwood, 2004; Hausman & Hurley, 1989; Pratt & Matthews, 2004; Reader's Digest, 1999; Stengler, 2001).

The last generation has seen the rise of alternative health self-appointed and self-anointed "gurus" who preach, rant, and rave against established medicine and the Federal Drug Administration agency. They report as facts possible conspiracies, contradictions, inadequacies, and rigidities in favor of more "natural" and easily available, inexpensive foods, vitamins, and alternative sources of nutrition and health. A recent brochure promoting a variety of miraculous nostrums in food- or pill-form, for instance, accused the medical profession of "...secretly using blacklisted alternative therapies on themselves" because these doctors don't get sick! In spite of all these raves, these gurus do cite what they conclude is research relevant to support their preferred nostrum of the day.

James F. Balch, MD, apparently a Board Certified urologist, for instance, in a large, expensive "Urgent Special Report" claims that "...popular cholesterol-lowering drugs can trigger a heart attack!" He blasted drug companies as liars (he may be right there), but, as is typical of self-appointed gurus, he offered remedies to "boost your brain power" as well as better erections, and "natural" cures for arthritis, high blood pressure, and diabetes, provided, of course that readers subscribe to "best value" 24 issues (just \$77.00) and receive as "free gifts" six additional reports. The free gift gimmick is one of the many enticements found in almost all advertisements (all suspiciously similar in format and style) of most gurus.

The literature spread by these gurus shares common, but questionable, characteristics: (1) lack of accountability, with sole reliance on anecdotally subjective testimonials by individuals who have been miraculously "cured" or apparently impressed by whatever food, vitamin, herb, or supplement or combination of the above, was provided by the guru; (2) a vast number of subscribers, who apparently allow supposedly credentialed gurus to survive and be heard through the circulation of a newsletter where the products they are promoting are for sale; (3) proprietary interests in businesses that sell the product(s) being promoted; and (4) failure to report failures in treatment, only successes are reported. Essentially, these gurus reject standard professional and scientific criteria other than their own whim and will, publishing their own newsletters, and taunting their own products commercially. How transparent can one be, and still be believed by a gullible, needy public that wants help but does not know any better!

One flyer about Featherspring Foot Supports, for instance, claims to reduce pain not only in feet, but also in toes, ankles, heels knees, hips, back, legs, veins, neck, and shoulders. Furthermore, the "Pain-Free Living Kit" is completely free-of-charge by just mailing a card. If mailed on time, the lucky subscriber will receive a "Mystery Gift"! What else can one ask for for free? Apparently, there *is* a free lunch in alternative medicine. This is what this literature wants readers to believe.

Subscription to a newsletter is obtained by adding a series of pamphlets that promise to "cure" practically any known or most common conditions known today. Usually, a very large, slick introductory, multiple page brochure describes the various conditions known to be cured by a particular product. However, the product itself, sometimes, is not described. The gullibly needy or vulnerably naïve respondent has to either subscribe to a newsletter and/or buy the product outright. Of course, the greater the amount of the subscription or purchase, the greater will be the savings. However, if the product possesses such curative powers, why should it be used continuously? Hence, these gurus are not different from the traveling, itinerant medicine men of the nineteenth century, who were selling nostrums which promised to cure everything but the common cold, and, if you did not have it, they would give it to you!

Let us look at some of these most prominent gurus and see what they promote. If what they promote is a matter of their opinion, then there should be contradictions among them in whatever product(s) they promote or sell, since evidence to support their use is lacking. Michael E. Rosenbaum, MD, for instance, offers a "simple solution" that is: "Doctors Little-Known Secret" for reviving their own health and feeling great.'' This miracle cure, designed to produce "remarkable results for cholesterol, joints, blood pressure, loss of energy, problem skin, immunity, liver, bladder and colon toxicity, stomach discomfort, memory, weight gain, and "so much more," is Sun Chlorella. "You receive a Free Gift for promptness in responding." The expensive, 24-page brochure is chock-full of testimonials and pictures depicting the lucky ones who benefited by this food. One testimonial by Randall E. Merchant, PhD, apparently Head of Neurosurgery at the Medical College of Virginia Commonwealth University, assures readers of good digestion and regularity, healthy cholesterol, and blood pressure levels, as well as support for stiff joints. The title and year of a paper published by Merchant et al., is given but the source or reference is lacking. Experimental use of this product by this writer produced constipation and no other noticeable change in body functions.

An advertisement for miraculous use of vinegar shows the picture of an elderly man in a white smock with a stethoscope around his neck proclaiming that "Scientific studies have shown vinegar to be an excellent natural source of healthful vitamins and minerals." Of course, commercially available vinegar won't do, only VinTabsPlus is "formulated to deliver the optimal amount of vinegar to your system each day to help you achieve maximum results." A Money-Saving Coupon is enclosed. How lucky can one be? Ridiculous and contradictory claims are made about drinking or not drinking tap water, consuming fat (good for you), sugar, and practically any food and minerals available commercially.

Jonathan V. Wright, MD, supposedly with credentials from prestigious universities, offers "Horse Urine" as another of the many cure-alls banned by the FDA. The lucky subscriber to a series of pamphlets describing miracle cures will receives a free-of-charge Library of Food and Vitamins Cure for any disease known to humanity. Mark Stengler, ND (?) is another guru supposedly consulted by Ivy-league universities, whose major claim to fame was to be interviewed by national TV networks, conferring a degree of legitimacy not found anywhere else.

Apparently, among many others, three seemingly professional, representative gurus, among many others, who share probably scientific information to their large numbers of readers and followers are: Robert J. Rowen, MD, Julian Whitaker, MD, and Dr. David G. Williams (type of degree not specified). In their prolific and supposedly professional newsletters, they do cite recent and reliable health and nutrition information gathered from peer-reviewed journals. Unfortunately, all three sell their own products, making their claims about their own products suspect, questionable, and unverified.

Names of alternative physicians with MD degrees could be added but their number is so great that it would fill too many precious pages that should be devoted to more serious pursuits. This list is practically unending but the issue remains. Why are all these quacks spending millions of dollars in expensive, seductive brochures and advertisements unless they are assured that there would be sufficient reader response to guarantee returns on investments? Apparently, there are sufficiently needy, gullible individuals who have not been helped, or, if helped, have not used, traditional medication to treat whatever ails them.

Perhaps one of the most telling characteristic of all these alternative practices is the promise of one magic cure for multiple, self-reported illnesses *without any pre-post test evaluation by sources external to the reader or to the promoter.* One single pill with multiple vitamins, minerals, and nostrums will do the trick. This writer knows of only one apparently serious commercial outfit that claims to produce a combined dose of vitamins, minerals, and supplements on the basis of a supposedly scientific examination of three urine samples performed by an external laboratory. Ideal Health, for instance, as far as this writer knows, not only relies on pre-post-evaluation, but also has a registered nurse available on the phone and online. Pills mailed monthly by this outfit supposedly are tailor-made to suit each subscriber's specific physical profile. A regular newsletter describes new products, supposedly based on new scientific information, That is more than any of the other health promoters do. However, whether all this information is reliable remains to be seen.

There is no regulatory agency to control or alert the public about the dangers of all these "free-for-all" cures. Any governmental effort to exercise control over what is a multi-billion-dollar industry would be expensive and unyielding, such as the creation of a regulatory agency akin to the Federal Drug Administration (FDA) to control alternative medicine and nutrition. Is there a solution to control the myriad cures offered in the mail every day? Will we need a sufficient number of deaths, like that of a famous ballplayer, by so-called alternative cures, before criteria to control this industry are found? How many deaths need to occur before a solution, if any exists, is found? How will the gullible, naïve, needy public be safeguarded by a literal flood of phony but solicitous advertisements?

Help is present in the publications of credible health newsletters by major universities (Harvard, Johns Hopkins, Minnesota, Berkley), by well-known *Consumer Reports*, and, perhaps less known but extremely relevant, the *Health Newsletter Nutrition Action* published by the Center for Science in the Public Interest in Washington, DC. Unfortunately, this information is available to a relatively small, well-educated section of the population that can afford to subscribe and understand whatever is contained in those newsletters. What about the larger and not-so-well informed or not-so-well-educated public that does not subscribe to this objective information, but receives seductive brochures full of exciting promises and quick (or quack?) cures? How is this public going to be reached, protected, and even safeguarded from quacks and gurus? How can the public in general be made aware of the difference between serious and reliable information from scientifically based sources and crassly commercial, greedy entrepreneurs? Unfortunately, over the last decade, inconsistencies in information given by these reliable sources have eroded the public trust in those very sources.

Recently (June 24–26, 2005), Harvard Medical School presented a program on "Natural Remedies for Psychiatric Disorders: Considering the Alternatives." Papers presented at this symposium covered: St. John's Worth for depression, Omega-3 Fatty Acids for bipolar and unipolar depression, SAMe, folate, B12 and depression, melatonin for insomnia, glycine and other natural agents for psychotic disorders, ginkgo-biloba, galantamine, growth hormone (GH), and dehydroe-iandrosterone (DHEA) for dementia, as well as maca, ginseng, ginkgo, and yohimbine for sexual dysfunction. A separate section was devoted to relaxation response therapy training, acupuncture, hypnosis, spirituality, and therapeutic touch. A symposium of this type at a leading medical institution went a long way to legitimize nontraditional nutrients and vitamins. This background serves as context for this section, as well as including Chapter 7 on self-administered alternatives to treat mental disorders.

The major, if only hope for progress in this field, lies in evidence-based research as the most effective tool to assess diets, supplements, minerals, vitamins, and herbs. Which are promoting health and which are dangerous? However, if physical and mental health professionals themselves do not know which product is supported by reliable evidence, how is the public to know? This is why it is so important to disseminate reliable, low-cost information to professional helpers, who will be able to practice and promote healthy diets and nutrition, not only for themselves and for their participants, but also for the public at large. This is the reason for the chapters included in this section.

References

Carwood, F. W. (Ed.). (2004). *Unleash the inner power of foods*. Peachthree City, GA: FC&A Medical Publishing.

Hausman, P., & Huley, J. B. (1989). *The healing foods: The ultimate authority on the curative power of nutrition*. Emmaus, PA: Rodale Press.

Pratt, S., & Matthews, K. (2004). *Superfoods: Fourteen foods that will change your life*. New York: Morrow.

Reader's Digest. (1999). *The healing power of vitamins, minerals, and herbs: The A–Z guide to enhancing your health and treating illness with nutritional supplements*. Pleasantville, NJ: Reader's Digest Association.

Stengler, M. (2001). *The natural physician's healing therapies: Proven remedies that medical doctors don't know about*. Stamford, CT: Bottom Line Books.

2

Diets, Health, and Weight Control: What Do We Know?

David L. Katz*, Ming-Chin Yeh, Meghan O'Connell and Zubaida Faridi

The prevalence of overweight and obesity has increased substantially in the past two decades and has become an epidemic in the US and around the world (Katz, 2003; Wang et al., 2002). According to a recent study based on National Health and Nutrition Examination Survey (NHANES) data, 65.1% of the adults aged 20 years or older in 1999–2002 were overweight or obese (Hedley et al., 2004). According to the same study, overweight children and adolescents have also increased markedly based on the Centers for Disease Control and Prevention's (CDC) growth chart. It is estimated that 31% of children aged 6 through 19 years in 1999 to 2002 were at risk of overweight or were overweight (Hedley et al., 2004).

The health consequences of obesity are well documented. Obesity is associated with increased risk of cardiovascular disease, diabetes, cancer, arthritis, and many other morbidities (Pi-Sunyer, 2002). The US Surgeon General's Report estimated the total economic burden associated with obesity to be $117 billion in the year 2000 (U.S. Department of Health and Human Services, 2001). The mortality toll of obesity is also staggering. An estimated 365,000 premature deaths each year are thought to result from direct and indirect effects of the obesity epidemic, second only to tobacco-related 435,000 annual deaths (Mokdad et al., 2004).

With the rates of obesity on the rise, Americans are obsessed with weight loss (Khan, Serdula, Bowman, & Williamson, 2001; Serdula et al., 1999). Over $33 billion were spent on weight loss related products and services annually in the US (Cleland et al., 2001). Based on data from a nationally representative sample of US adults, 24% of men and 38% of women were trying to lose weight (Kruger Galuska, Serdula, & Jones, 2004). Of those trying to lose weight, the most common strategies were eating fewer calories, eating less fat, and exercising more (58%, 49%, 54%, respectively for men; 63%, 56%, 52%, respectively for women); however, only one third (34%) of

* *Corresponding author*: David L. Katz, MD, MPH, FACPM, FACP. Associate Professor of Public Health, Director, Prevention Research Center, ***Yale University School of Medicine***, Medical Contributor, ***ABC News***, *Prevention Research Center*, 130 Division St., Derby, CT 06418, Katzdl@pol.net; david.katz@yale.edu, Administrative assistant: Helen Day: helen.day@yalegriffinprc.org

all those trying to lose weight reported using the recommended strategy of eating fewer calories and exercising more (Kruger et al., 2004). Other research demonstrates that women with higher body mass indices (BMIs) often started dieting at a younger age and diet more frequently compared to women with lower BMIs (Ikeda, Lyons, Schwartzman, & Mitchell, 2004). Dieting is also very common among young adults. A study of dieting behaviors among 324 college students showed that 38% and 13% of females and males respectively, were dieting to lose weight (Liebman, Cameron, Carson, Brown, & Meyer, 2001).

Thus, a comprehensive examination of weight loss strategies to promote weight loss or weight maintenance for overall health is important. This chapter will summarize the existing literature related to various approaches to weight loss and control, including dietary interventions and behavioral modifications. Related issues such as associations between dietary pattern and health outcomes, popular diet books used by the general public, effects of weight loss diets on body composition, and long-term sustainability of weight loss will also be discussed. The existing guidelines for health promotion and/or weight control are also provided.

Approaches to Weight Loss and Control

Dietary Interventions for Weight Loss and Control

The obesity epidemic has led to an influx of dietary approaches to prevent excess weight gain or to induce weight loss. There are numerous reviews on the subject of diet for weight loss (Astrup, 1999a; A. Astrup et al., 2000; Bedno, 2003; Cheuvront, 2003; Drewnowski, 2003; Jebb, 2005; Jequier & Bray, 2002; Moloney, 2000; Pirozzo, Summerbell, Cameron, & Glasziou, 2003; Plodkowski & Jeor, 2003; Rolls, Ello-Martin, & Tohill, 2004a; Vermunt Pasman, Schaafsma, & Kardinaal, 2003; Wadden & Butryn, 2003; Wing & Gorin, 2003). In the aggregate, however, this literature lends strongest support to diets abundant in fruits, vegetables and whole grains, and restricted in total fat. The following will discuss four common dietary approaches currently in use, namely, fat restricted diets, carbohydrate restricted diets, low glycemic diets, and Mediterranean diets.

Fat Restricted Diets (Low Fat Diets)

High dietary fat intake is a powerful predictor of weight gain (Schrauwen & Westerterp, 2000). Epidemiological studies have consistently shown that increasing dietary fat is associated with increased prevalence of obesity (Bray, Paeratakul, & Popkin, 2004). Transcultural comparisons dating back at least to the work of Ancel Keys consistently indicate that higher intake of dietary fat is associated with higher rates of obesity, and chronic disease (Keys, 1955; Keys et al., 1972; Keys et al., 1984). Most authorities concur that high intake of dietary fat contributes to obesity at the individual and population levels. The theoretical basis for weight loss through dietary fat restriction is strong, given the widely acknowledged primacy of calories in weight governance, and the energy density of fat (Katz, 2001a). Dietary fat is the most energy dense and least satiating of the macronutrient classes (Hill, Melanson, &

Wyatt, 2000; Peters, 2003; Schutz, 1995). When fat restriction is in accord with prevailing views on nutrition, i.e., achieved by shifting from foods high in fat to naturally low-fat foods, the results are consistently favorable with regard to energy balance and body weight. A review of the results from 28 clinical trials showed that a reduction of 10% in the proportion of energy from fat was associated with a decrease in weight of 16g per day (Bray & Popkin, 1998). The weight loss benefit of advice to follow fat-restricted diets is however, no more enduring than that of advice to restrict calories by any other means (Pirozzo, Summerbell, Cameron, & Glasziou, 2002).

Despite the extensive literature supporting dietary fat-restriction for weight loss and control, there are dissenting voices (Willett & Leibel, 2002). For the most part, dissent is predicated on the failure of dietary fat restriction to achieve population-level weight control in the United States. Recent trends in the US suggest that fat intake over recent decades was held constant, not reduced, and that intake of total calories has risen to dilute down the percent of food energy derived from fat. Increased consumption of highly processed, fat-reduced foods is the principal basis for these trends (Wright et al., 2004). Thus, the failure of dietary fat restriction to facilitate weight control is more a problem of adherence than effectiveness (Jequier, 2002).

In response to the public's interest in fat restriction, the food industry generated a vast array of low-fat, but not necessarily low-calorie, foods over the past two decades. The increase in calories was driven by increased consumption of calorie-dense, nutrient-dilute, fat-restricted foods, contemporaneous with a trend toward increasing portion sizes in general (Astrup, 1998; Harnack, Jeffery, & Boutelle, 2000; McCrory, Fuss, Saltzman, & Roberts, 2000; Nestle, 2003; Rolls & Miller, 1997). Lowering the fat content of processed foods while increasing consumption of simple sugars and starch is not consistent with the long-standing recommendations of nutrition authorities to moderate intake of dietary fat. Yet it is this distorted approach to dietary fat "restriction" that best characterizes secular trends in dietary intake at the population level, and that subtends the contention that dietary fat is unrelated to obesity.

Carbohydrate Restricted Diets (Low Carbohydrate Diets)

Although the popularity of carbohydrate-restricted diets for weight loss appears to be waning, they have been trendy for several years, so much so that they have reshaped the American food supply. Review of low-carbohydrate diets to date suggests that short-term weight loss is consistently achieved, but that neither weight loss sustainability, nor long-term effects on overall health, has yet been determined (Bravata et al., 2003). A recent systematic review published in Lancet, found that weight loss achieved while on low-carbohydrate diets is associated with the duration of the diet and restriction of energy intake, but not with restriction of carbohydrates (Astrup, Meinert Larsen, & Harper, 2004). Evidence supporting and refuting this claim and preliminary evidence related to the health impact of low-carbohydrate diets will be discussed in this section.

It is worth noting that interest in carbohydrate restriction for weight loss is not new; Atkins' "Diet Revolution" was first published in 1972 (Atkins, 1972). In 1978, Rabast and colleagues used isocaloric formula diets to compare fat– and carbohydrate– restricted approaches to weight loss in 45 obese adults

(Rabast, Kasper, & Schonborn, 1978). Carbohydrate restriction resulted in greater weight loss (14+/−7.2 kg vs. 9.8+/−4.5 kg) at 30 days. A recent study investigating carbohydrate and fat restriction diets on hunger perception in overweight premenopausal women suggested that short-term weight loss may due, in part, to increased cognitive eating restraint in both diets. However, a greater decrease in hunger perception may lead to a greater weight loss observed in carbohydrate restriction group (Nickols-Richardson, Coleman, Volpe, & Hosig, 2005).

Brehm and colleagues (Brehm, Seeley, Daniels, & D'Alessio, 2003) examined weight loss, cardiac risk factors, and body composition in 53 obese women randomly assigned to a very low carbohydrate diet, or a calorie-restricted, balanced diet with 30% of calories from fat. Subjects assigned to the very low carbohydrate diet group lost more weight (8.5+/−1.0 vs. 3.9+/−1.0 kg; $P<0.001$) and more body fat (4.8+/−0.67 vs. 2.0 +/− 0.75 kg; $P< 0.01$) than those assigned to the low fat diet group; cardiac risk measures improved comparably in both groups at 6 month follow-up.

Sondike et al. ran a 12-week weight loss trial comparing low-carbohydrate to moderately fat-restricted diets in 30 overweight adolescents. There was significantly greater weight loss with the low-carbohydrate assignment. LDL cholesterol levels improved with fat restriction, but not carbohydrate restriction (Sondike, Copperman, & Jacobson, 2003).

In 1999, Skov et al. reported an interesting variation on the low-carbohydrate diet theme by comparing two fat-restricted (30% of calories) diets, one high in carbohydrate (58% of calories), the other high in protein (25% of calories) (Skov, Toubro, Ronn, Holm, & Astrup, 1999). Subjects were 65 overweight adults followed for 6 months, and were provided diets strictly controlled with regard to nutritional composition, but unrestricted in calories. More weight was lost with high protein (8.9 kg) intake than with high carbohydrate (5.1 kg) intake; no weight loss occurred in a control group.

Two studies of low-carbohydrate diets that received widespread attention are those by Samaha et al. (2003) and Foster et al. (2003), published in the same issue of the *New England Journal of Medicine* in 2003. Samaha and colleagues compared a very low-carbohydrate diet (< 30 gm carbohydrate per day) to a fat-and calorie-restricted diet in 132 adults with a BMI of 35 or above over a 6-month period. The carbohydrate restricted diet resulted in greater weight loss at 6 months than the low-fat diet, but was also associated with a far greater reduction in daily calorie intake (a mean reduction of 271 kcal per day for the low fat diet, and 460 kcal for the low-carbohydrate diet). Foster et al. compared the Atkins' diet as described in *Dr. Atkins' New Diet Revolution* (Atkins, 1999) to a fat and calorie-restricted diet in 63 obese adults followed for 12 months. The low-carbohydrate diet produced significantly greater weight loss at 6 months, but not 12 months. Calorie intake was not reported. In both studies, attrition and recidivism were high; Samaha and colleagues noted that their trial was unblinded, whereas Foster et al. made no mention of blinding.

In a widely publicized recent study comparing the effectiveness and adherence rates of four popular weight loss diets among overweight subjects with hypertension, dyslipidemia or fasting hyperglycemia, Dansinger, Gleason, Griffith, Selker, & Schaefer (2005) found no significant difference in mean weight loss between groups at one-year (Dansinger et al., 2005).

Predictably, the study reported no significant differences in mean total calorie reduction between groups, lending support to the widely accepted notion that total calorie consumption, regardless of macronutrient content, is of prime importance in weight loss efforts. Further studies discussed in this section also support this contention. All diet groups (Atkins, Weight Watchers, Ornish and Zone) had poor adherence rates, with no significant difference between groups. In all diet groups, greater adherence to the diet resulted in improved weight outcomes; participants in the top tertile of adherence had a mean loss of 7% body weight. No significant differences in cardiac risk factors were noted between groups; in each group the amount of weight loss predicted improvements in several risk factors.

In a 6-month noncontrolled trial, Westman, Yancy, Edman, Tomlin, & Perkins (2002) assessed the effects of a very low-carbohydrate diet among 51 overweight or obese adults. Carbohydrate intake of less than 25 grams per day was recommended to start and was increased to 50 grams upon achievement of 40% of target weight loss. Mean daily calorie consumption at follow-up was 1447 ± 350, but was not measured at baseline. Calories restrictions were not prearranged; however, subjects were instructed to eat only until hunger was relieved. All subjects available for follow-up developed ketonuria; levels were used to verify self-reported carbohydrate intake. Subjects lost a mean of $10.3\% \pm 5.9\%$ body weight. Significant decreases in total cholesterol, LDL and trigylceride levels as well as increases in HDL were reported (Westman et al., 2002).

Yancy Olsen, Guyton, Bakst, & Westman (2004) compared a low-carbohydrate diet plus nutritional supplementation to low fat diet with calorie deficit of 500–1000 calories/day among 120 overweight, hyperlipidemic subjects. Both groups received exercise recommendation and attended group meetings. The low-fat diet group lost significantly less weight than the low-carbohydrate diet group at 6 months (mean change, -12.9% vs. -6.7%; $P < 0.001$). Reductions in fat mass were similar between groups. The low-carbohydrate group had lower attrition, yet the low-fat group appeared to have better adherence to the diet (Yancy et al., 2004).

Brinkworth et al. (2004) compared the effectiveness at 68 weeks of two calorie and fat controlled 12 week diets: a standard protein group (15% protein, 55% carbohydrate) and high-protein group (30% protein, 40% carbohydrate). Results indicated no significant difference in weight loss between groups; however neither group had high compliance to the diet. Both diets significantly increased HDL cholesterol concentrations ($P < 0.001$) and decreased fasting insulin, insulin resistance, sICAM-1 and CRP levels ($P < 0.05$) (Brinkworth et al., 2004).

In a small group of obese participants with type 2 diabetes that ate a usual diet for 7 days followed by a low-carbohydrate diet for 14 days, Boden, Sargrad, Homko, Mozzoli, & Stein (2005) found that the two-week low-carbohydrate diet resulted in spontaneous reduction in energy intake by almost one third (from 3111 kcal/d to 2164 kcal/d); weight loss during this period was completely accounted for by reduced caloric intake. This study highlighted a very important point in the low fat vs. low carbohydrate debate – that any diet program that reduces energy intake relative to energy expenditure will decrease body weight (Bray, 2005).

Several other studies comparing low-carbohydrate to low-fat or conventional diets with durations ranging from 6 to 12 weeks were reviewed. Studies using comparable energy intake among subjects across groups consistently reported no significant difference in weight loss regardless of the target population (Golay et al., 1996a 1996b; Meckling, O'Sullivan, & Saari, 2004; Miyashita et al., 2004; Segal-Isaacson, Johnson, Tomuta, Cowell, & Stein, but measured various other outcomes with some positive results attributed to low-carbohydrate intake.

The current preoccupation with carbohydrate restriction appears to be reactionary to the recent era during which fat restriction was prioritized. The popular press and media reports suggest that the public feels mislead by promises that fat restriction would lead to weight loss. In particular, the widely known USDA food guide pyramid has come under attack as a contributor to worsening obesity rates (Willet, 2001). The adulteration of messages in the pyramid under the influence of special interest groups is the subject of a recent book (Nestle, 2002). The competition between low-fat and low-carbohydrate diets for weight loss has in some ways polarized debate beyond the point of reason, or utility. "No diet *cures* obesity," as stated in one recent editorial from the Annals of Internal Medicine journal (Bray, 2005). The utility of different diets in the fight against obesity should be examined closely (Klein, 2004).

Low Glycemic Diets

Advocates of low-carbohydrate diets often share a common rationale pertaining to glycemic index (GI) or glycemic load (GL). The glycemic index of a food is a measure of how quickly its ingestion results in a rise in blood glucose levels, and the height of that response (Ludwig, 2002). Carbohydrate containing foods can be ranked according to their postprandial glycemic response (Colombani, 2004). It is only possible to apply GI analysis to foods containing at least 50 grams of available carbohydrates, while foods are commonly consumed in varying amounts and may not meet this threshold. Using GI alone, high GI foods that are consumed in small amounts (carrots, for example) can be labeled hazardous.

This deficit led to the development of the glycemic load. Taking both GI and reasonable serving sizes into account, the GL is the weighted average GI of a food multiplied by the percent of energy from carbohydrate (Moyad, 2004) and is believed to better predict the glycemic impact of foods (Colombani, 2004).

A recent trial by Ebbeling, Leidig, Sinclair, Hangen & Ludwig, (2003) reveals some of the potential distortions introduced when means of improving dietary intake pattern are considered as mutually exclusive of one another. This group of investigators compared a diet reduced in glycemic load, with 30 to 35% of calories from fat, to a diet termed "conventional" in which fat was restricted to 25 to 30% of calories, but the quality of the carbohydrate choices was unaddressed. The reduced glycemic load diet resulted in slightly greater weight loss, and control of insulin resistance, than the control diet in the 16 obese adolescents followed. What seems most noteworthy, however, is that the range of fat intake for the low-fat and low-glycemic load diets are actually contiguous. Thus, this study actually compared two diets that differed little with regard to fat content, one in which glycemic load was controlled, the other in which it was not. This is very much like comparing complex to simple carbohydrate, and finding that complex carbohydrate has preferable health effects. Regrettably, in the rush to defend competing dietary claims, this simple message is obscured.

In a 10-week trial, Sloth et al. (2004) investigated the role of glycemic index on energy intake, weight and risk factors for chronic disease in 45 healthy women by comparing a low-fat high-carbohydrate/high-GI diet to a low-fat high- carbohydrate/low-GI diet. No significant differences were observed between groups in energy intake, body weight or fat mass. Similarly, a 12-week randomized trail with a 24-week follow-up phase of comparing low-glycemic, high-glycemic or high-fat-hypocaloric diet did not find added benefit to energy restriction in promoting weight loss in obese men and women (Raatz et al., 2005).

In 2000, Spieth and colleagues reported the results of a retrospective cohort study comparing a low glycemic index to a low-fat diet for weight loss in 107 obese children (Spieth et al., 2000). Greater reduction in the BMI was observed at approximately 4 months in the low-GI group ($-1.53\,kg/m(2)$ [95% CI, -1.94 to -1.12]) as compared to the low-fat diet group ($-0.06\,kg/m(2)$ [-0.56 to $+0.44$], $P < .001$).

In a study by Heilbronn Noakes, & Clifton (2002), 45 overweight subjects with type II diabetes were randomly assigned to either a high or low GI diet following 4 weeks of high saturated fat diet. All diets were energy restricted. Weight loss did not differ between groups; however, a significantly greater reduction in LDL was observed in subjects on the low GI diet, with low glucose tolerance (Heilbronn et al., 2002).

A recent review paper has shown that low-glycemic load diets are associated with marked weight benefits and loss of adiposity in ad libitum studies in overweight or obese adults and children (Livesey, 2005). Some suggested that the primary mechanisms by which low-glycemic index foods may facilitate weight loss is through their ability to increase satiety and reduce subsequent food intake (Ludwig, Majzoub, Al-Zahrani, Dallal, Blanco, & Roberts, 1999; Warren, Henry, & Simonite, 2003). The relationship between glycemic index/ load diets and weight loss is a new area of research. More research is needed.

Mediterranean Diets

The Mediterranean diet differs from the typical American diet in the quantity and quality of fat, and the quantity of unrefined grains, vegetables, fruit, and lean protein sources (Simopoulos, 2001). The Mediterranean diet is low in saturated fat and high in monounsaturated fatty acids, high in antioxidants especially vitamin C and E, and high in fiber and folic acid (Kok & Kromhout, 2004). Olive oil is the dominant fat source, and consumption of fruit and vegetables, grains, fish and legumes are moderate to high. Wine is commonly served with meals (Kok & Kromhout, 2004). Although there is variation in the Mediterranean diet depending on country and region due to cultural, ethnic, religious, economic and agricultural production differences (Kris-Etherton, Eckel, Howard, St. Jeor, & Bazzarre, 2001; Simopoulos, 2001) and possibly even due to other elements that vary across culture, and are difficult to control for, such as stress, social bonds, familial support, and even spirituality, (Cukur, de Guzman & Carlo, 2004; DeJong et al., 2004) the dietary characteristics common to the region (described above) have been consistently associated with good health and longevity. Further, many of the Mediterranean populations enjoying good health have traditionally high rates of physical activity compared to Western societies; the effects of physical inactivity and high dietary fat intake may be synergistic with regard to weight gain (Astrup, 1999b).

The Mediterranean diet is relatively high in total fat. Some have expressed concerns that adherence to this diet may promote weight gain (Ferro-Luzzi, James, & Kafatos, 2002). However, because of the overall pattern of foods in this diet, it is not based largely on energy-dense foods as most higher-fat diets tend to be. According to a recent study from a large population-based investigation of 23,597 adult men and women, adherence to a traditional Mediterranean diet was found not related to BMI in both sexes, after adjusting for total energy intake. In fact, the authors concluded that the rise in obesity rates observed in Mediterranean populations is likely to be related to limited physical activity in conjunction with factors that lead to excess energy intake (Trichopoulou, Naska, Orfanos, & Trichopoulos, 2005). Evidence from other large cross-sectional studies has, however, found a beneficial association between weight status and the traditional Mediterranean dietary pattern (Schroder Marrugat, Vila, Covas, & Elosua, 2004; Shubair, McColl, & Hanning, 2005). For example, based on a sample of over 3,100 Spanish men and women, Schroder and colleagues found that obesity risk decreased in men and women with increasing adherence to the traditional Mediterranean dietary pattern ($p = 0.01$ and $p = 0.013$, respectively) (Schroder et al., 2004).

The evidence is convincing that energy-dense foods generally contribute to weight gain. However, it is also clear that when energy restriction can be achieved on a diet relatively high in fat content, weight loss is achieved (Shah & Garg, 1996). A Mediterranean diet which is high in monounsaturated fatty acids but overall not predominantly comprised of energy-dense foods may be more effective at long-term weight loss than a low total-fat diet, as it may be more palatable and therefore better sustained than a low-fat diet.

McManus, Antinoro & Sacks, (2001) evaluated a calorie-controlled moderate-fat Mediterranean diet compared to a standard low-fat diet (also calorie controlled). The Mediterranean diet resulted in superior long-term participation and adherence, leading to improvements in weight loss. The moderate-fat group lost a mean of 4.1 kg, body mass index of 1.6 kg/m^2, and waist circumference of 6.9 cm, compared to increases in the low-fat group of 2.9 kg, 1.4 kg/m^2 and 2.6 cm, respectively at 18 months; $P <$ or $= 0.001$ between the groups (McManus et al., 2001). A study by Flynn & Colquhoun (2004) demonstrated weight loss (and a strong reduction in cholesterol levels and increased feelings of well-being) among 115 postmenopausal women after 15 months of adopting the diet (Flynn & Colquhoun, 2004). The intervention involved a weekly cooking class for 1 year, with professional chefs providing training in the correct use of natural ingredients of the traditional Mediterranean diet.

There is some evidence that in addition to facilitating weight loss, a moderately hypocaloric Mediterranean diet may also improve body composition among obese subjects. Using a diet based on the Italian Recommended Dietary Allowances and elaborated using available nutritional indices, De Lorenzo et al demonstrated that a Mediterranean-style diet with energy content (mean 6.5 MJ/day) matching the resting metabolic rate and with macronutrient breakdown of 55% carbohydrate, 25% fat, 20% protein and 30 g fiber prevented loss of fat-free mass and improved metabolic parameters in 19 obese women. Following the diet, total and segmental fat mass decreased, while no significant loss of total and segmental lean body mass was observed. The study also resulted in significant improvements in metabolic profile (De Lorenzo et al., 2001).

It is worth noting that although many studies have demonstrated successful weight control and health improvements with adoption of the Mediterranean diet, only one weight loss study with greater than 6 months follow-up has been undertaken in the US (McManus et al., 2001). This study demonstrated positive weight related results and superior adherence to a Mediterranean diet compared to a low-fat diet. More research is needed to determine whether the diet can be implemented and sustained among free living populations in the US given the current state of ubiquitous access to and American affinity for energy-dense snacks and fast foods.

Behavioral Modifications for Weight Loss and Control

Similar to dietary interventions, behavioral modifications for weight loss and maintenance have been studied extensively. Strategies such as goal setting, self-monitoring, stimulus control, problem solving, cognitive restructuring, relapse-prevention, nutrition, and exercise are major features of a typical behavioral weight loss program (Berkel, Poston, Reeves, & Foreyt, 2005; Foster, Makris, & Bailer, 2005).

To achieve weight loss, behavioral modification strategies focus on changing current behaviors that lead to increased energy expenditure and decreased energy intake (Poston & Foreyt, 2000). Several behavioral strategies for controlling calorie intake have been devised. Some of the most exciting new research in the area focuses on how the properties of foods, namely energy density and portion size are important determinants of energy intake and can be manipulated to adjust intake.

Studies by Rolls and colleagues have demonstrated that increasing the volume of low-energy foods consumed prior to a meal leads to decreased consumption overall. In a study comparing energy intake among subjects provided with low-calorie salads in various sizes to those with no first course, inclusion of low-calorie salads resulted in reduced meal energy intake (by 7% for the small portion and 12% for the large) (Rolls, Roe, & Meengs, 2004c).

Other studies have shown that increasing the energy density of foods while keeping the volume constant does not influence energy intake. This suggests that the volume of food that is consumed has a greater influence on perceptions of a food's pleasantness and increases in volume may accelerate termination of eating (Bell, Roe, & Rolls, 2003). Increasing food volume while reducing or keeping calories constant can be accomplished by incorporating water (Rolls, Bell, & Thorwart, 1999) or air (Rolls, Bell, & Waugh, 2000a) into foods; however drinking water with or before meals may not result in similar reduced energy consumption. (Rolls et al., 1999) Incorporating fruits and vegetables into the diet may also decrease energy intake, given their low energy density and high concentration of water and fiber (Rolls et al., 2004a).

Evidence is clear that individuals underestimate the calorie content of foods (Anderson, Williamson, Johnson, & Grieve, 1999) and do not describe portion size accurately (Guthrie, 1984). Increases in the size of meals and snacks reliably results in increased consumption. In a study by Diliberti, Bordi, Conklin, Roe & Rolls (2004), restaurant customers who purchased oversized meals increased their calorie intake by 43% (Diliberti et al., 2004). Rolls et al., (2004d) investigated the effects of various portion size of sandwiches on calorie intake, showing that when served the 12-inch sandwich, compared with the 8-inch sandwich, females consumed 12% more energy (74 kcal) and males consumed 23% more energy (186 kcal). Importantly, increased consumption did not translate into differences in hunger and fullness ratings in this study (Rolls, Roe, Meengs, & Wall, 2004d) and others (Kral, Roe, & Rolls, 2004). Adults also overeat when snacks sizes are large. A study by Rolls et al. (2004) showed that intake of potato chips was greater among study subjects receiving larger snack bags compared to subjects receiving smaller bags. Results showed that snack intake increased significantly as the package size increased for both males and females (Rolls, Roe, Kral, Meengs, & Wall, 2004b). Rolls and colleagues have also demonstrated that children as young as five also overeat when served large portions, compared to smaller ones, as opposed to younger children who appear to rely on hunger as a cue for eating (Rolls et al., 2000b). Less conventional applications of behavior modification such as meal replacements, telephone and internet interventions have recently been shown to be effective in the treatment of obesity as well. For example, Noakes and coworkers compared meal replacements with a structured weight reduction diet (control diet) in 66 overweight and obese participants (Noakes, Foster, Keogh, & Clifton, 2004). The authors found that both meal replacement and control groups experienced significant weight loss compared to baseline data (9.0 ± 6.9 kg, $p < 0.001$; 9.2 ± 5.1 kg, $p < 0.001$, respectively). Although both groups produced comparable weight loss, participants in the meal replacement group found that their intervention was more convenient and easier to comply with than that of the control group.

Tate and colleagues conducted a study to investigate the effectiveness of an internet delivered weight loss program (Tate, Wing, & Winett, 2001). Participants were randomized into either a structured internet behavioral intervention group or a group that only received access to an educational web site about weight loss. The results showed that 45% of the behavioral group participants compared with 22% of those in the educational web site group lost at least 5% of their initial body weight ($p = 0.05$) by 6 months. Similar positive results of an internet-based weight loss program with the addition of a behavioral counseling component delivered through email were also reported (Tate, Jackvony, & Wing, 2003). The above studies point to the potential usefulness of the innovation in behavioral modifications in weight loss.

Associations between Dietary Patterns and Health Outcomes

There are close associations between dietary patterns, nutritional risks, and chronic disease profiles in men (Millen et al., 2005) and in women (Schulze et al., 2005). For example, a recent Nurses' Health Study results indicated that a diet that was high in sugar-sweetened and/or diet soft drinks, refined grains, processed meat and low in wine, coffee and vegetables was associated with an increased risk of diabetes (Schulze et al., 2005). In the Diabetes Prevention Program, a low-calorie, low-fat diet coupled with moderately intense physical activity for at least 150 minutes per week reduced the incidence of Type 2 diabetes by 58% (Knowler et al., 2002). Similarly, the Dietary Approaches to Stop Hypertension (DASH) Collaborative Research Group has shown that hypertension can be prevented and treated by reducing intake of saturated and total fat, and adopting a diet rich in fruits, vegetables, grains and low-fat dairy (Sacks et al., 2001) Cardiovascular disease prevention has been demonstrated with both fat- (Sacks et al., 2001) and Mediterranean dietary patterns (de Lorgeril et al., 1999). Weight loss is a common element in all of these successful interventions.

Reviews of diet for optimal health do not necessarily demonstrate complete accord on all points, but are nonetheless substantially confluent with regard to fundamentals. Diets rich in fruits, vegetables and whole grains; restricted in animal fats and trans fat from processed foods; limited in refined starches and sugar; providing protein principally from lean sources; and offering fat principally in the form of monounsaturated and polyunsaturated oils are linked to good health (Hu, 2003; Hu, Manson, & Willett, 2001; Hu & Willett, 2002; Katz, 2001c; Key et al., 2004; Mathers, 2003; Reddy & Katan, 2004; Willet, 2001). With regard to diet and optimal health, debate is substantially limited to variations on this basic theme, rather than any fundamental departures from it.

Popular Diet Books and Commercial Weight Loss Programs used by the General Public

Countless books and commercial programs on diet and weight loss/control have saturated the market. A search on Amazon.com using the terms "diet," "weight loss," and "weight control," yields bibliographies of 183,990; 250,704; and 264,163, respectively (www.amazon.com, accessed 11/18/05). The same terms entered into a web search on Google yield 92,600,000; 67,200,000; and 75,100,000 sites, respectively (www.google.com, accessed 11/18/05). Thus, it is far beyond the scope of this or any review, or even plausibility, to characterize even a representative sample of weight loss diets, programs, and products being promoted to the general public.

The best that can be done to characterize these myriad claims on the basis of evidence is to apply a process of exclusion. In a systematic review of the obesity prevention and control literature (Yale-Griffin Prevention Research Center, 10/00–8/03), strategies that emerge as most promising with regard to lasting weight control involve achieving an energy-controlled and balanced diet along with regular physical activity. Fundamentally, claims for virtually any other approach to sustainable weight loss are unsubstantiated. There is little or no scientific evidence to support the contentions of the most popular diets, including those based on carbohydrate restriction (e.g., the Atkins' diet), those based on food combination or food proportioning (e.g., the Zone diet), or those based on the glycemic index (e.g., the South Beach Diet; the GI Diet). There is, of course, no shortage of anecdotal support and testimonials for virtually all of the popular diets.

Worth noting is that a modest proportion of the books on the subject of diet address not so much the 'what' of weight loss, but the 'how,' describing strategies for achieving a diet and lifestyle the evidence indicates to be associated with both lasting weight control and good health. Among the offerings in this category are approaches based on energy density (Liebman et al., 2001; Vartabedian & Matthews, 1994); water and fiber content (Rolls & Barnett, 2000); and the array of skills and strategies needed to navigate through the modern, 'toxic' nutritional environment (Katz & Gonzalez, 2002). Related to these are books dedicated to the same goal for children &/or families (Sears, 1999).

Parallel to the popularity of the diet books, numerous commercial & self-help weight loss programs have also been introduced to the market (Clel& et al., 2001). Popular among them are (a) nonmedical commercial weight loss programs such as Weight Watchers, Jenny Craig, & LA Weight Loss, (b) medically supervised proprietary programs that use very-low-calorie diets such as OPTIFAST, health management Resources, & Medifast, (c) internet-based commercial weight loss programs such as eDiets.com, WebMD, & Nutrisystem.com, (d) organized self-help programs such as Take Off Pounds Sensibly (TOPS) and Overeaters Anonymous (Tsai & Wadden, 2005). According to a recent systematic review of major commercial weight loss programs in the US, the study results revealed that majority of the popular commercial weight loss programs were costly, had high attrition rates, and had low long-term weight loss maintenance rates (Tsai & Wadden, 2005). The treatment components and associated costs of the three largest commercial weight loss programs in the US are shown in Table 2.1.

Potential Hazards of Popular Weight Loss Diets

There is little to suggest that dietary fat restriction as a weight loss method is harmful. To the contrary, a rich and varied literature argues that restriction of dietary fat is both conducive to weight loss, and health-promoting (Astrup, 2001; Connor & Connor, 1997). Many cultures recognized for good health and longevity have native diets very low in fat (Drewnowski & Popkin, 1997); few free-living societies adhere to dietary patterns low in carbohydrates. The worst that can be said of fat restriction for weight loss is that if extreme, it may not be optimal for health (Katan, Grundy, S., & Willett, 1997). Even critics of dietary fat restriction appear to agree that low-fat diets offer health benefits relative to the typical American diet, which is high in saturated and trans fat.

Table 2.1. The treatment components and associated costs of the three largest commercial weight loss programs in the US.

	Treatment components			Costs	
Program	**Diet**	**Physical activity**	**Behavior modification**	**Membership fee or initial cost**	**Estimated cost of 3-month program**
Weight Watchers	Low-calorie, exchange diet; participants prepare own meals	"Get Moving" booklet	Behavioral weight control methods	$35 for first week (with membership fee)	$167.00
Jenny Craig	Low-calorie diet of prepackaged company meals only	Audiotapes for walking	Manual on weight loss strategies provided	$199 for 6 months, $364 for 1 year	$1249.00
LA Weight Loss	Low-calorie diet; participants prepare own meals	Optional walking videotape	Included in counseling sessions	$88	Data not available

Source: Adapted from Tsai, A. G., Wadden, T. A. (2005). Systematic review: an evaluation of major commercial weight loss programs in the United States. *Ann Intern Med*, 4 January; *142(1)*, 56–66.

Carbohydrate restriction, in contrast, is actually or potentially linked to an array of adverse health effects (Katz, 2003). There is evidence that weight loss attributable to carbohydrate restriction is in part body water loss. Gluconeogenesis consumes water along with glycogen, and ketone bodies cause increased renal excretion of sodium and water (Denke, 2001). Studies indicate dizziness, fatigue and headache are common side effects (Tapper-Gardzina, Cotugna, & Vickery, 2002) of ketosis.

Ketosis is potentially harmful, with possible long-term sequelae including hyperlipidemia, impaired neutrophil function, optic neuropathy, osteoporosis, and protein deficiency as well as alterations in cognitive function (Denke, 2001). Children on ketogenic diets as part of an antiseizure regimen have developed dehydration, constipation and kidney stones. In response to ketosis, renal calcium excretion increases. To make up for the loss of calcium in urine, it is mobilized from bone to circulation (Denke, 2001). One study of adolescents on a ketogenic diet showed decreased bone mineral density after just 3 months, despite vitamin D and calcium supplementation (Tapper-Gardzina et al., 2002). Sustained ketosis causes bone resorption, suggesting a risk for osteoporosis (Eisenstein, Roberts, Dallal, & Saltzman, 2002).

Comparison of eight high-protein, low-carbohydrate diets indicates that the Atkins diet had the highest level of total fat, saturated fat, and cholesterol (Tapper-Gardzina et al., 2002). Consuming a diet high in saturated fat may raise total and low-density lipoprotein cholesterol levels, both of which contribute to cardiovascular disease. A significant increase in LDL has been reported among subjects on the Atkins diet (Denke, 2001), although this finding is inconsistent. An increase in C-reactive protein (CRP) on the Atkins diet has been observed as well (Tapper-Gardzina et al., 2002), suggesting an inflammatory response. A high intake of saturated fat increases the risk of insulin resistance (Tapper-Gardzina et al., 2002), contradicting the contention of low-carbohydrate diet proponents that carbohydrates are to blame for insulin resistance (Atkins, 2002). High fat diets may also predispose to cancer (Katz, 2000).

High-protein intake may negatively affect renal function in healthy individuals, and certainly accelerates renal disease in diabetes. In participants with renal dysfunction on a high-protein diet, there is glomerular damage which causes spillage of plasma proteins and resultant tubular injury and fibrosis (Tapper-Gardzina et al., 2002). As noted, urinary calcium excretion is also increased and hypercalciuria may ensue, predisposing to calcium stone formation (Denke, 2001). High-protein intake imposes a metabolic burden on both the liver and kidneys, and requires additional excretion of urea and ammonia (Jeor et al., 2001).

Extreme carbohydrate restriction is potentially associated with increased risk of dysthymia, if not depression, through a serotonergic mechanism (Katz, 2001b). The production of serotonin in the brain requires delivery and uptake of tryptophan, which is influenced by both the availability of tryptophan and the actions of insulin. With very low carbohydrate intake and blunted insulin release, tryptophan delivery to the brain is impaired, serotonin production is limited, and mood instability has been reported to ensue (Benton, 2002); the public health significance of this mechanism remains uncertain.

Finally, high-protein, low-carbohydrate diets simply don't allow for adequate intake of fruits and vegetables, restricting nutrient and fiber-rich foods shown to be protective against cancer, cardiovascular disease, diabetes, diverticular disease, as well as constipation (Ornish, 2004; Terry, Terry, J. B., & Wolk, et al., 2001; Van Duyn & Pivonka, 2000; Weisburger, 2000). Fiber lowers cholesterol, reducing the risk for cardiovascular disease, and lowers insulin secretion after meals by slowing nutrient absorption (Chandalia et al., 2000; Tapper-Gardzina et al., 2002).

Effects of Weight Loss Diets on Body Composition

One of the most tantalizing claims of popular weight loss diets is that weight loss can be achieved or facilitated by means other than energy restriction. De-emphasizing calories is, in fact, quite characteristic of popular weight loss approaches. Proponents of carbohydrate restriction contend that limiting intake of carbohydrates allows for weight loss regardless of calorie intake (Atkins, 2002). At least one study reported at the 2003 meeting of the North American Association for the Study of Obesity (NAASO; http://www.naaso.org) suggested greater weight loss over a 12-week period among subjects on a low-carbohydrate diet than among those on a low-fat diet, despite 300 more calories per day on the carbohydrate restricted assignment.

However, only limited data are available to date on the effects of carbohydrate restriction on body composition. There is clear evidence of a dehydrating effect of very low-carbohydrate diets, and of ketosis, in the short term (Katz, 2003); thus, some of the early weight loss on low-carbohydrate diets is almost certainly water. An association between increasing dietary fat, and increasing body fat, has been noted (Larson et al., 1995). Nelson and colleagues reported a positive association between dietary fat and body fat, and negative associations with body fat for both total and complex carbohydrates (Nelson & Tucker, 1996).

Hays and colleagues recently reported that a diet rich in complex carbohydrates resulted in an increase in lean body mass, and a decrease in body fat, among 34 subjects with impaired glucose tolerance (Hays et al., 2004). Similar results have been observed by other groups (Siggaard, Raben, & Astrup, 1996). A recent study has shown that a high-fat diet might contribute to long-term detrimental effects of increased waist circumference, fat mass, triglycerides, and 2-hour blood glucose level among overweight insulin-resistant women (McAuley et al., 2006). Volek and colleagues, however, reported a loss of body fat, and an increase in lean body mass with carbohydrate restriction in 12 volunteers followed for six weeks (Volek et al., 2002). Thus, the independent effects of redistributing macronutrients on body composition remain the subject of controversy; more science is clearly required for closure. The effects of physical activity on body composition are, of course, clear and noncontroversial, with increased activity leading to relative increases in lean body mass at the expense of body fat (Kirk, Jacobsen, Gibson, Hill, & Donnelly, 2003; Racette Schoeller, Kushner, Neil, & Herling-Iaffaldano, 1995).

Overall, there is little evidence to support a claim that loss of body fat is achieved preferentially by redistributing macronutrients at isoenergetic levels. Worth noting is that a pound of body fat represents an energy reserve of over 4,000 kcal; a pound of muscle, a reserve of roughly 1,800 kcal; and a pound of water, no latent energy whatsoever. While each weighs a pound, each requires a markedly different energy deficit to be lost; water can be lost with no energy deficit. Thus until proved otherwise, the most plausible explanation for enhanced weight loss at any given level of energy intake is the loss of body compartments that represent lesser energy reserves. Such losses of water and muscle protein are undesirable.

Long-Term Weight Loss Maintenance

As opposed to most people who commit a lifetime to sequential dieting, the literature on long-term weight loss success is thin; frequency of dieting is a negative predictor of lasting weight control (Pasman, Saris, & Westerterp-Plantenga, 1999). Further, there is a general perception among public that weight loss maintenance is difficult to achieve. A *New England Journal of Medicine* editorial expressed the same pessimistic viewpoint by calling weight loss an "ill-fated new year's resolution." (Kassirer & Angell, 1998) According to prior literature, although inhomogeneous in definitions, between 15% to 20% of people in the general population are successful at long-term weight loss maintenance (Ayyad & Andersen, 2000; Wing & Phelan, 2005).

The best available data on long-term weight loss maintenance are from observational studies (Mattes, 2002), transcultural comparison, and the National Weight Control Registry (Wing & Hill, 2001). The Registry was established to characterize the behavioral patterns of individuals successful at long-term maintenance of considerable weight loss, defined as "intentionally losing at least 10% of initial body weight and keeping it off for at least 1 year" (Wing & Hill, 2001). According to the most recent data, members of the Registry have lost an average of 33 kg and maintained the loss for over 5 years (Wing & Phelan, 2005). Registry data indicate that eating a low-calorie, low-fat diet, having breakfast regularly, self-monitoring of weight, and keeping a consistent eating pattern are keys to successful weight maintenance, as is regular physical activity (Hill, Wyatt, Phelan, & Wing, 2005; Klem Wing, McGuire, Seagle, & Hill, 1997; McGuire, Wing, Klem, Seagle, & Hill, 1998; Shick et al., 1998; Wing & Phelan, 2005).

Existing Guidelines for Health Promotion and Weight Control

The 2005 Dietary Guidelines for Americans

The main tenets of the newly released Dietary Guidelines for Americans issued by the Departments of Health and Human Services (DHHS) and Agriculture (USDA) (US Department of Agriculture, 2005) are to choose a variety of nutrient-dense foods and beverages that limit the intake of saturated and trans-fats, cholesterol, added sugars, salt, and alcohol. Specific advice on appropriate consumption by food grouping for an average 2,000-calorie daily diet includes the following: two cups of fruit and 2½ cups of vegetables per day (including a wide variety of each weekly); three or more 1 ounce servings of whole-grain products per day (at least half of all grains should come from whole grains); three cups per day of fat-free or low-fat milk or equivalent dairy products; restriction of saturated and trans fatty acids to fewer than 10% of calories, with total fat intake less than 35% of calories (preferred fat sources are fish, nuts, and vegetable oils containing polyunsaturated and monounsaturated fatty acids) and lean, low-fat, or fat-free meats, poultry, dry beans are preferable protein sources. Additional recommendations to minimize added sugar, limit added salt in food preparation and consume less than 2,300 mg (approximately one teaspoon of salt) of sodium per day and limit alcohol to one and two drinks per day for women and men respectively, were provided. Following these guidelines while monitoring and balancing calories consumed with calories expended in physical activity, represent the most prudent means of weight control.

Other Governmental Guidelines, Agency Reports and Position Papers

On the basis of its review of evidence linking dietary pattern to health outcomes, *The United States Preventive Services Task Force* advises clinicians to endorse to all participants over the age of two a diet restricted in fat, particularly saturated fat, and one that is abundant in fruits, vegetables, and grains (U.S. Preventive Services Task Force, 1996). These recommendations are highly concordant with those of the National Heart Lung and Blood Institute at the National Institutes of Health (http://www.nhlbi.nih.gov/guidelines/obesity/prctgd_b.pdf, accessed, October, 2006). The *National Cancer Institute* sponsors the "5-a-day" program encouraging fruit and vegetable intake, and endorses dietary guidelines that include 20 to 35 grams of fiber per day, with 30% or less of calories from fat (National Cancer Institute, 2002). The *American Heart Association* offers dietary guidelines that call for 55% or more of calories from carbohydrate, 30% or less from fat (7 to 10% saturated/trans fat, 10% polyunsaturated and 15% monounsaturated fats), and 15 to 20% from protein (Krauss et al., 2000). The *American Dietetic Association* supports the USDA Dietary Guidelines and recommends a variety of grains, at least 5 servings of fruits and vegetables daily, restriction of saturated fat and cholesterol, and limited sugar and sweets consumption (American Dietetic Association, 2002). The *American Diabetes Association* advocates 55% of calories from carbohydrates, up to 30% from fat (10% saturated/trans-fat, 10% polyunsaturated fat), and 15 to 20% from protein (Franz et al., 2002). Differing only in detail, all of these recommendations are substantially congruent.

In 2002, The National Academies of Science' Institute of Medicine (IOM) released dietary guidelines calling for 45 to 65% of calories from carbohydrate, 20 to 35% from fat, and 10 to 35% from protein, in conjunction with 60 minutes each day of moderately intense physical activity (Food and Nutrition Board, 2002). The IOM guidelines further emphasize the restriction of saturated and trans-fat and their replacement with monounsaturated and polyunsaturated fat. Also in 2002, on the basis of consensus opinion, the *American College of Preventive Medicine* formally adopted a position in support of dietary recommendations within the IOM ranges, and in opposition to carbohydrate restriction for purposes of weight control (American College of Preventive Medicine Position Statement, 2002).

Conclusions

With obesity becoming an epidemic in the US and around the world, numerous studies with various approaches (e.g. dietary interventions and behavioral modifications) to weight loss and control have been conducted. Scientifically sound dietary approaches such as fat restriction diets consistently produce desirable health outcome that leads to safe and long-term weight loss. Behavioral modifications for weight loss also prove to be effective. Less-conventional behavior modification approaches including the use of meal replacements, phone or internet use are promising and need further investigation.

A substantial proportion of the US population is trying to lose weight currently (24% for men and 38% for women). It is not surprising that the market is saturated with fad diets and popular diet books. Many of them are questionable in their claims of effectiveness; some are even outright harmful to health. Concordance with the aggregate scientific literature, governmental guidelines such as the revised 2005 Dietary Guidelines for Americans are therefore important in setting recommendations for those who are seeking advice for healthy eating and weight loss.

Prior literature has suggested that long-term weight loss maintenance is suboptimal, with approximately 20% of people in the general population successful at losing weight and keeping it off for at least 1 year. Key features to successful weight loss maintenance include regular physical activity, eating a low-calorie, low-fat diet, having breakfast regularly, self-monitoring of weight, and keeping a consistent eating pattern.

Prevailing evidence to weight loss has been consistently shown to be associated with a diet rich in fruit and vegetables, unsaturated fats, lean protein,

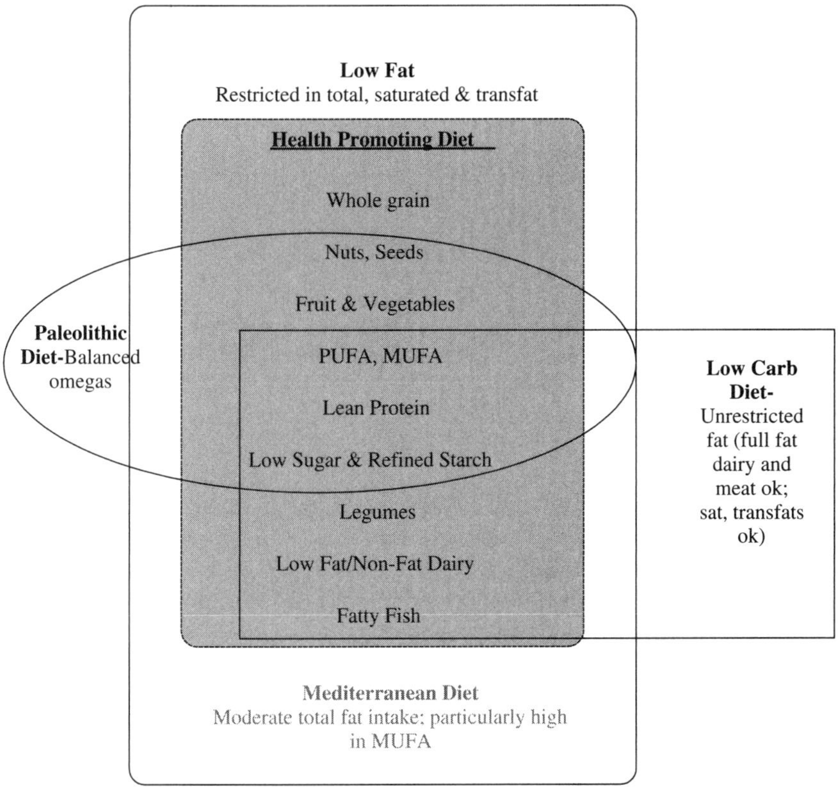

Figure 2.1. Identifying Common Ground. Key elements of a healthful diet for weight control are identifiable at the confluence of various dietary approaches.

low- or non-fat dairy and limited sugar and refined starches. See Figure 2.1 for commonalities shared by various diets for weight loss. Deviance from the scientifically sound dietary recommendations will lead to unsubstantiated health claims and unsustainable weight loss outcomes. The authors hope this chapter will help elucidate misconceptions regarding questionable dietary practices and promote effective strategies for weight loss and control in the general public.

References

American College of Preventive Medicine Position Statement. Diet in the prevention and control of obesity, insulin resistance, and type ii diabetes. Retrieved December, 2002

American Dietetic Association. (2002). Weight management – position of ADA. *J Am Diet Assoc, 102*, 1145–1155.

Anderson, D. A., Williamson, D. A., Johnson, W. G., & Grieve, C. O. (1999). Estimation of food intake: Effects of the unit of estimation. *Eat Weight Disord, 4*(1), 6–9.

Astrup, A. (1998). The American paradox: The role of energy-dense fat-reduced food in the increasing prevalence of obesity. *Curr Opin Clin Nutr Metab Care, 1*(6), 573–577.

Astrup, A. (1999a). Dietary approaches to reducing body weight. *Baillieres Best Pract Res Clin Endocrinol Metab., 13*, 109–120.

Astrup, A. (1999b). Macronutrient balances and obesity: The role of diet and physical activity. *Public Health Nutr., 2*, 341–347.

Astrup, A. (2001). The role of dietary fat in the prevention and treatment of obesity. Efficacy and safety of low-fat diets. *Int J Obes Relat Metab Disord, 25*(Suppl 1), S46–50.

Astrup, A., Meinert Larsen, T., & Harper, A. (2004). Atkins and other low-carbohydrate diets: Hoax or an effective tool for weight loss? *Lancet, 364*(9437), 897–899.

Astrup, A., Ryan, L., Grunwald, G. K., Storgaard, M., Saris, W., Melanson, E., et al. (2000). The role of dietary fat in body fatness: Evidence from a preliminary meta-analysis of ad libitum low-fat dietary intervention studies. *Br J Nutr, 83*, S25–32.

Atkins, R. (1999). *Atkins' new diet revolution*. New York, NY.: M. Evans & Company, Inc.

Atkins, R. (2002). *Dr. Atkins' new diet revolution*. New York, NY: HarperCollins Publishers, Inc.

Atkins, R. C. (1972). *Dr. Atkins' diet revolution*. New York, NY: Bantam Books.

Ayyad, C., & Andersen, T. (2000). Long-term efficacy of dietary treatment of obesity: A systematic review of studies published between 1931 and 1999. *Obesity Reviews, 1*(2), 113.

Bedno, S. A. (2003). Weight loss in diabetes management. *Nutr Clin Care, 6*, 62–72.

Bell, E. A., Roe, L. S., & Rolls, B. J. (2003). Sensory-specific satiety is affected more by volume than by energy content of a liquid food. *Physiol Behav, 78*(4–5), 593–600.

Benton, D. (2002). Carbohydrate ingestion, blood glucose and mood. *Neurosci Biobehav Rev, 26*, 293–308.

Berkel, L. A., Poston, W. S., Reeves, R. S., & Foreyt, J. P. (2005). Behavioral interventions for obesity. *J Am Diet Assoc, 105*(5 Suppl 1), S35–43.

Boden, G., Sargrad, K., Homko, C., Mozzoli, M., & Stein, T. P. (2005). Effect of a low-carbohydrate diet on appetite, blood glucose levels, and insulin resistance in obese patients with type 2 diabetes. *Ann Intern Med, 142*(6), 403–411.

Bravata, D. M., Sanders, L., Huang, J., Krumholz, H. M., Olkin, I., Gardner, C. D., et al. (2003). Efficacy and safety of low-carbohydrate diets: A systematic review. *JAMA, 289*, 1837–1850.

Bray, G. A. (2005). Is there something special about low-carbohydrate diets? *Ann Intern Med, 142*(6), 469–470.

Bray, G., & Popkin, B. (1998). Dietary fat intake does affect obesity! *Am J Clin Nutr, 68*, 1157–1173.

Bray, G. A., Paeratakul, S., & Popkin, B. M. (2004). Dietary fat and obesity: A review of animal, clinical and epidemiological studies. *Physiol Behav, 83*(4), 549–555.

Brehm, B. J., Seeley, R. J., Daniels, S. R., & D'Alessio, D. A. (2003). A randomized trial comparing a very low carbohydrate diet and a calorie-restricted low fat diet on body weight and cardiovascular risk factors in healthy women. *J Clin Endocrinol Metab, 88*, 1617–1623.

Brinkworth, G. D., Noakes, M., Keogh, J. B., Luscombe, N. D., Wittert, G. A., & Clifton, P. M. (2004). Long-term effects of a high-protein, low-carbohydrate diet on weight control and cardiovascular risk markers in obese hyperinsulinemic subjects. *Int J Obes Relat Metab Disord, 28*(5), 661–670.

Chandalia, M., Garg, A., Lutjohann, D., von Bergmann, K., Grundy, S. M., & Brinkley, L. J. (2000). Beneficial effects of high dietary fiber intake in patients with type 2 diabetes mellitus. *N Engl J Med, 342*(19), 1392–1398.

Cheuvront, S. N. (2003). The zone diet phenomenon: A closer look at the science behind the claims. *J Am Coll Nutr, 22*(1), 9–17.

Cleland, R., Graybill, D. C., Hubbard, V., Khan, L. K., Stern, J. S., Wadden, T. A., et al. (2001). Commercial weight loss products and programs: What consumers stand to gain and lose. A public conference on the information consumers need to evaluate weight loss products and programs. *Crit Rev Food Sci Nutr, 41*(1), 45–70.

Colombani, P. C. (2004). Glycemic index and load-dynamic dietary guidelines in the context of disease. *Physiology and Behavior, 83*, 603–610.

Connor, W., & Connor, S. (1997). Should a low-fat, high-carbohydrate diet be recommended for everyone? The case for a low-fat, high-carbohydrate diet. *N Engl J Med, 337*, 562–563.

Cukur, C. S., de Guzman M. R., & Carlo, G. (2004). Religiosity, values, and horizontal and vertical individualism-collectivism: A study of turkey, the united states, and the Philippines. *J Soc Psychol, 144*(6), 613–634.

Dansinger, M. L., Gleason, J. A., Griffith, J. L., Selker, H. P., & Schaefer, E. J. (2005). Comparison of the atkins, ornish, weight watchers, and zone diets for weight loss and heart disease risk reduction: A randomized trial. *JAMA, 293*(1), 43–53.

De Lorenzo, A., Petroni, M. L., Luca, P. P. D., Andreoli, A., Morini, P., Iacopino, L., et al. (2001). Use of quality control indices in moderately hypocaloric Mediterranean diet for treatment of obesity. *Diabetes Nutr Metab, 14*(4), 181–188.

de Lorgeril, M., Salen, P., Martin, J. L., Monjaud, I., Delaye, J., & Mamelle, N. (1999). Mediterranean diet, traditional risk factors, and the rate of cardiovascular complications after myocardial infarction: Final report of the lyon diet heart study. *Circulation, 99*(6), 779–785.

DeJong, M. J., Chung, M. L., Roser, L. P., Jensen, L. A., Kelso, L. A., Dracup, K., et al. (2004). A five-country comparison of anxiety early after acute myocardial infarction. *Eur J Cardiovasc Nurs, 3*(2), 129–134.

Denke, M. (2001). Metabolic effects of high-protein, low-carbohydrate diets. *The American Journal of Cardiology, 88*, 59–61.

Diliberti, N., Bordi, P. L., Conklin, M. T., Roe, L. S., & Rolls, B. J. (2004). Increased portion size leads to increased energy intake in a restaurant meal. *Obes Res, 12*(3), 562–568.

Drewnowski, A. (2003). The role of energy density. *Lipids, 38*, 109–115.

Drewnowski, A., & Popkin, B. M. (1997). The nutrition transition: New trends in the global diet. *Nutrition Reviews., 55*(2), 31–43.

Ebbeling, C. B., Leidig, M. M., Sinclair, K. B., Hangen, J. P., & Ludwig, D. S. (2003). A reduced-glycemic load diet in the treatment of adolescent obesity. *Arch Pediatr Adolesc Med, 157*, 773–779.

Eisenstein, J., Roberts, S. B., Dallal, G., & Saltzman, E. (2002). High-protein weight-loss diets: Are they safe and do they work? A review of the experimental and epidemiologic data. *Nutr Rev, 60*, 189–200.

Ferro-Luzzi, A., James, W. P., & Kafatos, A. (2002). The high-fat Greek diet: A recipe for all? *Eur J Clin Nutr, 56*(9), 796–809.

Flynn, G., & Colquhoun, D. (2004). Successful long-term weight loss with a Mediterranean style diet in a primary care medical centre. *Asia Pac J Clin Nutr, 13*, S139.

Food and Nutrition Board, I. o. M., National Academies of Science. (2002). *Dietary reference intakes for energy, carbohydrate, fiber, fat, fatty acids, cholesterol, protein, and amino acids (macronutrients)*. Washington, D.C.: National Academy Press.

Foster, G. D., Makris, A. P., & Bailer, B. A. (2005). Behavioral treatment of obesity. *Am J Clin Nutr, 82*(1 Suppl), 230S–235S.

Foster, G. D., Wyatt, H. R., Hill, J. O., McGuckin, B. G., Brill, C., Mohammed, B. S., et al. (2003). A randomized trial of a low-carbohydrate diet for obesity. *N Engl J Med, 348*(21), 2082–2090.

Franz, M. J., Bantle, J. P., Beebe, C. A., Brunzell, J. D., Chiasson, J., Garg, A., et al. (2002). Evidence-based nutrition. Principles and recommendations for the treatment and prevention of diabetes and related complications. *Diabetes Care, 25*, 148–198.

Golay, A., Allaz, A., Morel, Y., Tonnac, N. d., Tankova, S., & Reaven, G. (1996a). Similar weight loss with low- and high-carbohydrate diets. *Am J Clin Nutr., 63*, 174–178.

Golay, A., Eigenheer, C., Morel, Y., Kujawski, P., Lehmann, T., & Tonnac, N. d. (1996b). Weight-loss with low or high carbohydrate diet? *Int J Obes Relat Metab Disord., 20*, 1067–1072.

Guthrie, H. A. (1984). Selection and quantification of typical food portions by young adults. *J Am Diet Assoc, 84*(12), 1440–1444.

Harnack, L. J., Jeffery, R. W., & Boutelle, K. N. (2000). Temporal trends in energy intake in the united states: An ecologic perspective. *Am J Clin Nutr, 71*, 1478–1484.

Hays, N. P., Starling, R. D., Liu, X., Sullivan, D. H., Trappe, T. A., Fluckey, J. D., et al. (2004). Effects of an ad libitum low-fat, high-carbohydrate diet on body weight, body composition, and fat distribution in older men and women-a randomized controlled trial. *Arch Intern Med., 164*, 210–217.

Hedley, A. A., Ogden, C. L., Johnson, C. L., Carroll, M. D., Curtin, L. R., & Flegal, K. M. (2004). Prevalence of overweight and obesity among us children, adolescents, and adults, 1999–2002. *JAMA, 291*(23), 2847–2850.

Heilbronn, L. K., Noakes, M., & Clifton, P. M. (2002). The effect of high- and low-glycemic index energy restricted diets on plasma lipid and glucose profiles in type 2 diabetic subjects with varying glycemic control. *J Am Coll Nutr, 21*(2), 120–127.

Hill, J. O., Melanson, E. L., & Wyatt, H. T. (2000). Dietary fat intake and regulation of energy balance: Implications for obesity. *J Nutr, 130*, 284S–288S.

Hill, J. O., Wyatt, H., Phelan, S., & Wing, R. (2005). The national weight control registry: Is it useful in helping deal with our obesity epidemic? *J Nutr Educ Behav, 37*(4), 206–210.

Hu, F. B. (2003). Plant based foods and prevention of cardiovascular disease: An overview. *Am J Clin Nutr, 78*, 544S–551S.

Hu, F. B., Manson, J. E., & Willett, W. C. (2001). Types of dietary fat and risk of coronary heart disease: A critical review. *J Am Coll Nutr, 20*, 5–19.

Hu, F. B., & Willett, W. C. (2002). Optimal diets for prevention of coronary heart disease. *JAMA, 288*, 2569–2578.

Ikeda, J. P., Lyons, P., Schwartzman, F., & Mitchell, R. A. (2004). Self-reported dieting experiences of women with body mass indexes of 30 or more. *J Am Diet Assoc, 104*(6), 972–974.

Jebb, S. A. (2005). Dietary strategies for the prevention of obesity. *Proc Nutr Soc, 64*(2), 217–227.
Jequier, E. (2002). Pathways to obesity. *Int J Obes Relat Metab Disord, 26*, S12–17.
Jequier, E., & Bray, G. A. (2002). Low-fat diets are preferred. *Am J Med, 113*(Suppl 9B), 41S–46S.
Kassirer, J. P., & Angell, M. (1998). Losing weight – an ill-fated new year's resolution. *N Engl J Med, 338*(1), 52–54.
Katan, M., Grundy, S., & Willett, W. (1997). Should a low-fat, high-carbohydrate diet be recommended for everyone? Beyond low-fat diets. *N Engl J Med, 337*, 563–566.
Katz, D. L. (2000). Diet and cancer. In *Nutrition in clinical practice* (pp. 114–126). Philadelphia, PA: Lippincott Williams & Wilkins.
Katz, D. L. (2001a). Clinically relevant fat metabolism. In *Nutrition in clinical practice* (pp. 9–15). Philadelphia, PA: Lippincott, Williams & Wilkins.
Katz, D. L. (2001b). Diet, sleep-wake cycles, and mood. In *Nutrition in clinical practice* (pp. 243–247). Philadelphia, PA: Lippincott Williams & Wilkins.
Katz, D. L. (2001c). Dietary recommendations for health promotion and disease prevention. In *Nutrition in clinical practice* (pp. 291–298). Philadelphia, PA: Lippincott, Williams & Wilkins.
Katz, D. L. (2003). Pandemic obesity and the contagion of nutritional nonsense. *Public Health Rev, 31*, 33–44.
Katz, D. L., & Gonzalez, M. H. (2002). *The way to eat*. Naperville, Illinois: Sourcebooks. JACOBSON/NESTLE, ETC.
Key, T. J., Schatzkin, A., Willett, W. C., Allen, N. E., Spencer, E. A., & Travis, R. C. (2004). Diet, nutrition and the prevention of cancer. *Public Health Nutr, 7*, 187–200.
Keys, A. (1955). Relative obesity and its health significance. *Diabetes, 4*, 447–455.
Keys, A., Aravanis, C., Blackburn, H., Buchem, F. S. V., Buzina, R., Djordjevic, B. S., et al. (1972). Coronary heart disease: Overweight and obesity as risk factors. *Ann Intern Med, 77*, 15–27.
Keys, A., Menotti, A., Aravanis, C., Blackburn, H., Djordevic, B. S., Buzina, R., et al. (1984). The seven countries study: 2,289 deaths in 15 years. *Prev Med, 13*, 141–154.
Khan, L. K., Serdula, M. K., Bowman, B. A., & Williamson, D. F. (2001). Use of prescription weight loss pills among U.S. Adults in 1996–1998. *Ann Intern Med, 134*(4), 282–286.
Kirk, E. P., Jacobsen, D. J., Gibson, C., Hill, J. O., & Donnelly, J. E. (2003). Time course for changes in aerobic capacity and body composition in overweight men and women in response to long-term exercise: The Midwest exercise trial (met). *Int J Obes Relat Metab Disord, 27*, 912–919.
Klein, S. (2004). Clinical trial experience with fat-restricted vs. Carbohydrate-restricted weight-loss diets. *Obes Res, 12 Suppl 2*, 141S–144S.
Klem, M. L., Wing, R. R., McGuire, M. T., Seagle, H. M., & Hill, J. O. (1997). A descriptive study of individuals successful at long-term maintenance of substantial weight loss. *Am J Clin Nutr., 66*(2), 239–246.
Knowler, W. C., Barrett-Connor, E., Fowler, S. E., Hamman, R. F., Lachin, J. M., Walker, E. A., et al. (2002). Reduction in the incidence of type 2 diabetes with lifestyle intervention or metformin. *N Engl J Med, 346*(6), 393–403.
Kok, F. J., & Kromhout, D. (2004). Atherosclerosis – epidemiological studies on the health effects of a Mediterranean diet. *Eur J Nutr, 43*(Suppl1), 2–5.
Kral, T. V., Roe, L. S., & Rolls, B. J. (2004). Combined effects of energy density and portion size on energy intake in women. *Am J Clin Nutr, 79*(6), 962–968.
Krauss, R. M., Eckel, R. H., Howard, B., Appel, L. J., Daniels, S. R., Deckelbaum, R. J., et al. (2000). Aha dietary guidelines: Revision 2000: A statement for healthcare professionals from the nutrition committee of the American Heart Association. *Circulation, 102*(18), 2284–2299.

Kris-Etherton, P., Eckel, R. H., Howard, B. V., S. St. Jeor, & Bazzarre, T. L. (2001). Nutrition committee population science committee and clinical science committee of the American Heart Association. Aha science advisory: Lyon diet heart study. Benefits of a Mediterranean-style, national cholesterol education program/American Heart Association step I dietary pattern on cardiovascular disease. *Circulation, 103*(13), 1823–1825.

Kruger, J., Galuska, D. A., Serdula, M. K., & Jones, D. A. (2004). Attempting to lose weight: Specific practices among U.S. Adults. *Am J Prev Med, 26*(5), 402–406.

Larson, D., Tataranni, P., RT, R. F., & Ravussin, E. (1995). Ad libitum food intake on a "cafeteria diet" in native American women: Relations with body composition and 24-h energy expenditure. *Am J Clin Nutr, 62*, 911–917.

Liebman, M., Cameron, B. A., Carson, D. K., Brown, D. M., & Meyer, S. S. (2001). Dietary fat reduction behaviors in college students: Relationship to dieting status, gender and key psychosocial variables. *Appetite, 36*(1), 51–56.

Livesey, G. (2005). Low-glycaemic diets and health: Implications for obesity. *Proc Nutr Soc, 64*(1), 105–113.

Ludwig, D. S. (2002). The glycemic index: Physiological mechanisms relating obesity, diabetes, and cardiovascular disease. *JAMA, 287*, 2414–2423.

Ludwig, D. S., Majzoub, J. A., Al-Zahrani, A., Dallal, G. E., Blanco, I., & Roberts, S. B. (1999). High glycemic index foods, overeating, and obesity. *Pediatrics, 103*(3), E26.

Mathers, J. C. (2003). Nutrition and cancer prevention: Diet-gene interactions. *Proc Nutr Soc., 62*(3), 605–610.

Mattes, R. D. (2002). Feeding behaviors and weight loss outcomes over 64 months. *Eat Behav., 3*, 191–204.

McAuley, K. A., Smith, K. J., Taylor, R. W., McLay, R. T., Williams, S. M., & Mann, J. I. (2006). Long-term effects of popular dietary approaches on weight loss and features of insulin resistance. *Int J Obes (Lond), 30*(2), 342–349.

McCrory, M. A., Fuss, P. J., Saltzman, E., & Roberts, S. B. (2000). Dietary determinants of energy intake and weight regulation in healthy adults. *J Nutr, 130*, 276S–279S.

McGuire, M. T., Wing, R. R., Klem, M. L., Seagle, H. M., & Hill, J. O. (1998). Long-term maintenance of weight loss: Do people who lose weight through various weight loss methods use different behaviors to maintain their weight? *Int J Obes Relat Metab Disord., 22*(6), 572–577.

McManus, K., Antinoro, L., & Sacks, F. (2001). A randomized controlled trial of a moderate-fat, low-energy diet compared with a low fat, low-energy diet for weight loss in overweight adults. *Int J Obes Relat Metab Disord., 25*(10), 1503–1511.

Meckling, K. A., O'Sullivan, C., & Saari, D. (2004). Comparison of a low-fat diet to a low-carbohydrate diet on weight loss, body composition, and risk factors for diabetes and cardiovascular disease in free-living, overweight men and women. *J Clin Endocrinol Metab, 89*(6), 2717–2723.

Millen, B. E., Quatromoni, P. A., Pencina, M., Kimokoti, R., Nam, B. H., Cobain, S., et al. (2005). Unique dietary patterns and chronic disease risk profiles of adult men: The Framingham nutrition studies. *J Am Diet Assoc, 105*(11), 1723–1734.

Miyashita, Y., Koide, N., Ohtsuka, M., Ozaki, H., Itoh, Y., Oyama, T., et al. (2004). Beneficial effect of low carbohydrate in low caloric diets on visceral fat reduction in type 2 diabetic patients with obesity. *Diabetes Res Clin Pract., 65*(3), 235–241.

Mokdad, A. H., Marks, J. S., Stroup, D. F., & Gerberding, J. L. (2004). Actual causes of death in the united states, 2000. *JAMA, 291*(10), 1238–1245.

Moloney, M. (2000). Dietary treatments of obesity. *Proc Nutr Soc, 59*, 601–608.

Moyad, M. A. (2004). Fad diets and obesity-part ii: An introduction to the theory behind low-carbohydrate diets. *Urologic Nursing, 24*(3), 442–445.

National Cancer Institute. National cancer institute dietary guidelines. Retrieved September, 2002.

Nelson, L. H., & Tucker, L. A. (1996). Diet composition related to body fat in a multivariate study of 203 men. *J Am Diet Assoc, 96*, 771–777.
Nestle, M. (2002). *Food politics*. Berkeley, CA: University of California Press.
Nestle, M. (2003). Increasing portion sizes in American diets: More calories, more obesity. *J Am Diet Assoc, 103*(1), 39–40.
Nickols-Richardson, S. M., Coleman, M. D., Volpe, J. J., & Hosig, K. W. (2005). Perceived hunger is lower and weight loss is greater in overweight premenopausal women consuming a low-carbohydrate/high-protein vs. high-carbohydrate/low-fat diet. *J Am Diet Assoc, 105*(9), 1433–1437.
Noakes, M., Foster, P. R., Keogh, J. B., & Clifton, P. M. (2004). Meal replacements are as effective as structured weight-loss diets for treating obesity in adults with features of metabolic syndrome. *J Nutr, 134*(8), 1894–1899.
Ornish, D. (2004). Was dr. Atkins right? *Am J Diet Assoc, 104*, 537–542.
Pasman, W., Saris, W., & Westerterp-Plantenga, M. (1999). Predictors of weight maintenance. *Obes Res, 7*, 43–50.
Peters, J. C. (2003). Dietary fat and body weight control. *Lipids, 38*, 123–127.
Pi-Sunyer, F. X. (2002). The obesity epidemic: Pathophysiology and consequences of obesity. *Obes Res, 10*(Suppl 2), 97S–104S.
Pirozzo, S., Summerbell, C., Cameron, C., & Glasziou, P. (2002). Advice on low-fat diets for obesity. *Cochrane Database Syst Rev*, (2), CD003640.
Pirozzo, S., Summerbell, C., Cameron, C., & Glasziou, P. (2003). Should we recommend low-fat diets for obesity? *Obes Rev, 4*, 83–90.
Plodkowski, R. A., & Jeor, S. T. S. (2003). Medical nutrition therapy for the treatment of obesity. *Endocrinol Metab Clin North Am., 32*, 935–965.
Poston, W. S., 2nd, & Foreyt, J. P. (2000). Successful management of the obese patient. *Am Fam Physician, 61*(12), 3615–3622.
Raatz, S. K., Torkelson, C. J., Redmon, J. B., Reck, K. P., Kwong, C. A., Swanson, J. E., et al. (2005). Reduced glycemic index and glycemic load diets do not increase the effects of energy restriction on weight loss and insulin sensitivity in obese men and women. *J Nutr, 135*(10), 2387–2391.
Rabast, U., Kasper, H., & Schonborn, J. (1978). Comparative studies in obese subjects fed carbohydrate-restricted and high carbohydrate 1,000-calorie formula diets. *Nutr Metab, 22*, 269–277.
Racette, S. B., Schoeller, D. A., Kushner, R. F., Neil, K. M., & Herling-Iaffaldano, K. (1995). Effects of aerobic exercise and dietary carbohydrate on energy expenditure and body composition during weight reduction in obese women. *Am J Clin Nutr., 61*, 486–494.
Reddy, K. S., & Katan, M. B. (2004). Diet, nutrition and the prevention of hypertension and cardiovascular diseases. *Public Health Nutr, 7*(1A), 167–186.
Rolls, B. J., & Barnett, R. A. (2000). *The volumetrics weight-control plan: Feel full on fewer calories.*: Quill Publishing.
Rolls, B. J., Bell, E. A., & Thorwart, M. L. (1999). Water incorporated into a food but not served with a food decreases energy intake in lean women. *Am J Clin Nutr, 70*(4), 448–455.
Rolls, B. J., Bell, E. A., & Waugh, B. A. (2000a). Increasing the volume of a food by incorporating air affects satiety in men. *Am J Clin Nutr, 72*(2), 361–368.
Rolls, B. J., Ello-Martin, J. A., & Tohill, B. C. (2004a). What can intervention studies tell us about the relationship between fruit and vegetable consumption and weight management? *Nutr Rev, 62*, 1–17.
Rolls, B. J., Engel, D., & Birch, L. L. (2000b). Serving portion size influences 5-year-old but not 3-year-old children's food intakes. *J Am Diet Assoc, 100*(2), 232–234.
Rolls, B. J., & Miller, D. L. (1997). Is the low-fat message giving people a license to eat more? *J Am Coll Nutr, 16*, 535–543.

Rolls, B. J., Roe, L. S., Kral, T. V., Meengs, J. S., & Wall, D. E. (2004b). Increasing the portion size of a packaged snack increases energy intake in men and women. *Appetite, 42*(1), 63–69.

Rolls, B. J., Roe, L. S., & Meengs, J. S. (2004c). Salad and satiety: Energy density and portion size of a first-course salad affect energy intake at lunch. *J Am Diet Assoc, 104*(10), 1570–1576.

Rolls, B. J., Roe, L. S., Meengs, J. S., & Wall, D. E. (2004d). Increasing the portion size of a sandwich increases energy intake. *J Am Diet Assoc, 104*(3), 367–372.

S. St. Jeor, Howard, B., Prewitt, E., Bovee, V., Bazzarre, T., & Eckel, R. (2001). Dietary protein and weight reduction: A statement for healthcare professionals from the nutrition committee of the council on nutrition, physical activity, and metabolism of the American heart association. *Circulation, 104*, 1869–1874.

Sacks, F. M., Svetkey, L. P., Vollmer, W. M., Appel, L. J., Bray, G. A., Harsha, D., et al. (2001). Effects on blood pressure of reduced dietary sodium and the dietary approaches to stop hypertension (dash) diet. Dash-sodium collaborative research group. *N Engl J Med, 344*, 3–10.

Samaha, F. F., Iqbal, N., Seshadri, P., Chicano, K. L., Daily, D. A., McGrory, J., et al. (2003). A low-carbohydrate as compared with a low-fat diet in severe obesity. *N Engl J Med, 348*, 2074–2081.

Schrauwen, P., & Westerterp, K. R. (2000). The role of high-fat diets and physical activity in the regulation of body weight. *Br J Nutr, 84*, 417–427.

Schroder, H., Marrugat, J., Vila, J., Covas, M. I., & Elosua, R. (2004). Adherence to the traditional Mediterranean diet is inversely associated with body mass index and obesity in a Spanish population. *J Nutr, 134*(12), 3355–3361.

Schulze, M. B., Hoffmann, K., Manson, J. E., Willett, W. C., Meigs, J. B., Weikert, C., et al. (2005). Dietary pattern, inflammation, and incidence of type 2 diabetes in women. *Am J Clin Nutr, 82*(3), 675–684; quiz 714–675.

Schutz, Y. (1995). Macronutrients and energy balance in obesity. *Metabolism, 44*,7–11.

Sears, W. (1999). *The family nutrition book: Everything you need to know about feeding your children - from birth to age two.*: Little Brown & Company.

Segal-Isaacson, C. J., Johnson, S., Tomuta, V., Cowell, B., & Stein, D. T. (2004). A randomized trial comparing low-fat and low-carbohydrate diets matched for energy and protein. *Obes Res, 12*(Suppl 2), 130S–140S.

Serdula, M. K., Mokdad, A. H., Williamson, D. F., Galuska, D. A., Mendlein, J. M., & Heath, G. W. (1999). Prevalence of attempting weight loss and strategies for controlling weight. *JAMA, 282*(14), 1353–1358.

Shah, M., & Garg, A. (1996). High-fat and high-carbohydrate diets and energy balance. *Diabetes Care, 19*, 1142–1152.

Shick, S. M., Wing, R. R., Klem, M. L., McGuire, M. T., Hill, J. O., & Seagle, H. (1998). Persons successful at long-term weight loss and maintenance continue to consume a low energy, low fat diet. *J Am Diet Assoc, 98*, 408–413.

Shubair, M. M., McColl, R. S., & Hanning, R. M. (2005). Mediterranean dietary components and body mass index in adults: The peel nutrition and heart health survey. *Chronic Dis Can, 26*(2–3), 43–51.

Siggaard, R., Raben, A., & Astrup, A. (1996). Weight loss during 12 weeks ad libitum carbohydrate-rich diet in overweight and normal weight subjects at a Danish work site. *Obes Res, 347–356.*

Simopoulos, A. P. (2001). The Mediterranean diets: What is so special about the diet of Greece? The scientific evidence. *J Nutr, 131*, 3065S–3073S.

Skov, A., Toubro, S., Ronn, B., Holm, L., & Astrup, A. (1999). Randomized trial on protein vs. Carbohydrate in ad libitum fat reduced diet for the treatment of obesity. *Int J Obes Relat Metab Disord, 23*, 528–536.

Sloth, B., Krog-Mikkelsen, I., Flint, A., Tetens, I., Bjorck, I., Vinoy, S., et al. (2004). No difference in body weight decrease between a low-glycemic-index and a high-

glycemic-index diet but reduced ldl cholesterol after 10-wk ad libitum intake of the low-glycemic-index diet. *Am J Clin Nutr, 80*(2), 337–347.
Sondike, S. B., Copperman, N., & Jacobson, M. S. (2003). Effects of a low-carbohydrate diet on weight loss and cardiovascular risk factor in overweight adolescents. *J Pediatr, 142*(3), 253–258.
Spieth, L. E., Harnish, J. D., Lenders, C. M., Raezer, L. B., Pereira, M. A., Hangen, S. J., et al. (2000). A low-glycemic index diet in the treatment of pediatric obesity. *Arch Pediatr Adolesc Med, 154*(9), 947–951.
Tapper-Gardzina, Y., Cotugna, N., & Vickery, C. (2002). Should you recommend a low-carb, high-protein diet? *The Nurse Practitioner, 27*(4), 52–57.
Tate, D. F., Jackvony, E. H., & Wing, R. R. (2003). Effects of internet behavioral counseling on weight loss in adults at risk for type 2 diabetes: A randomized trial. *JAMA, 289*(14), 1833–1836.
Tate, D. F., Wing, R. R., & Winett, R. A. (2001). Using internet technology to deliver a behavioral weight loss program. *JAMA, 285*(9), 1172–1177.
Terry, P., Terry, J. B., & Wolk, A. (2001). Fruit and vegetable consumption in the prevention of cancer: An update. *J Intern Med, 250*, 280–290.
Trichopoulou, A., Naska, A., Orfanos, P., & Trichopoulos, D. (2005). Mediterranean diet in relation to body mass index and waist-to-hip ratio: The Greek European prospective investigation into cancer and nutrition study. *Am J Clin Nutr, 82*(5), 935–940.
Tsai, A. G., & Wadden, T. A. (2005). Systematic review: An evaluation of major commercial weight loss programs in the United States. *Ann Intern Med, 142*(1), 56–66.
U.S. Department of Agriculture. (2005). Dietary guidelines for Americans, 2005. Retrieved 11/19/05.
U.S. Department of Health and Human Services. (2001). *The surgeon general's call to action to prevent and decrease overweight and obesity*. Washington, DC: Centers for Disease Control and Prevention.
National Institutes of Health.
U.S. Preventive Services Task Force. (1996). *Guide to clinical preventive services*. Baltimore, MD: Williams & Wilkins.
Van Duyn, M. A., & Pivonka, E. (2000). Overview of the health benefits of fruit and vegetable consumption for the dietetics professional: Selected literature. *J Am Diet Assoc, 100*(12), 1511–1521.
Vartabedian, R. E., & Matthews, K. (1994). *Nutripoints: The breakthrough point system for optimal health*. (3rd ed.): Designs for Wellness Press.
Vermunt, S. H., Pasman, W. J., Schaafsma, G., & Kardinaal, A. F. (2003). Effects of sugar intake on body weight: A review. *Obes Rev, 4*, 91–99.
Volek, J. S., Sharman, M. J., Love, D. M., Avery, N. G., Gomez, A. L., Scheett, T. P., et al. (2002). Body composition and hormonal responses to a carbohydrate-restricted diet. *Metabolism, 51*, 864–870.
Wadden, T. A., & Butryn, M. L. (2003). Behavioral treatment of obesity. *Endocrinol Metab Clin North Am, 32*, 981–1003.
Wang, Y., Monteiro, C., & Popkin, B. M. (2002). Trends of obesity and underweight in older children and adolescents in the United States, Brazil, china, and Russia. *Am J Clin Nutr, 75*(6), 971–977.
Warren, J. M., Henry, C. J., & Simonite, V. (2003). Low glycemic index breakfasts and reduced food intake in preadolescent children. *Pediatrics, 112*(5), e414.
Weisburger, J. H. (2000). Eat to live, not live to eat. *Nutrition, 16*(9), 767–773.
Westman, E. C., Yancy, W. S., Edman, J. S., Tomlin, K. F., & Perkins, C. E. (2002). Effect of 6-month adherence to a very low carbohydrate diet program. *Am J Med, 113*(1), 30–36.
Willet, W. C. (2001). *Eat, drink, and be healthy*. NY, NY: Simon & Schuster Source.

Willett, W. C., & Leibel, R. L. (2002). Dietary fat is not a major determinant of body fat. *Am J Med, 113*(Suppl 9B), 47S–59S.
Wing, R. R., & Gorin, A. A. (2003). Behavioral techniques for treating the obese patient. *Prim Care, 30*, 375–391.
Wing, R. R., & Hill, J. O. (2001). Successful weight loss maintenance. *Annu Rev Nutr, 21*, 323–341.
Wing, R. R., & Phelan, S. (2005). Long-term weight loss maintenance. *Am J Clin Nutr, 82*(1 Suppl), 222S–225S.
Wright, J. D., Kennedy-Stephenson, J., Wang, C. Y., McDowell, M. A., Johnson, C. L., National Center for Health Statistics, et al. (2004). Trends in intake of energy and macronutrients—United States, 1971–2000. *MMWR, 53*, 80–82.
Yale-Griffin Prevention Research Center. (10/00 – 8/03). Obesity systematic review: Centers for Disease Control, Grant #U48-CCU115802.
Yancy, W. S., Olsen, M. K., Guyton, J. R., Bakst, R. P., & Westman, E. C. (2004). A low-carbohydrate, ketogenic diet versus a low-fat diet to treat obesity and hyperlipidemia: A randomized, controlled trial. *Ann Intern Med, 140*(10), 769–777.

3

Low-Cost Obesity Interventions: The Market for Foods

Michael S. Finke and Sandra J. Huston

Over the past two decades obesity rates in the United States have doubled for adults and nearly tripled for children. The direct costs of obesity are estimated to be approximately 7% of total health care costs in the United States (Colditz, 1999). Obesity has a greater impact on morbidity and disability than mortality, significantly increasing the number of unhealthy and potentially unproductive years of life. Although US government national health objectives for 2010 include reducing the obesity rate to less than 15%, recent obesity trends and current health data suggest the situation is not improving (Healthy People 2010).

It is estimated that obesity accounts for medical costs and lost productivity totaling more than $100 billion per year, with Medicare and Medicaid financing about half the medical costs associated with obesity. Not only does obesity carry a high personal cost when it threatens the quality and quantity of life, but also a social cost. The non-obese must bear a significant portion of increased expenses associated with treating the diseases of those who are obese. Does this social cost warrant government intervention? Clearly, a negative externality exists and a correction, whether personal or public, is required to eliminate or diminish its effect. Close scrutiny of obesity research provides some insight into appropriate low-cost interventions as well as the failure of current public intervention policies.

Two important economic factors have been forwarded to explain obesity trends. The first is that healthy, palatable foods are no longer affordable to lower-income consumers. Drenowski and Specter (2004) cite lower consumption of nutrient dense fruits and vegetables and increasing consumption of less expensive energy-dense foods such as added sugars, fats, and refined grains among lower socioeconomic status households. The second is that lower socioeconomic status is associated with less investment in future well-being through healthy behaviors such as good nutrition and regular exercise. Both the availability of inexpensive, convenient, high-calorie foods and the lack of a desire to eat a healthy diet may explain obesity trends. However, they imply different means of reversing these trends.

Obesity: Contributing Factors and Current Policies

The retail food marketplace in any large city is scattered with specialty supermarkets offering lower fat, organic, higher protein, high fiber foods that cater to a clientele of consumers who place a significant value on nutrition. There has never been a greater variety of good tasting, healthy, and convenient foods available to consumers. Within the same cities, and particularly in smaller cities and rural areas, there exist supermarkets that provide lower-cost choices where foods are often equally convenient and good tasting but where the customers generally place a lower value on nutrition. This clientele tends to be less educated, less knowledgeable about nutrition, lower income, rural, sedentary, black, Southern and Midwestern, and is more likely to be obese. Running a simple stepwise regression on the strongest predictors of obesity (BMI > 30) using the 1994–1996 USDA survey of food intakes by individuals (CSFII) yields the following results (see Table 3.1):

While many of the most significant predictors of obesity are correlated with income, income itself (measured as percent of poverty) is not among the strongest independent predictors of obesity – and neither is the importance placed on food price by the respondent. This seems to contradict the economic explanation of obesity trends, which cite the strengthening inverse relation between income and obesity during the 1980s and 1990s as evidence that the poor are less able to afford healthy foods. Healthy eating, although the fifth strongest predictor of obesity, trails energy expenditure proxies of exercise and television watching. Culture and physiology are also particularly strong predictors. Food label use, among the more potent tools of public nutrition policy, does make the list of statistically significant obesity predictors.

Taxes and Subsidies

The contemporary marketplace for food includes a remarkable variety of choices that are specifically tailored to provide satisfaction at the lowest possible cost. The ability of the modern agricultural system to provide this diversity of food that satisfies our immediate needs and wants, at a cost of roughly one seventh of the average American's budget, is the end result of producer response to the demand for better taste and convenience at the lowest possible price.

Table 3.1. Stepwise Regression Results.

Order	Variable	Cumulative R-squared
1	Black	0.0187
2	Hours of television per day	0.0313
3	Regular exercise (negative effect)	0.0388
4	Living in the Midwest	0.0429
5	Healthy eating index (negative effect)	0.0470
6	Smoking (negative effect)	0.0521
7	Female	0.0559
8	College degree (negative effect)	0.0591
9	Age 45–54	0.0628
10	Age 55–64	0.0688
11	Less than high school education	0.0711
12	Frequent use of food labels (negative effect)	0.0732

It is possible to modify food consumption by public intervention in food markets. Increasing the price of foods linked to obesity will result in reduced consumption, and subsidizing healthier foods will make them more attractive. Unfortunately, prices of healthier foods have risen in recent decades while less healthy foods have fallen in price.

Perhaps the most significant technological change related to the price of food in the late twentieth century is in technologies that allow producers to efficiently separate corn oil and fructose through the process of wet milling. Between 1970 and 1995, the volume of wet-milled corn increased from 238 million to 1.3 billion bushels. This resulted in a sharp decrease in the price of high fructose corn syrup relative to other sweeteners, and a sharp decrease in the price of vegetable oils. Annual consumption of high fructose corn syrup in the US increased from 8 ounces per person in 1970 to 62 pounds per person in 1997, a time period in which per capita non-diet soft drink consumption roughly doubled (Putnam & Allshouse, 1999). Consumption of total vegetable oils increased from 38 pounds per person in 1970 to 55 pounds per person in 1997.

That vegetable oils and sweeteners represent such a low-cost source of food energy is an unhappy accident of very well intentioned food engineering. Consider that in the 1960s the lowest cost sources of food energy were potatoes and grains, and low-income Americans tended to derive a greater share of food energy from tubers, legumes, and grain products. Due mainly to technological advances of corn milling, the lowest cost sources of food energy are now sweeteners and vegetable oils (Putnam & Allshouse, 1999; Raper, Zizza, & Rourke, 1992) (see Table 3.2).

It is also an unhappy accident of food production technology that cheap sugars and oils taste good, are not nearly as perishable as fruits and vegetables, and can be easily processed into convenient meals. These foods are now consumed in greater quantities by lower-income consumers, who not surprisingly gained greater excess body mass during the 1980s and 1990s than higher-income consumers. Nutrition researchers have only recently begun to uncover the links between high fructose corn syrup and obesity, while the links between high fat diets and obesity have received greater attention.

Taxing and subsidizing foods to meet diet composition goals is possible since foods are a normal good (as prices go up, quantity demanded goes down) and quantities demanded can be shifted by changing prices. Response to changes in food prices, however, is muted relative to other consumer goods. Price elasticities are low, particularly among the least expensive and least healthy food categories. The table below estimates the changes in quantity needed to align actual and recommended food intake based on the original food pyramid (see Table 3.3).

Table 3.2. Energy cost by food category.

Food category	Cents/kilocalorie
Red meats	0.31
Other protein foods	0.18
Dairy	0.21
Fats and oils	0.04
Grains	0.09
Fruits	0.57
Vegetables	0.33
Sweeteners	0.05

Table 3.3. Actual Food Disappearance vs. Recommended Consumption per Individual.

	1993 Actual intake		Recommended intake		
Commodity or food group	**Quantity (ounces)**	**Total calories (kilocalories)**	**Quantity (ounces)**	**Total calories (kilocalories)**	**Percent of actual**
Vegetables	9.88	159	9.92	160	100.6
Fruits	6.71	125	11.58	216	172.8
Dairy	20.01	267	19.24	230	86.1
Meat and alternatives	8.97	745	6.00	498	66.8
Breads, cereals, rice, pasta	7.46	779	6.12	639	82.0
Added fats and oils	2.86	647	1.16	263	40.6
Added sugars	6.13	450	1.69	124	27.6
All foods		3172		2130	67.2

Table 3.4. Food Price Changes Needed to Meet Recommended Diet.

Food category	**Quantity Change (%)**	**Price per pound ($) Initial price**	**New price**	**Total subsidy (tax) (millions of dollars)**
Red meat	-55	3.82	6.55	(86,790)
Dairy	-14	0.45	0.60	(34,343)
Fats and oils	-59	1.46	5.23	(41,499)
Grains	-18	1.45	2.43	(56,419)
Fruits	73	1.19	0.00	249,525
Sweeteners	-72	0.84	3.37	(36,292)

Combining the required quantity change with aggregate elasticity data from 1993 yielded the following estimated taxes and subsidies (see Table 3.4).

Since overall food consumption would need to decrease to meet recommended daily intake levels, most foods would need to be taxed heavily to reduce quantity demanded. The price of fats and oils would need to triple and the price of sweeteners to quadruple, while fruit would have to be given away for free in order to align diets with the original food pyramid. Taxes collected on the five taxed food categories would just cover the massive expense of providing free fruit.

The magnitude of price changes needed to meet nutrition objectives makes market intervention through tax policy impractical. If price policy does not qualify as a low-cost intervention, then perhaps improving diets by changing preferences for healthy foods is more practical. Increasing awareness of the links between diet and disease and providing information to guide consumers toward healthier food choices is the goal of information policy. For the most part, the primary intervention employed to improve nutrition and increase energy expenditure has been through information policy.

Information Policy

A goal established by the US Public Health Service in 1990 was a reduction in overweight rates to below 20% of all adults by the year 2000. By the end of the century, it became evident that the US had in fact moved further from this goal. A review of the possible policy interventions needed to improve nutrition and increase exercise emphasized providing increased "consistency of positive, reinforcing messages to the public on nutrition" and promoting "fruit and vegetable consumption and other healthful behaviors" (US Public Health Service, 1998).

When the government estimated the aggregate benefit from the Nutrition Labeling and Education Act of 1994, it based its estimate on an overall reduction in dietary fat through better food choices. Prior to the NLEA, just over half of all foods carried nutrition labels, and consumers often had to guess the nutrient content of unlabeled foods. For example, consumers deciding among lunch meats had to choose between ham (labeled) and bologna (unlabeled). They may have realized that the unlabeled foods were often less healthy than the labeled ones, but had to guess how unhealthy they were. This lack of information resulted in inefficient choice: a consumer may have used the ham label to guess the nutrient content of bologna which, in turn, led to a much higher-fat lunch than if foods were labeled consistently.

Subsequent analysis of the effects of the NLEA upon food choice suggest that those who used food labels after the Act were able to make better quality food choices with the new labels. Those who didn't use food labels (the majority of Americans) consumed a diet that was no different than the diet they ate before the NLEA. Since a slightly larger proportion of participants always used nutrition labels after the NLEA, there was an increase in the proportion of participants eating low-fat diets. The Act may have achieved the goal of improving food choices among consumers who valued nutrition by allowing them to more precisely choose foods that reflected the preference for nutrition. The following results compare the proportion of participants who ate a low-fat diet (< 30% of total calories from fat) prior to the NLEA (1989) and in 1995 (post-NLEA) using the Continuing Survey of Food Intakes by Individuals (CSFII) (see Table 3.5):

A much larger proportion of participants who always used food labels was able to eat a low-fat diet after the NLEA. This is consistent with a successful information policy. The information cost of choosing a low-fat diet was reduced by market intervention leading to improved choice, but only

Table 3.5. Proportion of participants who ate a low-fat diet (< 30% of total calories from fat) prior to the NLEA (1989) and in 1995 (post-NLEA).

	1989 Sample		1995 Sample	
Variables	**Low fat**	**Higher fat**	**Low fat**	**Higher fat**
Sample	32.73	67.27	36.79	63.21
Label Use				
Always	38.41	61.97	46.04	53.96
Sometimes	31.03	68.97	33.83	66.17
Rarely	30.72	69.27	30.28	69.72
Never	31.87	68.13	31.74	68.26
Education				
<High School	33.39	66.61	35.48	64.52
High School	29.27	70.73	35.98	64.02
Some College	34.27	65.72	32.25	67.75
College	38.20	61.80	43.64	56.36

among those who always use the label. participants who sometimes, rarely, or never use labels did not appear to change their diet behavior.

When the likelihood of eating a low-fat diet is estimated (which includes control variables) from a combined sample of participants in 1989 and 1995, only an interaction variable of always using the label in 1995 is a statistically significant predictor. Results are consistent with the hypothesis that label use after the NLEA was associated with an improved ability to choose a diet that meets the recommended threshold for fat content (see Table 3.6).

Those who often used these labels were more likely to eat a low-fat diet after the NLEA than they had been before the NLEA. The predicted probability of eating a low-fat diet was 13% higher for those who often, rather than rarely, used food labels in the 1989 sample, while often using food labels in the 1995 sample led to a 37% higher predicted probability of eating a low-fat diet.

In 1995 more consumers reported that they always used food labels than had been reported in 1989. The groups that increased their use of nutrition labeling information to the greatest degree were women, the more educated, those with a higher earned income, the young, and nonblacks. In particular, those who were aware of the relation between diet and disease and those with a college education increased label use frequency (see Table 3.7).

These data also suggest that demographic groups who were not motivated to eat a low-fat diet before the NLEA were not motivated to use labels after the NLEA despite the reduction in search cost. While the policy succeeded as a means of improving food choice among label users, the end result was a wider chasm between those who care about nutrition and those who don't. And those who don't are more likely to be of lower socioeconomic status.

Table 3.6. Analysis of Participants Eating a Low-Fat Diet Using Logistic Procedure.

Variable (N = 3856)	**Coefficient**	**Pr > Chi-square**	**Predicted probability (%)**
Label use (Sometimes reference category)			30.16
Always, 1995	+	***	40.87
Always, 1989	+		34.61
Rare, 1995	−		28.58
Rare, 1989	+		31.19
Never, 1995	+		30.44
Never, 1989	+		30.33

Table 3.7. Unweighted Frequencies of Participants Who Always Use Food Labels.

Variables	**1989**	**1995**	**% Change**	**Difference**
Aware of fat/disease				
Yes	24.07	37.51	55.84	***
No	16.96	15.54	(8.37)	
Education				
Less than high school	18.92	27.92	35.94	***
College	32.58	50.45	54.85	***

The problem with information policy is that it does not shift aggregate demand enough to substantively change the overall nutrient content of the American food supply. When a minority of consumers is able to avoid sugars and fats, increase their consumption of fruits and vegetables, and substitute healthier proteins for higher saturated fat alternatives, the increase in demand is negligible on the aggregate. However, within commodity markets prices increase for healthier food varieties. A review of food nutrients in the aggregate food supply illustrates the intractability of aggregate supply to changes in consumer demand (Putnam & Allshouse, 1999). Despite a strong trend toward consumption of lower-fat milk during the 1980s, total fat from dairy was exactly the same in 1994 as it had been in 1970. While fat consumption from meat declined slightly, fat consumption in the form of cooking fats and oils more than made up the difference. The only striking aggregate change in supply was an increase in carbohydrate consumption from sweeteners and grain products.

Perhaps the main problem of information policy is that agricultural supply cannot easily shift toward healthier variations of aggregate food categories. Until cows can be bred to produce lower-fat milk, information policy will simply shift demand for milk products. Those who value health will increase demand for lower-fat milk, leading to increased wholesale prices for milk protein and decreased prices for milk fat. An illustration of the regressive effects of information policy is the shift in demand for leaner meats during the 1980s. Ground beef is an ideal food from which to determine whether and to what extent consumers are willing to pay for the removal of fat.

Varieties of ground beef essentially differ only in content of fat and lean. Since millions of tons of grass-fed lean ground beef are imported from Australia to complement the supply of grain-fed American ground beef, supply of both lean and higher-fat ground beef is abundant. Both are easy to prepare, free of brand names, and contain essentially the same micronutrient (vitamin and mineral) content. Fat provides improved flavor and texture to ground beef, and both high- and low-income consumers enjoyed fat in ground beef prior to the increased awareness of the relation between heart disease and saturated fat consumption that occurred in the early 1980s. The table below illustrates a regression that models the fat content of ground beef as a function of price, income, race, and other controls (not listed) in the 1977–1978 and 1987–1988 Nationwide Food Consumption Surveys (see Table 3.8).

The relation between income and fat content of ground beef more than doubled in magnitude between the two time periods, as did the magnitude of race (all are statistically significant at $P < 0.01$). The relative impact of price

Table 3.8. Regression Results – Fat Content of Ground Beef as a Function of Price, Income, Race and Other Control Variables (not listed) in the 1977–1978 and 1987–1988 Nationwide Food Consumption Surveys.

Variable	1977–1978	1987–1988
Price	-0.076	-0.112
Log income	-0.011	-0.024
White	-0.028	-0.067

upon leanness of ground beef also increased during this period, consistent with a greater price disparity between leaner and fattier ground beef.

Overall fat consumption as a proportion of food energy in 1977 was highest in the middle-income categories and lowest in the bottom four income deciles. In 1987, the fat content of diets was lowest at the highest income categories and highest at the bottom income deciles. Information policy that stigmatized fat consumption during this time period resulted in a redistribution of fat from higher-income to lower-income consumers. This redistribution of less healthy foods within a relatively static food system is the inevitable result of information policy. The unhealthy foods, as well as the negative health outcomes associated with lower quality diets, are redirected to those who are either unwilling or unable to pay for healthier foods.

Paternalistic Interventions

The Women, Infants, and Children (WIC) program of targeted food subsidies represents a type of paternalistic nutrition policy that constrains food choice. By designating some (hopefully more nutritious) foods eligible for subsidy it is possible to force lower-income consumers to make better food choices. There is evidence that the WIC program can result in the achievement of diet objectives. For example, the children of parents receiving WIC support consume more milk and fewer soft drinks than other children in the same income category (Frazao, 2005).

In contrast, the Federal Food Stamp Program provides greater food choice autonomy. A closer examination of food stamp participation outcomes (through comparisons with nonparticipants who have comparable incomes) is inconsistent with the hypothesis that money serves as a barrier to healthy food consumption.

Food stamp participants appear to be less interested in health. Compared to non-participants, food stamp recipients are less likely to breast feed, exercise less frequently and vigorously, watch more television, and smoke tobacco with greater frequency (Fox & Cole, 2004). It is not surprising that when income is transferred to participants in the Food Stamp Program, they do not choose healthier diets nor are they less likely to be obese. Food stamp participants have lower healthy eating scores than higher-income nonparticipants, and even more surprisingly lower healthy eating scores than like income nonparticipants. It is possible that when given more money to spend on food, food stamp recipients eat worse and not better than if they had not received the transfer payment. Food stamp participants also had a higher mean body mass index than either higher- or like-income nonparticipants.

The negative relation between food stamps and diet quality raises the disturbing possibility that market intervention programs that provide more money to spend on food might result in higher rates of obesity, and result in a greater negative externality to be borne by society. If transfer programs that provide low-income households with more money to spend on higher-quality food are not an effective low-cost intervention to reduce obesity, then perhaps more paternalistic interventions hold greater promise.

Insight into these observed behavioral correlations between resource allocation and health-related behaviors is provided by the health production model, which describes the link between diet and other behaviors that reflect a willingness to make sacrifices in the present to gain longevity and higher quality of life in the future.

The Health Production Model

Why do people care about nutrition? What makes some take the time to research current information on the links between diet and disease, buy books on how to cook healthy meals, and spend time comparing the fat and cholesterol content of different foods? What makes some consciously forego flavor and cost in order to eat a healthy diet? Investment in health is like any other investment – it involves a conscious decision to reduce welfare in the present in order to improve well-being in the future. Choosing a nutritious diet is an investment in health capital, capital that is built up over time in order to realize a future return. Since the benefits of eating a less healthy diet accrue mainly in the present (flavor, convenience, satiety) while the benefits of eating a healthy diet accrue mainly in the future (increased longevity and future quality of life), the value individuals place on well-being over time may explain variation in diet choice.

Each individual is endowed with a stock of health capital, influenced by genetic and environmental factors, which is a component of overall human capital. While the quality of this endowment may differ among individuals, there is assumed to be at least some degree of health capital which can be manipulated by each individual. Grossman (1972) argues that health is endogenous and at least partly a function of activities undertaken over time to maintain and improve (or deteriorate) an individual's health capital. If this were not the case, and no choice existed, then economics could not be used to analyze behavior associated with the tradeoffs of one activity for another. Health stock is a compilation of utility-providing commodities (such as diet, exercise, medical care utilization, sleep, recreation, and abstention from smoking, excessive alcohol consumption, or drugs) that are produced with resource inputs of market goods and human effort measured through time.

The health production model views diet choice as a production process, an investment activity undertaken to maintain or enhance health capital. Diet choice depends on both an individual's willingness and his/her ability to invest. Individuals with lower rates of discounting future utility indicate higher proclivity for investment behavior through their preferences. Because these individuals are more prone to investment behavior they often have more accumulated assets and more productive human capital service flows to fund investment activities. That is, people with lower rates of time preference tend to be more educated, have higher incomes, and engage in health and savings behavior with a forward thinking approach – their preferences are realized through their ability to produce health capital. Some individuals may be inclined to be forward thinking but are unable to fully articulate their preferences because of affordability constraints, be it money or knowledge. Others who are more present oriented may have the resources to fund health capital investment activities, but choose not to. Still others are both unwilling and unable to make health capital investments for tomorrow at the expense of subverting utility available today.

As we have seen from the empirical evidence presented earlier in this chapter, when more information was made available through the NLEA it had the greatest impact on those who were already using this information. In other words, it helped those who were forward thinking make better diet choices at a lower cost by reducing the cost of information search. Evidence also suggests that those who exhibited behaviors consistent with a more present time orientation did not change behavior despite increased access to information aiding health capital investment.

It is possible that this information could have changed preferences, but income constraints prevented dramatic changes in dietary behavior. For example a lower income person now understands that increasing fruits and vegetables in her diet will help prevent cancer in the future, so she wants to consume more of these foods. However, given consumption needs in the present and the relatively high cost of fresh produce compared to products produced with refined oils and high fructose corn syrup, she cannot afford to purchase the diet she desires for long-term health. It is also possible that people preferring convenience and flavor in a market where these foods are cheap find this to be a corner solution. In either case, changing the environment to affect present consumption decisions by making nutrient-dense, lower-calorie foods relatively less expensive is a myopic policy intervention that can encourage better food choices among those who would not otherwise value health.

The health production model helps us to see that the most effective, low-cost intervention policies must take myopic utility into account. Instead of assuming that people will care about the future, an alternative strategy is to encourage people to make forward-thinking choices by altering incentives that increase that attractiveness or healthy choices in the present. Those with higher rates of time preference are unwilling to forgo utility in the present in order to gain utility in the future. This is consistent with observed correlations between dietary patterns and behaviors associated with higher rates of time preference including education, seat belt use, wealth accumulation, etc. People with high rates of time preference are not motivated by investment behavior. Policies encouraging investment behavior through eating a healthy diet, exercise, and nutrition education will not be effective for people who place little value on possible improvements in future welfare. Policies affecting utility in the present period by modifying present costs are much more likely to be successful. People with low rates of time preference are more likely to choose healthier foods anyway. With present costs higher, people with high rates of time preference will be more likely to make these same decisions, albeit for different reasons.

Myopic Policy Interventions

Heterogeneity in the value consumers place on health implies a clear benefit from information policy to forward-thinking consumers. These policies – for example nutrition labeling – may be efficient in that they reduce search costs for many at a low cost to food producers. However, information policy appears to have had no impact on aggregate food and nutrient consumption. Food stamps that transfer income to lower socioeconomic status households may be socially desirable; however there is no evidence that these transfers can positively impact obesity trends. What are the diet policy options available that account for myopic food choice?

Food intake patterns can be manipulated through different pricing structures, taxes, and subsidies for both producers and consumers. One example of a food pricing structure is multiple component product pricing. Increasing demand for healthier varieties of aggregate food categories, for example milk or ground beef, leads to higher prices for protein and lower market prices for fat. The market allocates healthier varieties to consumers who place greater value on health, while myopic consumers happily eat better tasting varieties that can now be bought at a lower cost. The end result is higher rates of obesity among myopic consumers and a transfer of wealth from healthier consumers to myopic consumers through public health care costs.

Careful identification of aggregate food categories that are composed of relatively healthier nutrients, for example grains that are higher in protein and fiber than corn or meats that are lower in fat than beef, will result in a healthier aggregate food supply and fewer unwanted fats and empty carbohydrates to be cheaply distributed. Current agricultural subsidy programs fail to account for the aggregate nutrient content of commodities, and may even favor variations that are less nutrient dense. Telling consumers to eat lower-fat varieties of milk or beef or grains while failing to enact policies that reduce the aggregate fat content of the American food supply will result in a predictable policy failure that inevitably hurts those who rely most on public health care programs.

The power of entrenched agricultural interests and the dispersion of beneficiaries (the obese and taxpayers) will reduce the feasibility of modifying subsidies to promote health. Food taxes are regressive (at least in terms of present welfare) and appear even less politically feasible. However, subjecting new commodity programs to an examination of public health consequences is a more rational and effective form of market intervention. Public investment in technologies that result in healthier varieties of agricultural commodities can also be justified as a means of increasing the quality of the food supply. Rather than investing in technology to more efficiently extract nutrients from grains that contain less favored nutrients, investment that improves the production efficiency of more nutrient-dense plants and animals is warranted.

Perhaps the greatest problem with taxing unhealthy foods is defining which foods are relatively healthy and the extent to which different foods contribute to obesity. Another problem is that taxes will have no impact on the aggregate food supply unless they stimulate production of healthier food varieties. Current agricultural policy, for example, restricts imports of sugar resulting in a much higher retail price. The market has responded by investing in technologies that reduce the prices of corn sweeteners that now substitute for cane sugar in many manufactured foods and beverages. One advantage of taxing sin foods, or common foods that have little nutritive merit, is that those who create an externality through unhealthy food choice now subsidize increased public health costs. Sin taxes may also be justified among excessively myopic consumers who prefer not to be obese yet who are not able to restrain themselves from making unhealthy choices (O'Donoghue & Rabin, 2005). Even if foods are taxed to produce a healthier food supply, the cost of tax policy may be greater than the amount society currently spends on treating obesity-related illnesses. The equity of imposing this cost on nonobese people who consume these foods in moderation is also questionable.

Another myopic intervention option is to make all food prices higher through a general food tax, the revenues from which could be used to finance the medical costs of obesity-related illness. In countries with higher food prices there are lower rates of obesity as people are induced to substitute other, cheaper goods that now provide more utility per dollar spent. Rather than deriving utility from eating, people are induced to spend more on other goods. The advantage is that people will eat fewer calories. The disadvantage is that this is a regressive policy that could lead to hunger among lower income individuals, especially children. Combining a general food tax with healthy food vouchers, similar to the WIC program, would improve diet quality while reducing aggregate consumption.

Recent studies provide ample evidence to suggest that gastric bypass surgery is a more cost-effective treatment for the severely obese (BMI > 40) than diet/exercise, pharmacological, and other medical interventions (Fang, 2003). In the short run, this surgery may present an extreme yet cost-effective intervention to treat obesity, however pricing policies and programs that alter food supply support an environment that encourages health capital investment and prevents obesity in the long run.

Conclusion

It can easily be argued that these myopic policy options are paternalistic in nature. Such approaches may be perceived as intrusive, but there are many paternalistic laws and policies (e.g., seat belts, child car seats, helmet laws, Social Security, age restrictions for purchasing alcohol and tobacco) enacted to achieve public health objectives. Many of these interventions are necessary because myopic individuals would otherwise place a long-term burden on society by ignoring social costs. If the current market does not result in a social welfare maximizing outcome, then obesity would deplete resources (human and financial) that could be used more productively. These types of paternalistic policies and laws do not disadvantage forward thinking individuals (because they act this way anyway) and do force present-oriented people into making a health investment in their future. This proscribed investment in health raises both individual and societal welfare by increasing longevity and decreasing health care costs associated with obesity-induced illnesses.

If obesity is associated with high rates of time preference, interventions should focus on changing the present costs and benefits. People with higher rates of time preference are not as willing to forgo satisfaction in the present for the promise of future health benefits. Increasing the cost of becoming obese today provides an incentive to make choices that reduce the likelihood of becoming obese. By changing the pricing and subsidy structure of foods produced and imported so that nutrient dense foods are relatively cheaper, all people, including those with higher rates of time preference, will demand healthier diets.

This approach is analogous to seatbelt laws. It is in the best interest of society to mandate that citizens wear seatbelts while driving cars because research has clearly indicated that seatbelt use results in lower health care costs and a higher quality/quantity of life for accident victims. Society has decided to increase the present cost of driving without seatbelts by fining individuals who do not adhere to seatbelt laws. Similarly, society needs to increase the present cost of becoming obese. Research on obesity clearly indicates that lower health care costs and a higher quality/quantity of life for individuals are realized by maintaining a healthy weight. While there is no practical way of making antiobesity laws, government regulation can support pricing and subsidy structures that are consistent with public health objectives.

References

Colditz, G. A. (1999). Economic costs of obesity and inactivity. *Medicine & Science in Sports & Exercise, 31*(11), Supplement 1, S663.

Drenowski, A., & Specter, S. (2004). Poverty and obesity: The role of energy density and energy consumption. *American Journal of Clinical Nutrition, 79*, 6–16.

Fang, J. (2003). The cost-effectiveness of bariatric surgery. *American Journal of Gastroenterology, 98*(9), 2097–2098.

Fox, M., & Cole, N. (2004). Nutrition and health characteristics of low-income populations: Volume I, Food Stamp Program participants and nonparticipants. E-FAN No. (04014–1), 393.

Frazao, E. (2005). Nutrition and health characteristics of low-income populations: Meal patterns, milk and soft drink consumption, and supplement use. *USDA ERS Agriculture Information Bulletin* 796–4.

Grossman, M. (1972). The demand for health. New York: Columbia University Press.

Healthy People 2010. Retrieved 10/29/05 from http://www.healthypeople.gov/Document/HTML/Volume2/19Nutrition.htm#_Toc490383122

O'Donoghue, E., & Rabin, M. (2005). Optimal sin taxes. *Working Paper*, University of California, Berkeley.

Putnam, J. J., & Allshouse, J. E. (1999). Food Consumption, Prices, and Expenditures, 1970–97. *Statistical Bulletin No. 965*, Washington, DC: Commodity Economics Division, ERS, US Department of Agriculture.

Raper, N. R., Zizza, C., & Rourke, J. (1992). Nutrient Content of the U.S. Food Supply, 1909–1988. *USDA Home Economics Research Report No. 50*, Washington, DC: US Department of Agriculture.

U.S. Public Health Service (1998). Healthy People 2000 Progressive Review: Nutrition. Retrieved 10/14/2005 from http://odphp.osophs.dhhs.gov/pubs/hp2000/PDF/prog_rvw/pr-nutri.pdf

4

Omega-3 Polyunsaturated Fatty Acids and Health*

John C. Umhau and Karl M. Dauphinais

Good health has been linked with healthy diet as far back as the sixth century B.C. when the clinical effects of a vegetarian diet on a group of Hebrew captives were documented in the Book of Daniel (Josephus, 1994). In this chapter, we will discuss diverse effects of an essential component of a healthy diet, long chain omega-3 polyunsaturated fatty acid (PUFA)(Burr & Burr, 1930). Because modern diets are relatively deficient in this special type of fat, there is a great potential for improving many aspects of health by adding it to the diet (Lands, 2003). For example, omega-3 fatty acids, especially eicosapentaenoic acid (EPA) and docosahexaenoic acid (DHA), are known to prevent heart attacks and sudden cardiac death in individuals with coronary artery disease (Albert et al., 2002). Greater omega-3 fat consumption has also been reported to reduce the risk for dementia (Morris et al., 2003; Tully et al., 2003), depression (Hibbeln, 1998), high triglycerides (Weber & Raederstorff, 2000), hypertension (Mori, Bao, Burke, Puddey, & Beilin, 1999), arthritis (Simopoulos, 2002), autoimmune diseases (Adam, 2003; Simopoulos, 2002), certain cancers (Terry, Rohan, & Wolk, 2003), and preterm delivery (Olsen & Secher, 2002). This chapter will examine diverse health risks due to omega-3 fatty acid deficiency and the reduction of this risk through the use of dietary supplements and food sources rich in omega-3 fatty acids, such as seafood.

What Are Omega-3 Polyunsaturated Fatty Acids and Why Are They Unique?

Fats are not only for storing energy, but they are also important components of cell membranes, hormones, and signaling molecules. Fats or fatty acids are long molecules composed of carbon atom chains with a particular ratio of hydrogen atoms attached. A saturated fat molecule holds a maximum number of carbon atoms, and is therefore "saturated" with hydrogen atoms. An unsaturated fat has one or more double bonds between carbon atoms on the fatty acid chain. Each double bond takes the place of two hydrogen atoms; thus

* Tricia H. Umhau, David Herbert, and Joseph Hibbeln provided thoughtful review of the manuscript.

these carbon chains are not "saturated" with hydrogen. Fat molecules are monounsaturated if they contain just one double bond and polyunsaturated if they contain more than one double bond. The number and position of double bonds in these molecules affect their physical properties and functional characteristics. The human body can make most fats from any source of calories consumed. However, there are some types of fats that the body can not make. These fats include the polyunsaturated omega-6 and omega-3 fatty acids, which are therefore termed "essential". The terms "omega-3" or "omega-6" signify that the first double bond in the carbon backbone of the fatty acid occurs at the third or the sixth carbon–carbon bond, respectively. Mammals lack the enzymes to introduce double bonds at the omega-6 or omega-3 position of a long fatty acid molecule, and therefore, these fats must be obtained from the diet. Humans can interconvert fats in the same omega family, but omega-6 fats cannot be converted to omega-3 fats. Many commonly consumed foods of industrialized countries are abundant in omega-6 fats, particularly linoleic acid (LA) found in soy and corn oils and arachidonic acid (AA) found in meat. Because of this, the American diet contains more than enough of the omega-6 fatty acids, a topic of concern addressed later in this chapter.

The 20- and 22-carbon long omega-3 fats, EPA and DHA, respectively, are critical to human health. These omega-3 fats must be obtained directly through the diet (i.e. from seafood) or manufactured in the body from precursor omega-3 fats such as the 18-carbon long omega-3 fatty acid, alpha-linolenic acid (ALNA) found in plant sources such as canola oil, walnuts, or flaxseed. Conversion of dietary ALNA to EPA is, however, limited, with conversion to DHA being minimal at best (Brenna, 2002; Pawlosky et al., 2003). The ratio between the omega-6 fats and the omega-3 fats in the tissue may be critical because of the 'competition' between these two essential fatty acid families for their entry into the enzymatic pathways, which convert them into bioactive metabolites. A low dietary ratio of omega-6 to omega-3 PUFAs increases the conversion of ALNA to EPA and DHA, while a high dietary ratio of omega-6 to omega-3 PUFA will accentuatea diet deficit in ALNA (Brenna, 2002). The limited conversion of ALNA to longer chain omega-3 fatty acids (EPA and DHA) establishes the importance of obtaining a diet rich in EPA and DHA omega-3 directly from the foods we eat. A simple schematic of the essential fatty acids and their metabolism is shown in Figure 4.1.

The Role of Omega-3 Fatty Acids in the Body

Omega-3 fatty acids have many important roles in the body. Polyunsaturated fatty acids such as omega-3 PUFA help to make up the phospholipids that are fundamental components of cell membranes. The particular type of PUFA in the phospholipid influences the biophysical properties of membranes (Martínez & Mougan, 1998; Niebylski & salem, 1994) and the peculiar properties of the DHA molecule make it a critical component of nerve and retinal cells (Anderson, Benolken, Dudley, Landis, & Wheeler, 1974). In the brain, DHA and the omega-6 PUFA, arachidonic acid (AA), are concentrated in the synapse where they function in phospholipid-mediated signal transduction (Jones, Toshanari, & Stanley, 1997). DHA is particularly important

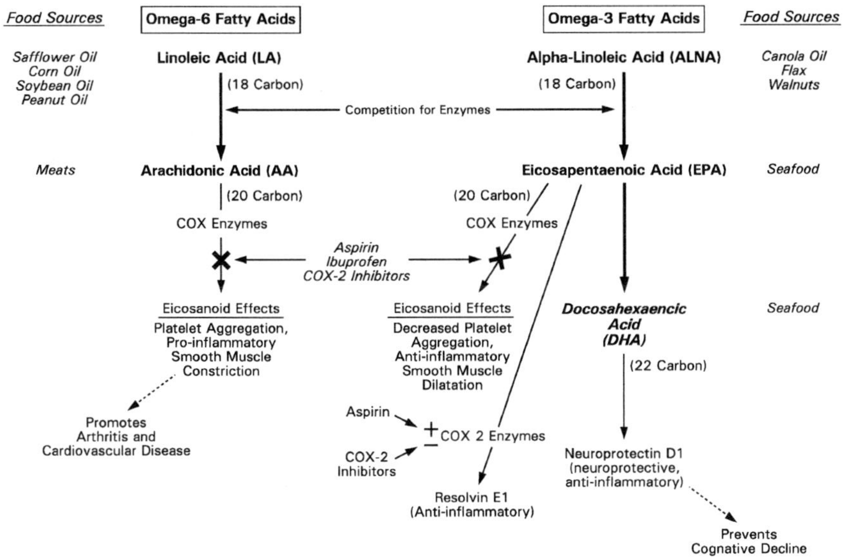

Figure 4.1. Basic enzymatic metabolism and products of the omega-6 and omega-3 PUFAs.

for ischemia-reperfusion injuries in the brain as it is metabolized into neuroprotectin D1, which regulates gene expression that promotes cell survival in stressed cells (Marcheselli et al., 2003).

In the 1960s it was found that molecules, which played a key role in cell signaling and inflammation, were derived from PUFA. These molecules, called eicosanoids, include leukotrienes, prostaglandins, and thromboxanes (Bergstrom, Danielsson, & Samuelsson, 1964; Van Dorp, Beerthuis, Nugteren & Vonkeman, 1964). Eicosanoids derived from the 20-carbon chain omega-6 fat, AA, are often proinflammatory while eicosanoids derived from the 20-carbon chain omega-3 fat, EPA, acids often moderate inflammation (Simopoulos, 2002; Van Epps, 2005). Omega-3 PUFAs can not only be metabolized into anti-inflammatory eicosanoids (particularly in the presence of aspirin), but they can compete with and replace omega-6 PUFA as precursors for the manufacture of inflammation-promoting molecules (Arita et al., 2005; Bannenberg et al., 2005; Serhan, Arita, Hong, & Gotlinger, 2004; Van Epps, 2005). The relative tissue concentrations of these omega-3 PUFA may be critical as omega-6 and omega-3 fats compete for entry into the same enzymatic pathways (Flower & Perretti, 2005; Lands, 2003). The same enzymatic pathways are also acted upon by anti-inflammatory drugs like ibuprofen, aspirin, and the COX-2 inhibitors. While aspirin blocks the conversion of AA into proinflammatory molecules, COX-2 inhibitors block the action of COX-2, an enzyme that promotes the conversion of AA into proinflammatory prostaglandins. By blocking this effect, COX-2 inhibitors reduce these proinflammatory prostaglandins and treat rheumatoid arthritis. However, COX-2 can also convert EPA to the anti-inflammatory eicosanoid, resolvin E1. When COX-2 inhibitors block this beneficial production of resolvin E1, the resulting effect may be the serious negative cardiovascular side effects associated with COX-2 inhibitors (Arita et al., 2005; Bannenberg et al., 2005; Serhan et al., 2004; Van Epps, 2005).

Evidence for the Health Benefits of Omega-3 Fatty Acids

Perinatal Effects

Omega-3 fatty acids are critical for pregnant women and their offspring. Pregnancy causes a decline in maternal DHA levels as DHA is transferred to the fetus. Maternal DHA levels continue to decline after birth as DHA is transferred via milk to the newborn. This decline in maternal DHA status may prove to result in deficient states, impairing maternal health after the pregnancy. Epidemiological data suggest that lower seafood consumption and levels of DHA are both associated with an increased risk of postpartum depression (Hibbeln, 2002). Other data suggest that DHA may have beneficial effects on pregnancy outcome. Neuronal membranes are highly enriched with long-chain PUFA, particularly DHA, which is critical for healthy development of the infant brain (Martínez & Mougan, 1998) and retina (Uauy, Hoffman, Mena, Llanos, & Birch, 2003). Low consumption of fish has been associated with preterm labor and low birth weight (Olsen & Secher, 2002) and DHA supplementation during pregnancy and lactation has been found to augment children's IQ (Helland, Smith, Saarem, Saugstad, & Drevon, 2003). DHA content of human milk varies and this variation is primarily a result of the mother's dietary intake. Thus, the low omega-3 diet of American mothers gives rise to some of the lowest worldwide levels of DHA in human milk (Hibbeln, 2002). Many researchers believe that pregnant women and women who are breastfeeding should consider supplementation with fish oil even though definitive studies have not yet been completed to evaluate the effect of such supplements. With the data available in 1999, one group of scientists and clinicians concluded that 300 mg of DHA per day was a reasonable amount recommended for pregnant women (Simopoulos, Leaf, & Salem, 1999). It is possible for infant formula to be supplemented with DHA, and beginning in 2002 in the United States, DHA was added to some brands of infant formula.

Psychiatric Benefits

Omega-3 fatty acids are thought to be important in psychiatric disorders not only because they are selectively concentrated in the brain, but also because they affect neurochemical pathways involved in the pathophysiology of psychiatric illnesses (Hibbeln & Salem, 1995). The proposition that depression and bipolar disorder are linked to a low omega-3 status is supported by diverse evidence. Many studies report that tissue concentrations of omega-3 fatty acids are lower among depressed subjects, and this finding is independent of alcohol abuse (Adams, Lawson, Sanigorski, & Sinclair, 1996; Edwards, Peet, Shay, & Horrobin, 1998a, 1998b; Maes et al., 1999, 1996; Peet, Murphy, Shay, & Horrobin, 1998). One large study found that subjects who consume fish twice or more a week have a lower risk of reporting depressive symptoms (Tanskanen et al., 2001), while results from double-blind, placebo-controlled studies show that omega-3 fatty acid supplements, particularly those higher in EPA than DHA, can reduce depressive symptoms in participants with mental illness (Frangou, Lewis, & McCrone, 2006; Peet & Horrobin, 2002; Stoll et al., 1999).

Perhaps the most intriguing health benefit of omega-3 fatty acids for the population is the possibility for a dramatic reduction in violence and aggression. Low blood levels of omega-3 fatty acids have been found in violent and impulsive offenders (Virkkunen, Horrobin, Jenkins, & Manku, 1987) and aggressive cocaine addicts (Buydens-Branchey, Branchey, McMakin, & Hibbeln, 2003). Double-blind, placebo-controlled intervention trials have demonstrated that omega-3 fatty acids can reduce hostility, an affective state closely related to anger and aggression (Hamazaki et al., 1996; Thienprasert et al., 2000; Weidner, Connor, Hollis, & Connor, 1992). Trials using omega-3s have also reduced aggression in women with borderline personality disorder (Zanarini & Frankenburg, 2003) and felony level violence in prisoners (who also received multiple vitamins) (Gesch, Hammond, Hampson, Eves, & Crowder, 2002). Rates of homicide mortality are twenty times higher in countries with little seafood consumption compared to those with the highest consumption (Hibbeln, 2001). The countries with the highest seafood have an average consumption of EPA + DHA, estimated to be approximately 1000 mg per day. These high levels of consumption contrast with the United States, which has an estimated daily intake of 180 mg of EPA + DHA per day. From these data, Hibbeln has estimated that approximately 1000 mg of EPA + DHA per day (along with a reduction of dietary omega-6 fat) may be sufficient to significantly decrease the risk of aggressive disorders in the general US population (Hibbeln, 2001; Hutchins, 2005).

Dementia

Lower levels of plasma DHA and the DHA metabolite neuroprotectin D1 have been associated with an increased risk of dementia (Conquer, Tierney, Zecevic, Bettger, & Fisher, 2000; Lukiw et al., 2005; Tully et al., 2003). In a prospective study of healthy individuals, eating one fish meal a week was associated with a 60% decreased risk of developing Alzheimer's disease (Morris et al., 2003). Although more randomized, controlled trials are needed, the data suggest that the consumption of 2.7 or more fish servings per week or 180 mg or more of DHA per day may be associated with as much as a 50% decrease in the risk of developing dementia (Hutchins, 2005; Schaefer, 2005).

Inflammatory and Autoimmune Benefits

Proinflammatory signals mediated by metabolites of omega-6 PUFA (i.e., AA), can be responsible for the inflammation that occurs in diseases such as rheumatoid arthritis, inflammatory bowel disease, and asthma. Omega-3 PUFA compete for the enzymes, which convert omega-6 PUFA into these proinflammatory signals, and it may have a profound beneficial impact on many disease processes. In rheumatoid arthritis, a number of randomized, placebo-controlled, double-blind studies of fish oil have shown a benefit from the use of a minimum of 3 g (combined) of EPA + DHA per day over a period of 12 weeks (Adam, 2003; Calder, 2005; Fortin et al., 1995; Kremer, 2000). There are also a number of promising reports of the use of omega-3 fatty acids in irritable bowel disease and asthma. For example, omega-3 fatty acids may decrease airway hyper-responsiveness in asthma (Black & Sharpe, 1997; Mickleborough, Ionescu, & Rundell, 2004). At this time, however, there are insufficient data available to draw firm conclusions regarding the clinical benefit of omega-3 fatty acids on asthma and bowel disorders (Balk et al., 2004; MacLean et al., 2004).

Cancer Benefits

EPA has been suggested to play a protective role in hormone-related cancers, particularly breast and prostate cancers. In animal experiments, EPA and DHA have consistently inhibited the proliferation of malignant breast and prostate cancers; however, epidemiological studies examining the role of omega-3 fats in cancer have not been consistent (Terry et al., 2003). Fish oils can have a benefit in reversing cancer-related cachexia by decreasing the protein degradation in cachectic muscle (Tisdale, 2003), suggesting that there may be a potential place for omega-3 PUFAs in cancer therapy as well as in prevention (Karmali, 1996).

Cardiovascular Benefits

Some of the strongest evidence for the health benefits of long-chain omega-3 fatty acids comes from research in cardiovascular disease (CVD) (Balk et al., 2004). In the 1970s, researchers first associated the low rates of heart disease in Greenland Eskimos with their higher consumption of fatty fish and sea mammals (Bang, Dyerberg, & Nielsen, 1971). Today, there are numerous studies including retrospective reviews and prospective randomized clinical trials, which support fish intake as a preventive measure in CVD, particularly to prevent sudden death (Albert et al., 2002; GISSI-Prevenzione-Investigators, 1999). In one large study, men who survived myocardial infarctions had 29% less overall mortality if they increased their fish intake to obtain 500–800 mg per day of omega-3 fatty acids. A subgroup from this study took 450 mg of EPA + DHA per day, and had 56% less overall mortality and 62% less CVD-related death (Burr et al., 1989).

Lipid Effects

Supplementation of omega-3 fatty acids has been shown to decrease triglyceride levels (Park & Harris, 2003; Weber & Raederstorff, 2000). Triglyceride reductions of 20% have been documented for intake of 4 g per day of EPA + DHA, but benefits have been noted with a dose as low as 1 g per day (Mori et al., 2000; Weber & Raederstorff, 2000). Reasons for this decrease appear related to both decreased hepatic production and increased clearance of triglycerides from the body (Nestel et al., 1984; Park & Harris, 2003). Recent evidence that high levels of triglycerides may be an independent risk factor for coronary heart disease further emphasizes the potential benefit of omega-3 PUFAs in these individuals (Eberly, Stamler, & Neaton, 2003).

Blood Pressure

Research suggests that blood pressure can be reduced by fish oil given in a dose of 3.7 g per day, while dosages less than 500 mg per day do not show this effect (Geleijnse, Giltay, Grobbee, Donders, & Kok, 2002). The statistically significant reduction in systolic blood pressure readings has ranged from 2 to 6 mmHg in hypertensive individuals (Bao, Mori, Burke, Puddey, & Beilin, 1998; Geleijnse et al., 2002; Mori et al., 1999). Greater reductions have been noted in older, hypertensive individuals and in individuals with concurrent weight loss (Bao et al., 1998; Geleijnse et al., 2002).

Historical Human Consumption of Omega-3 Fatty Acids

The modern diet has a very different fat composition compared to that of our ancestors. Throughout the early human history, humans consumed roughly equal amounts of omega-6 and omega-3 fat (Leaf & Weber, 1987). Today, the addition of omega-3-rich fish and seafood to the diet can be an expensive luxury, whereas at one time it was common in the diet (Simopoulos, Leaf, & Salem, 1999). Seed oil rich in omega-6 fat, particularly soy oil, is a mainstay of today's food industry. It is remarkable to note that between 1909 and 2000, the consumption of soy oil increased a thousand fold, from approximately 0.02 to 20% (expressed as a percentage of all food calories available) (Hibbeln, Nieminen, & Lands, 2004). Animals are fattened on omega-6 rich sources of feed and the result is meat that is higher in omega-6 PUFAs and lower in omega-3 PUFAs. These changes have resulted in a typical American diet that is now rich in omega-6 fats but depleted in omega-3. This change in the diet has changed the balance of omega-3 and omega-6 fats in the tissue, which has resulted in an imbalance of eicosanoid actions. Because this imbalance is reversible, scientists who study PUFAs are optimistic that by restoring an appropriate balance of omega-3 to the diet we can minimize human misery associated with many diseases (Lands, 2003).

Recommendations for the Intake of Omega-3 Fatty Acids

Based on its review of the literature, the FDA concluded that there is sufficient evidence to make a qualified health claim on the label of appropriate foods containing Omega 3 fatty acids (FDA, 2004a; Hubbard, 2004). It states: "Supportive but not conclusive research shows that consumption of EPA and DHA omega-3 fatty acids may reduce the risk of coronary heart disease." The Agency for Health Care Research and Quality (AHRQ) has noted that food sources of the 18-carbon long omega-3 fat, ALNA, may help to reduce deaths from heart disease, but to a much lesser extent than fish oil (Balk et al., 2004). The American Heart Association (AHA) recommends consumption of at least two servings of fish per week (particularly of fatty fish) along with food sources high in ALNA, based on the evident benefit from the omega-3 fatty acids. These guidelines further recommend that participants with documented coronary heart disease consume approximately 1 g of EPA + DHA per day and that participants with significantly elevated triglyceride levels take 2–4 g of EPA + DHA provided as capsules under a physician's care (Kris-Etherton, Harris, & Appel, 2002). The National Institutes of Health (NIH), the World Health Organization (WHO), and the United States Department of Agriculture (USDA) each have made specific recommendations (summarized in Table 4.1) for the dietary intake of omega-3 fatty acids, particularly for the intake of EPA and DHA.

Potential Risks of Omega-3 Fatty Acids

The FDA has determined that up to 3 g of EPA+DHA per day should be considered "Generally Recognized as Safe" (GRAS). While the addition of various sources of omega-3 fat to the diet is essentially without risk, it is always wise to examine potential drawbacks of such a recommendation. Perhaps the most common drawback of taking fish oil supplements occurs with less refined forms of fish oil, and is related to eructation, fishy aftertaste, or gastric upset. In an effort to minimize any fishy odor or gastric distress, some

Table 4.1. Summary of recommendations from key organizations and expert panels.

Organization	Recommendation
AHA, 2002 (Kris-Etherton et al., 2002)	Individuals without cardiovascular disease (CVD) should eat oily fish twice per week and foods rich in ALNA (walnuts, canola, soy, and flaxseed) Individuals with documented CVD should eat approximately 1 g of EPA + DHA per day from oily fish (preferable) or supplements For triglyceride lowering effects, 2–4 g of omega-3 fatty acids per day as a supplement under a physician's care
NIH-supported expert panel, 1999 (Simopoulos et al., 1999)	Recommends 650 mg of EPA + DHA per day and 2.2 g of ALNA per day for the average adult Recommends 300 mg DHA per day for pregnant or lactating females
WHO, 2003 (WHO, 2003)	Recommends 1–2 servings of fish per week (containing 200–500 mg of EPA + DHA per serving) to prevent heart disease and stroke
USDA Dietary Guidelines, 2005 (DHHS, 2005)	Recommends 8 oz per week (two servings) of fish high in EPA and DHA content to prevent CVD

AHA, American Heart Association; NIH, National Institutes of Health; WHO, World Health Organization; USDA, United States Department of Agriculture.

experts have advocated taking fish oil at bedtime or keeping fish oil capsules in the freezer. Swallowing frozen capsules may delay release of the oil until after it has passed through the stomach, but the gelatin capsules of some formulation may not withstand freezing. Although the weight of the evidence suggests that the benefit of eating fish outweighs potential risks, there is a concern regarding potential contaminants such as mercury and PCBs. Focusing primarily on the risks from mercury, the FDA advises that children as well as women who are pregnant or lactating should avoid fish which are high in mercury such as king mackerel, swordfish, shark, and tilefish. Seafood low in mercury includes salmon, caned light tuna, trout, Pollock, flounder, herring, catfish, halibut, cod, shrimp, crab, oysters, clams, and scallops (FDA, 2004b; Kris-Etherton, 2005). Significant contamination is not found in commercially available fish oil (Consumer Reports, 2003; Foran, Flood & Lewandrowski, 2003; Melanson, Lewandrowski, Flood, & Lewandrowski, 2005).

Omega-3 PUFAs have some hypothetical risks, which should be considered. Although there has been concern that omega-3 fatty acids could cause a problem by increasing the bleeding time, there is no documented case in the literature of serious bleeding caused by omega-3 fatty acids, and clinical trials, including trials of coronary artery bypass surgery, have not shown evidence of increased blood loss due to intake of omega-3s (Simopoulos, 1991). Increases in LDL cholesterol have been reported in individuals with extremely elevated triglyceride levels after treatment with omega-3 fatty acids, but the effect was not seen in individuals with normal or slightly elevated levels of blood lipids receiving omega-3 fats (Nestel et al., 1984; Weber & Raederstorff, 2000).

The effect of omega-3 fatty acids on LDL levels has been inconsistent, while the overall effect of omega-3 fatty acids on CVD has been positive (Balk et al., 2004; MacLean et al., 2004; Nestel et al., 1984). Although there has been suggestion that omega-3 fatty acids may increase fasting blood glucose and insulin resistance in diabetics (Mori et al., 2000), this was not supported by a meta-analysis, which did however show a beneficial decrease in triglyceride levels (MacLean et al., 2004). One recent report showed an increased risk of arrhythmias in participants with implantable cardiac defibrillators. In these participants, however, it was noted that there was no change in mortality with the increased firing of the device and increased episodes of ventricular tachycardia and fibrillation (Raitt et al., 2005). Because of these concerns, participants with extremely high triglyceride levels, implantable defibrillators, or who are taking blood-thinning agents should discuss the use of high doses (over 3 g per day) of omega-3 fatty acids with their doctor.

Sources of Omega-3 Fatty Acids in the Diet

Seafood, fish, and fish oil supplements are important sources of the long-chain omega-3 PUFAs, EPA, and DHA. The current average daily combined intake of EPA + DHA in a typical American diet comes from one fish serving every 10 days (i.e., about 150 mg per day) (Kris-Etherton et al., 2000). Consuming fish 2.5–3 times per week provides approximately 500 mg of EPA + DHA per day. Good sources of ALNA include canola oil, nuts (especially walnuts),flax, and green leafy vegetables. The circulating and tissue levels of omega-3 fatty acids depend on both the recent and long-term dietary consumption of these fatty acids. A long-standing diet that is high in omega-6 will be reflected in the composition of adipose tissue and continue to affect the balance of omega-6 to omega-3 fats throughout the body tissue for many years. Thus, the recommended daily intake of omega-3 fat should be higher or lower depending on the dietary history as well as on the current intake of omega-6 fats. For more details on sources of omega-3 and omega-6 fatty acids and how to generate a balanced dietary intake, a computer software package, KIM (Keep it Managed), has been developed, which can be downloaded free from http://ods.od.nih.gov/eicosanoids. Populations at risk for disease may have an increased requirement for omega-3 fatty acids. For example, reduced tissue levels of omega-3 fatty acids can result from heavy alcohol consumption (Pawlosky, Bacher, & Salem, 2001) and may be associated with folate deficiency (Umhau et al., 2006), obesity, diabetes, and youth (Sands, Reid, Windsor, & Harris, 2005).

Perhaps the most promising source of omea-3 fats for the general population is through fortified foods. There are a number of foods available that have been enriched by the addition of EPA and DHA. Eggs enriched with omega-3 fats are becoming commonly available in supermarkets and these eggs contain DHA, which is the result of feeding chickens with flaxseed meal, fish meal, or marine algae. One company has developed a line of omega-3-fortified fish products including salmon burgers, franks, and imitation crabmeat. Another new source is sandwich bread with omega-3s, which is claimed to supply up to 80 mg of omega-3 fatty acids in two slices of bread. Other foods fortified with omega-3s include margarine, peanut butter, chocolate milk, and spaghetti sauce. In the future, beef, chicken, and even soybeans may be developed with a higher proportion of omega-3 fats.

Fish Oil Supplements

In the eighteenth century, fish oil (i.e., cod liver oil) was taken for arthritis, and in the twentieth century, it was taken for respiratory infections, a use encouraged by controlled industrial studies demonstrating that a daily teaspoon of cod liver oil prevented colds and reduced absenteeism by half (Semba, 1999). Although traditionally associated with a fishy taste, modern manufacturing techniques can produce fish oil which is essentially tasteless. Capsules are readily available through many retail outlets, and for capsules containing 1 g of EPA + DHA, their cost ranged from $22 to $219 per year or $0.06 to $0.60 per day (Consumer Reports, 2003). A prescription strength formulation of 4 g of concentrated EPA+DHA is also available, which is specified for the reduction of high triglyceride levels and is marketed under the trade name Omacor®. It should be remembered that fish oil, however, does not provide all of the important nutrients contained in fish, such as selenium, calcium, iodine, and particularly vitamin D.

Summary

Our message is that omega-3 fats can contribute to a longer and healthier life and that seafood is a healthy food. For those who do not care to eat fish, omega-3 rich fish oils are a safe and inexpensive alternative to the pharmaceuticals used to treat diseases that fish oil might prevent. We recommend a diet rich in sources of long-chain omega-3 PUFA with reduced intake of omega-6 fat. Depending on the background diet and tissue levels of omega-6 fat, 1–2 g of EPA + DHA per day is likely to prevent most omega-3-related pathology in the Western countries. Sadly, the relatively low fish consumption in the United States may be further limited by mixed messages, as consumers hear more about harmful substances in fish than of the important nutrients it contains (FDA, 2001, 2004b; Lands, 2003; Verbeke, Sioen, Pieniak, Van Camp, & De Henauw, 2005). Thus, the maximum health benefit of omega-3s for the population may not be achieved until omega-3 fats are abundant in the food supply through fortification of appropriate and universally accepted foods.

References

Adam, O. (2003). Dietary fatty acids and immune reactions in synovial tissue. *European Journal of Medical Research, 8*(8), 381–387.

Adams, P. B., Lawson, S., Sanigorski, A., & Sinclair, A. J. (1996). Arachidonic acid to eicosapentaenoic acid ratio in blood correlates positively with clinical symptoms of depression. *Lipids, 31 Suppl*, S157–161.

Albert, C. M., Campos, H., Stampfer, M. J., Ridker, P. M., Manson, J. E., Willett, W. C., et al. (2002). Blood levels of long-chain $n-3$ fatty acids and the risk of sudden death. *New England Journal of Medicine, 346*(15), 1113–1118.

Anderson, R. E., Benolken, R. M., Dudley, P. A., Landis, D. J., & Wheeler, T. G. (1974). Polyunsaturated fatty acids of photoreceptor membranes. *Experimental Eye Research, 18*(3), 205.

Arita, M., Bianchini, F., Aliberti, J., Sher, A., Chiang, N., Hong, S., et al. (2005). Stereochemical assignment, antiinflammatory properties, and receptor for the omega-3 lipid mediator resolvin E1. *Journal of Experimental Medicine, 201*(5), 713–722.

Balk, E., Chung, M., Lichtenstein, A., Chew, P., Kupelnick, B., Lawrence, A., et al. (2004). *Effects of omega-3 fatty acids on cardiovascular risk factors and intermediate markers of cardiovascular disease. Evidence report/technology assessment. No. 93* (Prepared by Tufts-New England Medical Center Evidence-based Practice Center under Contract No. 290-02-0022). AHRQ Publication No. 04-E010-2. Rockville, MD: Agency for Healthcare Research and Quality.

Bang, H. O., Dyerberg, J., & Nielsen, A. (1971). Plasma lipid and lipoprotein pattern in Greenlandic West-coast Eskimos. *The Lancet, 297*(7710), 1143.

Bannenberg, G. L., Chiang, N., Ariel, A., Arita, M., Tjonahen, E., Gotlinger, K. H., et al. (2005). Molecular circuits of resolution: Formation and actions of resolvins and protectins. *Journal of Immunology, 174*(7), 4345–4355.

Bao, D. Q., Mori, T. A., Burke, V., Puddey, I. B., & Beilin, L. J. (1998). Effects of dietary fish and weight reduction on ambulatory blood pressure in overweight hypertensives. *Hypertension, 32*(4), 710–717.

Bergstrom, S., Danielsson, H., & Samuelsson, B. (1964). The enzymatic formation of prostaglandin E2 from arachidonic acid prostaglandins and related factors 32. *Biochimica et Biophysica Acta (BBA) – General Subjects, 90*(1), 207.

Black, P. N., & Sharpe, S. (1997). Dietary fat and asthma: Is there a connection? *European Respiratory Journal, 10*(1), 6–12.

Brenna, J. T. (2002). Efficiency of conversion of [alpha]-linolenic acid to long chain $n-3$ fatty acids in man. *Current Opinion in Clinical Nutrition & Metabolic Care, 5*(2), 127–132.

Burr, G. O., & Burr, M. M. (1930). On the nature and role of the fatty acids essential in nutrition. *Journal of Biological Chemistry, 86*(2), 587–621.

Burr, M. L., Gilbert, J. F., Holliday, R. M., Elwood, P. C., Fehily, A. M., Rogers, S., et al. (1989). Effects of changes in fat, fish, and fibre intakes on death and myocardial reinfarction: Diet and reinfarction trial (DART). *The Lancet, 334*(8666), 757.

Buydens-Branchey, L., Branchey, M., McMakin, D. L., & Hibbeln, J. R. (2003). Polyunsaturated fatty acid status and aggression in cocaine addicts. *Drug Alcohol Depend, 71*(3), 319–323.

Calder, P. (2005). *Omega-3 fatty acids and inflammation: Impact on heart disease, irritable bowel syndrome and asthma.* Paper presented at the Symposium Highlights – Omega 3 Fatty Acids: Recommendations for Therapeutics and Prevention, New York.

Conquer, J., Tierney, M., Zecevic, J., Bettger, W. J., & Fisher, R. H. (2000). Fatty acid analysis of blood plasma of patients with Alzheimer's disease, other types of dementia, and cognitive impairment. *Lipids, 35*, 1305–1312.

Consumer Reports (2003). Omega-3 oil: Fish or pills? *Consumer Reports* (July), 30–32.

DHHS (2005, August 19, 2004). *Department of Health and Human Services. Report of the Dietary Guidelines Advisory Committee on the Dietary Guidelines for Americans, 2005.* Retrieved December 1, 2005, from http://www.health.gov/dietaryguidelines/dga2005/report

Eberly, L. E., Stamler, J., & Neaton, J. D. (2003). Relation of triglyceride levels, fasting and nonfasting, to fatal and nonfatal coronary heart disease. *Archives of Internal Medicine, 163*(9), 1077–1083.

Edwards, R., Peet, M., Shay, J., & Horrobin, D. (1998a). Depletion of docosahexaenoic acid in red blood cell membranes of depressive patients. *Biochemical Society Transactions, 26*(2), S142.

Edwards, R., Peet, M., Shay, J., & Horrobin, D. (1998b). Omega-3 polyunsaturated fatty acid levels in the diet and in red blood cell membranes of depressed patients.

Journal of Affective Disorders, 48, 149–155.
FDA (2001). Highlights of FDA food safety efforts: Fruit juice, mercury in fish. *FDA Consumer.*
FDA (2004a). FDA news: FDA announces qualified health claims for omega-3 fatty acids. In FDA (Ed.) (Vol. Sept 8).
FDA (2004b). *What you need to know about mercury in fish and shellfish – 2004 EPA and FDA advice for: women who might become pregnant, women who are pregnant, nursing mothers, young children.* Retrieved December 14, 2005, from http://www.cfsan.fda.gov/~dms/admehg3.html
Flower, R. J., & Perretti, M. (2005). Controlling inflammation: A fat chance? *Journal of Experimental Medicine, 201*(5), 671–674.
Foran, S. E., Flood, J. G., & Lewandrowski, K. B. (2003). Measurement of mercury levels in concentrated over-the-counter fish oil preparations: Is fish oil healthier than fish? *Archives of Pathology and Laboratory Medicine, 127*(12), 1603–1605.
Fortin, P. R., Lew, R. A., Liang, M. H., Wright, E. A., Beckett, L. A., Chalmers, T. C., et al. (1995). Validation of a meta-analysis: The effects of fish oil in rheumatoid arthritis. *Journal of Clinical Epidemiology, 48*(11), 1379.
Frangou, S., Lewis, M., & McCrone, P. (2006). Efficacy of ethyl-eicosapentaenoic acid in bipolar depression: Randomised double-blind placebo-controlled study. *British Journal of Psychiatry, 188*, 46–50.
Geleijnse, J. M., Giltay, E. J., Grobbee, D. E., Donders, A. R., & Kok, F. J. (2002). Blood pressure response to fish oil supplementation: Metaregression analysis of randomized trials. *Journal of Hypertension, 20*(8), 1493–1499.
Gesch, C. B., Hammond, S. M., Hampson, S. E., Eves, A., & Crowder, M. J. (2002). Influence of supplementary vitamins, minerals and essential fatty acids on the antisocial behaviour of young adult prisoners. Randomised, placebo-controlled trial. *British Journal of Psychiatry, 181*, 22–28.
GISSI-Prevenzione-Investigators (1999). Dietary supplementation with $n-3$ polyunsaturated fatty acids and vitamin E after myocardial infarction: Results of the GISSI-Prevenzione trial. *The Lancet, 354*(9177), 447.
Hamazaki, T., Sawazaki, S., Itomura, M., Asaoka, E., Nagao, Y., Nishimura, N., et al. (1996). The effect of docosahexaenoic acid on aggression in young adults. A placebo-controlled double-blind study. *Journal of Clinical Investigation, 97*(4), 1129–1133.
Helland, I. B., Smith, L., Saarem, K., Saugstad, O. D., & Drevon, C. A. (2003). Maternal supplementation with very-long-chain $n-3$ fatty acids during pregnancy and lactation augments children's IQ at 4 years of age. *Pediatrics, 111*(1), e39-44.
Hibbeln, J. R. (1998). Fish consumption and major depression. *The Lancet, 351*(9110), 1213.
Hibbeln, J. R. (2001). Seafood consumption and homicide mortality. A cross-national ecological analysis. *World Review of Nutrition & Dietetics, 88*, 41–46.
Hibbeln, J. R. (2002). Seafood consumption, the DHA content of mothers' milk and prevalence rates of postpartum depression: A cross-national, ecological analysis. *Journal of Affective Disorders, 69*(1–3), 15–29.
Hibbeln, J. R., Nieminen, L. R., & Lands, W. E. (2004). Increasing homicide rates and linoleic acid consumption among five Western countries, 1961–2000. *Lipids, 39*(12), 1207–1213.
Hibbeln, J. R., & Salem, N., Jr. (1995). Dietary polyunsaturated fatty acids and depression: When cholesterol does not satisfy. *American Journal of Clinical Nutrition, 62*(1), 1–9.
Hubbard, W. K. (2004). Letter responding to health claim petition dated June 23, 2003 (Wellness petition): Omega-3 fatty acids and reduced risk of coronary heart disease (Docket No. 2003Q-0401). In FDA (Ed.). CFSAN/Office of Nutritional Products, Labeling, and Dietary Supplements.

Hutchins, H. (2005). Symposium Highlights – Omega-3 Fatty Acids: Recommendations for Therapeutics and Prevention. *Medscape General Medicine, 7*(4), 18.

Jones CR, Toshanari, A., & Stanley, R. (1997). Evidence for the involvement of docosahexaenoic acid in cholinergic stimulated signal transduction at the synapse. *Neurochemical Research, 22*(6), 663–670.

Josephus, F. (1994). *Josephus, the essential works* (P. Maier, Trans.). Grand Rapids: Kregel Publications.

Karmali, R. A. (1996). Historical perspective and potential use of $n-3$ fatty acids in therapy of cancer cachexia. *Nutrition, 12*(1 Suppl), S2-4.

Kremer, J. M. (2000). $n-3$ fatty acid supplements in rheumatoid arthritis. *American Journal of Clinical Nutrition, 71*(1 Suppl), 349S–351S.

Kris-Etherton, P. M. (2005). *How much omega-3 fatty acid is enough and from when should it come?* Paper presented at the Symposium Highlights – Omega 3 Fatty Acids: Recommendations for Therapeutics and Prevention, New York.

Kris-Etherton, P. M., Harris, W. S., & Appel, L. J. (2002). Fish consumption, fish oil, omega-3 fatty acids, and cardiovascular disease. *Circulation, 106*(21), 2747–2757.

Kris-Etherton, P. M., Taylor, D. S., Yu-Poth, S., Huth, P., Moriarty, K., Fishell, V., et al. (2000). Polyunsaturated fatty acids in the food chain in the United States. *American Journal of Clinical Nutrition, 71*(1), 179S–188.

Lands, W. E. (2003). Diets could prevent many diseases. *Lipids, 38*(4), 317–321.

Leaf, A., & Weber, P. C. (1987). A new era for science in nutrition. *American Journal of Clinical Nutrition, 45*, 1048–1053.

Lukiw, W. J., Cui, J.-G., Marcheselli, V. L., Bodker, M., Botkjaer, A., Gotlinger, K., et al. (2005). A role for docosahexaenoic acid-derived neuroprotectin D1 in neural cell survival and Alzheimer disease. *Journal of Clinical Investigation, 115*(10), 2774–2783.

MacLean, C., Mojica, W., Morton, S., Pencharz, J., Hasenfeld, G. R., Tu, W., et al. (2004). *Effects of omega-3 fatty acids on lipids and glycemic control in type ii diabetes and the metabolic syndrome and on inflammatory bowel disease, rheumatoid arthritis, renal disease, systemic lupus erythematosus, and osteoporosis. Evidence report/technology assessment. No. 89*. Rockville, MD: Agency for Healthcare Research and Quality.

Maes, M., Christophe, A., Delanghe, J., Altamura, C., Neels, H., & Meltzer, H. Y. (1999). Lowered omega-3 polyunsaturated fatty acids in serum phospholipids and cholesteryl esters of depressed patients. *Psychiatry Research, 85*(3), 275–291.

Maes, M., Smith, R., Christophe, A., Cosyns, P., Desnyder, R., & Meltzer, H. (1996). Fatty acid composition in major depression: Decreased omega 3 fractions in cholesteryl esters and increased C20: 4 omega 6/C20:5 omega 3 ratio in cholesteryl esters and phospholipids. *Journal of Affective Disorders, 38*, 35–46.

Marcheselli, V. L., Hong, S., Lukiw, W. J., Tian, X. H., Gronert, K., Musto, A., et al. (2003). Novel docosanoids inhibit brain ischemia–reperfusion-mediated leukocyte infiltration and pro-inflammatory gene expression. *Journal of Biological Chemistry, 278*(44), 43807–43817.

Martínez, M., & Mougan, I. (1998). Fatty acid composition of human brain phospholipids during normal development. *Journal of Neurochemistry, 71*(6), 2528–2533.

Melanson, S. F., Lewandrowski, E. L., Flood, J. G., & Lewandrowski, K. B. (2005). Measurement of organochlorines in commercial over-the-counter fish oil preparations: Implications for dietary and therapeutic recommendations for omega-3 fatty acids and a review of the literature. *Archives of Pathology and Laboratory Medicine, 129*(1), 74–77.

Mickleborough, T. D., Ionescu, A. A., & Rundell, K. W. (2004). Omega-3 fatty acids and airway hyperresponsiveness in asthma. *Journal of Alternative & Complementary Medicine, 10*(6), 1067–1075.

Mori, T. A., Bao, D. Q., Burke, V., Puddey, I. B., & Beilin, L. J. (1999). Docosahexaenoic acid but not eicosapentaenoic acid lowers ambulatory blood pressure and heart rate in humans. *Hypertension, 34*(2), 253–260.

Mori, T. A., Burke, V., Puddey, I. B., Watts, G. F., O'Neal, D. N., Best, J. D., et al. (2000). Purified eicosapentaenoic and docosahexaenoic acids have differential effects on serum lipids and lipoproteins, LDL particle size, glucose, and insulin in mildly hyperlipidemic men. *American Journal of Clinical Nutrition, 71*(5), 1085–1094.

Morris, M. C., Evans, D. A., Bienias, J. L., Tangney, C. C., Bennett, D. A., Wilson, R. S., et al. (2003). Consumption of fish and $n-3$ fatty acids and risk of incident Alzheimer disease. *Archives of Neurology, 60*(7), 940–946.

Nestel, P. J., Connor, W. E., Reardon, M. F., Connor, S., Wong, S., & Boston, R. (1984). Suppression by diets rich in fish oil of very low density lipoprotein production in man. *The Journal of Clinical Investigation, 74*(1), 82.

Niebylski, C., & Salem, N. (1994). A calorimetric investigation of a series of mixed-chain polyunsaturated phosphatidylcholines: effect of sn-2 chain length and degree of unsaturation. *Biophysical Journal, 67*(6), 2387–2393.

Olsen, S. F., & Secher, N. J. (2002). Low consumption of seafood in early pregnancy as a risk factor for preterm delivery: Prospective cohort study. *BMJ, 324*(7335), 447–450.

Park, Y., & Harris, W. S. (2003). Omega-3 fatty acid supplementation accelerates chylomicron triglyceride clearance. *Journal of Lipid Research, 44*(3), 455–463.

Pawlosky, R. J., Bacher, J., & Salem, N., Jr. (2001). Ethanol consumption alters electroretinograms and depletes neural tissues of docosahexaenoic acid in rhesus monkeys: Nutritional consequences of a low $n-3$ fatty acid diet. *Alcoholism, Clinical and Experimental Research, 25*(12), 1758–1765.

Pawlosky, R. J., Hibbeln, J. R., Lin, Y., Goodson, S., Riggs, P., Sebring, N., et al. (2003). Effects of beef- and fish-based diets on the kinetics of $n-3$ fatty acid metabolism in human subjects. *American Journal of Clinical Nutrition, 77*(3), 565–572.

Peet, M., & Horrobin, D. F. (2002). A dose-ranging study of the effects of ethyl-eicosapentaenoate in patients with ongoing depression despite apparently adequate treatment with standard drugs. *Archives of General Psychiatry, 59*(10), 913–919.

Peet, M., Murphy, B., Shay, J., & Horrobin, D. (1998). Depletion of omega-3 fatty acid levels in red blood cell membranes of depressive patients. *Biology and Psychiatry, 43*(5), 315–319.

Raitt, M. H., Connor, W. E., Morris, C., Kron, J., Halperin, B., Chugh, S. S., et al. (2005). Fish oil supplementation and risk of ventricular tachycardia and ventricular fibrillation in patients with implantable defibrillators: A randomized controlled trial. *JAMA, 293*(23), 2884–2891.

Sands, S. A., Reid, K. J., Windsor, S. L., & Harris, W. S. (2005). The impact of age, body mass index, and fish intake on the EPA and DHA content of human erythrocytes. *Lipids, 40*(April), 343–347.

Schaefer, A. (2005). Omega-3 fatty acids and dementia. *Omega-3 fatty acids: Recommendations for therapeutics and prevention symposium.*

Semba, R. D. (1999). Vitamin A as "anti-infective" therapy, 1920–1940. *Journal of Nutrition, 129*(4), 783–791.

Serhan, C. N., Arita, M., Hong, S., & Gotlinger, K. (2004). Resolvins, docosatrienes, and neuroprotectins, novel omega-3-derived mediators, and their endogenous aspirin-triggered epimers. *Lipids, 39*(11), 1125–1132.

Simopoulos, A. (1999). Genetic variation and evolutionary aspects of diet. *In: A.M. Papas (ed). Antioxidant status, diet, nutrition and health* (pp. 65–88). Boca Raton, FL: CRC Press.

Simopoulos, A. P. (1991). Omega-3 fatty acids in health and disease and in growth and development. *American Journal of Clinical Nutrition, 54*(3), 438–463.

Simopoulos, A. P. (2002). Omega-3 fatty acids in inflammation and autoimmune diseases. *Journal of the American College of Nutrition, 21*(6), 495–505.
Simopoulos, A. P., Leaf, A., & Salem, N., Jr. (1999). Workshop on the Essentiality of and Recommended Dietary Intakes for Omega-6 and Omega-3 Fatty Acids. *Journal of the American College of Nutrition, 18*(5), 487–489.
Stoll, A. L., Severus, W. E., Freeman, M. P., Rueter, S., Zboyan, H. A., Diamond, E., et al. (1999). Omega 3 fatty acids in bipolar disorder: A preliminary double-blind, placebo controlled trial. *Archives of General Psychiatry, 56*, 407–412.
Tanskanen, A., Hibbeln, J. R., Tuomilehto, J., Uutela, A., Haukkala, A., Viinamaki, H., et al. (2001). Fish consumption and depressive symptoms in the general population in Finland. *Psychiatric Services, 52*(4), 529–531.
Terry, P. D., Rohan, T. E., & Wolk, A. (2003). Intakes of fish and marine fatty acids and the risks of cancers of the breast and prostate and of other hormone-related cancers: A review of the epidemiologic evidence. *American Journal of Clinical Nutrition, 77*(3), 532–543.
Thienprasert, A., Hamazaki, T., Kheovichai, K., Samuhaseneetoo, S., Nagasawa, T., & Wantanabe, S. (2000). The effect of docosahexaenoic acid on aggression/hostility in elderly subjects: A placebo-controlled double blind trial *(abstract)* (pp. 189). Tsukuba, Japan: 4th Congress of the International Society for the Study of Lipids and Fatty Acids.
Tisdale, M. J. (2003). Pathogenesis of cancer cachexia. *The Journal of Supportive Oncology, 1*(3), 159–168.
Tully, A. M., Roche, H. M., Doyle, R., Fallon, C., Bruce, I., Lawlor, B., et al. (2003). Low serum cholesteryl ester-docosahexaenoic acid levels in Alzheimer's disease: A case-control study. *British Journal of Nutrition, 89*(4), 483–489.
Uauy, R., Hoffman, D. R., Mena, P., Llanos, A., & Birch, E. E. (2003). Term infant studies of DHA and ARA supplementation on neurodevelopment: Results of randomized controlled trials. *The Journal of Pediatrics, 143*(4, Supplement 1), 17.
Umhau, J. C., Dauphinais, K. M., Patel, S. H., Nahrwold, D. A., Hibbeln, J. R., Rawlings, R. R., et al. (2006). The relationship between folate and docosahexaenoic acid in men. *European Journal of Clinical Nutrition, 60*(3), 352–357.
Van Dorp, D. A., Beerthuis, R. K., Nugteren, D. H., & Vonkeman, H. (1964). The biosynthesis of prostaglandins. *Biochimica et Biophysica Acta (BBA) – General Subjects, 90*(1), 204.
Van Epps, H. L. (2005). Inflammation control gets fishy. *Journal of Experimental Medicine, 201*(5), 662.
Verbeke, W., Sioen, I., Pieniak, Z., Van Camp, J., & De Henauw, S. (2005). Consumer perception versus scientific evidence about health benefits and safety risks from fish consumption. *Public Health Nutrition, 8*(4), 422–429.
Virkkunen, M. E., Horrobin, D. F., Jenkins, D. K., & Manku, M. S. (1987). Plasma phospholipid essential fatty acids and prostaglandins in alcoholic, habitually violent, and impulsive offenders. *Biology and Psychiatry, 22*, 1087–1096.
Weber, P., & Raederstorff, D. (2000). Triglyceride-lowering effect of omega-3 LC-polyunsaturated fatty acids – A review. *Nutrition Metabolism & Cardiovascular Diseases, 10*(1), 28–37.
Weidner, G., Connor, S. L., Hollis, J. F., & Connor, W. E. (1992). Improvements in hostility and depression in relation to dietary change and cholesterol lowering. *Annals of Internal Medicine, 117*, 820–823.
WHO (2003). Diet, nutrition and the prevention of chronic diseases: Report of the joint WHO/FAO expert consultation, Geneva.
Zanarini, M. C., & Frankenburg, F. R. (2003). Omega-3 Fatty acid treatment of women with borderline personality disorder: A double-blind, placebo-controlled pilot study. *American Journal of Psychiatry, 160*(1), 167–169.

5

Vitamins, Minerals and Health

Edward Giovannucci

Classic examples of vitamin deficiency diseases are scurvy, rickets, beriberi, and pellagra. However, evidence over the past several decades clearly shows that suboptimal intakes of some vitamins and minerals may contribute to risk for some chronic diseases, including major causes of mortality and morbidity such as cardiovascular disease, cerebrovascular disease, cancer, osteoporosis, and hypertension. On the other hand, consuming excess amounts of vitamins and minerals may be deleterious in some circumstances. At the opposite end of clear deficiency is overt toxicity, but there could also be adverse effects in a range that does not produce clear toxicity, but that in the long-term, could be deleterious to health in more subtle ways.

This chapter will provide an overview of the major established or highly suspected associations between vitamins and minerals and the development and prevention of major chronic disease states. Unlike the establishment of a clear deficiency state and reversal of the condition, such as vitamin C to cure scurvy, studying the relationship between the range of vitamins and minerals and chronic diseases is fraught with many difficulties. Thus, the relationships are likely to generate less consensus and more scientific controversy. Nonetheless, a large body of evidence is currently available for many of the relationships, and sensible recommendations to optimize benefit while minimizing risk can be made. However, as science and research evolve, and the strength of evidence for a specific relationship waxes and wanes, these recommendations will also evolve. In addition, new relationships are likely to be discovered, and these could alter existing recommendations.

In the first part of this chapter, the major research approaches utilized in this field will be summarized, and the major strengths and limitations will be addressed. Then, specific nutrient-disease relationships will be discussed. This chapter will only examine vitamins and minerals for which there are a sufficient amount of human data for effects of long-term, suboptimal intakes and a major health consequence. The classic vitamin deficiency syndromes will not be reviewed. The focus will be on studies in which apparently healthy individuals are followed, and the influence of specific vitamins and minerals is studied before a disease occurs. Whether these nutrients influence the course of an existing disease will not be addressed in this chapter. In the final section, recommendations will be made.

Research Approaches

Three factors make study of vitamin/mineral and chronic disease difficult to conduct and interpret. First, chronic diseases typically develop over a long time period. For example, colorectal cancer may develop 40 years or more after the initial carcinogenic insult. In contrast, for the classical vitamin deficiency diseases, reversal of the conditions occurs a very short time after the administration of the active compound. Secondly, chronic diseases involve multiple factors. Unlike scurvy, which is only caused by vitamin C deficiency, chronic diseases have multiple factors involved, which often interact. Moreover, nutrients tend to interact with other nutrients and factors, and thus may be beneficial or deleterious only under specific conditions. For example, a specific nutrient may only be relevant for individuals who have a certain behavior, such as those who smoke cigarettes or drink alcohol, or who are deficient in another nutrient, or who have a genetic susceptibility. The importance of a particular factor may vary across populations depending on the constellation of co-factors.

To establish a benefit of a nutrient, human studies are required. Animal studies may in some cases be quite complementary in understanding mechanisms and biologic plausibility, but metabolic differences among species, and sometimes even among individuals within the same species, make it infeasible to base recommendations strictly on animal data. While many subtleties exist in the design and conduct of human studies of nutrient-disease associations, two critical distinctions are most important to consider. First, it is important to note whether the study is based on a randomized design or is observational, and second, among observational studies, whether the study design is prospective or retrospective. In principle, causality of an association can only be established using a randomized design, in which the exposure of interest or a placebo is randomly assigned to study subjects. Thus, if an association is observed, it can be attributed strictly to the compound, assuming adequate statistical power and execution of the study. In observational studies, we observe an association between a certain factor and an outcome, for example, vitamin C and cancer risk, but because the vitamin C is based on the subjects' self-selected diet, confounding factors could potentially account for the association. Well-designed observational studies are those that are designed to best account for confounding factors. One of the important factors that influences reliability in observational studies is whether information is collected prospectively or retrospectively relative to the disease outcome. If the disease has occurred prior to collection of exposure information, as in a case-control study, the likelihood for biased and unreliable results is typically increased.

Although in principle, randomized controlled studies are the gold standard, these studies are expensive and difficult to conduct. In fact, chronic diseases are known to have a relatively long period for development, and most randomized trials conducted are typically only over a period of several years. Thus, if an observational study that assessed diet for a 20-year period provides an apparently conflicting answer from a randomized trial conducted over a 3-year period, the differences in results could be because the results from the observational study are biased, or that the randomized trial was not conducted for a sufficient time. Of course, many other factors could have contributed to the differences, such as underlying population differences in the prevalence of cofactors for the disease. Because of these complexities, the consensus of the likelihood of an association being causal is based on the integration of a combination of the following: (1) randomized trial data if available, (2) epidemiologic (observational) data, and (3) complementary mechanistic data.

Antioxidants

Vitamins C and E

Free radicals are generated from normal metabolism, smoking, or from chronic inflammation. Free radicals can damage DNA, protein and lipids, and thus could potentially influence many chronic diseases and perhaps even ageing in general. The body has evolved a host of antioxidant defenses; for example, repair enzymes efficiently repair damage caused by free radicals to DNA (Ames, Gold, & Willett, 1995). Micronutrients could be beneficial in one of two ways: some micronutrients such as selenium and manganese are part of enzymes involved in antioxidant defense, and other small molecules may help neutralize reactive oxygen species or free radicals. Two vitamins are of most importance. Vitamin C is the major water-soluble antioxidant, and α-tocopherol or vitamin E is the major lipid-soluble, membrane-localized antioxidant in humans. Despite much initial promise, however, studies have not consistently supported roles for vitamins C and E on lowering cancer risk (World Cancer Research Fund, American Institute for Cancer Research, 1997). In the Alpha-Tocopherol Beta-Carotene (ATBC) trial, a large randomized trial conducted among Finnish male smokers, no association between supplemental α-tocopherol and lung cancer was found, but a 34% lower incidence of prostate cancer among was observed (Anonymous, 1994). Subsequent epidemiologic analyses of vitamin E supplements, usually in the form of α-tocopherol, or levels of vitamin E in prostate cancer, support a possible role of this nutrient limited to smokers, but not in nonsmokers (Gann et al., 1999). In several studies, individuals with long-term use of vitamin E supplements had a lower risk of bladder cancer (Michaud et al., 2002). The doses in these studies were generally much higher than the recommended daily intakes.

Antioxidants have also been proposed to be related to lower risk of heart disease because oxidized LDL-cholesterol is believed to be particularly atherogenic. A number of apparently well-conducted earlier epidemiologic studies suggested that vitamin E could lower risk of coronary heart disease. These studies led to more rigorous randomized trials to provide a more definitive answer. The randomized trials have not been supportive, though the fact that the trials tended to be of short duration and limited to secondary cardiovascular events tended to limit conclusions. However, two recent trials provided strong null results. In one large trial, participants with cardiovascular disease or diabetes received no risk reduction for cardiovascular disease or cancer from 400 IU of vitamin E. Moreover, a borderline statistical significant increase in the risk of heart failure was observed (Lonn et al., 2005). In another study of apparently healthy women, 600 IU of natural source vitamin E on alternate days did not lower risk of cancer or cardiovascular disease, though a borderline significant 24% reduction in risk of cardiovascular death was observed (Lee et al., 2005). Finally, a meta-analysis of randomized trials found an increase in total mortality among individuals who received more than 150 IU/day of vitamin E. These trials were largely conducted in participants with chronic disease so it is difficult to generalize to healthy populations (Miller et al., 2005). Thus, the randomized trials do not support an appreciable benefit of supplementary vitamin E on health.

Recently, a pooled analysis of nine prospective epidemiologic or observational studies was conducted on vitamins E and C and cardiovascular disease (Knekt et al., 2004). This study was based on 10 years of follow-up, and 4647 major incident coronary heart disease events that occurred in almost 30,000 study participants who were free of coronary heart disease at baseline. In contrast to the earlier epidemiologic studies, no appreciable benefit of vitamin E was noted. However, compared with participants who did not take supplemental vitamin C, those who took > 700 mg supplemental vitamin C had a statistically significant 25% reduction in risk of coronary heart disease. There are no "definitive" randomized trials on vitamin C to date to support or refute this finding.

B-Vitamins

Three important B vitamins may influence the risk of developing major chronic diseases. These are vitamins B6, B12, and folate (in supplements, folate is usually provided as folic acid). Two major benefits have been proposed, one on cancer risk and the other on cardiovascular risks. More recently, a potential benefit on osteoporosis has been suggested. The benefit on cardiovascular disease extends from the ability of these nutrients to lower circulating homocysteine levels. Homocysteine is a nonprotein forming amino acid that is derived from the loss of the methyl group found in the amino acid methionine. Hyperhomocysteinemia or plasma homocysteine levels above 150 μmol/L is believed to be an independent risk factor for cardiovascular disease. Levels of plasma homocysteine are determined by both genetic and nutritional factors. In terms of nutrition, the B-vitamins folate, B-12 and B-6 are the most important for homocysteine metabolism. Approximately two thirds of all cases of hyperhomocysteinemia are apparently due to an inadequate status of one or all of these vitamins, especially folate (Ward, 2001). Increasing intakes of these three B-vitamins typically normalizes homocysteine levels. Attaining the current recommended doses of 400 μg of folic acid, 2 mg for vitamin B6 and 6 μg of vitamin B12 will reduce homocysteine. However, folate at 800 μg/day might be necessary to minimize homocysteine levels (Wald et al., 2001). Alcohol has well-established antifolate effects, and modifies the relationship between folate and homocysteine (Chiuve et al., 2005), that is, alcohol consumers may require more folate to optimally lower homocysteine levels.

There is no question that folate, vitamins B6 and B12 are critical in minimizing homocysteine levels, but the important question is whether they ultimately would lower risk of heart disease. Most available epidemiologic evidence suggests that hyperhomocysteinemia increases risk of coronary heart disease (Eikelboom et al., 1999). Epidemiologic studies also suggest that folate and vitamin B6, including from supplements, may reduce risk of coronary heart disease (Rimm et al., 1998). These results are promising, though definitive answers require randomized trials. Initial randomized trials are not promising, though these have focused on prevention of secondary cardiac events and less on healthy people. Interestingly, the effects of these nutrients on lowering heart disease risk appear to be more important in alcohol drinkers, which is consistent with the antagonistic effect of alcohol on homocysteine metabolism.

These B vitamins may also be important for cancer risk. Adequate folate is critical for DNA methylation, repair and synthesis (Duthie et al., 2000). Epidemiologic studies have linked low folate intake with higher risk of several cancers, most notably colorectal (Giovannucci, 2002), breast (Eichholzer, Luthy, Moser, & Fowler, 2001), and possibly cervical cancer (Eichholzer et al., 2001). Long-term use of folic acid-containing multivitamin supplements is associated with a 20–70% reduction in risk of colon cancer (Giovannucci et al., 1995). Isolated studies in other cancers, including esophageal cancer (Prasad et al., 1992) and leukemia (Thompson, Gerald, Willoughby, & Armstrong, 2001), also suggest that inadequate folate intake or metabolism may contribute to carcinogenesis in other sites. Supporting an anti-cancer role of folate is that genotypes for methylene tetrahydrofolate reductase (MTHFR), an enzyme known to be involved in folate metabolism, predict risk of colon cancer dependent on folate intake or status (Chen et al., 1996; Giovannucci, 2002). As for homocysteine lowering and effects on cardiovascular disease, the influence of folate in lowering cancer risk may be particularly important in alcohol drinkers.

Vitamin B6 has been less studied in relation to cancer than folate. However, recent studies suggest that vitamin B6 may be an important factor for colorectal cancer (Larsson, Giovannucci, & Wolk, 2005). These effects could be related to one-carbon metabolism as for folate, but vitamin B6 participates in more than 100 enzymatic reactions, and a number of mechanisms have been proposed for anti-cancer benefits (Matsubara, Komatsu, Oka, & Kato, 2003).

Recent evidence also suggests that bone fractures (especially of the hip) may be a consequence of higher serum homocysteine levels. Presumably, high serum homocysteine levels may weaken bone by interfering with collagen cross-linking. In a study based on 825 men and 1174 women in the Framingham Study, men in the highest quartile of plasma homocysteine had a four-fold greater risk of hip fracture than those in the lowest quartile, and women in the highest quartile had almost twice the risk as those in the bottom quartile (McLean et al., 2004). In the same issue of the *New England Journal of Medicine*, quite similar results were found in the Longitudinal Aging Study of Amsterdam (van Meurs et al., 2004). In that study, during 11,253 person-years of follow-up, osteoporotic fractures occurred in 191 subjects. A homocysteine level in the highest age-specific quartile was associated with an almost doubling of the risk of fracture, and the association appeared to be independent of bone mineral density and other risk factors for fracture. The B vitamins, especially folate, are known to lower homocyteine levels. Thus, it is reasonable to conclude that adequate intake of B vitamins may lower risk of osteoporotic fractures, although this has not been definitively demonstrated to date.

Although no untoward effects of folate have been established, one study found that women who consumed more than 400 μg/day of supplemental folic acid had 23% lower natural killer cell toxicity in the serum (Troen et al., 2006). The health consequence of this reduction in an index of immunity is unknown, but suggests that some caution is warranted in exceeding recommendations for folate intake.

Vitamin K

Vitamin K is a fat-soluble vitamin that is essential for normal blood clotting. Serious vitamin K deficiency can lead to blood clotting abnormalities and to hemorrhage. Dietary sources of vitamin K include dark-green vegetables, such as spinach, but vitamin K can also be synthesized by intestinal bacteria. Vitamin K deficiency may arise from long-term low intake of these vegetables, perhaps coupled with long-term use of antibiotics which may alter the intestinal bacteria. Individuals who are anticoagulated with warfarin must monitor their vitamin K intake because warfarin acts through disrupting vitamin K-dependent reactions. For individuals on warfarin therapy, intake of dark-green vegetables should remain relatively constant over time.

Regarding chronic disease, another role of vitamin K may be more relevant. Vitamin K is essential in chemical reactions that cross-link important bone proteins, and thus deficiency of vitamin K may contribute to increased risk of osteoporosis (Binkley & Suttie, 195). Lower levels of vitamin K have been associated with lower bone mass density (Kanai et al., 1997) and an increased risk of fractures (Hodges et al., 1993). Two recent prospective cohort studies have found that higher intakes of vitamin K are associated with a reduced risk of hip fractures (Feskanich et al., 1999). In the Nurses' Health Study report, women who ate a serving of lettuce or other green leafy vegetable per day had about half the risk of a hip fracture as those consuming these only once per week (Feskanich et al., 1999). The recommended intakes are 80 μg for men and 65 μg per women. It is not proven that getting additional supplemental vitamin K over an adequate diet would lower risk of hip fracture. Individuals with inadequate dietary vitamin K may be most likely to benefit from supplements.

Vitamin A

Vitamin A is critical for a number of important functions, including vision, helping to maintain the cells that line the body's interior surfaces (epithelial cells), and the immune response. In the diet, vitamin A comes in two forms, one from plant sources and one from animal sources. From plant sources we only get the precursor form of vitamin A (pro-vitamin A), from a group of substances that are called carotenoids. Some carotenoids, most notably beta-carotene, can be converted within the body to vitamin A. The animal form of vitamin A (retinol, or preformed vitamin A) comes from liver, fish liver oil, eggs and dairy products. If one does not consume liver, which is by far the most highly concentrated source of retinol, then the intake of preformed vitamin A will be relatively low. Supplements could contain either beta-carotene or retinol as a source of vitamin A. Thus, an individual may potentially get much higher doses of retinol from supplements (even from multivitamins) than one could get from most natural diets (unless liver is a substantial item in the diet).

Vitamin A deficiency is a serious problem in many parts of the world, particularly in poverty-stricken areas. However, there is little evidence that acquiring additional vitamin A from supplements in a generally well-fed population such is in the United States would confer any health benefits. Some evidence suggests that avoiding low vitamin A may have some benefits on risk of some cancers, but this is not proven. On the other hand, a potentially important downside of getting too much retinol exists. High retinol intake has been associated with a reduction in bone mineral density (Promislow, Goodman-Gruen, Slymen, & Barrett-Connor, 2002), and an increase in hip fractures (Feskanich, Singh, Willett, & Colditz, 2002), and serum retinol levels have been correlated with an increased risk of fracture (Michaelsson, Lithell, Vessby, & Melhus, 2003). This potential downside of retinol may be due to potential antagonistic effects of retinol on vitamin D actions. These adverse effects may occur at levels not much higher than the RDA. Thus, if one uses multivitamins, it is preferable to select those that use beta-carotene rather than retinol as the source of vitamin A, as these specific effects have not been observed with beta-carotene.

Vitamin D

Technically, vitamin D is not actually a vitamin as we can make adequate levels of vitamin D through skin exposure to solar UV-B radiation. However, many individuals are at risk for vitamin D deficiency because they do not make adequate vitamin D through solar radiation. There are various reasons for this: dark skin tends to block the conversion of the precursor into vitamin D in the skin, low sun exposure yields insufficient vitamin D, obesity lowers blood vitamin D levels, and the elderly have reduced capacity to make this vitamin. Thus, those with darker skin, the elderly, individuals living in Northern latitudes, individuals who avoid sun exposure, and those who are obese tend to be deficient in vitamin D. Vitamin D deficiency is indeed highly prevalent.

Why is vitamin D important? An undisputed role of vitamin D relates to bone health. The deficiency state for vitamin D is rickets, a disease of bone formation. Although this disease had become relatively rare following the discovery of vitamin D, it has begun to reemerge, especially in dark-skinned individuals living in countries that receive minimal sunlight. However, rickets may represent the extreme end of vitamin D deficiency. Suboptimal vitamin D in adulthood, especially in the elderly, increases risk of osteoporotic fractures. The evidence for this relationship is strong and is based on randomized trials. A systematic review and meta-analysis of randomized trials that examined vitamin D supplementation use in relation to risk of hip and nonvertebral fractures in older persons was conducted recently (Bischoff-Ferrari et al., 2005). The analysis included only double-blind randomized controlled trials of oral vitamin D supplementation with or without calcium supplementation that examined hip or nonvertebral fractures in older persons (≥ 60 years). The risk of fracture in those receiving vitamin D was compared to those who received only calcium supplementation or placebo. A vitamin D dose of 700–800 IU/day reduced the relative risk of hip fracture by 26% and any nonvertebral fracture by 23% versus calcium or placebo. Interestingly, no significant benefit was observed for studies with 400 IU/day vitamin D for hip fracture or for any nonvertebral fracture. Thus, vitamin D supplementation between 700 and 800 IU/day appears to reduce the risk of hip and any nonvertebral fractures in ambulatory or institutionalized elderly persons, but a dose of 400 IU/day does not appear to be sufficient for fracture prevention. It is unknown whether higher doses of vitamin D would reduce fracture risk further. Moreover, these trials only assessed the influence of vitamin D for several years; potentially, much more benefit could occur with long-term use over the lifespan.

Much of the benefit of vitamin D on fracture risk reduction is believed to be related to the bone strengthening effects of vitamin D, but vitamin D has another well-established function in the elderly. Vitamin D deficiency is related to muscle weakness, especially lower extremity weakness, and thereby with a higher likelihood of falling. Randomized trials indicate that supplementation with 800 IU/day of vitamin D reduces the number of falls in the elderly, including falls that lead to fractures (Bischoff et al., 2003). Having weak bones and a greater propensity to fall due to lower extremity weakness are both obvious risk factors for bone fractures.

If vitamin D were only related to rickets, increased risk of falling, and fractures, that would be important enough. However, a developing body of evidence has been accumulating indicating that deficient or suboptimal levels of vitamin D may predispose to a number of seemingly diverse disorders. Although the evidence is not definitive for these, the affected conditions include a variety of cancers, some autoimmune diseases such as type 1 diabetes, rheumatoid arthritis and multiple sclerosis, high blood pressure, periodontal disease, and bone pain (Holick, 2004). Why should vitamin D influence so many conditions? In the past two decades, researchers have discovered and documented that many cell types have the capacity to utilize vitamin D for many specific cellular functions, so vitamin D may be thought of as an ubiquitous "local hormone", termed a paracrine or autocrine factor. If vitamin D levels are low, diverse cellular functions in different tissues may be disrupted, which could have a whole range of consequences for the body.

It is important to emphasize that other than the role of bone formation and muscle strength, the conditions attributed to deficient or suboptimal vitamin D have not been definitively established. The evidence is strongest for some cancers. Some of the evidence relating low vitamin D status to higher rates of cancer incidence and mortality is based indirectly on data linking higher average regional solar UV-B radiation, which is required to make vitamin D in the skin, with lower cancer mortality rates, with the strongest association for colorectal cancer (Grant, 2002). Solar radiation, however, can be related to factors other than vitamin D, so this association does not prove that vitamin D is the critical factor. However, a number of studies now show that individuals with lower blood vitamin D levels have a much higher of colorectal cancer or its precursor, the colorectal adenoma or adenomatous polyp (Feskanich et al., 2004). In general, those with vitamin D levels in the top 20% have a 40–50% lower risk of colorectal cancer as do those in the lowest 20%. Additionally, a number of studies indicate that higher total vitamin D intake (diet plus supplements) is associated with lower colorectal cancer risk (Giovannucci, 2005). A recent analysis of the Nurses' Health Study found that high blood levels of vitamin D were associated with a reduced risk of breast cancer in postmenopausal but not premenopausal women (Bertone-Johnson et al., 2005).

A complicating factor for making recommendations for optimal vitamin D intake is that for most people, most of the vitamin D is made from sun exposure. In fact, in less than half an hour sunbathing at the beach, a light-skinned person may make upwards of 20,000 IU of vitamin D. For comparison, a glass of milk contains only 100 IU. Supplements that contain vitamin D usually contain 400 IU, but a further complication is that many supplements may use a form of vitamin D (D2 or ergocalciferol) which is weaker by a factor of three than the natural form (D3 or cholecalciferol). The optimal dose for overall health is not known and may vary by individual depending on sun exposure. However, for most people, 1000 IU/day may be the minimum required. For safety, 2000 IU/day should not be exceeded for prolonged time periods.

Calcium

Having adequate calcium, an essential mineral, is important for health, but questions remain on what is the long-term intake level required for optimal health. Calcium is important for bone health, but it is one of many relevant factors. It is unclear how important getting high levels of calcium is as the body appears able to compensate over a wide degree of intakes to achieve calcium balance. Recent epidemiologic studies (and some randomized trial evidence) suggest roles for vitamin D, vitamin K, and possibly B vitamins, by lowering serum homocysteine, in fracture prevention. The effect of exercise in keeping bones strong is also important. The role of calcium has been greatly emphasized in the media, but it remains unclear if it is the most important factor. In fact, some of the populations with the highest rates of fractures tend to have high, rather than low calcium intakes. While factors other than calcium may account for the high fracture rates in these populations, the fact that some populations with the lowest calcium intakes have among the lowest fracture rates suggests that factors other than low calcium intake are likely to be of paramount importance in the high fracture rates in some Western countries.

Although the role of calcium on bone health has been emphasized, calcium has been shown to have other effects on common chronic diseases. In most epidemiologic studies, low calcium intake has been associated with higher risk of colorectal cancer (Platz & Giovannucci, 1999) and adenoma, the cancer precursor (Baron et al., 1999). Prospective studies have shown a relatively consistent inverse association between low calcium intake, including that from supplements, and increased colorectal and colon cancer risk (McCullough et al., 2003). A role of calcium on colorectal carcinogenesis has also been supported by randomized intervention trials of colorectal adenomas as the outcome (Baron et al., 1999). The optimal dose and form of calcium that may be most protective is not known, but prospective studies suggest that benefits may plateau at 1000 mg per day or less (McCullough et al., 2003). Few studies on calcium and breast cancer have been reported. One hospital-based case control study reported a statistically significant lower risk (20%) of breast cancer with high versus low calcium intakes (Negri et al., 1996) while results in three others were not significant (Katsouyanni et al., 1988; Levi, Pasche, Lucchini, & La Vecchia, 2001; Negri et al, 1996; Potischman et al., 1999). A recent prospective study reported a significant inverse association between calcium and breast cancer but only in premenopausal women (Shin et al., 2002). The relationship between calcium and breast cancer needs more study.

On the other hand, some data suggest an increased risk of prostate cancer with higher calcium intake (Chan et al., 2001), particularly above 1500 mg/day and for advanced (metastatic) prostate cancer (Giovannucci et al., 1998). A recent meta-analysis that combined the results of all prospective studies shows that high calcium intake may increase the risk of prostate cancer, especially of advanced or aggressive prostate cancer (Gao, LaValley, & Tucker, 2005).

The data suggest, but cannot definitively show, that it is calcium rather than some other component in dairy foods that increases risk. Why calcium should increase risk of prostate cancer appears puzzling, but very high calcium intakes could suppress the active component of vitamin D in the serum (Giovannucci et al., 1998), and vitamin D could be a potentially protective factor for prostate carcinogenesis.

The bottom line is that we need more study to determine the optimal calcium intake. Certainly going from very deficient intakes (for example, below 500 mg/day) to higher levels is likely to do some good, perhaps for bone health and colorectal cancer risk. However, especially for prostate cancer risk in men, going too high may be harmful. Until more definitive data are available, aiming for approximately 1000 mg/day seems to be a reasonable target. For those who consume little or no dairy products, use of a calcium supplement is a reasonable option, although men especially should be careful not to substantially exceed 1000 mg/day from supplements and diet combined.

Potassium

Potassium is an important mineral for many cellular functions, and its levels are thus tightly regulated by the body. In regard to chronic disease, the most important role of potassium is for blood pressure. Low potassium intake, especially combined with high sodium, may contribute to elevated blood pressure. Probably mostly due to the effect on blood pressure, high potassium intake could lower risk of stroke (Srinath Reddy & Katan, 2004). Eating lots of fruits and vegetables and low quantities of processed foods is optimal in keeping the relative amounts of potassium to sodium high. In addition, use of potassium salt, in which part of the sodium is replaced by potassium, may be useful for some individuals, especially those with high blood pressure. It is advisable to avoid the use of specific potassium supplements without discussing this with a physician, as these could induce serious sides effects and even fatalities when kidney function is compromised. The amount of potassium in multivitamins that include it is relatively low.

Selenium

Selenium is a trace metal that functions through selenoproteins, including selenium-dependent glutathione peroxidases that defend against oxidative stress. The selenium content of food varies depending on the selenium content of soil where plants are grown or animals are raised. Because soil selenium content can vary more than 10-fold, nutrient databases for selenium are unreliable. It is difficult to reliably recommend specific food sources for selenium because of the variability of selenium content in various foods. The current recommended levels are 55 μg per day for women and 70 μg per day for men. In the United States, most though not all people achieve these levels, though there are areas in the world where the selenium content in soil (and thus foods) is very low and some individuals may be deficient. Most epidemiologic evidence on the anti-carcinogenic role of selenium stems from biomarker (for example, measuring selenium level in serum or toenails) and intervention studies. Selenium has been strongly associated with reduced prostate cancer risk in one trial of selenium supplementation originally designed to study skin cancer (Clark et al., 1996), and some studies indicate that individuals with low selenium body stores as assessed in serum or toenails have an increased risk of prostate cancer (Nomura, Lee, Stemmermann, & Combs, 2000). However, not all data are supportive. In Finland, an area with very low selenium levels in the soil, selenium was added to fertilizer in the 1980s. The blood levels in the population were shown to increase dramatically, but this was not followed by a decrease in prostate cancer incidence or mortality. For now, there is insufficient evidence to recommend selenium supplementation for individuals (unless they are determined to be deficient). However, a large ongoing supplement trial funded by the National Cancer Institute (The SELECT trial) is examining supplemental selenium, vitamin E, or a combination of these, compared to placebo, on primary prevention of prostate cancer. The results of this trial may yield useful information regarding selenium supplementation.

Iron

Iron deficiency is common in many parts of the world. Inadequate iron can lead to anemia and to growth and developmental problems in children. In the United States, iron deficiency is relatively rare due to the wide consumption of meat and iron-fortified grain products. Primarily infants and menstruating women are susceptible to iron deficiency, so some iron supplementation may be advisable in these groups. For most adults in the US (except possibly for some menstruating women and vegetarians), the potential for excess iron may be more of concern than problems associated with deficiency. A relatively small percentage of individuals have the genetic tendency to accumulate very high levels of iron, which can lead to a serious condition called hemochromatosis. Another sizable group can accumulate relatively high iron stores, but not high enough to cause overt problems. However, excess iron could be a pro-oxidant and a source of free radicals. Although nothing definitive can be said, limited evidence suggests that moderately elevated iron levels could be a risk factor for heart disease, diabetes and some cancers. Serious iron deficiency in adults is typically caused by bleeding abnormalities, such as in the gastrointestinal tract, rather than insufficient intake. Thus, it is generally not advisable to routinely take iron supplements, especially above the RDA levels.

Zinc

Zinc is an important mineral that is involved in numerous important reactions in the body. These involve antioxidation, vision, blood clotting, wound healing, sperm production and possibly prostate function. The recommended daily intakes are 15 mg for men and 12 mg for women. Zinc supplements are often taken to prevent colds, or to lessen cold symptoms. However, benefits of zinc supplements in this regard have not been definitively proven.

For chronic diseases, there is little evidence that additional zinc from supplements may be beneficial. It is noteworthy that symptoms of excess zinc can arise at doses not much above 15 mg/day. These symptoms may include a depressed immune system, reduced wound healing, hair loss, taste, smell disturbances, and skin problems. It is advisable not to take doses of zinc much above the RDA, as little evidence of benefit exists. On the contrary, one observational study found that men taking high doses of zinc for long periods of time had almost a 3-fold higher risk of advanced prostate cancer than those not taking supplements (Leitzmann et al., 2003). Although this study could not definitively prove that zinc, rather than some other correlated factor, was the culprit, it does raise some concern over the prolonged use of high-dose zinc supplements.

Practical Applications

Most individuals in the US obtain sufficient amounts of vitamins in their diet to prevent overt vitamin deficiency diseases. However, chronic diseases could develop from long-term imbalances or suboptimal intakes of vitamins and minerals in the diet. Although it is often assumed that vitamin deficiency in the American diet is relatively rare, the prevalence of suboptimal intakes may be much higher. Supplementation with vitamins and minerals has potential benefits in regard to chronic diseases, but also presents some risks when intake is excessive. A well-balanced diet based on consumption of a wide array of foods is likely to provide many benefits, both in terms of supplying vitamins and minerals, but also in providing other dietary constituents that are important for health (e.g. fiber, essential fatty acids). The overall dietary pattern will also determine some important aspects that relate to health (e.g. polyunsaturated to saturated fat ratio, relative amounts of potassium to sodium, glycemic index or load). Finally, diets may contain many potentially beneficial items but nonestablished nutrients (e.g. carotenoids other than beta-carotene, acting as antioxidants). For these reasons, supplements should never be considered as a replacement for a healthful diet. If one has an unhealthful diet, supplementation could only help offset some of a number of negative consequences. Nonetheless, the wise use of supplements can complement even a generally sound dietary plan because it may be difficult to obtain optimal amounts of all micronutrients.

There are a number of specific cases where supplements may be particularly helpful. Alcohol consumption has a depleting effect of folate, so it may be reasonable for alcohol consumers to get an additional multivitamin equivalent of folate. However, going much above the RDA may not necessarily be better or safer. Many older individuals with digestive problems may have problems absorbing vitamin B12 from foods, so extra vitamin B12 may be warranted for the older population. Vegetarians may also require additional B12. Individuals who consume little or no meat may also benefit from more vitamin B6, as some recent evidence suggests higher levels of B6 may help prevent colon cancer.

The situation for vitamin E is complex. The current recommended intake is 20 mg (30 IU). High-dose supplements (400 or 800 IU) are available and widely used, but the evidence is mixed. It is possible that some individuals may benefit (e.g. men at risk for prostate cancer; primary prevention for coronary heart disease), but some negative consequences have been observed in secondary prevention of coronary heart disease trials. Thus, some caution is advisable before taking high dose supplements of vitamin E, especially among those already with underlying heart disease.

For vitamin A, obtaining recommended intakes of it in the form of beta-carotene is unlikely to be harmful. However, it is important to remember that many of the benefits attributed to beta-carotene are actually from carotene-rich diets, which essentially means diets rich in diverse fruits and vegetables. Mega-doses of beta-carotene in a pill form increase lung cancer risk in smokers. Supplements with retinol as the source of vitamin A are probably best avoided, and individuals should certainly avoid consuming much more than the recommended intake of vitamin A in the form of retinol.

For most individuals, 800 IU/day of vitamin D, in the form of cholecalciferol or vitamin D3, is likely to be beneficial. The full picture of the potential benefits of vitamin D is far from clear. It may turn out that even higher intakes of vitamin D may be required for optimal benefits. The upper limit dose for safety is set at 2000 IU/day, though many researchers question this and believe that 2000 IU/day may be well within the safe range. Some individuals, such as lifeguards at the beach, may make up to 20,000 IU/day and there has never been a documented case of vitamin D toxicity from sun exposure. Until more definitive data are available, it is advisable not to exceed greater than 2000 IU/day for prolonged time periods.

For minerals, for nonconsumers of dairy products, obtaining some supplemental calcium is a reasonable choice. Aiming for a total calcium intake of about 1000 mg/day appears sensible, but men especially should not exceed this substantially due to a potentially higher risk of aggressive prostate cancer. High-dose zinc supplements should also be avoided, especially by men, again because of a possible increased risk of prostate cancer. Except possibly in menstruating women, supplemental iron beyond the RDA should be avoided. Selenium is a potentially beneficial trace element in regards to cancer risk, though this has not been proven. Most Americans probably get the RDA doses of selenium from their diet.

In general, taking a multivitamin with vitamins within the RDA may be considered a safety net for individuals. This practice is unlikely to do much harm, and may help fill in some nutrient gaps that may develop in individuals with even relatively healthful diets. Preferably, the supplement should have beta-carotene instead of retinol as the source of vitamin A, and vitamin D3 or cholecalciferol as the vitamin D form. Obtaining additional vitamin D may be reasonable, as multivitamins generally have 400 IU or less. Benefits of mega-doses of vitamins are not established, and there is evidence of harm for a number of vitamins and minerals at doses substantially higher than the RDA, but below doses that are typically associated with toxicity. Thus, the indiscriminate use of doses of vitamins and minerals well above the RDA is discouraged.

References

Ames, B. N., Gold, L. S., & Willett, W. C. (1995). The causes and prevention of cancer. *Proceedings of the National Academy of Sciences of the United States of America, 92*, 5258–5265.

Anonymous. (1994). The effect of vitamin E and beta carotene on the incidence of lung cancer and other cancers in male smokers. The Alpha-Tocopherol, Beta Carotene Cancer Prevention Study Group. *New England Journal of Medicine, 330*, 1029–1035.

Baron, J. A., Beach, M., Mandel, J. S., van Stolk, R. U., et al. (1999). Calcium supplements for the prevention of colorectal adenomas. *The Calcium Polyp Prevention Study Group. New England Journal of Medicine, 340*, 101–107.

Bertone-Johnson, E., Chen, W. Y., Holick, M. F., Hollis, B. W., et al. (2005). Plasma 25-hydroxyvitamin D and 1,25-dihydroxyvitamin D and risk of breast cancer. *Cancer Epidemiology, Biomarkers and Prevention, 14*, 1991–1997.

Binkley, N. C., & Suttie, J. W. (1995). Vitamin K nutrition and osteoporosis. *Journal of Nutrition, 125*, 1812–1821.

Bischoff, H. A., Stahelin, H. B., Dick, W., Akos, R., et al. (2003). Effects of vitamin D and calcium supplementation on falls: a randomized controlled trial. *Journal of Bone and Mineral Research, 18*, 343–351.

Bischoff-Ferrari, H. A., Willett, W. C., Wong, J. B., Giovannucci, E., et al. (2005). Fracture prevention with vitamin D supplementation: a meta-analysis of randomized controlled trials. *JAMA, 293*, 2257–2264.

Chan, J. M., Stampfer, M. J., Ma, J., Gann, P. H., et al. (2001). Dairy products, calcium, and prostate cancer risk in the Physicians' Health Study (comment). *American Journal of Clinical Nutrition, 74*, 549–554.

Chen, J., Giovannucci, E., Kelsey, K., Rimm, E. B., et al. (1996). A methylenetetrahydrofolate reductase polymorphism and the risk of colorectal cancer. *Cancer Research, 56*, 4862–4864.

Chiuve, S. E., Giovannucci, E. L., Hankinson, E. E., Hunter, D. J., Stampfer, M. J., Willett, W.C., Rimm, E. B. (2005). Alcohol intake and methylenetetrahydrofolate reductase polymorphism modify the relation of folate intake to plasma homocysteine. *American Journal of Clinical Nutrition, 82(1)*: 155–62.

Clark, L. C., Combs, G. F., Jr., Turnbull, B. W., Slate, E. H., et al. (1996). Effects of selenium supplementation for cancer prevention in patients with carcinoma of the skin. A randomized controlled trial. Nutritional Prevention of Cancer Study Group. *JAMA, 276*, 1957–1963.

Duthie, S. J., Narayanan, S., Blum, S., Pirie, L., et al. (2000). Folate deficiency in vitro induces uracil misincorporation and DNA hypomethylation and inhibits DNA excision repair in immortalized normal human colon epithelial cells. *Nutrition and Cancer, 37*, 245–251.

Eichholzer, M., Luthy, J., Moser, U., & Fowler, B. (2001). Folate and the risk of colorectal, breast and cervix cancer: the epidemiological evidence. *Swiss Medical Weekly, 131*, 539–549.

Eikelboom, J. W., Lonn, E., Genest, J., Jr., Hankey, G., et al. (1999). Homocyst(e)ine and cardiovascular disease: a critical review of the epidemiologic evidence. *Annals of Internal Medicine, 131*, 363–375.

Feskanich, D., Ma, J., Fuchs, C. S., Kirkner, G. J., et al. (2004). Plasma vitamin D metabolites and risk of colorectal cancer in women. *Cancer Epidemiology, Biomarkers and Prevention, 13*, 1502–1508.

Feskanich, D., Singh, V., Willett, W. C., & Colditz, G. A. (2002). Vitamin A intake and hip fractures among postmenopausal women. *JAMA, 287*, 47–54.

Feskanich, D., Weber, P., Willett, W. C., Rockett, H., et al. (1999). Vitamin K intake and hip fractures in women: a prospective study. *American Journal of Clinical Nutrition, 69*, 74–79.

Gann, P. H., Ma, J., Giovannucci, E., Willett, W., et al. (1999). Lower prostate cancer risk in men with elevated plasma lycopene levels: results of a prospective analysis. *Cancer Research, 59*, 1225–1230.

Gao, X., LaValley, M. P., & Tucker, K. L. (2005). Prospective studies of dairy product and calcium intakes and prostate cancer risk: a meta-analysis. *Journal of the National Cancer Institute, 97*, 1768–1777.

Giovannucci, E. (2002). Epidemiologic studies of folate and colorectal neoplasia: a review. *Journal of Nutrition, 132*, 2350S–2355S.

Giovannucci, E. (2005). The epidemiology of vitamin D and cancer incidence and mortality: a review (United States). *Cancer Causes and Control, 16*, 83–95.

Giovannucci, E., Rimm, E. B., Ascherio, A., Stampfer, M. J., et al. (1995). Alcohol, low-methionine-low-folate diets, and risk of colon cancer in men. *Journal of the National Cancer Institute, 87*, 265–273.

Giovannucci, E., Rimm, E. B., Wolk, A., Ascherio, A., et al. (1998). Calcium and fructose intake in relation to risk of prostate cancer. *Cancer Research, 58*, 442–447.

Grant, W. B. (2002). An estimate of premature cancer mortality in the U.S. due to inadequate doses of solar ultraviolet-B radiation. *Cancer, 94*, 1867–1875.

Hodges, S. J., Akesson, K., Vergnaud, P., Obrant, K., et al. (1993). Circulating levels of vitamins K1 and K2 decreased in elderly women with hip fracture. *Journal of Bone and Mineral Research, 8*, 1241–1245.

Holick, M. F. (2004). Sunlight and vitamin D for bone health and prevention of autoimmune diseases, cancers, and cardiovascular disease. *American Journal of Clinical Nutrition, 80*, 1678S–1688S.

Kanai, T., Takagi, T., Masuhiro, K., Nakamura, M., et al. (1997). Serum vitamin K level and bone mineral density in post-menopausal women. *International Journal of Gynaecology and Obstetrics, 56*, 25–30.

Katsouyanni, K., Willett, W., Trichopoulos, D., Boyle, P., et al. (1988). Risk of breast cancer among Greek women in relation to nutrient intake. *Cancer, 61*, 181–185.

Knekt, P., Ritz, J., Pereira, M. A., O'Reilly, E. J., et al. (2004). Antioxidant vitamins and coronary heart disease risk: a pooled analysis of 9 cohorts. *American Journal of Clinical Nutrition, 80*, 1508–1520.

Larsson, S. C., Giovannucci, E., & Wolk, A. (2005). Vitamin B6 intake, alcohol consumption, and colorectal cancer: a longitudinal population-based cohort of women. *Gastroenterology, 128*, 1830–1837.

Lee, I. M., Cook, N. R., Gaziano, J. M., Gordon, D., et al. (2005). Vitamin E in the primary prevention of cardiovascular disease and cancer: the Women's Health Study: a randomized controlled trial. *JAMA, 294*, 56–65.

Leitzmann, M. F., Stampfer, M. J., Wu, K., Colditz, G. A., et al. (2003). Zinc supplement use and risk of prostate cancer. *Journal of the National Cancer Institute, 95*, 1004–1007.

Levi, F., Pasche, C., Lucchini, F., & La Vecchia, C. (2001). Dietary intake of selected micronutrients and breast-cancer risk. *International Journal of Cancer, 91*, 260–263.

Lonn, E., Bosch, J., Yusuf, S., Sheridan, P., et al. (2005). Effects of long-term vitamin E supplementation on cardiovascular events and cancer: a randomized controlled trial. *JAMA, 293*, 1338–1347.

Matsubara, K., Komatsu, S., Oka, T., & Kato, N. (2003). Vitamin B6-mediated suppression of colon tumorigenesis, cell proliferation, and angiogenesis (review). *Journal of Nutritional Biochemistry, 14*, 246–250.

McCullough, M. L., Robertson, A. S., Rodriguez, C., Jacobs, E. J., et al. (2003). Calcium, vitamin D, dairy products, and risk of colorectal cancer in the cancer prevention study II nutrition cohort (United States). *Cancer Causes and Control, 14*, 1–12.

McLean, R. R., Jacques, P. F., Selhub, J., Tucker, K. L., et al. (2004). Homocysteine as a predictive factor for hip fracture in older persons. *New England Journal of Medicine, 350*, 2042–2049.

Michaelsson, K., Lithell, H., Vessby, B., & Melhus, H. (2003). Serum retinol levels and the risk of fracture. *New England Journal of Medicine, 348*, 287–294.

Michaud, D. S., Spiegelman, D., Clinton, S. K., Rimm, E. B., et al. (2002). Prospective study of dietary suppplements, macronutrients, micronutrients, and risk of bladder cancer in US men. *American Journal of Epidemiology, 152*, 1145–1153.

Miller, E. R. r., Pastor-Barriuso, R., Dalal, D., Riemersma, R. A., et al. (2005). Meta-analysis: high-dosage vitamin E supplementation may increase all-cause mortality. *Annals of Internal Medicine, 142*, 37–46.

Negri, E., La Vecchia, C., Franceschi, S., D'Avanzo, B., et al. (1996). Intake of selected micronutrients and the risk of breast cancer. *International Journal of Cancer, 65*, 140–144.

Nomura, A. M. Y., Lee, J., Stemmermann, G. N., & Combs, G. F., Jr. (2000). Serum selenium and subsequent risk of prostate cancer. *Cancer Epidemiology, Biomarkers and Prevention, 9*, 883–887.

Platz, E. A., & Giovannucci, E. (1999). Vitamin D and calcium in colorectal and prostate cancers. In D. Heber, G. L. Blackburn, & V. L. Go (Eds.), *Nutritional Oncology* (pp. 223–252). San Diego, CA: Academic Press.

Potischman, N., Swanson, C. A., Coates, R. J., Gammon, M. D., et al. (1999). Intake of food groups and associated micronutrients in relation to risk of early-stage breast cancer. *International Journal of Cancer, 82*, 315–321.

Prasad, M. P., Krishna, T. P., Pasricha, S., Krishnaswamy, K., et al. (1992). Esophageal cancer and diet–a case-control study. *Nutrition and Cancer, 18*, 85–93.

Promislow, J. H., Goodman-Gruen, D., Slymen, D. J., & Barrett-Connor, E. (2002). Retinol intake and bone mineral density in the elderly: the Rancho Bernardo Study. *Journal of Bone and Mineral Research, 17*, 1349–1358.

Rimm, E. B., Willett, W. C., Hu, F. B., Sampson, L., et al. (1998). Folate and vitamin B_6 from diet and supplements in relation to risk of coronary heart disease among women. *JAMA, 279*, 359–364.

Shin, M. H., Holmes, M. D., Hankinson, S. E., Wu, K., et al. (2002). Intake of dairy products, calcium, and vitamin D and risk of breast cancer. *Journal of the National Cancer Institute, 94*, 1301–1310.

Srinath Reddy, K., & Katan, M. B. (2004). Diet, nutrition and the prevention of hypertension and cardiovascular diseases. *Public Health Nutrition, 7*, 167–186.

Thompson, J. R., Gerald, P. F., Willoughby, M. L., & Armstrong, B. K. (2001). Maternal folate supplementation in pregnancy and protection against acute lymphoblastic leukaemia in childhood: a case-control study. *Lancet, 358*, 1935–1940.

Troen, A. M., Mitchell, B., Sorensen, B., Wener, M. H., et al. (2006). Unmetabolized folic acid in plasma is associated with reduced natural killer cell cytotoxicity among postmenopausal women. *Journal of Nutrition, 136*, 189–194.

van Meurs, J. B., Dhonukshe-Rutten, R. A., Pluijm, S. M., van der Klift, M., et al. (2004). Homocysteine levels and the risk of osteoporotic fracture. *New England Journal of Medicine, 350*, 2033–2041.

Wald, D. S., Bishop, L., Wald, N. J., Law, M., et al. (2001). Randomized trial of folic acid supplementation and serum homocysteine levels. *Archives of Internal Medicine, 161*, 695–700.

Ward, M. (2001). Homocysteine, folate, and cardiovascular disease. *International Journal for Vitamin and Nutrition Research, 71*, 173–178.

World Cancer Research Fund, American Institute for Cancer Research. (1997). *Food, nutrition and the prevention of cancer: a global perspective*. Washington, DC: American Institute for Cancer Research.

6

Herbal Medicines in the Treatment of Psychiatric and Neurological Disorders

Shahin Akhondzadeh*

Herbal medicines include a range of pharmacologically active compounds: in some cases it is not well understood which ingredients are important for a therapeutic effect. The supporters of herbal medicine believe that isolated ingredients in the majority of cases have weaker clinical effects than whole plant extract, a claim that would obviously require proof in each case. Generalizations about the efficacy of herbal medicines are clearly not possible. Each one needs systematic research including a variety of animal studies and also randomized clinical trials. Indeed, clinical trials of herbal medicines are feasible much in the same way as for other drugs (Schulz, Hansel & Tyler, 1998). Numerous randomized clinical trials of herbal medicines have been published and systematic review and meta-analyses of these studies are available. Many of today's synthetic drugs originated from the plant kingdom, and only about two centuries ago the major pharmacopoeias were dominated by herbal drugs. Herbal medicine went into rapid decline when basic and clinical pharmacology established themselves as leading branches of medicine. Nevertheless, herbal medicine is still of interest in many diseases in particular psychiatric and neurological disorders. There are some reasons for this: (1) participants are dissatisfied with conventional treatment, (2) participants want to have control over their healthcare decisions, and (3) participants see that herbal medicine is congruent with their philosophical values and beliefs (Astin, 1998). It has been reported that most participants with a mental disorder sought herbal medicine treatment for somatic problems rather than for their mental and emotional symptoms and the best example is somatic symptoms of depression.

Physicians need to understand the biochemical and evidential bases for the use of herbs and nutrients to diagnose and treat participants safely and effectively, to avoid interactions with standard medications, and to provide participants with the benefits of alternative treatments (Schulz et al., 1998).

* Correspondence: Professor. Shahin Akhondzadeh, Ph.D., FB Pharmacols, Psychiatric Research Center, Roozbeh Hospital, Tehran University of Medical Sciences, South Kargar Street, Tehran 13337, Iran. Tel: +98-21-88281866, Fax: +98-21-55419113, Email: s.akhond@neda.net.

Although a multitude of pharmaceutical agents are available for the treatment of mental disorders, physicians find that many participants cannot tolerate the side effects, do not respond adequately, or eventually lose their response. In comparison, many therapeutic herbs have far fewer side effects. They can provide an alternative treatment or be used to enhance the effect of prescription medications.

This chapter will indicate the quality of the evidence supporting the clinical effects of a number of commonly used types of herbal medicines for the psychiatric and neurological disorders which follow:

1- Alzheimer's disease
2- Depression
3- Anxiety
4- Insomnia
5- Substance use disorders
6- Attention deficit and hyperactivity disorder (ADHD)
7- Migraine

The highest level of confidence derives from well-designed, randomized, double-blind controlled studies.

Alzheimer's Disease

Alzheimer's disease (AD) is the most common cause of severe mental deterioration (dementia) in the elderly (Evans, Funkenstein, & Albert, 1989; Geldmacher & Whitehouse, 1997). AD was known to occur occasionally in families, but was not necessarily related to the more frequent occurrence of cognition impairment in late life. The latter condition was known as senile dementia. When results of careful pathology studies emerged in the 1970s and 1980s showing that the pathology of the brains of participants with early-onset (before the age of 65 years) and late-onset AD was the same, research into the pathologic process as well as the clinical manifestations accelerated (Evans et al., 1989; Geldmacher & Whitehouse, 1997). The incidence and prevalence of AD rose with increasing age, especially for those over the age of 65 years. The incidence of AD ranges from 1 to 4% of the population per year, rising by half a decade from its lowest level at ages 65–70 years to rates that may approach 6% over the age of 85 years. Prevalence of AD has been a subject of discussion. Prevalence rates of AD also increase by half decade or decade; reports in the literature of how many cases exist at any one period vary. Estimate of the prevalence of AD range from 3% of the population between the ages of 65 and 75 years to the highest reported estimate of 47% of people over the age of 85 years. In general, all studies report a progressive increase in the prevalence of dementia as a function of age between 65 and 85 years. More conservative estimates at the higher end are in the range of 30–35% which is still a significant number. Whatever the current estimates are, all researchers agree that the number of AD cases will probably triple over the next 30–40 years (Evans et al., 1989; Geldmacher & Whitehouse, 1997).

Definitions of AD

There are three widely used criteria-based approaches to the diagnosis of AD: the International Classification of Diseases, 10th revision (ICD-10), the Diagnostic and Statistical Manual of Mental Disorders, fourth edition (DSM-IV), and the National Institute of Neurological and Communicative Disorders and Stroke-Alzheimers's Disease and Related Disorders Association (NINCDS-ADRDA) work group criteria (McKhann et al., 1984). Not surprisingly, the three definitions share many common features.

There are three common misconceptions regarding AD: (1) that it is a global disorder, (2) that it is a diagnosis of exclusion, and (3) that it can be a diagnosed only at autopsy. All are challenged by the three diagnostic frameworks, which require that attention be sufficiently intact to exclude delirium as the cause of the mental status changes, whereas a global disorder would include attention abnormalities. All the definitions specify expected findings (i.e., memory impairment) thus utilizing inclusionary criteria in the diagnosis rather than approaching the disorder as a diagnosis of exclusion. All definitions are predicted on the feasibility of clinical diagnosis, and most series find accuracy rates of 85–90% based on these criteria. Diagnosing AD should begin with detailed interviews of both the patient and an informant who is familiar with the patient. The medical history can provide relevant information, such as the timing of onset of symptoms, level of functional impairment, rate of deterioration, and any alterations in mood (Geldmacher & Whitehouse, 1997). A complete physical examination should include an in-office cognitive assessment, such as the Mini-Mental State Examination, and a brief neurological examination. The presence of depression should also be evaluated; useful screens include the Geriatric Depression Scale and the Zung Self Rating Scale for Depression. Laboratory evaluations should include blood chemistries, a complete blood cell count; and tests for neurosyphilis, thyroid, kidney and liver function, and serum levels of vitamin B_{12}. Some neuroimaging is generally recommended. Computerized tomography is usually sufficient to eliminate subdural hematoma or tumors as a potential cause; however, Magnetic Resonance Imaging may be necessary to detect the presence of white matter ischemic lesions. Positron Emission Tomography or Single Photon Emission Computed Tomography are useful in distinguishing AD from other dementias through quantifying metabolism or assessing general blood flow (Geldmacher & Whitehouse, 1997).

Pathophysiology of AD

Neuroimaging of the patient with AD or other dementias may reveal atrophy of the brain, such as enlarged ventricles and sulci, and narrowed gyri, although these features are not always present (Geldmacher & Whitehouse, 1997). Neuronal loss is the main neuropathologic feature underlying the symptoms of AD. Microscopically, AD is characterized by the presence of senile plaques and neurofibrillary tangles (NFTs). Plaques are extracellular deposits of filamentous ß-amyloid, a protease cleavage product of amyloid precursor protein (Geldmacher & Whitehouse, 1997).

NFTs are formed intracellulary by the abnormal rearrangement of microtubule-associated proteins, such as tau. Both NFTs and senile plaques, although diagnostic of AD when observed in large numbers, are also present to some degree in the brains of normal elderly persons. However, the plaques seen in normal brains or early-stage AD are diffuse and relatively benign deposits of ß-amyloid, whereas at later stages, the plaques assume a compact b-pleated conformation and subsequently become associated with dystrophic neuritis. These later-stage plaques are thought to represent a more neurotoxic form (Geldmacher & Whitehouse, 1997).

The Cholinergic Hypothesis

The first neurotransmitter defect discovered in AD involved acethylcholine (Ach). As Cholinergic function is required for short-term memory, the cholinergic deficit in AD was also believed to be responsible for much of the short-term memory deficit (Francis, Palmer, Snape, & Wilcock, 1999). Markers for cholinergic neurons, such as choline acetyltransferase (ChAT) and acetylcholinestrase (AChE), which are enzymes responsible for synthesis and degradation of Ach, respectively, are decreased in the cortex and hippocampus, areas of the brain involved in cognition and memory. The earliest loss of neurons occurs in the nucleus basalis and the entorhinal cortex where cholinergic neurons are preferentially affected. As the illness progresses, up to 90% of cholinergic neurons in the nucleus basalis of Mynert may be lost. Preclinical studies have demonstrated that loss of cholinergic functions in these areas is associated with declines in learning capacity and memory. The resultant decrease in Ach-dependent neurotransmission is thought to lead to the functional deficits of AD, much as dopaminergic deficits underlie Parkinson's disease and its clinical manifestations (Francis et al., 1999). Clinical drug trials in participants with AD have focused on drugs that augment levels of Ach in the brain to compensate for losses of cholinergic function in the brain. These drugs have included acetylcholine precursors, muscarinic agonists, nicotinic agonists, and AChEIs (Livingston & Katona, 2000). The most highly developed and successful approaches to date have employed AChE inhibition. The first drug approved for general clinical use in AD was tacrine, followed a few years later by donepzil. Most recently, rivastigmine has been used in several countries around the world, and was released in the US in 2000. Another released AChEI is galantamine, and metrifonate was being developed by Bayer Corp as an AChE inhibitor (Bullock, 2001, 2002) and were approved by FDA. All of these drugs have been tested primarily in participants with AD, with most trials studying treatment in participants with mild to moderately severe illness.

Pharmacolological Treatment

Pharmacological treatment strategies in AD include three classes of agents: (a) mechanism based disease-modifying therapies such as vitamin E and selegiline, (b) mechanism-based therapies that compensate for transmitter deficits such as AchEIs, and (c) psychotropic agents administered to relieve behavioral symptoms of AD (Akhondzadeh & Noroozian, 2002). Various other agents have been used in an attempt to modify the course or improve the symptoms of AD, including Ginkgo biloba and anti-inflammatory agents (Akhondzadeh & Noroozian, 2002). The majority of FDA-approved drugs for Alzheimer's disease (AD) (e.g., tacrine, donepezil, rivastigmine, and galantamine) act by countering the cholinergic deficit associated with the cognitive dysfunction and are based on inhibition of the AChE (Akhondzadeh & Noroozian, 2002). Peripheral cholinergic (gastrointestinal) adverse effects for currently used cholinesterase inhibitors are common as well as other side effects such as hepatotoxicity (tacrine). More recently, the uncompetitive NMDA (N-methyl-aspartate) antagonist memantine that improves functioning and behavioral symptoms in participants with AD has been approved. Other targets, which include anti-inflammatory, antioxidative and estrogenic mechanisms, nicotinic receptors, nerve growth factors and the formation of neurofibrillary tangles and plaques, are the most important research activities in this field (Akhondzadeh & Noroozian, 2002). There are several studies and documents that indicate a unique role of herbal medicines in the treatment of Alzheimer's disease.

Ginkgo Biloba

Ginkgo biloba is an herbal medicine that has been used to treat a variety of ailments for thousands of years in China. An extract of Ginkgo biloba has been found in several studies to improve the symptoms and slow the progression of Alzheimer's disease. A study of 309 participants with mild dementia was performed. The participants were given either 120 mg of Ginkgo biloba extract or placebo every day for up to a year (Kanowski & Hoerr, 1997). At the 6-month point, 27% of those using ginkgo had moderate improvement on a variety of cognitive tests. Only 14% of those using placebo had an improvement on these tests. In a separate trial, 112 participants with chronic cerebral insufficiency received 120 mg per day of ginkgo biloba extract (Le Bars et al., 1997). The researchers found that the use of this extract led to significant improvements in blood and oxygen flow. Restricted blood and oxygen flow to the brain may be an important factor in the development of Alzheimer's. Ginkgo biloba extract (GBE) appears to be most effective in the early stages of Alzheimer's. This could potentially mean that participants with early Alzheimer's may be able to prevent being placed in a nursing home and to maintain a reasonably normal life. GBE has been shown to have the ability to normalize the acetylcholine receptors in the hippocampus area of the brain (the area most affected by the disease) in aged animals (De Feudis, 1991). GBE has also demonstrated the ability to increase cholinergic activity and to provide improvements in other aspects of the disease (Kleijnen, 1992). A double-blind study of 216 Alzheimer's participants or dementia caused by small strokes found that 240 mg of GBE daily led to significant improvements in a variety of clinical parameters when compared to placebo. The most effective form of GBE is one that is standardized to a concentration of 24% Ginkgo flavoglycosides.

A study compared the effectiveness of the most common Alzheimer's drugs, such as donepezil and rivastigmine, to that of a Ginkgo extract called EGb 761. The researchers determined that EGb 761 was as effective as any of these commonly prescribed drugs in treating the symptoms of Alzheimer's participants. In general, various forms of Gingko have been found to be safe, but in individuals who take aspirin or other anticoagulant drugs, Gingko should be taken with great caution and with the advice of a physician. Ginkgo is sold as a drug and regulated in Germany, and it is used in many other parts of the world to slow the progression of various forms of dementia. EGb 761 is the most commonly sold form of Gingko in Europe (Le Bars, Kieser, & Itil, 2000; Schulz, 2003).

A different study found that EGb 761 prevents beta-amyloid toxicity to brain cells, a key part of the development of the disease. All forms of Gingko need to be taken consistently for at least 12 weeks, a potentially difficult task for Alzheimer's participants, to determine whether the supplement is working. A recent double-blind, placebo-controlled randomized study of participants with Alzheimer's found that EGb 761 produced significant improvements in cognitive function compared to a placebo group. Other recent comprehensive surveys of multiple clinical trials found similar results with EGb 761 in participants with Alzheimer's diseases. An additional study found that EGb 761 produced cognitive improvement compared to placebo over a 26-week period using a variety of research measures. This study also demonstrated that EGb 761 was as safe as placebo during the study period (Le Bars et al., 2000; Schulz, 2003).

Huperzine A

Huperzine A is a chemical derived from a particular type of club moss (*Huperzia serrata*). Like caffeine and cocaine, huperzine A is a medicinally active, plant-derived chemical that belongs to the class known as alkaloids. This substance is really more a drug than an herb, but it is sold over the counter as a dietary supplement for memory loss and mental impairment. According to three Chinese double-blind trials enrolling a total of more than 450 people, use of huperzine A can significantly improve symptoms of Alzheimer's disease and other forms of dementia. One double-blind trial failed to find evidence of benefit, but it is relatively small study (Zhang, Tang, & Han, 1991; Xu, Gao, & Weng, 1995).

Vinpocetine

Vinpocetine is a chemical derived from vincamine, a constituent found in the leaves of common periwinkle (*Vinca minor*) as well as in the seeds of various African plants. It is used as a treatment for memory loss and mental impairment.

Developed in Hungary more than 20 years ago, vinpocetine is sold in Europe as a drug under the name Cavinton. In the US it is available as a "dietary supplement," although the substance probably doesn't fit that category by any rational definition. Vinpocetine doesn't exist to any significant extent in nature. Producing it requires significant chemical work performed in the laboratory. Several double-blind studies have evaluated vinpocetine for the treatment of Alzheimer's disease and related conditions. Unfortunately, most of these suffered from significant flaws in design and reporting. A review of the literature found three studies of acceptable quality, enrolling a total of 728 individuals. Perhaps the best of these was a 16-week, double-blind, placebo-controlled trial of 203 people with mild to moderate dementia, which found significant benefit in the treated group. However, even this trial suffered from several technical limitations, and the authors of the review concluded that vinpocetine cannot yet be regarded as a proven treatment. Currently, several better quality trials are underway (Szatmari & Whitehouse, 2003).

Galantamine

An alkaloid ChEI originally derived from European daffodils, or common snowdrops, this drug is a competitive and selective AchE inhibitor. Galantamine also allosterically modifies nicotinic Ach receptors, potentiating the presynaptic response to Ach. Like donepezil and rivastigmine, galantamine is brain selective. Galantamine has a half-life of 5–6 hours and is metabolized by the same CYP 450 enzymes as donepezil. Galantamine has not been associated with hepatotoxicity in clinical trials (Akhondzadeh & Noroozian, 2002).

Melissa officinalis and Salvia officinalis

It has been reported that *Melissa officinalis* (lemon balm) improves cognitive function and reduces agitation in participants with mild to moderate Alzheimer's disease. *Melissa officinalis* is known to have acetylcholine receptor activity in the central nervous system with both nicotinic and muscarinic binding properties (Perry, Pikering, Wang, Houghton, & Perry, 1998, 1999). A recent study has shown that this plant modulates mood and cognitive performance when administered to young healthy volunteers (Kennedy, Scholey, Tildesley, Perry, & Wesnes, 2002). In addition, a parallel, randomized, placebo-controlled study assessed the efficacy and safety of *Melissa officinalis* in 42 participants with mild to moderate AD (Akhondzadeh, Noroozian, Mohammadi, & Ohadinia, 2003a). Subjects were treated for 4 months. The main efficacy measures were the cognitive subscale of Alzheimer's Disease Assessment Scale (ADAS-cog) and the Clinical Dementia Rating-Sum of the Boxes (CDR-SB) scores. The CDR-SB provides a consensus-based global clinical measure by summing the ratings from 6 domains: memory, orientation, judgment, problem solving, community affairs, home, and hobbies, and personal care. The results revealed that participants receiving *Melissa officinalis* extract experienced significant improvements in cognition after 16 weeks of treatment. Improvements were seen on both the ADAS-cog and CDR-SB scores. The researchers observed no significant difference in the frequency of side-effects between the placebo group and those receiving the herb extract. However, the frequency of agitation was higher in the placebo group compared to those receiving active treatment (Akhondzadeh et al., 2003a). Moreover, another study showed that participants with mild to moderate Alzheimer's disease receiving *Salvia officinalis* (sage) extract experienced statistically significant benefits in cognition after 16 weeks of treatment (Akhondzadeh, Noroozian, Mohammadi, & Ohadinia, 2003b). The clinical relevance of these findings was emphasized by the improvements seen in both the ADAS-cog and CDR-SB measures in the *S. officinalis* extract group on both observed case and Intention to treat analyses. The side-effects associated with Salvia in this study were generally those expected from cholinergic stimulation, and similar to those reported with cholinesterase inhibitors (Wake et al., 2000). Frequency of agitation appeared higher in the placebo group and this may indicate an additional advantage for *Salvia officinalis* in the management of participants with Alzheimer's disease.

Depression

Depression is a serious disorder in today's society. With estimates of lifetime prevalence as high as 21% of the general population in some developed countries. As defined by the American Psychiatric Association, depression is a heterogeneous disorder often manifested with symptoms at the psychological, behavioral and physiological levels. Such participants are often reluctant to take synthetic antidepressants in their appropriate doses due to their anticipated side-effects including inability to drive a car, dry mouth, constipation and sexual dysfunction. As a therapeutic alternative, effective herbal drugs may offer advantages in terms of safety and tolerability, possibly also improving patient compliance (Richelson, 1994). The advent of the first antidepressants – the Monoamine Oxidase Inhibitors (MAOIs) and Tricyclic Antidepressants (TCAs) in the 1950s and 1960s represented a dramatic leap forward in the clinical management of depression. The subsequent development of the Selective Serotonin Reuptake Inhibitors (SSRIs) and the Serotonin Norepinephrine Reuptake Inhibitor (SNRI) venlafaxine in the past decade and a half has greatly enhanced the treatment of depression by offering participants medications that are as effective as the older agents but are generally more tolerable and safer in an overdose. The introduction of atypical antidepressants, such as bupropion, nefazadone, and mirtazapine, has added substantially to the available pharmacopoeia for depression. Nonetheless, rates of remission tend to be low and the risk of relapse and recurrence remains high. Thus, there is a need for more effective and less toxic agents (Richelson, 1994). Plant extracts are some of the most attractive sources of new drugs, and have produced promising results for the treatment of depression (Akhondzadeh, Kashani, Fotouhi, & Jarvandi, 2003).

Hypericum perforatum (St. John's Wort)

As one of the best-studied botanicals of all time, St. John's Wort (SJW) is notable for its ability to treat mild-to-moderate depression and is also known to be safe and effective for children. As a result, SJW has become very popular in the US where it is available over the counter. In Germany, physicians prescribe SJW to participants with mild-to-moderate depression (Gaster & Holroyd, 2000; Kim, Streltzer, & Goebert, 1999). The possible action of SJW stems in part from its hypericin and hypericin-like constituents, which may act on acetylcholinesterase by decreasing the degradation rate of acetylcholine. Sedative actions come from the hypericins, biflavones, and hyperforin. Other reports demonstrate a serotonergic activity, by which it can act as a weak serotonin-reuptake inhibitor (SSRI) that leads to fewer side-effects. In addition, sigma 1 receptors, which are affected by antidepressant medications in animal studies, may also be affected by SJW. Most likely, the demonstrated efficacy of this botanical in treating depression is through its synergistic effects, orchestrated by the multitude of components in the whole herb working both within and peripheral to the central nervous system (Hansgen, Vesper, & Ploch, 1994; Lieberman, 1998; Linde, Ramirez, & Mulrow, 1996; Wheatley, 1999).

A meta-analysis of 23 randomized trials which included 1757 outpatients with mainly mild or moderately severe depressive symptoms found that *Hypericum* extracts were significantly superior to placebo and similarly effective as standard antidepressants. Side effects occurred in 19.8% of participants on *Hypericum* and 52.8% of participants on standard antidepressants [23], and data analysis revealed a dropout rate of 0.8% for SJW and 3.0% for standard antidepressant drugs due to side-effects (Gaster & Holroyd, 2000; Kim et al., 1999). The action of SJW has been well characterized in direct comparisons with leading antidepressant medications. In a randomized controlled double-blind trial, 70 participants suffering from mild-to-moderate depression received one tablet of either SJW extract or fluoxetine twice a day for 6 weeks. participants were rated by the 17-item Hamilton Rating Scale for Depression (HAMD) and the von Zerssen Depression Scale (ZDS). HAMD scores significant decreased ($p < 0.001$) in the SJW group (50%) and in the fluoxetine group (58%), and ZDS also decreased in both treatments (42% and 52%, respectively). Assessments by physicians and participants indicated considerable improvement with no between-treatment differences. The conclusion of that study is that SJW was therapeutically equivalent to fluoxetine and is therefore a reasonable alternative to synthetic antidepressants. *Hypericum* extract has similarly been tested and showed an efficacy similar to that of sertraline in the treatment of mild-to-moderate depression in a small group of outpatients. Efficacy and tolerability of SJW was also compared with imipramine and was equivalent to that of the drug in treating mild-to-moderate depression. In addition, participants tolerated SJW better than imipramine (Gaster & Holroyd, 2000; Kim et al., 1999). In a review of over 3000 depressed participants spanning 34 double-blind trials, the effective dosage level of SJW for mild-to-moderate depression was between 500 and 1000 mg of standardized alcohol extract per day (Gaster & Holroyd, 2000). For participants with preexisting conductive heart dysfunction or elderly participants, high-dose *Hypericum* extract has been found to be safer with respect to cardiac function than tricyclic antidepressants. The side-effect profile of SJW extract is minor, especially when compared to the well known side effects of antidepressant medications. Due to its lack of monoamine oxidase (MAO) inhibition, SJW is not considered to interact negatively with MAO-inhibiting drugs or tyramine-containing foods. However, it has been shown that important SJW–drug interactions may occur. SJW can reduce the circulating levels of certain drugs. Synergistic therapeutic effects may also lead to complications and unfavorable treatment outcome. SJW is a potent inducer of cytochrome P450 (CYP) enzymes, particularly CYP 3A4 and/or P-glycoprotein, and it may also inhibit or induce other CYPs (Gelenberg, 2000). Although SJW induces photosensitivity in some participants, this not likely to happen with standard dosages; it has occurred mainly in HIV participants using larger than normal quantities for an antiviral effect. SJW is not recommended for use during pregnancy, because its safety in pregnancy has not been studied (Gelenberg, 2000).

Lavendula angustifolium (lavender)

Lavender is used principally as an aromatic essential oil for relaxation. In a single-blind randomized control trial, 80 women who took daily baths with lavender oil experienced improved mood, reduced aggression, and a more positive outlook (Akhondzadeh et al., 2003). Furthermore, the combination of lavender (60 drops/day of a lavandula tincture) and imipramine (100 mg/day) was found to be more effective in the treatment of depression than either treatment alone, according to a double-blind randomized control trial. The findings of this study suggested that taking a moderate amount of lavender may help reduce the amount of tricyclic antidepressants needed to treat depression, leading to fewer side-effects (Akhondzadeh et al., 2003).

Crocus sativus (Saffron)

Saffron is the world's most expensive spice and apart from its traditional value as a food additive recent studies indicate its potential as an anti-cancer agent and memory enhancer (Abdullaev, 2002; Abe & Saito, 2000; Rios, Recio, Giner, & Manez, 1996). The value of saffron (dried stigmas of *Crocus sativus L.*) is determined by the existence of three main secondary metabolites: (1) crocin and its derivatives which are responsible for color, (2) picrocrocin, responsible for taste, and (3) safranal responsible for odor. This plant belongs to the Iridaceae family and as is considered an excellent aid for stomach ailments and an antispasmodic, helps digestion and increases appetite. It is also relieves renal colic, reduces stomach ache and relieves tension (Hosseinzadeh and Younesi, 2002; Rios et al., 1996). Saffron is used for depression in Persian traditional medicine (Akhondzadeh, Fallah Pour, Afkham, Jamshidi, & Khalighi-Cigarodi, 2004). Indeed, it is a Persian herb with a history as long as the Persian Empire itself. Iran, the world's largest producer of saffron, has been investing in research into saffron's potential medicinal uses. Much of the work surrounds its traditional application for alleviating depression. The clinical findings suggest that saffron is a safe and effective antidepressant. For example, in a randomized, double-blind study, 30 mg of saffron extract (in capsules) given for 6 weeks resulted in significant alleviation of depression compared to those on placebo, and did so without evident side-effects. This study was a follow-up to a preliminary trial in which the same saffron preparation performed as well as imipramine for treating depression in a double-blind trial. In further preliminary work, when saffron was compared to the drug fluoxetine, saffron performed as well as fluoxetine in the treatment of depression. (Akhondzadeh et al., 2004, 2005a; Noorbala, Akhondzadeh, Tamacebi-pour, & Jamshidi, 2005).

Anxiety

Generalized Anxiety Disorder (GAD) is the most common anxiety disorder but is generally less severe than panic disorder. GAD is probably the disorder most often found with a coexisting mental disorder, usually another anxiety disorder or a mood disorder. The ratio of women to men is about 2 to 1. The cause of GAD is not known. The primary symptoms of GAD are anxiety, motor tension, autonomic hyperactivity and cognitive vigilance. DSM-IV employs the following criteria for GAD: excessive anxiety and worry, occurring more days than not for at least 6 months, about a number of events or activities that are difficult to control (Akhondzadeh et al., 2001a). Autonomic symptoms are no longer required for diagnosis. The principal neurotransmitter systems thought to modify anxiety are the gamma-aminobutyric acid (GABA) system, and the noradrenergic, serotonergic, dopaminergic and histaminergic system. The most effective treatment of participants with GAD is probably one that combines psychotherapeutic, pharmacotherapeutic and supportive approaches. Because of the long-term nature of the disorder, a treatment plan must be carefully thought out. The two major drugs to be considered for the treatment of GAD are buspirone and the benzodiazepines. Benzodiazepines are the drugs most frequently prescribed for the treatment of anxiety disorders. They act through the benzodiazepines-GABA receptor, where they inhibit neuronal activity by increasing the chloride ion influx into neurons. This includes hyperpolarization of the nerve cell, a condition that leads to decreased responsiveness to incoming stimuli (Akhondzadeh et al., 2001a). Several problems are associated with the use of benzodiazepines (BZDs) in

GAD. About 25–30% of all participants fail to respond, and tolerance and dependence may occur. Some participants also experience impaired alertness while taking the drugs. In addition, there are several reports that indicate cognition impairment induced by benzodiazepines. The cessation of use of benzodiazepines can induce a withdrawal syndrome, characterized by: (1) psychological symptoms of anxiety such as apprehension and irritability, (2) physiological symptoms of anxiety such as tremor and palpitation, and (3) perceptual disturbances such as hypersensivity to light, sounds, touch or motion. Only one-third of participants who have GAD seek psychiatric treatment. Many participants go to general practioners, internists, cardiologists and also use herbal medicine like passiflora (Akhondzadeh et al., 2001a).

Passiflora incarnata

Passionflower (*Passiflora incarnata*) is a woody, hairy, climbing vine and is reputed to have sedative/anxiolytic properties. It has been used widely as an ingredient of herbal remedies, chiefly in the form of a liquid extract tincture. The commission E approved the internal use of passionflower for nervous restlessness. The British Herbal Compendium indicates its use for sleep disorders, restlessness, nervous stress, and anxiety [26–29]. A double-blind and randomized trial showed that that passiflora extract is an effective drug for the management of generalized anxiety disorder, and the low incidence of impairment of job performance with passiflora extract compared to oxazepam is an advantage (Akhondzadeh et al., 2001a).

Kava

Kava is a ceremonial and social drink in the South Pacific, containing approximately 250 mg of kava lactones. Its use is constrained by elaborate rituals in Fiji, Samoa, and Tonga where it has also been used for analgesia. Kava contains alpha-pyrones, a recently discovered class of potent skeletal muscle relaxants. In Germany, doses of 70–80 mg kava lactones are given t.i.d. for stress and muscle spasms. For milder symptoms, a dose of 60–70 mg kava lactones q.d. is usually sufficient. When 6 of the 9 major alpha-pyrones found in Kava extract are administered together in animal studies, they create a synergistic effect. Whether or not Kava affects benzodiazepine or GABA-A receptors is controversial. However, it has anticonvulsant properties in animal models. Kava exerts some serotonin blocking activity and sodium channel blocking. In preclinical studies, the primary calming effect is mediated through the amygdale (Lehmann, Kinzler, & Friedmann, 1996; Lindenberg & Pitule-Schodel, 1990; Pittler and Ernst, 2000). Kava's traditional use as an analgesic was confirmed in preclinical studies. Naloxone, when administered in doses that blocked morphine-induced analgesia, did not reverse Kava's antinociceptive effects. The intriguing finding that the analgesia induced by Kava occurs by way of nonopiate pathways deserves further study. Some double-blind, placebo-controlled studies support the efficacy of Kava for anxiety. In participants with generalized anxiety disorder, Kava worked as well as oxazepam without producing any cognitive dysfunction. "Menopause related" anxiety in 20 women improved on kava by week 1 compared with no improvement in 20 women on placebo. Anxious participants receiving 70 mg kava lactones t.i.d. improved compared to a placebo group by week 1. They became increasingly better over 28 days, as measured by Hamilton Anxiety ratings, CGI, and self-ratings, with no side-effects reported. In the longest study to date, 108 participants were randomized to 70 mg kava lactones t.i.d. or to placebo. By week 25, Hamilton Anxiety scores dropped from 31 to 10 in the 59 participants on kava and fell from 30 to 15 in the 49 participants on placebo; 75% of the kava group attained significant global improvement with no evidence of dependency compared to 50% in the placebo group. Although the participants had clinically significant anxiety, this study, like the Lehmann et al. (1996) study, suffered from lack of precise diagnoses. Recent reviews concluded that kava extract is relatively safe and more effective than placebo. Only three of the studies met criteria for meta-analysis, including the selection of participants by HAM-A>19 and treatment with kava extract WS1490 100 mg t.i.d. (210 kavapyrones/day). Because of methodological questions in the studies, the authors suggested more rigorous risk-benefit trials (Lehmann et al., 1996; Lindenberg & Pitule-Schodel, 1990; Pittler and Ernst, 2000). Dosage and side-effects: Two postmarketing studies of over 3000 participants found a 1.5% and a 2.3% incidence of side-effects. Gastrointestinal complaints, allergic skin reaction, headache, and photosensitivity were the most common side-effects. Other complaints included restlessness, drowsiness, lack of energy, and tremor. Schelosky et al. described 4 cases in which kava induced symptoms suggestive of central dopaminergic antagonism, including dystonic reactions (eyes, neck, and trunk), oral/lingual dyskinesias, and one case of worsening Parkinsonian symptoms in a woman on levodopa (Schelosky, Raffauf, & Jendroska, 1995). Until more information is available, kava should be avoided in participants with Parkinson's disease and in those at risk for dystonia or dyskinesia. No studies of long-term safety, teratogenicity, or mutagenicity beyond 6 months have been done. Kava should not be combined with alcohol or other sedatives (Lehmann et al., 1996; Lindenberg & Pitule-Schodel, 1990; Pittler and Ernst, 2000).

Sleep Disorders

Herbal medicines are used extensively as sleep aids. A study of the use of nonprescription sleep products in an ambulatory elderly population found that 27% of total participants had used a nonprescription sleep product in the past year (Sproule, Busto, & Buckle, 1999).

Valerian

Valerian (*Valeriana officianalis*) is probably the best known herbal sedative. However, there is only weak research support for its mechanism of action and efficacy. Valerian is thought to act by potently binding to GABA-A receptors. Four small double-blind trials in insomnia and five studies in otherwise healthy people with sleep disturbance have been done. It may require 2–4 weeks for valerian to work. In one study, which compared valerian and hops used together (hops has estrogenic effects) with flurazepam, a benzodiazepine, the researchers concluded that valerian and hops did not cause the deficits in attention and reaction time seen with benzodiazepines. There have been some reports of dystonia and hepatitis from valerian, but the preparations most likely contained a mixture of ingredients making it difficult to place the onus on valerian. Patient compliance is a problem since valerian tea and tablets often have the odor of "old gym socks" (Balderer and Borbely, 1985; Connor & Davidson, 2002; Donath, Quispe, & Diefenbach, 2000).

Lavandula angustifolia (English Lavender)

English Lavender is approved by Germany's Commission E for nervousness and insomnia, as well as for loss of appetite, circulatory disorders and dyspeptic complaints (PDR for Herbal Medicines, 2000). Like hops, lavender is sometimes put into a pillow or beneath the pillow to promote sleep. There are some preclinical studies suggesting the sedative qualities of English Lavender (Delaveau, Guillemain, Narcisse, & Rousseau, 1989).

Substance Use Disorders

Many existing pharmacological and psychosocial interventions for substance use disorders are solidly evidence-based. Yet, there is a need to identify additional treatments. The use of natural and complementary therapies fits well within a range of existing theoretical frameworks for understanding and treating drug dependence. They could fulfil a variety of roles:

(1) As adjunctive treatments to existing pharmacological or psychosocial interventions.
(2) As treatment alternatives for substance users who are not eligible for existing treatments, who are nonresponsive to existing treatments, or who refuse existing treatments.
(3) As treatment options in countries or regions where evidence-based interventions are not routinely available.
(4) As treatment options for disorders where there is no current gold standard treatment.

It has been estimated that up to 45% of substance users employ natural and complementary therapies. Surveys suggest that more than three-quarters of substance users contacting treatment services find complementary or alternative treatments acceptable (Dean, 2005).

Substance Withdrawal Syndrome

The traditional aim of detoxification is to achieve a safe and humane withdrawal from a drug of dependence. Although unlikely to produce long-term abstinence in itself, detoxification is an attractive treatment option for many substance users, and may permit individuals to reduce their drug use, or prepare them for other treatment programs.

Pharmacological Interventions

Pharmacological management of substance withdrawal is standard practice in many countries, and an important component of comprehensive treatment provision. Use of complementary medicines with relevant pharmacological properties fits well within existing models of withdrawal management (Dean, 2005).

Hypericum (Hypericum perforatum)
Hypericum has also been investigated for its effects on nicotine withdrawal. Similar pharmacological effects to existing treatments such as bupropion has partly contributed to the interest in hypericum. In a clinical study, 45 adult smokers were randomized to receive an oral spray containing hypericum or placebo spray, in addition to brief counseling sessions and nicotine replacement patches. Although abstinence rates were similar in each group after 1 month, hypericum was associated with lower craving scores, and less anxiety, restlessness and sleeplessness compared with controls (Becker, Bock, & Carmona-Barros, 2003). An animal study also reports that high doses of hypericum attenuated effects of nicotine withdrawal in mice. This effect was greatest when hypericum was initiated prior to nicotine cessation rather than delayed until emergence of withdrawal symptoms (Catania, Firenzuoli, & Crupi, 2003).

Other Herbs
Numerous complementary medicines are utilized for their putative sedative properties. Some, such as valerian (*Valeriana officinalis*), have evidence to support their use in insomnia. Sedative compounds have a potential role in the management of agitation, insomnia or anxiety associated with substance withdrawal. Pilot studies have reported beneficial effects of passionflower (*Passiflora incarnata*) for opiate withdrawal (Dean, 2005) or melatonin for benzodiazepine or nicotine cessation (Akhondzadeh et al., 2001b; Dean, 2005). However, there are few recent clinical studies of these agents focusing on withdrawal management. One review discusses the mechanisms of passionflower in the treatment of substance use disorders, focusing on one particular constituent, a benzoflavone moiety, which animal studies have shown to reduce withdrawal severity from various substances (Akhondzadeh et al., 2001b). Unfortunately, this review does not address the comparative effects between this constituent and whole plant preparations typically utilized for sedative and anxiolytic effects. Morphine withdrawal signs in mice has been reported for rosemary (Rosmarinus officinalis) and the corn poppy (Papaver rhoeas), which may possess opioid and anticholinergic effects. Positive effects in animal studies do not necessarily translate to clinical effectiveness. These studies may contribute to our understanding of the pharmacology of these compounds; however, without ongoing research, they provide little to inform treatment (Dean, 2005).

Attention Deficit and Hyperactivity Disorder (ADHD)

ADHD is a loosely defined assemblage of neuropsychiatric symptom clusters that emerge in childhood and often persist into adulthood. Though the means to its diagnosis is only empirical, ADHD increasingly is being employed as a diagnostic label for individuals who display a wide range of symptoms, such as restlessness, inability to stay focused, mood swings, temper tantrums, problems completing tasks, disorganization, inability to cope with stress, and impulsivity (Brue & Oakland, 2002).

The etiology of ADHD is not understood, yet potent drugs are being employed for its medical management while safe and effective alternatives are being neglected. Neurochemical studies suggest alterations in catecholaminergic-mainly dopaminergic and noradrenergic-transmitter functions markedly contribute to the symptoms of ADHD. The symptoms of ADHD are significantly ameliorated by agents that specifically influence these neurotransmitter systems, and animal studies implicate areas of the brain in which these neurotransmitters are most dominant (Brue & Oakland, 2002). ADHD is the most prevalent behavioral disorder in children and frequently its symptoms are commingled with learning problems, oppositional conduct, and depression, which altogether compound the family's emotional burden. Psychostimulant medications are generally the first choice in medication of ADHD. Approximately 70% of the children treated show improvement in the primary ADHD symptoms and in comorbidity such as conduct disorder, although the benefits may not hold beyond two years. Despite the well-established efficacy and safety of stimulants for ADHD, alternative medicines are still needed for several reasons. About 30% of children and adolescents with ADHD may not respond to stimulants or may be unable to tolerate potential adverse events such as decreased appetite, mood lability and sleep disturbances. Although stimulants do not increase risk for later substance abuse in ADHD, concerns have been raised about special prescription rules, and a potential for abuse by persons other than the ADHD subjects (Akhondzadeh, Mohammadi, & Momeni, 2005b; Brue & Oakland, 2002). Herbal medicines have been shown to ameliorate ADHD related behaviors in individuals without this disorder. For example, Ginkgo biloba is somewhat effective for disorders dementia and memory impairment. A review of 40 controlled trials found at least a partial positive outcome in nearly all subjects who had cerebral insufficiency (e.g., difficulties of concentration and memory, absentmindedness). This finding may help to provide support for using Ginkgo in children with ADHD, especially those who are primarily inattentive. Moreover, Ginkgo improves cerebrovascular blood flow and attention may help to reduce hyperactivity due to boredom and lack of focus (Brue & Oakland, 2002). A recent study showed that Passiflora may be a novel therapeutic agent for the treatment of attention deficit hyperactivity disorder. In addition, a tolerable side-effect profile may be considered as one of the advantages of Passiflora in the treatment of attention deficit hyperactivity disorder (Akhondzadeh et al., 2005b).

Migraine

Migraine prevalence studies have indicated that the condition is suffered by more than 17% of the female and six percent of the male population in the United States. In addition to the debilitating effect of a migraine attack, sufferers report a significant impact on their quality of life between attacks. Many migraine participants report that the fear of getting a headache totally disrupts their ability to plan social events, vacations, and other family activities. Available research on the treatment of migraine focused in acute treatment and prophylactic medications. Advances in acute treatment are well documented. Sumatriptan, a serotonin-1 agonist administered subcutaneously, orally, or intranasaly, is effective in alleviating the pain and associated symptoms of the acute migraine attack. In contrast there has been limited progress in the prophylactic treatment of migraine. Herbal medicine approaches to migraine prevention have shown some promise (Sensenig, Marrongelle, Johnson, & Staverosky, 2001).

Feverfew

There is significant comorbidity of migraine with mood and anxiety disorders. Three out of four double-blind, placebo-controlled trials found that feverfew reduces the frequency and severity of migraines and the associated nausea and vomiting. The negative outcome of the fourth study was due to its use of a preparation standardized for parthenolide (thought to be the key compound with sesquiterpine lactones), instead of the whole leaf extract of feverfew used by other researchers. Parthenolide is unstable and needs other components for its activity. In fact, the Canadian Regulatory Commission will only certify whole leaf extract of feverfew as an effective medication. Spurred by uncertainty about the ideal preparation and concerned about what effects previous exposure to feverfew has on patient expectations, a recent study reduced the possibility of this bias by selecting only those participants who had never taken feverfew before. In this 4-month, three-phase, crossover study, 57 participants were divided into two groups. The feverfew group experienced significant reduction in migraine pain only when they were on feverfew. The mechanism of activity is uncertain. However, participants who are not able to obtain relief on standard prescription medications, many of which have undesirable side-effects, could benefit from feverfew. Feverfew is generally well tolerated with very few side-effects. However, feverfew can affect bleeding time and should not be used with warfarin. Feverfew should be discontinued 2–3 weeks prior to surgery. Doses range from 100–200 mg/day (2–4 pills) (Sensenig et al., 2001). Feverfew has additional uses including treatment of menstrual irregularities and arthritis. Feverfew plants from different parts of the world contain different substances. For example, the variety in Guatemala is without parthenolide and has not yet been tested in the study of migraine (Sensenig et al., 2001). This is an example of the different contexts in which experience by accomplished herbalists is needed to guide further scientific research.

Butterbur

Petadolex contains an extract of *Petasites hybridus* (Butterbur root) with demonstrated benefits for the prophylaxis of migraines. A randomized, double blind, placebo controlled study of 58 migraine sufferers found a significant reduction in the frequency of headaches (46% at week 4, 60% at week 8, and 50% at week 12) in the group given Petadolex 50 mg b.i.d. compared to those given placebo (24%, 17%, and 10%, respectively) (Sensenig et al., 2001).

Conclusion

Many factors underlie the growing popularity of herbal treatments for a variety of chronic conditions. Interestingly, people who use alternative therapies are not necessarily uninformed. If anything, they are more "culturally creative" (i.e., comfortable with cultural changes) and more highly educated (Astin, 1998).

Many people using herbal medicines find the healthcare alternatives are more congruent with their own values, beliefs, and philosophical orientations toward health and life. Similarly, it seems likely that many people feel that herbal medicines are empowering by allowing them to treat themselves without seeing a physician. (This same attitude may be behind the growing popularity of patient-initiated diagnostic scanning procedures such as whole body scans). The danger is that many people believe that herbal medicines have no toxicity problems or even side effects. In addition, they are not aware of many possible interactions of herbal medicine with concurrent prescribed medications.

References

Abdullaev, F. I. (2002). Cancer chemopreventive and tumoricidal properties of saffron (Crocus sativus L.). *Experimental Biology and Medicine, 227*, 20–25.

Abe, K., & Saito, H. (2000). Effects of saffron and its constituent crocin on learning behavior and long-term potentiation. *Phytotherapy Research, 14*, 149–152.

Akhondzadeh, S., Naghavi, H. R., Vazirian, M., Shayeganpour, A., Rashidi, H., & Khani, M. (2001a). Passionflower in the treatment of generalized anxiety: A double-blind and randomized trial with oxazepam. *Journal of Clinical Pharmacy and Therapeutics, 26*, 363–367.

Akhondzadeh, S., Kashani, L., Mobaseri, M., Hosseini, S. H., Nikzad, S., & Khani, M. (2001b). Passionflower in the treatment of opiates withdrawal: a double-blind randomized controlled trial. *Journal of Clinical Pharmacy and Therapeutics, 26*, 369–373.

Akhondzadeh, S., & Noroozian, M. (2002). Alzheimer's disease: pathophysiology and Pharmacotherapy. *Idrugs, 4*, 1167–1172.

Akhondzadeh, S., Noroozian, M., Mohammadi, M., & Ohadinia, S. (2003a). Melissa officinalis extract in the treatment of patients with mild to moderate Alzheimer's disease: a double blind, randomised, placebo controlled trial. *Journal of Neurology, Neurosurgery and Psychiatry, 74*, 863–866.

Akhondzadeh, S., Noroozian, M., Mohammadi, M., & Ohadinia, S. (2003b). Salvia officinalis extract in the treatment of patients with mild to moderate Alzheimer's disease: a double blind, randomized and placebo-controlled trial. *Journal of Clinical Pharmacy and Therapeutics, 28*, 53–59.

Akhondzadeh, S., Kashani, L., Fotouhi, A., & Jarvandi, S. (2003). Comparison of Lavandula angostofolia Mill. tincture and imipramine in the treatment of mild to moderate depression: a double-blind, randomized pilot study. *Progress in Neuropsychopharmacology and Biological Psychiatry, 27*, 123–127.

Akhondzadeh, S., Fallah Pour, H., Afkham, K., Jamshidi, A. H., & Khalighi-Cigarodi, F. (2004). Comparison of Crocus sativus L. and imipramine in the treatment of mild to moderate depression: a pilot double-blind randomized trial [ISRCTN45683816]. *BMC Complementary and Alternative Medicine, 4*, 12.

Akhondzadeh, S., Tamacebi-pour, N., Noorbala, A. A., Amini, H., Fallah Pour, H., Jamshidi, A. H., & Khani, M. (2005a). *Crocus sativus L.* in the treatment of mild to moderate depression: A double-blind, randomized and placebo controlled trial. *Phytotherapy Research, 19*, 25–29.

Akhondzadeh, S., Mohammadi, M. R., & Momeni F. (2005b). *Passiflora incarnata* in treatment of attention-deficit hyperactivity disorder in children and adolescents. *Therapy, 2*, 609–614.

Astin, J. A. (1998). Why patients use alternative medicine: results of a national study. *Journal of the American Medical Association, 279*, 1548–1553.

Balderer, G., & Borbely, A. A. (1985). Effect of valerian on human sleep. *Psychopharmacology, 87*, 406–409.

Becker, B., Bock, B., & Carmona-Barros, R. (2003). St John's Wort oral spray reduces withdrawal symptoms during quitting smoking. In: *Society for Research on Nicotine and Tobacco 9th Annual Meeting*, New Orleans, Louisiana.

Brue, A. W., & Oakland, T. D. (2002). Alternative treatments for attention deficit hyperactivity disorders: Does evidence support their use. *Alternative Therapy Medicine, 8*, 68–74.

Bullock, R. (2001). Drug treatment in dementia. *Current Opinion in Psychiatry, 14, 349–353.*

Bullock, R. (2002). New drugs for Alzheimer's disease and other dementias. *British Journal of Psychiatry, 180*, 135–139.

Connor, K. M., & Davidson, J. R. (2002). A placebo-controlled study of Kava kava in generalized anxiety disorder. *International Clinical Psychopharmacology, 17, 185–188.*

Catania, M. A., Firenzuoli, F., & Crupi, A. (2003). Hypericum perforatum attenuates nicotine withdrawal signs in mice. *Psychopharmacology, 169*, 186–189.

Dean, A. J. (2005). Natural and complementary therapies for substance use disorders. *Current Opinion in Psychiatry, 18*, 271–276.

Delaveau, P., Guillemain, J., Narcisse, G., & Rousseau, A. (1989). Neurodepressive properties of essential oil of lavender. *Comptes Rendus des Seances de la Societe de Biologie et de ses Filiales, 183*, 342–348.

De Feudis, F. V. (1991). Gingko biloba extract (EGb761): pharmacological activities and clinical applications. Paris: Elsevier.

Donath, F., Quispe, S., & Diefenbach, K. (2000). Critical evaluation of the effect of valerian extract on sleep structure and sleep quality. *Pharmacopsychiatry, 33*,47–53.

Evans, D. A., Funkenstein, H. H., & Albert, M. S. (1989). Prevalence of Alzheimer's disease in a community population of older persons: higher than previously reported. *Journal of the American Medical Association, 262*, 2551–2556.

Francis, P. T., Palmer, A. M., Snape, M., & Wilcock, G. K. (1999). The cholinergic hypothesis of Alzheimer's disease: a review of progress. *Journal of Neurology, Neurosurgery and Psychiatry, 54*, 137–147.

Gaster, B., & Holroyd, J. (2000). St. John's wort for depression: A systematic review. *Archive of Internal of Medicine, 160*, 152–156.

Geldmacher, D. S., & Whitehouse, P. J. (1997). Differential diagnosis of Alzheimer's disease. *Neurology, 48*(Suppl. 6), S2–S9.

Gelenberg, A. J. (2000). St. John's Wort update. *Biological Therapies in Psychiatry, 23*, 22–24.

Hansgen, K. D., Vesper, J., & Ploch, M. (1994). Multicenter double-blind study examining the antidepressant effectiveness of the hypericum extract L160. *Journal of Geriatric Psychiatry and Neurology, 7*, S15–S18.

Hosseinzadeh, H., & Younesi, H. (2002). Petal and stigma extracts of Crocus sativus L. have antinociceptive and anti-inflammatory effects in mice. *BMC Pharmacology, 2*, 7.

Kanowski, S., & Hoerr, R. (1997). Proof of the efficacy of the gingko biloba special extract egb761 in outpatients suffering from mild to moderate primary degenerative dementia of the Alzheimer type of multi-infarct dementia. *Phytomedicine, 4*, 215–222.

Kennedy, D. O., Scholey, A. B., Tildesley, N. T. J., Perry, E. K., & Wesnes, K. A. (2002). Modulation of mood and cognitive performance following acte administration of Melissa officinalis (lemon balm). *Pharmacology and Biochemistry and Behavior, 72*, 953–964.

Kim, H. L., Streltzer, J., & Goebert, D. (1999). St. John's wort for depression: A meta-analysis of well-defined clinical trials. *Journal of Nervous and Mental Disease, 187*, 532–539.

Kleijnen, J. (1992). Gingko biloba. *Lancet, 340*, 1136–1139

Le Bars, P. L., Katz, M. M., Berman, N., Itil, T. M., Freedman, A. M., & Schatzberg, A. F. (1997). A placebo-controlled, double-blind, randomized trial of an extract of Ginkgo biloba for dementia. North American EGb Study Group. *Journal of the American Medical Association, 278*, 1327–1332.

Le Bars, P. L., Kieser, M., & Itil, K. Z. (2000). A 26-week analysis of a double-blind, placebo-controlled trial of the ginkgo biloba extract EGb 761 in dementia. *Dementia, Geriatric and Cognition Disorder, 11*, 230–237.

Lehmann, E., Kinzler, E., & Friedmann, J. (1996). Efficacy of a special Kava extract (Piper methysticum) in patients with states of anxiety, tension, excitedness of non-mental origin: A double-blind, placebo-controlled study of four weeks treatment. *Phytomedicine, 3*, 113–119.

Lieberman, S. (1998). Nutriceutical review of St. John's wort (hypericum perforatum) for the treatment of depression. *Journal of Women's Health, 7*, 177–182.

Linde, K., Ramirez, G., & Mulrow, C. D. (1996). St. John's wort for depression: An overview and meta-analysis of randomised clinical trials. *BMJ, 313*, 253–258.

Lindenberg, D., & Pitule-Schodel, H. (1990). Kava in comparison with oxazepam and anxiety disorders: A double- blind study of clinical effectiveness. *Fortschr Medicine, 108*, 49–54.

Livingston, G., & Katona, C. (2000). How useful are cholinesterase inhibitor in the treatment of Alzheimer's disease? A number needed to treat analysis. *International Journal of Geriatric Psychiatry, 15*, 203–207.

Medical Economics. (2000). PDR (Physicians' Desk Reference) for Herbal Medicines (2nd edn). Montvale, NJ: Medical Economics Company.

McKhann, G., Drachman, D., Folstein, M., Katzman, R., Price, D., & Stadlan, E. M. (1984). Clinical diagnosis of AD: Report of NINCDS-ADRDA work group under the auspices of department of health and human services task force on AD. *Neurology, 34*, 939–944.

Noorbala, A. A., Akhondzadeh, S., Tamacebi-pour, N., & Jamshidi, A. H. (2005). Hydro-alcoholic extract of *Crocus sativus L.* versus fluoxetine in the treatment of mild to moderate depression: A double-blind, randomized pilot trial. *Ethnopharmacology, 97*, 281–284.

Perry, E. K., Pikering, A. T., Wang, W. W., Houghton, P. J., & Perry, N. S. (1998). Medicinal plants and Alzheimer's disease: integrating ethnobotanical and contemporary scientific evidence. *Journal of Alternative and Complementary Medicine, 4*, 419–428.

Perry, E. K., Pikering, A. T., Wang, W. W., Houghton, P. J., & Perry, N. S. (1999). Medicinal plants and Alzheimer's disease: from etnobotany to phytotherapy. *Journal of Pharmacology, 51*, 527–534.

Pittler, M. H., & Ernst, E. (2000). Efficacy of kava extract for treating anxiety: Systematic review and meta-analysis. *Journal of Clinical Psychopharmacology, 20*, 84–89.

Richelson, E. (1994). Pharmacology of antidepressants-characteristic of the ideal drug. *Mayo Clinic Proceeding, 69*, 1069–1081.

Rios, J. L., Recio, M. C., Giner, R. M., & Manez, S. (1996). An update review of saffron and its active constituents. *Phytotherapy Research, 10*, 189–193.

Schelosky, L., Raffauf, C., & Jendroska, K. (1995). Kava and dopamine antagonism [letter]. *Journal of Neurology, Neurosurgery and Psychiatry, 58*, 639–640.

Schulz, V. (2003). Gingko extract or cholinesterase inhibitors in patients with dementia: what clinical trials and guidelines fail to consider. *Phytomedicine, 14*(Suppl. 10), 74–79.

Schulz, V., Hansel R., & Tyler, V. E. (1998). *Rational phytotherapy: a physicians' guide to herbal medicine* (3rd ed.). Berlin, Germany: Springer-Verlag.
Sensenig, J., Marrongelle, J., Johnson, M., & Staverosky, T. (2001). Treatment of migraine with targated nutrition focused on improved assimilation and eliminiation. *Alternative Medicine Review, 6*, 488–494.
Sproule, B.A., Busto, U.E., & Buckle, C. (1999). The use of non-prescription sleep products in the elderly. International Journal of Geriatric Psychiatry 14, 851–857.
Szatmari, S. Z., & Whitehouse, P. J. (2003). Vinpocetine for cognitive impairment and dementia (Cochrane Review). Cochrane Database Systematic Review CD003119.
Wake, G., Court, J., Pikering, A., Lewis, R., Wilkins, R., & Perry, E. (2000). CNS acetylcholine receptor activity in European medicinal plants traditionally used to improve failing memory. *Journal of Ethnopharmacology, 69*, 105–114.
Wheatley, D. (1999). Hypericum in seasonal affective disorder (SAD). *Current Medical Research Opinion, 15*, 33–7.
Xu, S. S., Gao, Z. X., & Weng, Z. (1995). Efficacy of tablet huperzine-A on memory, cognition, and behavior in Alzheimer's disease. *Zhongguo Yao Li Xue Bao, 16, 391–395.*
Zhang, R. W., Tang, X. C., & Han, Y. Y. (1991). Drug evaluation of huperzine A in the treatment of senile memory disorders [in Chinese; English abstract]. *Zhongguo Yao Li Xue Bao, 12*, 250–252.

Section III

Primary Nonverbal Approaches

Rosenbaum's (2005) recent paper about the neglect of motor control as the pariah of psychology finds definite parallels in the neglect of the nonverbal medium in psychotherapy and prevention. Rosenbaum documented this neglect in textbooks, journals, and in the Social Science Citation Index. He developed some hypotheses about this neglect: (1) there aren't celebrities in the science of motor control while there are many in the cognitive area, (2) talk is human while motor control is animal, (3) motoric activities do not need the same kind of intelligence that is needed for talking, (4) motor behavior is too hard to study, (5) we think before we act, therefore why worry about what seem to be automatic actions? (6) motor control is the baby but talk is the bath water, and (7) motor behavior should be studied by neuroscientists and not by psychologists.

By the same token, we can find the same neglect in psychotherapy as well as in prevention treatises. Rather than accept this conclusion as a given, this writer made a summary check on samples of psychotherapy journals and textbooks to search for how many among these sources included nonverbal motor therapies. He found none. There are no references to nonverbal therapies in psychotherapy textbooks and journals. This area, however, has journals of its own but they are not read by the prevention and psychotherapy communities. They are a separate area of intervention independent of talk-based therapy.

The nonverbal medium is just not mentioned or used in psychotherapy. L'Abate and Baggett (1997, pp. 315–322) reviewed many of the nonverbal methods to improve behavior, and concluded: "The use of nonverbal behavior for therapeutic and para-therapeutic purposes has had, thus far, limited applications in clinical circles" (p. 315). L'Abate and Baggett mentioned some of the leaders who stressed the importance of using nonverbal techniques in psychotherapy, like Virginia Satir, Frits Perls, Albert Pesso, Ida Rolf, William Schults, and many others. L'Abate and Baggett also offered a rationale for the use of nonverbal techniques in psychotherapy (pp. 316–317) and gave examples of nonverbal exercises for groups of individuals, couples, and families (pp. 318–321). Unfortunately, as far as this writer knows, the literature on nonverbal approaches to psychotherapy has not been validated by research as much as the verbal medium, to the point that if positive results are shown, they have been ignored by the prevention and psychotherapy professions. A great many nonverbal techniques received validation by the influence and mystique of a guru rather than by controlled evaluation. That state of affairs is unfortunate because it decreases the options that can be given to those who need help.

Why has this area been neglected by prevention and psychotherapy oriented professionals? In addition to the hypotheses raised by Rosenbaum (2005), some possible answers come to mind. First, the history of psychotherapy started with talk, and talk continued to be the preferred, if not the only, medium of communication and healing over the last century, and spilled over into this century. Second, it is easier to talk with someone in an office than to exhibit behavior that would be contextually inappropriate, i.e., one would not dance with a patient in one's office. Third, while nonverbal methods of therapy need to be integrated into the psychotherapeutic process, they, by definition, do not fit into the promotional approaches. They are based on a prolonged interaction with a professional, are expensive, and there is no knowledge about how many of these techniques become self-administered, independently of the presence and direction of a professional. Fourth, nonverbal behavior is for children, and while therapies for children do stress the nonverbal medium, adults do not need to be bothered with "childish" behavior.

In spite of these conclusions, there are indeed many nonverbal approaches, as shown in this section. They are easy to learn, become self-administered once the learning is completed, and last a lifetime.

References

L'Abate, L., & Baggett, M. S. (1997). *The self in the family: A classification of personality, criminality, and psychopathology*. New York: Wiley.

Rosenbaum, D. A. (2005). The Cinderella of psychology: The neglect of motor control in the science of mental life and behavior. *American Psychologist, 60*, 308–317.

7

Daily Practices for Mindful Exercise

Rachel Calogero and Kelly Pedrotty

The idea that participation in physical exercise is essential for a healthy body and mind has been espoused in Eastern and Western cultures for thousands of years (Dalleck & Kravitz, 2002). Contemporary scientific research has supported this idea demonstrating that physical exercise can play a significant role in the primary and secondary prevention of certain physiological and psychological conditions including cardiovascular disease (Bassuk & Manson, 2003; Lee, Hsieh, & Paffenbarger, 1995), Type II diabetes (Chipkin, Klugh, & Chasan-Taber, 2001), cancer (Knols, Aaronson, Uebelhart, Fransen, & Aufdemkampe, 2005), osteoporosis (Kohrt, Snead, Slatopolsky, & Birge, 1995), sleep disturbances (Montgomery & Dennis, 2002), negative mood (Arent, Landers, & Etnier, 2000), depression (Byrne & Byrne, 1993; Dunn, Trivedi, Kampert, Clark, & Chambliss, 2005), anxiety (Byrne & Byrne, 1993; Long & van Stavel, 1995), psychological stress (Norris, Carroll, & Cochrane, 1992; Throne, Bartholomew, Craig, & Farrar, 2000), low self-esteem (Fox, 2000), and all-cause morbidity and mortality (Blair et al., 1989; Manson et al., 2002).

Despite this wealth of evidence that physical exercise can protect against a wide variety of human ailments, the relationship between exercise behavior and health is not always so positive. There is a dark side to exercise that is often masked by its social and scientific sanctioning as *good* for health. When an unhealthy relationship with exercise develops, physical and mental health can be compromised instead of optimized. This chapter presents a broadened conceptualization of unhealthy exercise that extends previous definitions of the phenomenon. First, the nature of unhealthy exercise as mindless exercise is considered, and its concomitant dangers are delineated. Second, the nature of healthy exercise as mindful exercise, and programmatic efforts to foster it, are described. Finally, this chapter concludes by offering some guidelines and techniques for the practice of healthy, mindful exercise at the individual and community level.

What is Unhealthy Exercise?

"I work at 100% all the time... push as long and as hard as I can."

Previous research on unhealthy exercise has applied such labels as "exercise addiction" (Adams & Kirkby, 2002), "exercise dependence" (Hausenblaus & Downs, 2002), "obligatory exercise" (Davis, Brewer, & Ratusny, 1993), or "excessive exercise" (Shroff et al., 2006) to describe the maladaptive or disordered behavior. A common quality shared by these conceptualizations is a compulsion to exercise, which often stem from addiction/abuse models (Steinberg, Sykes, & LeBoutillier, 1995; Veale, 1995) or individual psychopathology (Davis et al., 1993; Pasman & Thompson, 1988). If we compare unhealthy exercise patterns to other behavioral disorders such as pathological gambling, indeed the similarities are apparent. Table 7.1 lists the criteria for pathological gambling modified for unhealthy exercise based on the fourth edition of the Diagnostic and Statistical Manual for Mental Disorders (DSM-IV; American Psychiatric Association, 1994). Based on these modified criteria, it is clear that unhealthy exercise can follow patterns of addiction, dependence, obligation, and excessiveness (Davis, 2000).

We propose, however, that unhealthy exercise can take many other forms. Unhealthy exercise extends beyond frequency/intensity-based descriptions of activity to include a variety of other contexts in which exercise may or may not be undertaken (e.g., Robison, 2000; Taylor, Baranowski, & Sallis, 1994; Trost, Owen, Bauman, Sallis, & Brown, 2002). These contexts refer to the particular nature, meaning, and purpose of exercise for the individual, and they consider the social and cultural forces influencing exercise behavior. Engagement in exercise behaviors encompasses psychological and social components as well as physical components. Individuals' thoughts, feelings, and behaviors related to exercise are shaped by a multitude of social and cultural influences that act upon them all the time (Otis & Goldingay, 2000; Rejeski & Thompson, 1993). Thus, instead of pathologizing the individual in regard to their exercise, we emphasize the various contexts in which this "pathology" has arisen and is maintained.

Unhealthy Exercise in Context

Exercise-relevant contexts can include, but are not limited to, an individual's exercise history, physical condition, emotional experiences, belief systems, social relationships, ecological factors, and sociocultural pressures. For example, exercising without proper nourishment and hydration or in

Table 7.1. DSM-IV criteria for pathological gambling modified for unhealthy exercise

- Feel preoccupied with exercise (think about it when not exercising).
- Feel a need to exercise with increasing amounts of time in order to achieve satisfaction.
- Have an inability to control your exercise use.
- Feel restless or irritable when attempting to cut down or stop exercising.
- Use exercise as a way of escaping from problems or of relieving a poor mood (feelings of helplessness, guilt, anxiety, or depression).
- Lie to family members or friends to conceal the extent of involvement with exercise.
- Jeopardize or risk the loss of a significant relationship, job, educational, or career opportunity because of exercise.
- Keep returning to exercise after spending an excessive amount of money on exercise-related expenses.
- Go through withdrawal when not exercising (increased depression, anxiety).
- Exercise longer than originally intended.
- Why don't I want to go to dancing with my friends?

unsafe environmental conditions would be considered *physical* contexts that constitute unhealthy exercise. This is demonstrated by an avid cyclist who reported cycling in a severe rain storm because he could not continue his day without his scheduled workout. Avoiding exercise because of feelings of shame or guilt would be considered an *emotional* and *social* context that constitutes unhealthy exercise. This is demonstrated by an avid exerciser who reported that she no longer exercised because she had lost her "ideal" body shape and "ruined" her exercise regimen, and therefore could not face others who knew her as the "exerciser." Exercising for the sole purpose of weight loss would be considered a *cognitive* and *sociocultural* context that constitutes unhealthy exercise. This is demonstrated by a woman who reported doing calisthenics in the bathroom of an airplane after she ate because she believed she would gain weight otherwise.

This broadened conceptualization of unhealthy exercise that considers various contexts for exercise behavior is necessary for identifying patterns of unhealthy exercise and the development of intervention and treatment protocols. First, asking questions about these various contexts, and not only about the quantity of exercise, can provide a more comprehensive picture of an individual's experience with exercise. Second, by following a context-based model, treatment efforts can focus on changing the contextual factors contributing to the unhealthy exercise, and actually use the exercise itself as a therapeutic tool as it becomes redefined over time (Hays, 1999). This is in contrast to behavioral treatment protocols that tend to focus on reducing and ultimately eliminating the abusive behavior. Third, these contextual factors can be applied to understand the unhealthy exercise behavior and particular exercise issues of people across age, ethnic, and weight spectrums. Finally, this approach does not ignore the pervasive, overarching cultural context perpetuating beliefs and/or myths about exercise. Currently, in many Western cultures, particularly American culture, there exists an almost religious fervor toward *being fit*, which has essentially normalized unhealthy exercise attitudes and behaviors (Otis & Goldingay, 2000; Robison, 2000). Media messages are saturated with promises of achieving the ultimate combination of weight loss, health, and happiness by performing the "right" exercise program: "Six-Pack in Six Days!" or "Lose 10 lbs. in 10 days!" or "Tone Your Way to Happiness!" These messages about fitness and exercise are distorted, confusing, and dangerous, and they do not consider the specific needs of individuals. Even the exercise prescriptions put forth by established authorities on fitness can be considered arbitrary and change regularly (Corbin, LeMasurier, & Franks, 2002). Not surprisingly, however, individuals consider these valid sources for determining their exercise goals, practices, and possibilities. It seems virtually impossible to disentangle the influences of the multiple contexts contributing to unhealthy exercise behavior. In order to understand the scope and impact of unhealthy exercise, we cannot ignore the historical, psychological, social, and cultural contexts that foster it.

Unhealthy Exercise is Mindless Exercise

Drawing from the work of Ellen Langer (1989), we have come to identify many of these exercise-relevant contexts as fostering "mindless" exercise. Individuals who mindlessly exercise approach it with particular beliefs about why and how they should exercise that are based heavily on outcomes. According to Langer this outcome orientation develops early, "From kindergarten on, the focus of schooling is usually on goals rather than on the process by which they are achieved" (p. 33). A focus on outcomes fuels mindless exercise by keeping individuals focused narrowly "out there" on what can be gained, lost, fixed, numbed, or undone. Attention is directed toward the outcome, and not the process of exercise itself.

An outcome orientation may explain the considerable dependence people seem to have on fitness "experts" to tell them how to exercise. There is an assumption that someone else (e.g., magazine models, people at the gym, personal trainers) is more knowledgeable about what our bodies need, how they should look, and how they should feel regarding exercise. Importantly, this reliance on others for how we should exercise fosters mistrust of our own bodies' preferences and needs related to exercise. Certainly, there are fitness professionals who consider individual needs and promote mindful exercise, but many people do not have direct or safe access to these resources (Wilson, Kirtland, Ainsworth, & Addy, 2004). An outcome orientation may also explain people's adherence to rigid definitions for what constitutes exercise, thereby contributing to individuals' fundamentally distorted reasons for *why* they should exercise and *how* they will exercise.

Mindless exercise as described throughout this chapter includes any of the following experiential patterns: exercising solely for weight loss or reshaping the body, self-punishment, affect regulation, acquiring "permission" to eat, identity maintenance, in all or nothing patterns, in obsessive, rigid patterns, surreptitiously, to avoid social interactions, when sick, in pain, injured, physically fatigued, malnourished, undernourished, and/or dehydrated, avoiding exercise completely, being consumed with thoughts of exercise whether one actually exercises or not, dreading it or feeling it to be a "chore," and when exercise presides over all other experiences. Together, the patterns described above represent an overuse/misuse of the body and a disconnection between the body and mind, which is referred to as "mindless" exercise.[1]

Based on this broadened definition, it is clear that mindless exercise can be completely unrelated to the actual frequency or volume of exercise undertaken. In fact, recent research has demonstrated that individuals who experience frequent negative thoughts and feelings about exercise, but do not actually exercise, report lower self-esteem, more depression, and more disordered eating compared to individuals who frequently engage in exercise without these negative thoughts and feelings (Ackard, Brehm, & Steffen, 2002). Thus, it is not the amount of exercise per se that contributes to an

---

[1] In determining the extent or severity of unhealthy exercise, it is important to consider the consistency of the patterns and the length of time they have been experienced. For example, individuals may have thoughts such as "I must go to the gym today to make up for what I ate last night" or "I need to run to alleviate my stress" or "I just need to do 10 more stomach crunches even though my back hurts." Not everyone who has had these thoughts practices unhealthy exercise. While these thoughts are not part of a healthy, mindful mindset (to be discussed shortly), they may not reflect the individuals' overall approach to exercise, and should be considered along with the other aspects of their exercise experience. However, depending on the context these thoughts can lead to a distorted, mindless approach to exercise over time, and thus should be considered seriously in the identification of unhealthy exercise.

unhealthy relationship with exercise, but rather the particular mindset by which the exercise is guided. Mindless forms of exercise may account for the relatively low participation rate in regular physical activity despite its highly popularized usage and promoted health benefits (Centers for Disease Control and Prevention, 1995; Rosenberg, 1998).

To further illustrate this point, consider the exercise programs of the following individuals: Case 1: Swimming, weight training, and cycling 4 hours per day, 6 days per week. Case 2: Treadmill for 30 minutes and 200 stomach crunches before bed, 7 days per week. Case 3: Yoga, weight training, and racquetball or running, 4 days per week. Case 4: Aerobics classes, running, and spinning 3 hours per day, 5 days per week. Case 5: Dance class 1 day per week, walking 5 days per week, stretching most days per week. Can you identify the unhealthy exerciser? Now, consider these cases again with the following additional information. Case 1: History of being a competitive athlete, no injuries, prioritizes proper nutrition, and "athlete" is not the primary identity. Case 2: Severe anxiety and guilt if exercise is missed, no rest days or variety, and dreads doing it. Case 3: Enjoys the activities, incorporates variety, exercises with others, and no known negative affect associated with it. Case 4: Exercise is primary focus, no rest days, no enjoyment, never feels like it is enough, inadequate caloric intake to support the activities, and uses it to avoid other social interactions. Case 5: Enjoys the activities, previous history of exercise avoidance, feels good moving in body, and the focus is not weight loss.

When presenting this simple illustration in workshops, Case 2 is most often identified as the healthiest and Case 4 is most often identified as the unhealthiest when the quantity of exercise is used to make the diagnosis. However, the additional information tells a different story and in fact, Case 2 is just as unhealthy as Case 4 even though their quantities are not comparable. Case 3 and Case 5 are actually the healthiest based on the overall quality of their exercise experience. Case 1 also appears healthy, but it is critical to probe athletes about their genuine pleasure and enjoyment, which is often assumed just because they continue to participate in a sport. In sum, the nature, meaning, and purpose of the exercise expands the scope and impact of unhealthy exercise considerably (Calogero & Pedrotty, 2004; Cox & Orford, 2004), and warrants the development and implementation of more specific intervention efforts.

Prevalence and Consequences of Mindless Exercise

"I like the pain. I want to feel the pain. If I can't exercise, I cut."

The generally accepted views of exercise as good and beneficial place exercise in a different category from other types of behaviors, thus making it difficult to identify a problem (de la Torre, 1995; Tanji, 2000). In fact, unhealthy exercise practices are often viewed as disciplined and not disordered. In addition, the literature is plagued with different labels and definitions for the phenomenon (Hausenblas & Downs, 2002). However, some evidence does exist from community and clinical samples suggesting that other factors besides quantity constitute unhealthy exercise, and that unhealthy exercise is a significant problem.

Emphasizing the multidimensional nature of obligatory exercise, Ackard, Brehm, & Steffen (2002) demonstrated an association between negative emotionality and exercise as the best predictor of disordered eating, depression, and self-esteem. Based on self-reports of the exercise frequency, exercise fixation, and exercise commitment among 586 college women, a remarkable 42 % of this sample were identified as having a dysfunctional or unhealthy relationship with exercise: Almost half of this sample of college-aged women engaged in mindless forms of exercise. Recent research by Jon Mond and colleagues has attempted to refine the definition of "excessive exercise" for the purposes of the treatment and prevention of eating disorders. In a community sample of women aged 18–45, exercise related to (a) changing appearance or body tone and (b) feeling guilty about missing an exercise session were the two qualities most strongly associated with eating disordered behavior and reduced quality of life (Mond, Hay, Rodgers, Owen, & Beumont, 2004). Based on these criteria, 14.2 % of 169 women were identified as excessive exercisers. Notably, the self-reported frequency of exercise was unrelated to disordered eating and quality of life. Replicating these findings in a larger general population sample, 17 % of 3,472 women aged 18–42 reported either exercising solely to influence appearance (i.e., weight, shape, or body tone), guilt about missing an exercise session, or both of these qualities, indicating their "excessive exercise" (Mond, Hay, Rodgers, & Owen, 2006). Again, notably, the self-reported frequency of exercise was unrelated to disordered eating and physical and mental health.

This research underlies the importance of the quality of the exercise, and in particular people's motivations for participating in exercise. Research examining the relationships between exercise motives and psychological well-being has demonstrated that extrinsic (or outcome-based) exercise motives (e.g., social recognition, changing appearance) are significantly related to poorer psychological well-being whereas intrinsic (or process-based) exercise motives (e.g., feeling revitalized, personal enjoyment) are significantly related to better psychological well-being (Maltby & Day, 2001). Adkins and Keel (2005) examined the distinction between the quality versus the quantity of exercise as they relate to disordered eating symptoms in a sample of college students. These researchers demonstrated that appearance-based motives for exercising were associated with higher levels of drive for thinness, bulimic symptoms, body dissatisfaction, and other disordered eating patterns compared to nonappearance-based motives (Adkins & Keel, 2005). Furthermore, in appearance-based exercisers, it was the quality of the exercise behaviors, and not the quantity of the exercise itself, that was associated with eating pathology. For nonappearance-based exercisers, neither compulsive nor excessive exercise predicted eating pathology. An additional interesting finding in this research revealed that health and fitness motives for exercising were associated with less disordered eating, but a greater compulsion to exercise. While health and fitness motives may be considered intrinsic motives, it is clear from this research that these intrinsic motives do not foster better psychological well-being with regard to exercise attitudes and behaviors. Thus, at first glance, intrinsic motives for exercise may seem "healthy," but may actually stem from an outcome-based orientation toward exercise that can be masked by the ubiquitous messages that link "exercise" and "health." Together, these findings suggest that outcome-based exercise motives such as exercising for the purpose of weight loss, changing appearance, or social approval negatively affect people's psychological well-being and contribute to disordered eating patterns.

Pathological patterns of exercise have been implicated in the etiology, development, and maintenance of eating disorders since the early 1970s (Beumont, Arthur, Russell, & Touyz 1994; Brewerton, Stellefson, Hibbs, Hodges, & Cochrane, 1995; Bruch, 1973; Davis, 2000; Davis et al., 1997; le Grange, & Eisler, 1993; Shroff et al., 2006; Thompson & Sherman, 1992; Yates, 1991). Clinical studies have estimated that the prevalence of "excessive" or high-level exercise in individuals diagnosed with inpatient eating disorder populations varies between 33 and 100% (Calogero & Pedrotty, 2004; Davis, Kennedy, Ravelski, & Dionne, 1994; Davis et al., 1997; Katz, 1996). In a 10-year follow-up study of 95 participants with anorexia nervosa, the compulsion to exercise at discharge predicted earlier relapses and chronic pathological outcomes (Strober, Freeman, & Morrell, 1997). High levels of total and aerobic exercise reported by participants with eating disorders have been significantly related to high levels of drive for thinness and longer periods of hospitalization (Solenberger, 2001). In a sample of 254 women in residential treatment for eating disorders, 40% of the women reported that their unhealthy exercise behavior preceded the onset of their eating disorder, with some identifying the onset of excessive types of exercise as early as 11 years old (Calogero & Pedrotty, 2004). In a sample of 1,857 women across subtypes of eating disorders, 39% of the entire sample met criteria for excessive exercise (Shroff et al., 2006), which was defined as interference with important activities, exercising more than 3 hours per day, inappropriate times and places for exercise, and exercising despite injury, pain, or illness. In this sample, the highest prevalence of excessive exercisers (54%) was observed in the purging subtype of anorexia nervosa. Thus, although the definitions vary, mindless forms of exercise appear to be prevalent to varying degrees in both community and clinical populations.

Other Negative Consequences

It is perhaps not surprising that engaging in mindless exercise places individuals at risk for a multitude of physical injuries. A non-exhaustive list of these dangers includes stress fractures (Burr, 1997), non-fatal, often disabling, injuries (Plugge, Stewar-Brown, Knight, & Fletcher, 2002), decreased immune function (Fry et al., 1994), osteopenia and osteoporosis (Golden, 2002), and even death (Davis 1997). Anecdotal reports from women communicated to the authors illustrate the permanent physical damage that can result from mindless exercise. For example, a collegiate runner who continued to run every day despite persistent knots and cramps in her legs damaged her leg muscles so severely that she will never be able to run again. A middle-aged woman reported doing thousands of stomach crunches every day in an effort to obtain a flat stomach, and eventually damaged the protective skin surrounding her spine to the point of causing permanent damage to her lower back.

Beyond the direct influence of mindless exercise on the body, when the focus of the exercise is outcome-based compared to process-based it can place people in dangerous or unsafe situations. Although there is little to no documented research about these physical dangers related to unhealthy exercise, the case example below illustrates their significance in the lives of mindless exercisers.

> Robin often woke up at 4 a.m. and went for a 5–10 mile run. Instead of staying in bed with her husband who she rarely saw because of their work schedules, Robin would run, regardless of the weather or season. Although the paths and streets she ran were not completely desolate, she said that it was almost always dark when she began running, and she felt uneasy being alone. She remembers her heart racing many times when she heard a car slow down behind her. On several occasions, men, presumably intoxicated, yelled obscene remarks or whistled/called to her. She admitted that more than once she barely avoided being hit by a drunk driver. However, she believed firmly that nothing "bad" would actually happen to her.

By rigidly adhering to the same routine for purposes clearly unrelated to genuine physical health and well-being, the case of Robin and many others illustrates the serious effects of mindlessness on personal safety and awareness of environmental threats and/or dangers.

Although lacking in empirical research, individuals have provided anecdotal reports to the authors describing the deleterious effects of mindless exercise on their social relationships, including relationships with partners, children, parents, siblings, friends, and/or co-workers. For example, a woman reported that she exercised for 3 hours every day on her honeymoon. When prevented from exercising, she became irritable and fought with her spouse. In another example, a married couple admitted that they spend most of their day exercising, and they prioritize it over spending time with their daughter. In sum, considering both the qualitative and quantitative evidence presented here, mindless patterns of exercise constitute a significant problem that warrants direct treatment independent of any concomitant eating-related problems (Beumont et al., 1994; Calogero & Pedrotty, 2004; Solenberger, 2001).

What is Healthy Exercise?

"I have far more strength than I expected, and I have better access to that strength."

Healthy exercise is conceptualized here as "mindful exercise," which is based on process and not outcomes (e.g., Douillard, 2001). The practice of mindful exercise should adhere to the four basic principles outlined here. First, exercise should be used to rejuvenate the body, not exhaust or deplete it. Second, exercise should enhance mind–body connection and coordination, not confuse or dis-regulate the mind–body relationship. Third, exercise should alleviate mental and physical stress, not contribute to and exacerbate stress. And finally, exercise should provide us with genuine enjoyment and pleasure, not provide pain and be dreaded. Approaching exercise with a mindful orientation should lead to feelings of control, greater freedom of action, and less burnout (Langer, 1989).

The original development of these conceptions about healthy (mindful) and unhealthy (mindless) exercise emerged out of a need to directly identify and address the exercise issues of women in residential treatment for eating disorders. Despite the significant struggles with exercise that women with eating disorders often experience, disordered patterns of exercise have been viewed often as symptoms that will subside with general eating disorders treatment. As indicated above, Strober and colleagues (1997) have demonstrated that this is clearly not the case. However, this common wisdom has prevailed and it has prevented exercise issues from being treated specifically and systematically over time. The exercise program developed by the first two authors (see Calogero & Pedrotty, 2004) provides women with eating disorders the opportunity to experience, practice, and process exercise in new ways. With guidance and supervision from Exercise Coordinators, the women in the program are challenged in weekly group settings to sense, support, and strengthen themselves through a variety of physical activities. One key focus of the program is to enable the women to identify the differences between mindful and mindless patterns of exercise, and actually practice new ways of being physically active and moving in their bodies. A second key focus is to raise their awareness of the various contexts that foster mindless exercise, and how to change these contexts. A third key focus is to enable the women to distinguish between what they like to do and what they experience as fun, as opposed to what their eating disorder/unhealthy mindset "likes" to do, or "tells" them to do. Normalizing an exercise program so that it is healthy and beneficial requires a capacity to address internal needs rather than external concerns. Over time, by learning to rely upon adequate rest and nutrition, and working to develop self-respect and self-care, many of the women have been able to make healthier, more *mindful* choices about their exercise.

The exercise principles and interventions utilized in populations with eating disorders are applicable to everyone's exercise experience, and therefore can be extended to the broader population. Generally, almost any community member can use these daily practices to challenge, change, and ultimately circumvent unhealthy exercise in their own lives and the lives of others. The remainder of this chapter describes the basic guidelines and techniques that we have found to be most effective for promoting mindful exercise in people's lives.

The Practice and Process of Healthy Exercise

Sensing the Self

The first fundamental element of healthy exercise includes sensing the self. Individuals who engage in mindless exercise are not utilizing exercise to *sense* and stay connected to the body. Instead, exercise activities and environments are selected that direct people's attention away from themselves and not to how they feel during the activity itself. Individuals who are not sensing themselves do not focus on breathing, do not know when to stop certain movements or activities, and often compare themselves to others during exercise. It is important that individuals pay attention to their own bodies, which allows them to be aware of themselves experientially during periods of physical activity. Sensing the self requires paying attention to how the body feels while it is in action, and not only after it has acted.

Supporting the Self

The second fundamental element of healthy exercise includes supporting the self. Individuals who engage in mindless exercise are not utilizing exercise to *support* the body in a way that maintains their psychological and physical balance. Instead, individuals adopt exercise practices that often serve only one purpose or need, which is often the attainment of the goal (usually weight loss). When balance is absent from an exercise program, it is difficult to know how much exercise to do, which exercises are most appropriate for us, when other social experiences should take priority, or how to fuel ourselves with appropriate amounts of food. This, in turn, increases reliance on external sources to guide our bodies instead of our internal experiences. For example, Zoe, a former dancer, only considered dance-related activities to be exercise, and her main goal was to be able to do a split again. She declined opportunities to be active with friends (e.g., biking) because it was a waste of time for her – it did not count as exercise. Attaining balance requires making mindful choices about what activities (exercise and non-exercise) to incorporate into our lives. Variety, flexibility, and enjoyment are key elements to supporting the body with healthy exercise.

Strengthening the Self

The third fundamental element of healthy exercise includes strengthening the self. Individuals who engage in mindless exercise are not utilizing exercise to *strengthen* the body and mind. For some individuals, exercising is a way to punish the body or to "beat up" the self. For other individuals, the exercise performed does not foster their natural strengths, which can hinder the potential for genuine enjoyment and satisfaction in the activity. And still for other individuals, the label "exerciser" becomes the primary identity (Anderson & Cychosz, 1995), which renders them vulnerable to feelings of invalidity and inadequacy if they stray from their exercise routines. This mindset serves to weaken, not strengthen, the body and mind over time. For example, Ava belonged to the track team in high school and identified herself as a runner. In college, Ava did not make the track team and decided to continue running on her own. She admitted that running always felt like a punishment, but she had to do it because she was a runner. Running interfered with other social activities and she was often too exhausted to complete her coursework. In this way, exercise served to drain and weaken her mind and body over time. Individuals should be encouraged to engage in activities because they strengthen them, not because they define them.

A Prescription for a Mindful Exercise Program

There is no magic number of calories, minutes, miles, laps, repetitions, or classes. In fact, it would be contradictory to prescribe mindful exercise in terms of numbers. Mindful exercise does not need to be counted. Instead, building on the elements of sensing, supporting, and strengthening the self, we prescribe that activities be selected based on the four components described below: Function, Feeling, Fun, and Fuel. In order to self-monitor exercise patterns and identify mindless exercise activities, it is helpful to create a personalized exercise checklist. This checklist can be created by generating a list of questions about one's specific exercise activities. These questions should address specific issues regarding whether the exercise works toward sensing, supporting, and strengthening the self as well as identify how these activities do or do not incorporate function, feeling, fun, and fuel in mindful ways. Reviewing the checklist before and after exercise may help individuals stay present and connected to their bodies, and avoid using exercise for

Table 7.2. Examples of items for an exercise Checklist

- Do I want to exercise because of what I ate today?
- Is there another activity I would rather be doing today instead of exercise?
- What exactly would I like to be doing right now?
- Is today a rest day? What exactly would I like to do with my day?
- Am I feeling guilty because I do not think I am exercising enough?
- Am I avoiding exercise today because I am uncomfortable in my body?
- Do I want to go exercise alone so no one will interfere with what I do?
- Do I feel that if I cannot do everything I planned for exercising than I do not want to do any of it?
- Did I enjoy this exercise the last time I did it?

unhealthy or mindless reasons. At the very least, asking questions related to specific exercise issues before exercising requires a moment of pause. Even if individuals continue to exercise in an unhealthy way, it may not be to the same degree. The key to its effectiveness is answering honestly and following through with behaviors that keep the self safe and strong. This checklist should be reviewed regularly if struggling with unhealthy exercise patterns and kept in a place where it is easily retrieved. Table 7.2 provides examples of questions for an exercise checklist based on different types of exercise issues.

Function

Why we exercise determines and guides *how* we exercise. An important message to propagate in the community is that the sole purpose of exercise should not be weight loss (Burgard & Lyons, 1994; Gaesser, 2002). Research has shown that not all exercising individuals will significantly reduce their body weight (Gaesser, 2002). More recently, it was shown that exercise can decrease total and abdominal body fat without observing corresponding changes in measures of relative weight such as body mass index (Janssen et al., 2004). Furthermore, debunking the "thinner is better" doctrine, researchers have found that weight has little bearing on living a long life; it is about being physically fit, not physically fat (Barlow, Kohl, Gibbons, & Blair, 1995). Thus, the function of exercise in people's lives should necessarily focus on purposes other than weight loss. It is essential to shift from a passive weight loss mindset to a more mindful reflection about what exercise can and cannot bring to one's life overall. Physical activities should be selected that support a wide spectrum of physical and mental functioning, bring pleasure, and enhance feelings of strength and self-competence.

Feeling

How we exercise determines and guides *what* we feel when we exercise. An important message to propagate in the community is that physical activity should connect us to our bodies, not disconnect us (Douillard, 2001). It is especially important to select activities that minimize feelings of body dissatisfaction, body shame, comparisons with others, guilt, and punishment; instead, physical activities should foster natural strengths and abilities, and not require self–other comparisons to feel good or worthwhile. By paying attention to how the body feels, and how the exercise experience makes us feel, safer decisions can be made in the moment about if and how we should exercise on a particular day.

Fun

Being able to explore how *we* like to move in our bodies and what makes *us* feel healthy and strong can be very empowering, and change our relationship with exercise. An important message to propagate in the community is that physical activity should bring pleasure, not pain. Many individuals do not consider exercise to be fun. As we suggested earlier, this is partly because the exercise being performed is not truly self-chosen and not a preferred way of moving in one's body. However, participation in exercise, particularly sports participation, has been associated with personal enjoyment, personal growth, and improved social integration (Wankel & Berger, 1991). By challenging and changing our rigid categories, or "preconceived cognitive commitments" (Langer, 1989), about what constitutes real exercise, endless possibilities for physical activity become available to us. Ultimately, greater enjoyment can lead to greater adherence (Wankel, 1993) and reduced dependence on numbers to tell us when to stop. See Table 7.3 for examples of fun exercises suggested by former mindless exercisers.

Fuel

The dangers of exercising when the body is not properly fueled, hydrated, or rested can include fatigue, injury, fainting, major organ failure, and even death. Often individuals feel that exercising gives them permission to eat, which reflects the outcome orientation of mindless exercisers. Being "in shape" includes getting adequate nutrition (Otis & Goldingay, 2000). In order to be safe and obtain the most physical and mental benefits from periods of physical activity, the selected physical activities should include appropriate nutritional support.

General Guidelines for Challenging and Changing Mindless Exercise

In reality, we recognize that it can be difficult to incorporate the missing pieces of sensing, supporting, and strengthening the self into our exercise practices, and to challenge the barrage of societal messages and pressures about what is and is not exercise. We offer some suggestions below about how to begin identifying and challenging mindless exercise behavior in

Table 7.3. List of fun physical activities generated by former mindless exercisers

Biking	Roller blading	Kite flying
Hiking	Skiing	Trampoline
Rock climbing	Making snowpeople	Nature walks
Playgrounds	Apple picking	Dancing
Gardening	Walking pet	Bowling
Yoga	Swimming	Kickboxing
Flag football	Horseback riding	Canoeing
Intramurals	Ice skating	Playing with kids
Jump rope	Walking tours	Volleyball
Raking Leaves	Karate	Tai Chi

ourselves and others. Each suggestion is accompanied by references to actual techniques that can be found in Tables 7.4 and 7.5 . Individual-level interventions are indicated with an "I" and group-level interventions are indicated with a "G." These guidelines can be modified to fit the needs of specific participants, specific persons, or broader groups and communities. It is important to remember that the overarching focus should be to help individuals reclaim exercise for themselves by redefining and rediscovering it in a mindful way.[2]

Explore exercise history to determine past and present experiences with exercise. Examine individual reasons for exercising in the past and present, which will help to understand the present mindset guiding the exercise. Questions to ask include: What are your earliest memories of being physically active? How would you describe your relationship to exercise up to this point? After a workout, do you feel refreshed & energized? Do you feel present and connected to how your body feels when you exercise? What types of exercise do you do and what is the usual setting? Are you looking forward to the activity again? The answers to these questions are important for determining if exercise is undertaken for unhealthy reasons (#2I, 3I, 12G).

Educate about the specific dangers of mindless exercise and exercise myths. It is necessary to discuss basic information about how the body uses food as fuel for the heart, brain, and muscles – food is energy and we need it. Plan activities around meals to insure proper fueling and refueling of the body. Remember, we should eat to exercise, not exercise to eat! It is also necessary to challenge exercise myths. It is important to consider the words that people use to describe their exercise goals and experiences. We suggest deleting these words from one's exercise vocabulary: tone, sculpt, firm, shape, lift, and tighten. These words reflect media hype and distort rather than clarify our understanding about the actual structure and function of our bodies. Perhaps one of the most pervasive exercise myths is that we can get "toned." It is important to understand that muscle tone refers to a muscle's level of fullness or firmness. Therefore, to be toned is to have muscle. It is often eye-opening to tell individuals that if you are able to walk and do activities of daily living your muscles already have tone. It should be stressed that *everybody has tone*. This usually leads to challenging another pervasive exercise myth – that muscle can turn into fat and fat can turn into muscle. Muscle and fat are two separate types of body tissues and cannot be converted into the other (e.g., Otis & Goldingay, 2000). Educating ourselves and others about exercise facts and myths is essential to changing unhealthy exercise practices (#7I, 9I, 1G–13G).

Serve as a role model for safe and healthy exercise behavior. As members of families, peer groups, communities, workplaces, and society, we transmit

[2] It is important to emphasize that it is not safe or appropriate for *all* individuals who engage in unhealthy exercise to continue exercising. If individuals have been diagnosed with an eating disorder or have reported disordered eating, are medically compromised, not adhering to appropriate nutritional guidelines, or not changing their mindless exercise behavior, then they may not be ready to benefit from participation in the practices we have described here. In addition, exercise should not be provided for the sake of exercising itself. This may actually contribute to the belief that exercise is absolutely necessary despite weight or other health concerns, and thus may further exacerbate the unhealthy exercise.

Table 7.4. Examples of individual-level interventions to challenge mindless exercise practices

Intervention	Description	Example
1. Exercise World	Draw the people, places, things, feelings, thoughts, actions related to exercise. Provides powerful, nonverbal expression of exercise experience and identifies specific targets for change.	
2. Exercise Journal	Record thoughts and feelings before, during, and after exercise. Provides check-in and can redirect to healthier behavior. Record thoughts about specific topics or questions related to exercise.	Reflect on questions such as: what have I missed in my life because of exercise? what do I feel unwilling to change and why? what exercise issue did I struggle with the most today?
3. Checklist	Self-generated questions to ask before exercise that are specific to the exercise issues. Provides check-in and can redirect to healthier behavior. Should leave checklist next to sneakers or in gym bag.	See Table 7.2.
4. Mindful Reminders	Post positive, informative, individualized notes in strategic places to remind about purpose of mindful exercise.	"I stop exercising when tired." "I will support my mind and body with fun physical activity." "I do not exercise to burn calories." "If I look at the time more than 3 times I stop."
5. Healthy Buddy	Exercising with a healthy person encourages mindful exercise choices and provides a role model.	Walk with friends, play volleyball, bring buddy to gym. Be careful that you choose someone who you will not compare to.
6. Reframe Goals	Setting realistic goals that incorporate mindful exercise principles can reduce mindless exercise.	Make your physical activity goals about enhancing your life overall instead of just your physical self. Take a dance class instead of running if you are not a runner. Start a garden if you like to be outdoors.
7. Ripped	Rip out pages of fitness magazines that contain triggering images (ads, tips, interviews) and see what information is left that would help guide healthy exercise. Identify mindless exercise messages. Reduce reliance on mindless exercise information.	Magazines such as *Shape, Fitness*, or *Men's Health* work well here. They depict unrealistic images of men and women and offer conflicting and unhealthy exercise tips. Be prepared to offer evidence and information to support your critiques.
8. Avoid Triggers	Identify activities that lead to mindless exercise and stay away from them. Selecting alternative, pleasurable physical activities and contexts enhances adherence to mindful exercise principles.	Do not run on the treadmill if there is constant competition between you and the time or you and the person next to you. Explore how you like to move in different ways.
9. Fuel Up	Fueling the body properly will reduce fatigue and overall mindless exercise tendencies, allowing the healthy exerciser to feel more pleasurable.	Place snacks next to checklist, in car, in gym bag, so they are easily accessible before exercise.
10. Slow Pace	Slowing the pace of activity, if possible, when triggered by environmental cues (e.g. other bodies, gym) can re-focus attention to self and staying connected to the body.	Close eyes whenever possible to focus on the self. Change activity or stop it completely if mindless thoughts and feelings do not relent. Move more slowly and intentionally, paying attention to all body sensations. Remind self of personal, mindful goals to keep focused.

Table 7.5. Examples of group-level exercise interventions to challenge mindless exercise practices

Intervention	Description	Example
1. Trust Exercises	Creates connection with self and others through group and partner work.	Partner squat, partner yoga, kneeling on exercise ball.
2. Balance Exercises	Directs attention toward being calm and present while increasing mind and body strength.	Bicep curls on a bosu ball, standing on one foot, yoga.
3. Channel Aggression	Provides safe outlet for negative feelings so they are not directed toward the self and can be shared with others.	Ball slap, kickboxing, karate, tug of war, yoga.
4. Conscious Cardio	Use different senses to notice surroundings and be present during activity.	Smell flowers, listen to different sounds, focus on the breath.
5. Cross-Training	Creates variety and enjoyment while strengthening body and mind.	Basketball, swimming, gardening, yoga, bike riding, dance, change activities when you can.
6. Circuit Training	By moving through different exercises consecutively it reduces time, can be at home or with friends, adds variety.	Swimming, squats, kicks, core work, jumping jacks, jump rope, yoga poses, dance.
7. Touching Muscles	Touching a muscle to feel it engaged during exercise increases connection to physical and overall self.	Touch upper leg while sitting against wall to feel quad muscles working.
8. Slow and Steady	Moving with purpose and control increases connection and focus on form rather than momentum and numbers.	Try to kneel on exercise ball.
9. Fun in the Sun	Be active outside whenever possible to increase fun and stay connected to social world.	Take a long walk, play catch, rollerblade.
10. Recess	Engage in activities that have positive associations to enhance enjoyment and get out of ruts.	Play on a playground, swing, jump rope, run the bases, tag.
11. Numbers and Colors	When doing repetitions, count random numbers or use colors to avoid obsessing.	17, 80, 44, 2, 53 or purple, red, green, blue, yellow.
12. Process	Talk to others before and after physical activity about thoughts and feelings experienced during the activity.	After a run or playing ball, talk about what thoughts/feelings arose and what to repeat or change next time.
13. Breathe	Creates mind–body connection by maintaining a focus on the breath throughout activity.	Practice watching and noticing breath to monitor exertion and be mindful.

and reinforce social information about exercise. If we are uncomfortable with our bodies, exercise mindlessly, or believe that exercise is really about weight loss, then we cannot expect others to trust new experiences or new information about exercise that we provide to them. In order to address mindless exercise at a community level, it is first imperative to attain a shift in the individual's approaches to exercise. Expect resistance to debunking the myths such as "no pain, no gain", "more is better", "cardio is the best form of exercise," or "If I take a day off I will loss my fitness level." We cannot just tell others that these are myths; we have to actually practice and model something different for them to observe directly. By working alongside others, it is possible to direct their attention to how their body moves and feels; and thus to how healthy, mindful exercise feels. In the case with exercise groups, a disingenuous leader can be counterproductive to facilitating a new experience with exercise (see Calogero & Pedrotty, 2004) (#6I, 1G–13G).

Raise awareness about societal pressures to attain unrealistic body ideals and give permission to challenge these dangerous messages. Acknowledging and addressing the societal contexts that promote thinness and obsessive exercise is imperative. Practice critiquing sources of fitness information. If others choose to continue reading fitness magazines, encourage them to use a healthy filter. This may be difficult because a large portion of the information presented is focused on weight loss and achieving unrealistic body shapes. Remind them that the exercise tips and workout programs offered do not consider individual needs, especially if the individual struggles with an eating disorder. Individuals need to be aware that not all fitness professionals are trained to identify unhealthy patterns of exercise and/or eating disorders. Again, distinguishing between fact and fiction regarding exercise can help us make better choices for our bodies and minds (#7I, 8I).

Incorporate the elements described above into your program of activity. Expand the variety of activities that "count" as exercise. Remember – there is no "best" exercise, only what is best for us. Visiting parks, dancing, hiking, biking, walking, yoga, or just being outside, playing with children, or doing yard work constitute exercise. Attempt to create a program that is fun, and includes a variety of activities and other people. A mindful exercise program allows for the unexpected so "workouts" can be missed (#1G–10G). Plan rest days and stick to them! Rest is an essential component to a healthy exercise program. The guidelines put forth by the American College of Sports Medicine (ACSM) may provide a starting point if needed in regard to "appropriate" amounts of exercise, but remember that general guidelines cannot address specific exercise issues. These recommendations should be modified to fit the needs of the individual, especially in regard to what exercise activities bring the most pleasure (#1I, 3I, 4I, 6I, 8I, 9I, 1G–11G).

Identify triggering and non-triggering activities and environments. Triggers can be any number of people, places, or activities that lead individuals to mindlessly exercise. In these cases, the context needs to be changed. For example, if the gym triggers unhealthy exercise thoughts and behaviors, individuals should seek out other places for physical activity. These can be wide-ranging and include yoga studios, dance classes, playgrounds, games of kickball or softball, outdoor hikes, biking, sledding, playing with kids, gardening, or walking. Recess-like activities are less likely to trigger unhealthy exercise. We cannot enjoy recess and simultaneously count calories or minutes or feel inadequate too – at least not very easily. For another example, if conversations about weight loss and obsessive exercising trigger negative thoughts, find other people to converse with and seek out alternate places to meet people who do not share this mindless mindset (#1I, 8I, 1G–13G).

Practice mindful exercise practices daily. Individuals will benefit from listening to their bodies before, during, and after exercise. This will help guide them toward what activities they want to do in the first place. Thoughts and feelings can be recorded in an exercise journal and utilized to determine if and how to exercise on any particular day. Individuals should also practice avoiding comparison with others about exercise. Remember that focusing on others leads to minimizing one's own skills, achievements, and body's needs. Closing one's eyes can help redirect attention to the self and away from comparison with others. An emphasis should be placed consistently on redefining and re-experiencing exercise. Individuals should be encouraged to experiment with what activities make them feel good and to try new things (#2I, 5I, 8I, 10I, 5G, 9G, 10G).

Conclusion

"My whole life I have been used to killing myself. It feels so good to know I can stop."

This chapter extends previous definitions of unhealthy exercise by incorporating the role of multiple contexts into the conceptualization of unhealthy exercise. Furthermore, unhealthy exercise is recast as mindless exercise, with an emphasis on being outcome-oriented versus process-oriented in our approach to exercise. Considerable evidence exists demonstrating that mindless exercise can compromise physical and mental health. We may reduce these dangerous exercise patterns by (a) recognizing the contexts in which mindless exercise is fostered and change them, (b) redefining healthy exercise as mindful, and (c) re-experiencing exercise in a way that sustains the body and mind. Efforts toward increasing mindful approaches to exercise may reduce unhealthy exercise practices as well as improve health and exercise adherence across diverse groups and communities.

References

Ackard, D.M., Brehm, B.J., & Steffen, J.J. (2002). Exercise and eating disorders in college-aged women: Profiling excessive exercisers. *Eating Disorders, 10,* 31–47.

Adams, J. & Kirkby, R.J. (2002). Excessive exercise as an addiction: A review. *Addiction Research & Theory, 10,* 415–438.

Adkins, E.C., & Keel, P.K. (2005). Does "excessive" or "compulsive" best describe exercise as a symptom of bulimia nervosa? *International Journal of Eating Disorders, 38,* 24–29.

American Psychiatric Association. (1994). *Diagnostic and statistical manual of mental disorders.* Washington, DC: Author.

Anderson, D.F., & Cychosz, C.M. (1995). Exploration of the relationship between exercise behavior and exercise identity. *Journal of Sport Behavior, 18,* 159–163.

Arent, S., Landers, D., & Etnier, J.L. (2000). The effects of exercise on mood in older adults: A meta-analytic review. *Journal of Aging & Physical Activity, 8,* 407–430.

Barlow, C.E., Kohl, H.W., Gibbons, L.W., & Blair, S.N. (1995). Physical fitness, mortality, and obesity. *International Journal of Eating Disorders, 19,* S41–S44.

Bassuk, S.S., & Manson, J.E. (2003). Physical activity and cardiovascular disease prevention in women: How much is good enough? *Exercise Sport Sciences Reviews, 31,* 176–181.

Beumont, P.J.V., Arthur, B., Russell, J.D., & Touyz, S.W. (1994). Excessive physical activity in dieting disorder patients: Proposals for a supervised exercise program. *International Journal of Eating Disorders, 15,* 21–36.

Blair, S.N., Kohl, H.W., Paffenbarger, R.S., Clark, D.G., Cooper, K.H., & Gibbons, L.W. (1989). Physical fitness and all-cause mortality. A prospective study of healthy men and women. *Journal of the American Medical Association, 262,* 2395–2401.

Brewerton, T.D., Stellefson, E.J., Hibbs, N., Hodges, E.L., & Cochrane, C.E. (1995). Comparison of eating disorder patients with and without compulsive exercising. *International Journal of Eating Disorders, 17,* 413–416.

Bruch, H. (1973). *Eating disorders: Obesity, anorexia nervosa, and the person within.* New York: Basic Books.

Burgard, D., & Lyons, P. (1994). Alternatives in obesity treatment: Focusing on health for fat women. In P. Fallon, M.A. Katzman, & S. Wooley (Eds.), *Feminist perspectives on eating disorders* (pp. 212–230). New York, NY: Guilford Press.

Burr, D.B. (1997). Bone, exercise, and stress fractures. *Exercise & Sport Sciences Reviews, 25,* 171–194.

Byrne, A.E., & Byrne, D.G. (1993). The effect of exercise on depression, anxiety, and other mood states: A review. *Journal of Psychosomatic Research, 37,* 565–574.

Calogero, R.M., & Pedrotty, K.N. (2004). The practice and process of healthy exercise: An investigation of the treatment of exercise abuse in women with eating disorders. *Eating Disorders, 12,* 273–291.

Centers for Disease Control and Prevention. (1995). *Physical Activity and Health: A Report of the Surgeon General.* Pittsburgh, PA: U.S. Dept of Health and Human Services.

Chipkin, S.R., Klugh, S.A., & Chasan-Taber, L. (2001). Exercise and diabetes. *Cardiology Clinics, 19,* 489–505.

Corbin, C.B., LeMasurier, G., & Franks, B.D. (2002). Making sense of multiple physical activity recommendations. *President's Council on Physical Fitness and Sports Research Digest, 3(19),* 1–8.

Cox, R., & Orford, J. (2004). A qualitative study of the meaning of exercise for people who could be labeled as 'addicted' to exercise-can 'addiction' be applied to high frequency exercising? *Addiction Research and Theory, 12,* 167–188.

Dalleck, L.C., & Kravitz, L. (2002). The history of fitness. *IDEA Health & Fitness Source, 20,* 26–33.

Davis, C. (1997). Eating disorders and hyperactivity: A psychological perspective. *Canadian Journal of Psychiatry, 42,* 168–175.

Davis, C. (2000). Exercise abuse. *International Journal of Sport Psychology, 31,* 278–289.

Davis, C., Brewer, H., & Ratusny, G. (1993). Behavioral frequency and psychological commitment: Necessary concepts in the study of excessive exercising. *Journal of Behavioral Medicine, 16,* 611–628.

Davis, C., Katzman, D.K., Kaptein, S., Kirsh, C., Brewer, H., Kamlbach, K., Olmstead, M.P., Woodside, D.B., & Kaplan, A.K. (1997). The prevalence of high-level exercise in the eating disorders: etiological implications. *Comprehensive Psychiatry, 38,* 321–326.

Davis, C., Kennedy, S.H., Ravelski, E., & Dionne, M. (1994). The role of physical activity in the development and maintenance of eating disorders. *Psychological Medicine, 24,* 957–967.

de la Torre, J. (1995). Mens sana in corpore sano, or exercise abuse? Clinical considerations. *Bulletin of the Menninger Clinic, 59,* 15–31.

Douillard, J. (2001). *Body, mind, and sport.* New York: Three Rivers Press.

Dunn, A.L., Trivedi, M.H., Kampert, J.B., Clark, C.G., & Chambliss, H.O. (2005). Exercise treatment for depression: Efficacy and dose response. *American Journal of Preventive Medicine, 28,* 1–8.

Fox, K.R. (2000). Self-esteem, self-perceptions and exercise. *International Journal of Sport Psychology, 31,* 228–240.

Fry, R.W., Grove, J.R., Morton, A.R., Zeroni, P.M., Gaudieri, S., & Keast, D. (1994). Psychological and immunological correlates of acute overtraining. *British Journal of Sports Medicine, 28,* 241–246.

Gaesser, G.A. (2002). *Big fat lies: The truth about your weight and your health.* Carlsbad, CA: Gurze Books.

Golden, N.H. (2002). A review of the female athlete triad (amenorrhea, osteoporosis and disordered eating). *International Journal of Adolescent Medicine & Health, 14,* 9–17.

Hausenblas, H.A., & Downs, D.S. (2002). Exercise dependence: A systematic review. *Psychology of Sport & Exercise, 3,* 89–123.

Hays, K.F. (1999). *Working it out: Using exercise in psychotherapy* (pp. 59–71). Washington, DC, US: American Psychological Association.

Janssen, I., Katzmarzyk, P.T., Ross, R., Leon, A.S., Skinner, J.S., Rao, D.C., Wilmore, J.H., Rankinen, T., & Bouchard, C. (2004). Fitness alters the associations of BMI and waist circumference with total and abdominal fat. *Obesity Research, 12,* 525–537.

Katz, J. (1996). Clinical observations on the physical activity of anorexia nervosa. In W.F. Epling, & W.D. Pierce (Eds.), *Activity anorexia: Theory, research, and treatment* (pp. 199–207). Mahwah, NJ: Lawrence Erlbaum Associates.

Kohrt, W.M., Snead, D.B., Slatopolsky, E., & Birge, S.J. (1995). Additive effects of weight-bearing exercise and estrogen on bone mineral density in older women. *Journal of Bone Mineral Research, 10,* 1303–1311.

Knols, R., Aaronson, N.K., Uebelhart, D., Fransen, J., & Aufdemkampe, G. (2005). Physical Exercise in Cancer patients During and After Medical Treatment: A Systematic Review of Randomized and Controlled Clinical Trials. *Journal of Clinical Oncology, 23,* 3830–3842.

Langer, E.J. (1989). *Mindfulness.* Reading, MA: Perseus Books.

Lee, I.M., Hsieh, C.C., & Paffenbarger, R.S. (1995). Exercise intensity and longevity in men: The Harvard alumni health study. *Journal of the American Medical Association, 273,* 1179–1184.

le Grange, D., & Eisler, I. (1993). The link between anorexia nervosa and excessive exercise: A review. *European Eating Disorders Review, 1,* 100–119.

Long, B.C., & van Stavel, R. (1995). Effects of exercise training on anxiety: A meta-analysis. *Journal of Applied Sport Psychology, 7,* 167–189.

Maltby, J., & Day, L. (2001). The relationship between exercise motives and psychological well-being. *The Journal of Psychology, 135,* 651–660.

Manson, J.E., Greenland, P., LaCroix, A.Z., Stefanick, M.L., Mouton, C.P., Oberman, A., Perri, M.G., Sheps, D.S., Pettinger, M.B., & Siscovick, D.S. (2002). Walking compared with vigorous exercise for the prevention of cardiovascular events in women. *New England Journal of Medicine, 347,* 716–725.

Mond, J.M., Hay, P.J., Rodgers, B., & Owen, C. (2006). An update on the definition of "excessive exercise" in eating disorders research. *International Journal of Eating Disorders, 39,* 147–153.

Mond, J.M., Hay, P.J., Rodgers, B., Owen, C., & Beumont, P.J.V. (2004). Relationships between exercise behavior, eating-disordered behavior and quality of life in a community sample: When is exercise "excessive"? *European Eating Disorders Review, 12,* 265–272.

Montgomery, P., & Dennis, J. (2002). Physical exercise for sleep problems in adults aged 60+. *Cochrane Database of Systematic Reviews, 4,* CD003404.

Norris, R., Carrol, D., & Cochrane, R. (1992). The effects of physical activity and exercise training on psychological stress and well-being in an adolescent population. *Journal of Psychosomatic Research, 36,* 55–65.

Otis, C., & Goldingay, R. (2000). *The athletic women's survival guide.* Champaign, IL: Human Kinetics.

Pasman, L., & Thompson, J.K. (1988). Body image and eating disturbance in obligatory runners, obligatory weightlifters, and sedentary individuals. *International Journal of Eating Disorders, 7,* 759–769.

Plugge, E., Stewar-Brown, S., Knight, M., & Fletcher L. (2002). Injury morbidity in 18–64-year-olds: Impact and risk factors. *Journal of Public Health Medicine, 24,* 27–33.

Rejeski, W.J., & Thompson, A. (1993). Historical and conceptual roots of exercise psychology. In P.Seraganian (Ed.), *Exercise psychology: The influence of physical exercise on psychological processes* (pp. 3–35). New York: Wiley.

Robison, J.I. (2000). Do we really need to exercise and eat low fat to get into heaven? *Healthy Weight Journal, Sept/Oct,* 74–75.

Rosenberg, I.H. (1998). Let's get physical. *Annals of Internal Medicine, 129,* 133–134.

Shroff, H., Reba, L., Thornton, L.M., Tozzi, F., Klump, K.L., Berrettini, W.H., et al. (2006). Features associated with excessive exercise in women with eating disorders. *International Journal of Eating Disorders, 39,* 454–461.

Solenberger, S.E. (2001). Exercise and eating disorders: A 3-year inpatient hospital record analysis. *Eating Behaviors, 2,* 151–168.

Steinberg, H., Sykes, E.A., & LeBoutillier, N. (1995). Exercise addiction: Indirect measures of 'endorphins'? In J. Annett, B. Cripps, & H. Steinberg (Eds.), *Exercise addiction: Motivation for participation in sport and exercise.* Leicester: The British Psychological Society.

Strober, M., Freeman, R., & Morrell, W. (1997). The long-term course of severe anorexia nervosa in adolescents: Survival analysis of recovery, relapse, and outcome predictors over 10–15 years in a prospective study. *International Journal of Eating Disorders, 22,* 339–360.

Tanji, J.L. (2000). The benefits of exercise for women. *Clinics in Sport Medicine, 19,* 175–185.

Taylor, W.C., Baranowski, T., & Sallis, J.F. (1994). Family determinants of childhood physical activity: A social-cognitive model. In R.K. Dishman (Ed.), *Advances in exercise adherence* (pp. 249–290). Champaign, IL: Human Kinetics Publishers.

Thompson, R.A., & Sherman, R.T. (1992). *Helping athletes with eating disorders.* Champaign, IL: Human Kinetics Publishers.

Throne, L.C., Bartholomew, J.B., Craig, J., & Farrar, R.P. (2000). Stress reactivity in fire fighter: An exercise intervention. *International Journal of Stress Management, 7,* 235–246.

Trost, S.G., Owen, N., Bauman, A.E., Sallis, J.F., & Brown, W. (2002). Correlates of adults' participation in physical activity: Review and update. *Medicine and Science in Sports and Exercise, 34,* 1996–2001.

Veale, D. (1995). Does primary exercise dependence really exist? In J. Annett, B. Cripps, & H. Steinberg (Eds.), *Exercise Addiction: Motivation for participation in Sport and Exercise.* Leicester: The British Psychological Society.

Wankel, L.M. (1993). The importance of enjoyment to adherence and psychological benefits from physical activity. *International Journal of Sport Psychology, 24,* 151–169.

Wankel, L.M., & Berger, B.G. (1991). The personal and social benefits of sport and physical activity. In B.L. Driver, P.J. Brown, & G.L. Peterson (Eds.), *Benefits of leisure* (pp. 121–144). State College, PA: Venture Publishing.

Wilson, D.K., Kirtland, K.A., Ainsworth, B.E., & Addy, C.L. (2004). Socioeconomic status and perceptions of access and safety for physical activity. *Annuals of Behavioral Medicine, 28,* 20–28.

Yates, A. (1991). *Compulsive exercise in the eating disorders: Toward an integrated theory of activity.* New York: Bruner-Mazel.

8

Relaxation and Meditation

Angele McGrady

In one form or another, ancient traditions included times of contemplation, peacefulness, quiet and solitude. Much of what we know about relaxation and meditation derives from the practices of non Western cultures, religious groups, and spiritual healers, where contemplation was a part of everyday life (Sharma, 1996). Popular interest in mind-body therapies and Alternative Medicine has grown dramatically during the past several decades. However, it is frequently assumed that relaxation and meditation are quick fixes for 21st century malaise, an assumption not based on fact. It is true that relaxation and meditation can produce powerful effects on health, well-being and quality of life, but time, practice and commitment are necessary to obtain those benefits.

Some understanding of the stress response is necessary to facilitate the application of meditation and relaxation to stress reduction and prevention of stress-related illness. Therefore, this chapter will begin with a brief discussion of the stress response as a normal, effective response to certain situations and the transformation of this set of physiological and emotional reactions into stress-related disorders. Preparation for personal change, goal setting, beginning the process, and enhancing the experience with additional tools such as imagery applies to both relaxation and meditation, so these topics will be discussed in the same sections. Then, specifics of relaxation and meditation and support from scientific research for the use of each of the techniques will be considered. Finally, risk factors and determining the need for providers of relaxation or meditation will be explained.

Effects of Stress

Stress impacts individuals in physiological, psychological, cognitive or spiritual ways, with all domains interrelated. In some individuals, one organ or one function such as digestion in the stomach may be sensitive to stress, while in others, the effects of stress may manifest in diverse, multiple symptoms, such as chewing, swallowing and digestion in the stomach and small intestine. The nervous system (central and autonomic) forms the neural network that allows the body to react to physical and emotional stresses. The endocrine system and the immune system are other key players in organizing the individual's response to stress, forming a triad of systems that is superbly organized to react to short-term situations in a largely physical manner

(Widmaier et al., 2004). This pattern of responses is found throughout the animal kingdom, and still exists today because it is necessary for survival. Typical acute physiological reactions to stressful situations include increased blood pressure, heart rate, shunting of blood away from the gastrointestinal system, and tense muscles. Emotionally the person may experience feelings of anxiety, worry, sadness or anger. Emotional and physical responses are closely related (Kroenke, Jackson, & Chamberlin, 1997; Sternberg, 2001). For example, hyperventilation (rapid, shallow breathing) brings about dizziness, tingling in the limbs, and chest pain of noncardiac origin, all of which increase anxiety. In turn, worry and anxious thoughts lead to a further increase in cardiovascular and respiratory activity (Gevirtz & Schwartz, 2003). With repeated stressors, the normal response becomes maladaptive, out of proportion to the severity of the situation. For example, a person may react to a minor hassle, such as being stuck in slowly moving traffic, as if he or she were in a traffic accident. The stress response system is further designed to recover or return to baseline or prestress levels after the stressful situation is over, yet that does not always happen, leaving the systems over-activated for too long (Cacioppo, 1994).

In the case of chronic stress, the triad of systems may continue to respond, upsetting the balance of physiological systems. Stress hormones in the blood and tissues produce damage over time, and increase the risk for stress-related diseases, such as high blood pressure, chronic headaches and diabetes (Björntop, Holm, & Rosmond, 1999). Individuals faced with stressful circumstances over the course of their lives have activated the stress response hundreds or thousands of times. Even relatively minor situations mobilize the entire system, automatically. The stress response has evolved into the default response system. The person may report that he/she has reacted without thinking; this can be explained by the existence of preprogrammed emotional, cognitive or behavioral reactions elicited without conscious awareness.

Recent discoveries in the field of neuroscience highlight the capacity of nerve cells to make new connections even in the adult brain. Logic tells us that based on this demonstration of nerve plasticity, modification of maladaptive patterns is possible through learning and practice (Sapolsky, 2003). When relaxation is performed on a consistent basis, the relaxation response is conditioned in place of the stress response and becomes the default mode. Repetition builds self-confidence and belief that the techniques will be of benefit in most stressful circumstances (Bourne, 1998).

Another consequence of chronic stress is a breakdown in self care, which has variable consequences depending on the person's current state of health. Daily stretching for back pain, exercise after a myocardial infarction and meal planning for the person with diabetes are behaviors necessary to prevent worsening of the illness, or keeping pain at manageable levels. Anxiety may prevent persons from attending to their own needs and disrupt their usual health maintaining behavior, so that they do not devote the time to stretching or cooking healthy meals. As explained by Cohen and Rodriguez (1995), affective disturbances or certain personality traits modify physical health and illness behaviors through cognitive, emotional, and social pathways. The person who has lost sight of their health goals because of anxiety or depression resulting from stress is at risk for one of the stress related diseases.

Development of Stress Related Disorders

As discussed previously, normal stress reactions may develop into sustained excessive responses. Later, simple maladaptive responses to stress become ingrained into the person's system (McGrady, 2002). The normal, life saving, adaptive stress responses transform into life shortening, maladaptive responses. Understanding allostasis and allostastic load will clarify the concept of maladaptive transformation (McEwen, 2002). Allostasis refers to a process whereby physiological systems keep the body stable because they are able to change in response to stimulation. Allostatic load refers to a build up of maladaptive responses to stress, such as frequent daily stressful situations, inability to recover from stress and over- and under-activity of physiological and emotional systems. These stress responses have become chronic and have led to physical or emotional illnesses, such as high blood pressure, muscle tension headaches, migraine headaches, irritable bowel syndrome, generalized anxiety disorder, panic disorder and chronic depression (McEwen, 1998).

Some disorders were not originally due to stress but have been complicated by current stress. When a person has an accident, he/she may recover from the acute injury. Despite objective evidence of tissue healing, pain may continue for months or years, at the same or reduced levels. Over time, pain becomes the center of the person's life: it exerts psychological and social effects, which affects relationships with family, significant others and job performance. It is likely that the person with chronic pain will benefit from a multimodal treatment package, which includes physical exercise, medication and mind-body therapy.

Preparation for Relaxation

There are many different types of relaxation strategies, but all share three components: (1) a passive attitude towards intruding thoughts, (2) repetition, and (3) a quiet and peaceful mind (Benson, 1975). Individuals can begin all of the relaxation strategies on their own at relatively low cost, but some of the more advanced techniques require the assistance of a professional. Relaxation is a structured process which cannot be learned by occasional practice. It will not eliminate stress, but rather the person learns to perceive situations differently, and to change behavior during and after stress. Although the techniques seem simple, the assumption that a person will be able to "just relax" or "not let it bother me" is not a realistic approach to beginning to learn to relax. Frequently, healthcare providers recommend stress management to their participants with the advice to "get rid of stress," yet little information regarding implementation accompanies the directive. This worsens frustration and anxiety.

Most people need guidance in choosing relaxation techniques and finding resources (Lehrer, 1996). The choice of technique depends on several factors: the levels of distress that the person is experiencing, the personal goals for self-relaxation and how much time the individual can put into the process. As is common in learning other self care behaviors such as healthy eating or exercise, people are more likely to drop out in the early weeks and months. If some effects are felt quickly, the naïve student of relaxation is more likely to continue. Therefore it is recommended that the neophyte begin with simple techniques and front load the practice time to increase the probability of experiencing the relaxation response.

Needs Assessment

Before beginning relaxation, the person must perform an honest self- appraisal and assessment of the present state of mind, body and spirit (Bourne, 2005). A visit to a physician or a licensed mental health provider may be necessary to determine the nature of the physical or emotional problems. A body scan will serve to identify areas of tension, discomfort or pain, at different times during the day and in various locations. Thus, the environments generating the most stress can be identified, as well as the times and places where a sense of quiet and peacefulness is usually experienced. Next, assessment of personal capacity to respond to stressful situations should be made, including analysis of successful or unsuccessful attempts to cope with past and present stress (Burns, 1999). Input can be sought from loving significant others to complete the assessment; however, the person's own appraisal is the most important (Sobel & Ornstein, 1996). Questionnaires and inventories are available to aid in the appraisal process of determining what body system, or mental state is most susceptible to stress effects, as well as the severity and frequency of stress responses.

Goal Setting

The personal assessment establishes the foundation for goal setting, which in turn is based on readiness for change. How much time and effort is the person willing to devote to learning the relaxation process? Is the person just thinking about changing behavior or actually committed to action? The model of change elaborated by Prochaska, Norcross, & Diclemente (1994) defines precontemplation as the stage where a commitment is unlikely, followed by contemplation when serious thought is directed to the process of change. Preparation entails actually making a plan and setting goals for change. Then, the plan is implemented and the results evaluated. Once change has taken place, the new behaviors must be maintained to avoid relapse. The stages of change model is appropriate to weight loss and smoking cessation (Zimmerman et al., 2000) and can similarly be applied to initiating relaxation or meditation. Having a detailed plan and recognizing potential barriers to change increases the chances of maximum benefit.

Expectations and projected time commitment should be realistic; otherwise, discontinuation of the program will be more likely if initial goals are not met. The starting point determines the short term goals and how quickly progress can be anticipated. Similarly, in weight loss programs, short-term goals are the main driver of change. Thinking about loosing 100 pounds is often overwhelming for the person, so weight loss goals of 10 or 20 pounds are set for the short term. In the case of relaxation, the person who has multiple symptoms of stress and genuinely wants to change may give up if too lofty goals are set, such as removing all effects of stress or learning relaxation quickly.

The categories of personal goals consist of first: achieving wellness for the individual who is healthy but wishes to be optimally well. Secondly, for stress management, the individual recognizes that stress is affecting them and wishes to decrease the impact of stress. Thirdly, the individual with a chronic illness needs to decrease maladaptive responses to stress that may have led them to illness. Fourth, the person can choose to use relaxation techniques as therapy for the illness itself. Lastly, chronic illnesses that are psychophysiological in nature can be targets for intervention. For example, the tension headache sufferer should focus on reduction of muscle tension with relaxation.

Case Example

"Cody" is a 36-year-old roofer. He is divorced, has a 12-year-old son, and works 50 hours a week during the spring, summer and fall. He has suffered from back pain since a fall 10 years ago. At his last check-up his physician told him he was in good health. The back pain remains mild as long as he exercises three times per week. His girlfriend of three years recently told him that she needed time away from him to think over their relationship. Cody recognizes that despite exercise, his back pain has been worse since that time and he is worried about it. Without his girlfriend, he is nervous during social situations and when he feels anxious his back pain is more noticeable. He also avoids confrontation as long as possible and this sometimes causes problems in dealing with his preteen son, Jake. Cody has multiple needs: to relax back muscles, reduce pain, lessen anxiety, gain a sense of control in social situations and hasten recovery after difficult situations. Since there are multiple potential sources of stress, Cody is well advised to have a repertoire of more than one technique of stress management.

Beginning the Process

Beginning the process of relaxation requires preparation, willingness to experience something new, and an understanding that dramatic effects are unlikely. However, learning relaxation involves building on a foundation that already exists. The relaxation response is natural to newborns and infants, as evidenced by youngsters falling asleep in any position and at any time. Later, children in the early years of education "unlearn" the natural relaxation response so that tension and anxiety become the norm, as discussed earlier.

The first step in learning relaxation is to become accustomed to being alone and still, in one's own mind. Many people are accustomed to living with constant noise from the radio, television or visual stimulation from the computer. The mind is usually filled with continuous thoughts, worries, and attending to physical sensations. The person learning relaxation can use props such as music or white noise or a cue that produces a hypnotic effect until a certain comfort level is achieved. Cody would be advised to begin by claiming 15 minutes every day for himself. He can choose a time after work or before bedtime when the house is quiet. His stomach should be moderately full, not swollen after a large meal, but not so empty that it becomes a distraction. Motivation does not mean insisting that Cody spend the total time relaxing. Nothing negative or associated with punishment should be associated with the relaxation experience.

Second, the person proceeds to create an atmosphere in his or her home where he/she can learn relaxation techniques. He/she should find a quiet area of his/her home, an entire room or a portion of the room where he/she is surrounded by pleasing sights, perhaps a favorite picture on the wall, a beautiful book that he/she can use to bring his/herself into the proper frame of mind. The area chosen for relaxation should be one of calm beauty. One or two words that are associated with a calming, positive visual image, such as *breath, silence*, and *heal* can be used to direct and maintain attention (Goldman, 2001).

Types of Relaxation

Breathing, Progressive and Autogenic

It is fair to say that breathing is a foundation for relaxation therapy as it is for meditation. "Controlled breathing is one of the oldest and certainly the single most efficient acute intervention for the mitigation and treatment of excessive stress" (Everly & Lating, 2002). Whatever type of relaxation is most beneficial, deep diaphragmatic breathing should be incorporated into regular practice.

Progressive and autogenic relaxations were developed many years ago in a format requiring months of training before achieving mastery. The modified versions that are in current usage carry similar power, but are shorter and easier to learn (Anselmo & Kolkmeier, 2000; Lehrer & Woolfolk, 1993a; Linden, 1990; Smith, 2005). Progressive relaxation entails structured tensing and relaxing of muscle groups in the lower, central and upper body, ending with the face. The person is instructed to tense each muscle group for several seconds at a moderate level of tension, never strong enough to produce pain. Tension is followed by a longer period of relaxation. The goal of this type of relaxation is to differentiate tension from relaxation and to learn to consciously produce muscle relaxation.

Autogenic relaxation fosters decreased sympathetic nervous system activity and lower muscle tension. Instead of tensing and relaxing muscles, the person learning autogenic relaxation repeats words and phrases designed to passively relax the muscles, and to warm the hands. Autogenic relaxation scripts contain the words: heavy, warm, relaxed, peaceful and comfortable. These words and associated phrases ("I feel heavy and relaxed" or "my hands are warm") are repeated slowly while attention is focused on the parts of the body to which the phrases are directed (Davis, Eshelman, & McKay, 1995).

When Cody is experiencing severe anxiety, he chooses the progressive relaxation technique which seems easier for him compared to a passive relaxation format that would require him to sit motionless. He is also advised to practice deep breathing multiple times during the day to keep his stress level manageable.

Coping Skills Training

Coping skills training is often integrated into stress reduction programs that utilize relaxation or meditation in order to facilitate incorporation of relaxation into daily life (Kabat-Zinn, 1990). The type of stress that is the most difficult to handle is a stressor that has not been anticipated and for which there is no plan, a situation that comes at the person without warning. Thus, ideal stress management is composed of techniques that the person can use if they have been affected by an unplanned or unanticipated stressor in addition to techniques that are useful in lessening the impact of stress. Perception of stress (termed appraisal) strongly influences the type, magnitude, and duration of the stress response (Lazarus, 1984). If the actual minimal stress is deemed to be beyond personal capability, vigorous stress responses will occur. Thus, part of coping skills training involves changing the person's perception of what is actually stressful. Cody will be assisted to reframe social situations or think about them in a different way so that he feels more comfortable going to a social event without his girlfriend. Once his expectations of the social situation are modified, his anxiety is likely to decrease.

The following example will clarify the concept of multidimensional coping. In physics and in physiology, there are two types of mechanisms that control or help to regulate physiological mechanisms. These are feed forward and feedback, both are necessary to maintain healthy regulation of cardiovascular, digestive, respiratory systems, as examples. Feedback is a process by which the effects of a disturbance in a system are decreased once they have occurred. This is like coping with a stressor after the physiological, psychological, cognitive effects are identified. A good analogy is of the thermostat in one's house that turns the heat on when the house is too cold and turns the air conditioning on when the house is too hot. Feed forward allows the system to anticipate a disruption of a controlled system. In the human body, the temperature regulation system is built on both feedback and feed forward principles. Skin temperature receptors allow the brain to anticipate a change in temperature. Receptors in the brain control center, called the hypothalamus measure the temperature of the blood. Sensing an elevation or decrease in temperature in the brain will immediately activate a compensatory response. In response to cold temperatures, the body may shiver, constrict the blood vessels in the periphery; in contrast, the body will initiate the sweating response and increase circulation to peripheral blood vessels (Widmaier et al., 2004). Cody must learn to anticipate potential stressful situations so that he can prepare in advance. He will also benefit by minimizing the impact of stressful situations as they occur by thinking about the stress and his own capabilities in a more positive manner.

Relaxation Aids

Materials and Classes

Scripts for relaxation are available in workbooks and guides to relaxation (Davis et al., 1995; Sobel & Ornstein, 1996) and can be purchased at major bookstores, found on the internet, or checked out of the library. Some books include worksheets that are useful in assessment, tracking progress, mood, anxiety behavior checklists (Barlow, 1994; Bourne, 1998; Burns, 1999). Relaxation tapes can be purchased, or the person can make a relaxation tape for themselves, or ask a friend to read a script into a tape recorder. They can purchase a workbook to guide them through the relaxation response. Many cities offer community education classes, seminars or get away weekends. The YMCA, YWCA, hospitals, senior centers, local high schools, colleges and some churches offer adult education. Examples of audiovisual and text materials are listed at the end of this chapter; these can also help create an atmosphere that facilitates the relaxation process (Table 8.1).

Table 8.1. Suggested helpful materials.

Bourne, E. (1998). Healing fear. Oakland, CA: New Harbinger.
Burns, D.D. (1999). The feeling good handbook (2nd ed.). New York: Plume.
Carrington, P. (1998). The book of meditation. London: Element Books.
Davis, M., Eshelman, E.R., and McKay, M. (1995). The relaxation & stress reduction workbook, 4th ed. (Chapters 3, 4, 5, 9, 15). Oakland, CA: New Harbinger Publications.
George, M. (1998). Learn to Relax. San Francisco: Chronicle Books.
Goldman, C. (2001). Healing words for the body, mind and spirit. New York: Marlowe & Company.
Kabat-Zinn, J. (2000). Mindfulness & Meditation video. Wellspring Media. Website: www.mindfulnesstapes.com
Time Life books. The book of calm (ways to manage stress), 1997.
Wellness Productions Publishing. Mental Health & Wellness Resources www.wellness-resources.com. Workbooks, guided imagery videos and CDs on relaxation.

Biofeedback

Small, inexpensive feedback devices are also available to monitor the physiology of the relaxation response. Biofeedback is a process by which an instrument is used to provide information to a person about the level of activity of a physiological function. For example, sensors are placed across the forehead and a digital display or fluctuating sound indicates the amount of tension that the person carries in the muscles around the forehead. The use of feedback can facilitate the relaxation response, since the person becomes aware of subtle changes in physiological activity and is encouraged to reproduce the same sensations in home practice. Some biofeedback devices are quite sophisticated research instruments, while others are simple and inexpensive. Skin temperature monitors, skin conductance meters, pulse rate monitors and breathing rate monitors are simple biofeedback instruments (Peek, 2003). The devices are set to reinforce a physiological change in the direction of relaxation, such as lower muscle tension, less sweating, lower heart rate and warmer hands. A specific example is an instrument called Resperate which provides information on breathing rate; the data reinforces slower, deeper breathing. With slowed breathing, heart rate and respiratory rate become coherent, and heart rate slows, contributing to decreased blood pressure (Elliot et al., 2004).

Imagery

Imagery or visualization directs the central and autonomic systems in a negative, maladaptive way or in a manner that promotes relaxation or healing. Worrying about something that may or may not have occurred produces negative images of possible consequences that in turn produce the physiological stress response. Imagery as a therapeutic relaxation technique uses the same hard wiring to direct the brain towards positive, healing images. Sense imagery consists of visualization, producing a visual image or focusing on a sound, or a feeling in addition to the mental picture. The mind presents a detailed picture that is associated with a positive experience and fosters relaxation. All senses are used to capture the total pleasant experience in as much detail as possible, so that the person feels as though the pleasant scene is all around them. Narrative imagery involves visualization of a relaxing scene in which the person is walking along a beach, petting a cat, or floating in warm water, directing the attention to the sensations of relaxation. Interactive guided imagery with a therapist involves the participant and the therapist dialoguing throughout the imagery session to assist the participant in developing insight or in solving problems (Schaub & Dossey, 2000; Smith, 2005).

Scientific Basis for the Benefits of Relaxation

It is important for the reader to understand how the benefits of relaxation are validated by scientific research. For the individual not accustomed to reading science, a statement such that this technique has a 40% success rate or even a 60% success rate may seem as if it is not worth undertaking. In most research studies, the expected level of benefit is preset. For example, in research studying the effects of relaxation on migraine headache, it is common to preset the standard for success as a 50% reduction in average pain (Blanchard & Diamond, 1996). A 60% success rate means that 6 of 10 individuals who used the technique on a regular basis reduced their average pain by 50%. If the participants followed the directions and used the techniques as directed, they had a good chance of being one of the 6, instead of the 4 who did not meet the criterion. Also, some participants may have achieved decreased pain, but not enough to meet the criterion for success. Perhaps 2 of the 4 "failures" received some benefit also. Nonetheless, it is important, when reading the scientific literature to determine if the therapy harmed any individuals or made their symptoms worse.

Regular practice of relaxation was found to decrease anxiety, lower high blood pressure, reduce stress, lessen the chronic pain of headaches and minimize muscle spasms (Freeman, 2001). Physiological effects of relaxation "desensitize" the nervous system, facilitating more rapid recovery after stress. The person begins to feel more in control of stress, defined as improved self efficacy (Everly & Lating, 2002). Relaxation therapy is a major part of behavioral approaches to management of chronic headache and back pain (Gevirtz, Hubbard, & Harpin, 1996; Holroyd, 2002). In the case of low back pain specifically, a multidimensional approach that combines medical and psychological-behavioral therapies produces the best outcomes of reduced pain and less dependence on medication (Argueta-Bernal, 2004). Migraine and muscle tension headache decrease in frequency, intensity and duration in approximately 50% of participants treated with relaxation combined with biofeedback (McGrady, Andrasik, & Davies, 1999). Regular practice of deep breathing will also facilitate significant reductions in blood pressure in persons with essential hypertension (Elliott et al., 2004). Management of participants with elevated blood pressure can combine relaxation with other forms of therapy in a format tailored to the specific needs of each participant (Linden, Lenz, & Con, 2001). In another common chronic illness, type 2 diabetes mellitus, relaxation combined with biofeedback was shown to decrease blood glucose and help participants develop a greater sense of control over their illness (McGinnis, McGrady, Cox, & Grower-Dowling, 2005).

Meditation

Types of Meditation

The introduction of meditation as a path to improved quality of life in mind, body and spirit dates from the 1970s. Benson's "relaxation response" was in fact a nonreligious type of meditation designed to produce a physiological response opposite to the stress response (Anselmo & Kolkmeier, 2000; Benson, 1975). Types of meditation include transcendental meditation (TM), mindfulness meditation, breathing meditation and walking meditation. Breathing meditation consists of inhaling while focusing on affirmations and exhaling to rid oneself of tension and anxiety. The self is observed during this process, but in a passive way, without distress if pain or tension is identified (Bourne, 1998). Mindfulness consists of taking a focal point on day-to-day activities, observing and experiencing the moment without judgment (Smith, 2005). Walking meditation (Kabat-Zinn, 1990) involves paying attention to each element of the walk, how do the arms and legs feel, the whole body moving, the breathing, the heart rhythm that makes it go. Slow walking is recommended because if the pace is too fast, the walker cannot attend to all of the sensations.

Kabat-Zinn (1994) defined mindfulness as "paying attention in a particular way: on purpose, in the present moment, and nonjudgmentally". The practice is learned during an 8–10 week course or an intensive 5-day course. Practice sessions of 45 minutes each day 6 days per week is recommended. The person learns to become aware of what is going on, the experience of the moment in an accepting frame of mind. The process is framed as if the person is an observer of the self and the experience. Many people are bound to time and schedules; although they fulfill their responsibilities, they do not enjoy anything that they are doing (Dunn, Hartigan, & Mikulas, 1999). This technique directly confronts the slavery of time, as each moment is worthy of attention. According to Kabat-Zinn, there needs to be more "being" in human beings and less human "doings" (Kabat-Zinn, 1990).

TM is based on Indian Vedic philosophy and was brought to the United States by Maharishi Mahesh Yogi in the sixties (Sharma, 1996). TM emphasizes concentration on a single word or words. The untrained mind labels and organizes information and experience according to the rules that have been set up. Sometimes the rules are inflexible, rigid and inappropriate and result in negative judgments of the self, others or the future. Instead, meditation encourages the person to be open to each moment in a nonjudgmental, noncategorizing way. The "beginners' mind" is cultivated so that the person sees the world as if for the first time. Negative thoughts that filter into the meditation process can be observed similarly to other thoughts. The person is encouraged to move away from the negative state of mind to concentration on the word(s) in order to achieve a calm and orderly mind.

Before Cody learned relaxation and meditation, he experienced a serious aftermath when he had to discipline his son. He did not notice tension or pain in his back during the conversation. However, after his son stormed out of the house, he became aware of pain in the neck, shoulders and back that took about three hours to decrease. Sometimes a nonsteroidal antiinflammatory agent was needed to decrease the pain so he could sleep. Cody learned mindfulness meditation and after two months, he does not raise his voice or lose his temper while discipling his son. When the interaction is over, he experiences tension in the neck, shoulders and back, but he no longer has pain. He recovers physically and emotionally from the incident within 30 minutes with no medication.

Scientific Basis for the Benefits of Meditation

Recall the effects of stress explained early in the chapter so that it will be easier to understand the significance of the benefits of meditation. Regular practice of meditation has been shown to reduce oxygen consumption, decrease heart rate and respiration rate, and blood lactate levels through mechanisms that are different than simply sitting with eyes closed (Dillbeck & Orme-Johnson, 1987). The habitual meditators, who practice regularly for months, change the ways in which they respond to stress. So not only does the baseline, usual, daily stress level decrease, but persons are less responsive to stressful situations (Freeman, 2001). Meditation facilitates mobilization of internal healing neural, endocrine and immune systems, builds emotional and spiritual strength, and increases personal resources. Long-term benefits also include decreased blood pressure, alleviation of chronic pain, less anxiety and improved mood (Grossman, Niemann, Schmidt, & Walach, 2004).

Based on findings from research studies, meditation programs are frequently incorporated into medical settings where participants are treated for physical illnesses. Equally important as exercise and nutritional counseling, participants learn a type of meditation as part of their treatment. Significant benefits are found in participants undergoing cardiac rehabilitation after a myocardial infarction; benefits are also found in those who have congestive heart failure and heart disease (Barnes, Treiber, Turner, Davis & Strong, 1999; Linden, 1990; Ornish, 1990; Schneider et al., 2005). Meditation has also been included in therapeutic management of emotional illness, particularly anxiety and depression (Miller, Fletcher, & Kabat-Zinn, 1995; Teasdale et al., 2000). Mindfulness is the essential component of several psychotherapies, for example, Mindfulness based Stress reduction (Kabat-Zinn, 1990), Acceptance and Commitment Therapy (Hayes, Strosahl, & Wilson, 1999) and Mindfulness based Cognitive Behavioral Therapy (Borkovec & Sharpless, 2004).

Choice of Technique

How can the person choose the technique that is most likely to produce benefit? Meditation practices, like relaxation practices are not the same and produce different effects (Lehrer & Woolfolk, 1993b; Travis & Wallace, 1997). However, the reader should be aware that there is no single best type of relaxation/meditation that will work all of the time for every purpose. The person seeking a specific benefit is advised to read the scientific literature or the popular press and note the particular type of intervention that is described and the length and frequency of practice that was utilized. Several different styles of relaxation or meditation may produce calming of the mind and relaxation of the body, but for each individual, one or two techniques will emerge as the most helpful in specific stressful situations (Smith, 2005). A sense of familiarity with several techniques will help the person to find those that match his or her personality, needs and available time (George, 1998; Nichol & Birchard, 2001).

Risks and Limitations

Are there any risks to learning relaxation on one's own? Can relaxation response mask serious symptoms? There are small and relatively infrequent side-effects such as a paradoxical anxiety response to relaxation. The person should at that point back off of practice and go about it much more gradually (Lehrer, 1996). Individuals with limited cognitive functioning may lack the capacity to understand the mind-body relationship. Lack of motivation and unwillingness to follow through may cause the individual to give up practice before any benefit is achieved. Some religious groups may find the concept of meditation against their religious beliefs. In that case, breathing training is a good starting point. The practice of relaxation and deep breathing can temporarily mask the symptoms of a true anxiety disorder. People with very high anxiety may have difficulty focusing long enough to practice and may stop prematurely. Repeated occurrences of increased anxiety during relaxation or failure of relaxation to provide any benefit despite regular practice may signal the presence of a true anxiety disorder. In this case, the person may need professional intervention to handle underlying problems that are interfering with the relaxation response.

When Self Help is Not Enough

Are there situations when self-help or the low cost interventions are not enough? The person has tried to help himself/herself using a relaxation tape, a workbook, and has taken the classes at the local YWCA. The sense of malaise worsens, the symptoms remain or worsen. Coping is not easier and recovery time from stressful situations is not decreasing appreciably. It is important for the person to deter thoughts of self blame. Recall that some stress-related illnesses are multifactorial and have other etiologies besides stress. In the case of essential hypertension, the increase in blood pressure is expected to continue for biological reasons not due to personal failure. Sometimes the frequency of stressful situations accelerates, such as caring for a loved one whose dementia is worsening and requires more time and effort on the part of the caregiver. The person may need medical management or psychological help, neither of which eliminates the possibility of using relaxation or meditation.

There are several different types of providers in most communities that can assist the person who is suffering the ill effects of stress. A physician can provide medical management if medication is required. The psychologist can provide testing of the person's personality structure and how that may be affecting unhealthy reactions to stress. A social worker or counselor as well as a psychologist and psychiatrist can provide counseling therapy to help the person understand how background, upbringing and environment has affected his/her stress response. Some of these clinicians can also teach the relaxation response, provide guided imagery, biofeedback in a comprehensive approach to stress related disorders.

Summary

This chapter discusses relaxation and meditation techniques as methods to counter the short-term and chronic effects of stress. Scientific research supports the use of relaxation and meditation as beneficial for physical and emotional illness. Individuals can use available resources and adjunctive tools, such as biofeedback or imagery to learn the relaxation response on their own. Suggestions for getting started, making the commitment, and monitoring progress are summarized. The chapter ends by exploring the risks of relaxation techniques and suggestions for finding professional assistance if necessary.

References

Anselmo, J., & Kolkmeier, L. G. (2000). Relaxation: the first step to restore, renew and self-heal. In B. M. Dossey, L. Keagan, & C. Guzzetta (eds.), *Holistic nursing A handbook for practice* (3rd ed., pp. 497–538). Gaithersburg, Maryland: Aspen Publishers Inc.

Argueta-Bernal, G. (2004). Behavioral approaches for chronic low back pain. *Seminars in Pain Medicine, 2*, 197–202.

Barlow, D. H. (1994). *Clinical handbook of psychological disorders: A step-by-step treatment manual*. New York: Guilford.

Barnes, V. A., Treiber, F. A., Turner, R., Davis, H., & Strong, W. B. (1999). Acute effects of transcendental meditation on hemodynamic functioning in middle-aged adults. *Psychosomatic Medicine, 61*, 525–531.

Benson, H. (1975). *The relaxation response*. New York: Marrow.

Björntop, P., Holm, G., & Rosmond, R. (1999). Hypothalamic arousal, insulin resistance and type 2 diabetes mellitus. *Diabetic Medicine*, 373–383.

Blanchard, E. B., & Diamond, S. P. (1996). Psychological treatment of benign headache disorders. *Professional Psychology: Research and Practice, 6*, 541–547.

Borkovec, T., & Sharpless, B. (2004). Generalized anxiety disorder. In S. C. Hayes, V. M. Follette, & M. M. Linehan (Eds.), *Mindfulness and acceptance* (pp. 209–242). New York: The Guilford Press.

Bourne, E. J. (1998). *Healing fear*. Oakland, CA: New Harbinger Publications, Inc.

Bourne, E. J. (2005). *The anxiety and phobia workbook* (4th ed.). Oakland, CA: New Harbinger Publications.

Burns, D. D. (1999). *The feeling good handbook*. New York: Plume.

Cacioppo, J. T. (1994). Social neuroscience: autonomic, neuroendocrine and immune responses to stress. *Psychophysiology, 31*, 113–128.

Cohen, S., & Rodriguez, M. S. (1995). Pathways linking affective disturbances and physical disorders. *Health Psychology, 14*(5), 374–380.

Davis, M., Eshelman, E. R., & McKay, M. (1995). *The relaxation & stress reduction workbook* (4th ed., pp. 91–100). Oakland, CA: New Harbinger Publications.

Dillbeck, M. C., & Orme-Johnson, D. W. (1987). Physiological differences between transcendental meditation and rest. *American Psychologist, 42*, 879–881.

Dunn, D. R., Hartigan, J. A., & Mikulas, W. L. (1999). Concentration and mindfulness meditations: Unique forms of consciousness? *Applied Psychophysiology and Biofeedback, 24*(3), 147–165.

Elliott, W., Izzo Jr., J., White, W. B., Rosing, D., Snyder, C. S., Alter, A., Gavish, B., & Black, H. R. (2004). Graded blood pressure reduction in hypertensive outpatients associated with use of a device to assist with slow breathing. *Journal of Clinical Hypertension, 6*(10), 553–559.

Everly Jr., G. S., & Lating, J. M. (2002). *A clinical guide to the treatment of the human stress response* (2nd ed.). New York: Kluwer.

Freeman, L. W. (2001). Meditation. In L. Freeman, & G. F. Lawlis (Eds.), *Mosby's complementary & alternative medicine* (pp. 166–195). St. Louis: Mosby.
Gevirtz, R. N., Hubbard, D., & Harpin, E. (1996). Psychophysiologic treatment of chronic low back pain. *Professional Psychology: Research and Practice, 27*(6), 561–566.
Gevirtz, R. N., & Schwartz, M. S. (2003). The respiratory system in applied psychophysiology. In M. Schwartz, & F. Andrasik (Eds.), *Biofeedback A practitioner's guide* (pp. 212–244). New York: Guilford Press.
Goldman, C. (2001). *Healing words for the body, mind and spirit* (pp. 22–24; 76–78; 164–166). New York: Marlowe & Company.
Grossman, P., Niemann, L., Schmidt, S., & Walach, H. (2004). Mindfulness-based stress reduction and health benefits – a meta-analysis. *Journal Psychosomatic Research, 57*, 35–43.
Hayes, S. C., Strosahl, K., & Wilson, K. G. (1999). *Acceptance and commitment therapy: an experimental approach to behavior change*. New York: Guilford Press.
Holroyd, K. A. (2002). Assessment and psychological management of recurrent headache disorders. *Journal Consulting and Clinical Psychology, 70*(3), 656–677.
Kabat-Zinn, J. (1990). *Full catastrophe living*. New York: Dell Publishing.
Kabat-Zinn, J. (1994). *Wherever you go, there you are*. New York: Hyperion.
Kroenke, K., Jackson, J. L., & Chamberlin, J. (1997). Depressive and anxiety disorders in participants presenting with physical complaints: Clinical predictors and outcome. *American Journal of Medicine, 103*(5), 339–347.
Lazarus, R. S. (1984). On the primacy of cognition. *American Psychologist, 39*, 124–129.
Lehrer, P. M. (1996). Varieties of relaxation methods and their unique effects. *International Journal of Stress Management, 3*(1), 1–15.
Lehrer, P. M. & Woolfolk, R. L. (1993a). *Principles and practice of stress management* (2nd ed.). New York: Guilford.
Lehrer, P. M., & Woolfolk, R. L. (1993b). Specific effects of stress management techniques. In P. M. Lehrer, & R. I. Woolfolk (Eds.), *Principles and practice of stress management* (pp. 481–520). New York: Guilford.
Linden, W. (1990). *Autogenic training: A clinical guide*. New York: Guilford.
Linden, W., Lenz, J. W., & Con, A. H. (2001). Individualized stress management for primary hypertension: A randomized trial. *Archives of Internal Medicine, 161*, 1071–1080.
McEwen, B. S. (1998). Protective and damaging effects of stress mediators. *The New England Journal of Medicine, 338*, 171–179.
McEwen, B. S. (2002). *The end of stress as we know it*. Washington, DC: The Dana Press.
McGinnis, R., McGrady, A., Cox, S., & Grower-Dowling, K. (2005). The effects of biofeedback assisted relaxation in Type 2 diabetes mellitus. *Diabetes Care, 28*(9), 2154–2149.
McGrady, A. (2002). Psychophysiological foundations of the mind-body therapies. In D. Moss, A. McGrady, T. C. Davies, & I. Wickramasekera (Eds.), *Handbook of mind-body medicine for primary care* (pp. 43–55). Thousand Oaks: Sage Publications, Inc.
McGrady, A., Andrasik, F., & Davies, T. (1999). Psychologic therapy for chronic headache in primary care. *Primary Care Companion to the Journal of Clinical Psychiatry, 1*, 96–102.
Miller, J., Fletcher, K., & Kabat-Zinn, J. (1995). Three year follow-up and clinical implications of a mindfulness-based stress reduction intervention in the treatment of anxiety disorders. *General Hospital Psychiatry, 17*, 192–200.
Nichol, D., & Birchard, B. (2001). *The one-minute mind meditator: Relieving stress and finding meaning in everyday life*. Cambridge, MA: Perseus Publishing.
Ornish, D. (1990). *Dr. Dean Ornish's Program for Reversing Heart Disease*. New York: Random House.

Peek, C. (2003). A Primer of Biofeedback Instrumentation. In M. Schwartz, & F. Andrasik (Eds.), *Biofeedback A practitioner's guide* (pp. 43–87). New York: Guilford Press.

Prochaska, J. E., Norcross, J. C., & Diclemente, C. C. (1994). *Changing for good: The revolutionary program that explains the six stages of change and teaches you how to free yourself from bad habits*. New York: Morrow.

Sapolsky, R. M. (2003). Stress and plasticity in the limbic system. *Neurochemical Research, 28*, 1735–1742.

Schaub, B. G., & Dossey, B. M. (2000). Imagery: Awakening the inner healer. In B. Dossey, L. Keagan, & C. Guzzetta (Eds.), *Holistic nursing: A handbook for practice* (pp. 539–581). Gaithersburg, MD: Aspen Publishers Inc.

Schneider, R. H., Alexander, C. N., Staggers, F., Rainforth, M., Salerno, J. W., Hartz, A., Arndt, S., Barnes, V. A., & Nidich, S. I. (2005). Long-term effects of stress reduction on mortality in persons $\geq$ 55 years of age with systemic hypertension. *The American Journal of Cardiology, 95*, 1060–1064.

Sharma, H. M. (1996). Maharishi Ayurveda. In M. S. Micozzi, & C. E. Koop (Eds.), *Fundamentals of complementary and alternative medicine* (pp. 243–258). New York: Churchill Livingstone.

Smith, J. C. (2005). *Relaxation, meditation, & mindfulness*. New York: Springer Publishing Co., Inc.

Sobel, D. S., & Ornstein, R. (1996). Chapter 6: Relaxation and Chapter 7: Imagery. In *The healthy mind, healthy body handbook* (pp. 81–96 and 97–108). Los Altos, CA: DR_X Publishing.

Sternberg, E. M. (2001). *The balance within. The science connecting health and emotions*. New York: W. H. Freeman & Company.

Teasdale, J. D., Segal, Z. V., Williams, J. M. G., Ridgeway, V. A., et al. (2000). Prevention of relapse/recurrence in major depression by mindfulness-based cognitive therapy. *Journal Consulting Clinical Psychology, 68*, 615–623.

Travis, F., & Wallace, R. K. (1997). Autonomic patterns during respiratory suspensions: Possible Markers of transcendental consciousness. *Psychophysiology, 34*(1), 39–46.

Widmaier, E. P., Raff, H., & Strang, K. T. (2004). The adrenal glands and the response to stress. In Vander, Sherman & Luciano's Human Physiology, (9th ed., pp. 360–363). Boston: McGraw Hill.

Zimmerman, G. L., Olsen, C. G., & Bosworth, M. F. (2000). A "stages of change" approach to helping patients change behavior. *American Family Physician, 61*(5), 1409–1416.

9

Expressive Movement

Dianne Dulicai and Ellen Schelly Hill

Expressive movement is at the heart of the practice of dance/movement therapy, a profession that integrates both the art and science of dance/movement and psychotherapy. Dance/movement therapy is defined by the American Dance Therapy Association as "the psychotherapeutic use of movement in a process which furthers the emotional, social, cognitive, and physical integration of the individual" (www.adta.org/about/factsheet.cfm, 2006). As body and psyche interplay in expressive movement, body and psyche also interplay in movement throughout human development to inform an individual's experience, interaction, and functioning. The dance/movement therapist applies this holistic understanding of movement in a therapy relationship process to foster growth and health.

Dance/movement therapists view all human movement as expressive. Expressive movement encompasses a turning spin in a creative dance as well the exuberant leap of a gleeful child and the inward turned attention and diminished movement vitality in depression. The following chapter provides an outline of how dance/movement therapists understand, facilitate, and respond to the movement expressions of the people with whom they work to support their physical and psychological health. Many mental and physical health disorders are expressed in both physiological and psychological symptoms. The effectiveness of dance/movement therapy may lie in its ability to address both aspects of illness. Dance/movement techniques may also mobilize and support the strengths of the participant for more effective coping with psychological or physical distress. And dance/movement techniques may be used to augment other treatment methods for a more effective and efficient comprehensive treatment approach. Whether one chooses private dance movement therapy consultation or dance/movement therapy as a part of a comprehensive system participants can access cost-effective services. Within the outline of the dance/movement therapy research and clinical practice presented here, there are some suggestions as to how the reader may make use of dance/movement as a personal resource for health in daily life. Taking responsibility for health is one of the most effective ways of curtailing the costs of illness.

A number of movement disciplines and dance artists that contribute complementary expertise to the use of expressive movement for physical and mental health will be referenced in this chapter in addition to dance/movement therapy resources. The next paragraph includes information concerning the professional organization, credentialing, and scope of practice of dance/movement therapists, related dance/movement specialists, and dance educators. The appendix at the end of the chapter provides contact information for the organizations identified and other resources the reader can tap for additional information and location of services.

The American Dance Therapy Association (ADTA) is the professional organization and credentialing body for dance/movement therapy. The credential for entry-level practice in dance/movement therapy is Dance Therapist Registered (DTR). The DTR credential requires graduate education in dance/movement theory and practice, movement observation and assessment, psychological foundation coursework, clinical fieldwork, a 700-hour supervised clinical practice internship, and adherence to ADTA Ethics and Standards. Following an additional two years of supervised clinical practice the registered dance/movement therapist is eligible to apply for the Academy of Dance Therapists Registered credential (ADTR) which signifies the dance/movement therapist is qualified to work privately and provide clinical supervision. Dance/movement therapists at the ADTR credential level are also eligible to sit for the National Counselor Exam (NCE) and in many states are eligible to apply for the Licensed Professional Counselor (LPC) credential.

Dance/movement therapists practice in inpatient psychiatric and medical hospitals, in early intervention settings, in schools and special education settings, in community mental health centers, in community/wellness programs, in social service agencies, prisons, and in facilities serving older adults. Dance/movement therapy may be an integrated component of treatment and support in these settings. At other times dance/movement therapy services are available by request or can be obtained through referral to a dance/movement therapist in private practice. Dance/movement therapists in private practice provide both psychotherapy and consultation services.

Graduate study in dance movement therapy includes an introduction to Laban Movement Analysis (LMA). Laban Movement Analysis is a rich and comprehensive system for understanding the language of movement. It provides a framework for movement observation, description, analysis, and notation. The Certified Movement Analyst (CMA) credential, awarded by the Laban/Bartenieff Institute of Movement Studies in NYC and several satellite locations, and the Graduate Certificate in Laban Movement Analysis (GCLMA), awarded by Columbia College in Chicago, are credentials that signify completion of a graduate level certificate program in Laban Movement Analysis. A number of dance/movement therapists have completed this specialized training in addition to their dance/movement therapy education. Movement specialists with this credential apply movement analysis skills in a variety of fields, including nonverbal communication research, dance education and performance, theater, physical education, rehabilitation, and dance/movement therapy. A number of assessments tools used by dance/movement therapists have a foundation in LMA. These include the Movement Psychodiagnostic Inventory (MPI) (Davis, 1991), the Nonverbal Assessment of Families (Dulicai, 1997), and the Kestenberg Movement Profile (KMP) (Kestenberg, 1965a, 1965b, 1967).

The National Dance Educators Association (NDEO) is a professional organization that "promotes dance as an artistic process which broadens and deepens human experience" (http://www.ndeo.og/ToMove.pdf, 2001). Given this broad mission for dance education, the NDEO advocates for the inclusion of the arts in all K-12 educational curricula. The NDEO promotes dance education research and sets standards for K-12 dance education, dance schools, and the university training of dancers and dance educators. Member educators of the NDEO may be involved in the challenging technical and artistic training of young girls and boys who hope to become professional dancers. However, other dance educators may create dance experiences for "non-dancers" who learn about cooperation, creativity, and valuing themselves through a community dance experience. Still other dance educators may collaborate with classroom teachers to bring class assignments to life through arts-based learning approaches. Encompassed within NDEO's mission is a recognition of dance/movement as life enrichment valuable to all.

Dance/Movement Therapy History and Theory

The profession of dance/movement therapy began in the United States during the era of World War II. A number of World War II veterans who returned home with war trauma symptoms, now known as Posttraumatic Stress Disorder, received treatment at Saint Elizabeth's Hospital, a federal hospital in Washington D.C. Many participated in the dance therapy sessions of Marian Chace, a dance/movement therapy pioneer. Chace was a dancer who received her formal dance training at the New York School of Denishawn. Following years of teaching, performing, and developing choreography, Chace became an "artist in residence" at Saint Elizabeth's. At Saint Elizabeth's Hospital, Chace developed fundamental concepts of dance with psychiatric participants that still influence dance/movement therapy practice and education today. Components of Chace technique include body action, rhythmic group activity, symbolism, and the therapeutic movement relationship (Chaiklin & Schmais, 1979).

In the same era, several other dancers independently were involved in an exploration of the application of dance to therapy. Blanche Evan originated an approach to dance therapy that utilized movement improvisation to help neurotic urban adults. She was also involved in creative dance intervention with children. Liljan Espenak brought her extensive dance training to the United States, after first fleeing her German homeland for England. In the United States she studied at the Alfred Adler Institute and later worked with participants and taught dance therapy at New York Medical College. Espenak developed a dance/movement therapy approach in which she used both free movement and specific exercises in an approach she called psychomotor therapy. West coast dance/movement therapy pioneers included Mary Whitehouse, founder of the discipline of Authentic Movement, which she developed as she worked in her dance studio with normal neurotic adults. Mary Whitehouse (1979) integrated principles from Jungian depth psychology in her dance therapy approach. Trudi Schoop (Schoop & Mitchell, 1974) worked with the seriously mentally ill in inpatient psychiatric treatment in California through a creative dance process. A very full description and detailing of dance/movement therapy history and theory is available in the book *Dance/Movement Therapy: A Healing Art* (Levy, 2005) for readers who are interested in a more comprehensive overview. The field of dance/movement therapy has become increasingly sophisticated in theory and technique. However, much of dance/movement therapy theory, and the techniques described later in the Dance/Movement Therapy Practice section of this chapter, have their genesis in the work of dance/movement therapy pioneers.

Dance/movement therapy theory, introduced in an early publication, Dance Therapy: Focus on Dance VII has stood the test of time (Schmais, 1974). The primary premises of dance/movement therapy theory that were identified in the early publication were:

1. Movement reflects personality.
2. The relationship established between the therapist and patient through movement supports and enables behavioral change.
3. Significant changes occur on the movement level that can affect total functioning (p. 10).

These early premises developed out of therapist reflection on the dance/movement therapy experience. They can now be substantiated through reference to anthropological, psychological, and biological study and developments.

The premise that movement reflects personality was relatively new to science when the dance/movement therapy profession was initiated in the 1960s. Anthropological investigation of individual and collective dance expression as an expression of persons and cultures supports this premise (Lomax et al., 1968). Neuroscience and genetic findings now confirm that characteristics of personality are a part of our genetic endowment displayed through movement (Bates & Malhorta, 2002; Plomin & DeFries, 1998). An expansion of the premise that movement reflects personality is the understanding that expressive movement has personal meaning.

Psychotherapy theorists and practitioners have long understood the importance of relationship as a significant factor in the change process of therapy (Lambert, 1992). The significance of relationship in the therapy process is the second dance/movement therapy premise. The dance/movement therapy relationship is a movement relationship. The 1960s and 1970s were a period of groundbreaking nonverbal communication research. Understanding of the role of movement in communication was advanced through the work of scientists such as Birdwhistell (1963); Condon (1968); and Scheflen (1972). Their work found that over 50% of communication is nonverbally expressed through gestures, postures, and interactional reciprocals of movement. Birdwhistell also studied the phenomenon of interactional synchrony, in which people are engaged in interaction move "in sync" with one another. The dance/movement therapist intentionally initiates the rhythmic synchrony of dance to facilitate relationship and group cohesion. Recent findings in neuroscience are also relevant to the dance/movement therapy relationship. A basic component of the dance/movement relationship is movement "mirroring" or "empathic reflection" through which the therapist experiences and communicates empathy, joins with, and engenders the trust of the client. Recent discoveries in neuroscience have established the existence of "mirror neurons" that provide a basis for attachment in the human relationship. The research shows excitation in the brain areas appropriate to emotional expression when the subject observes another displaying movement appropriate to that emotion (Gallese et al., 2004). Berrol (2006) discusses the significance of these findings as providing a neurological basis for understanding empathic reflection in the movement relationship.

The third premise of dance/movement therapy addresses the power of changes in movement to effect changes in functioning and experience. Some of the rationale for this lies in the understanding of body and mind unity. The bidirectional relationship between body and mind mean that changes in one initiate changes in the other. In dance/movement therapy a participant may find that a change in movement shifts his/her perspective and experience. At the same time, the dance/movement therapist elicits the participant's cognitive understanding and clarification of movement expression verbally. This insight may enable behavioral change and become manifest in movement changes. An expansion of an individual's movement repertoire reflects a broader behavioral repertoire through which the individual interacts with the world (Davis, 1970).

Dance/movement therapy theory is grounded in the dance training and experience of its practitioners. The working vocabulary of the dancer and choreographer involves sensitivity to capturing the essential form and specific quality of gesture to project an emotion. Dance/movement therapists bring this vocabulary and sensitivity to understanding movement in the dance/movement therapy session and to supporting the movement expression of the dance/movement therapy participant. Dance/movement therapists also align themselves with various verbal therapy orientations and incorporate elements of other theories of therapy in their work. They borrow from Winnicott's concept of the holding environment and play theory, Freud's and Jung's understanding of symbolism and the unconscious, Sullivan's interpersonal therapy approach, appreciation for caregiver/child "object relations theory" and humanistic therapy's attention to the here-and-now experience in therapy, among others. However, the three premises of dance/movement therapy identified by Schmais continue to provide a unifying foundation for all dance/movement therapy practice, whatever the individual orientation of the dance/movement therapist.

A range of dance/movement techniques have developed which the dance/movement therapist applies in practice to meet the varied needs of dance/movement participants. Some dance/movement applications are outlined below. The route from theory to practical application is informed by ongoing research. Dance/movement therapy research is reviewed in the next section of this chapter.

Dance/movement techniques are designed to:

- Increase grounded and sequenced movements of the body
- Improve sense of control of one's body
- Help participants organize their thoughts and actions through rhythmic action
- Provide validation and build, relationship through the mirroring of movement responses
- Support social connection by supporting engagement in synchronous movement and movement interaction
- Offer a venue for self-awareness
- Provide an outlet for self-expression
- Expand options of behavior through the development of an expanded movement repertoire
- Make meaning by clarifying symbolic images and relevant themes expressed in movement
- Improve recognition of sensory feedback about feelings, needs, and relationships

- Improve children's ability to focus directly, restrain impulses, and improve perception
- Help families work toward fulfilling each member's potential through movement interaction

Research

Early psychological researchers interested in the meaning of movement relied on observational methods of testing hypotheses. A great deal of research in this arena took place from the late nineteenth century through the middle twentieth century. Darwin's (1872) work was a great leap toward understanding the role of movement in human behavior through observation of animal behavior. Freud's early work cited the movement of participants' during analysis (Freud, 1938). Allport and Vernon (1933) presented work based on their hypothesis that movement patterns were consistent over time and were the most direct way to study personality. Other works emerged from analyst Deutsch (1947), who studied the postures of his participants and Reich (1949), who developed character analysis through observation of the physical tensions and expressions of his participants.

The development of new scientific methods for testing theories in psychology and other areas of science has advanced our theoretical understanding in many areas of science and art. Dance/movement therapy theory was initially based on untested hypotheses, and has benefited from an ongoing development of scientific methods of measurement. The establishment of graduate programs in dance/movement therapy in the 1970s paralleled the first scientific research methods in the profession. Beth Kalish (1976) was a pioneer in developing scientific assessment methods. Her movement scale for the assessment of autistic children was included in the final Behavior Rating Instrument for Autistic and other Atypical Children (Ruttenberg, Kalish, Wenar, & Wolf, 1978). An early documentation of scientific investigation into the effectiveness of dance/movement therapy with children was the dissertation of Cynthia Berrol (1978), *The effects of two movement remediation programs on selected measures of perceptual-motor ability, academic achievement and behavior on first-grade children manifesting learning and perceptual-motor problems*. This was followed by a number of additional scientific investigations of dance/movement therapy by Berrol (Berrol & Katz, 1985; Berrol, 1992; Berrol, Ooi & Katz, 1997). Dianne Dulicai (1977) piloted the nonverbal assessment of families. This study was followed, in the next two decades, by investigations of the nonverbal assessment of family interaction patterns in 18 families. The assessment has been used in numerous publications in understanding family interactions in a wide sample of family circumstances. Nathan Schappin (2003), developed the Functional Assessment of Movement Scale (FAM) a movement-based assessment tool of nonverbal interaction and interpersonal behavior. Used as an outcome measure and research tool, the FAM Scale allows the collection of clinical data relevant for all creative arts therapies.

A number of movement researchers in other fields directly contributed to dance/movement therapy through their research. The early studies of psychologist Martha Davis on the movement behavior of hospitalized participants and her development of a number of movement assessments contributed enormously to the understanding of movement and behavior and research methodology in the field of dance/movement therapy (Davis, 1970, 1975). Marion North, a movement analyst and founder of the Laban Centre for Movement Studies in London, contributed knowledge of how movement characteristics of children reflect personality through her book, *Personality Assessment through Movement* (North, 1972). Additionally, the original research of psychoanalyst Judith Kestenberg, MD contributed to our understanding of movement in children and their families. A series of published works, which addressed the role of movement patterns in development, began in the Psychoanalytic Quarterly (Kestenberg, 1965a, b, 1967) and was later summarized and elaborated by her students and colleagues (Amighi, Loman, Lewis & Sossin, 1999). Dance/movement therapy theory was tested and refined with the assistance of these related research contributions.

In the last ten years, as graduate programs have emerged in Europe, so has research developed there. In 2004, dance/movement therapists Iris Brauninger and Sabine Koch, chaired the first International Research Colloquium in Dance/Movement Therapy. An impressive array of researchers representing 11 countries reported on a wide range of research projects, some state-sponsored, others university-sponsored. Brauninger and Koch were thrilled by the dance/movement therapy international community spirit ignited by this professional gathering. The progressive evolution of dance/movement therapy in Europe is consistent with globalization of dance/movement therapy in 37 countries across the world, reported in international survey results by Dulicai and Berger (2005).

Many of the clinically oriented studies in dance/movement therapy continue to take place in dance/movement therapy graduate programs by students meeting thesis requirements. American Dance Therapy Association approved programs in dance/movement therapy consist of graduate programs at Antioch New England Graduate School, Columbia College, Drexel University, Naropa Institute, and Pratt Institute. The Chace Foundation publishes a compendium of thesis and dissertation research abstracts every five years, available from the American Dance Therapy Association. The profession of dance/movement therapy has an ongoing commitment to building the research base for its practice and contributing research to the larger psychotherapy community. Additional references to dance/movement therapy research relevant to clinical practice are cited in the Practice section which follows.

Practice

Since its inception, dance/movement has served persons interested in movement as a medium for personal growth as well as those who suffer from severe and persistent mental illness. In practice, dance/movement therapists offer services, in both primary and allied health roles, which respond to a broad range of interests and needs.

The section that follows describes clinical and wellness applications of dance/movement therapy and related approaches. Some of the dance/movement techniques that dance/movement therapists use to promote health are described. The dance/movement therapist carefully assesses the participant, establishes goals, and responsively selects and works with dance/movement techniques that support the strengths and meet the needs of the participant in the dance/movement process. As noted earlier, as in any psychotherapy approach, the dance/movement process is a relationship process. Whatever the techniques employed, the relationship is a significant agent in treatment and growth. However, at the foundation of dance/movement is the intrinsic healing power of creativity and movement in an expressive dance experience.

Dance/Movement for Adults

Before the saving advent of psychotropic medications, Marian Chace pioneered dance/movement therapy in the inpatient psychiatric back wards of Saint Elizabeth's Hospital in Washington, D.C. She reached participants who the traditional therapies of the time were often unable to serve.

Medication prescribed by a physician is often the first line of treatment defense in psychiatric crisis or severe mental illness in current times. The dance/movement therapist as a member of the treatment team helps establish a coordinated treatment plan that augments medication benefits and contributes to the health of the patient through psychotherapeutic support. Dance/movement therapist Sheila Stone, currently Interim Director of Dance/Movement Therapy at Saint Elizabeth's Hospital, says, "Dance/Movement Therapy remains an integral part of a modernized approach to inpatient psychiatric treatment at Saint Elizabeth's Hospital. Integrating concepts of the Recovery Model, dance/movement therapy contributes to numerous treatment programs at the hospital: Geriatric, Psychosocial Rehabilitation, Substance Abuse, Behavior Modification, Cognitive Remediation programs and services for the medically ill. Dance/movement therapy continues to support participants by providing an outlet for self-expression and a venue for interpersonal connection and self-awareness. It is a particularly effective form of therapy for participants with severe mental illness who struggle with verbal therapies" (personal communication, August 2005). Today dance/movement therapy can be found in psychiatric settings in many urban centers. Marian Chace created the basic group movement structure that many dance/movement therapists continue to use in inpatient and community mental health settings today (Sandel, Chaiklin, & Lohn, 1993).

A Chacian dance/movement session begins with the grounded and sequential movements of a body warm-up and rhythmic movement to music that may help participants organize their thoughts and actions. The modulation of tempo and dynamic in the music and dance support the self-regulation of the participant. Participating with others in the synchronous movement of the developing group dance may permit an experience of social connection for persons withdrawn or who require structure for successful interaction. The social affiliation of synchronous group movement is perhaps akin to the solidarity experienced participating in the rhythmic unison movement of a folk dance circle or the sequential movement of a movement wave at an athletic event. However, the dance/movement technique is an improvisation in which the leader of the group observes, responds to, and incorporates the sometimes subtle movement initiations of the group participants in the group dance. The participants' movements, which may reflect intense inner experiences and feelings, are mirrored by the leader and shaped in the group dance. Mirroring is a basic technique that involves matching and replicating the essence of another's expression in movement (Sandel, 1993b). Mirroring has a basis in foundations of human interaction and development in mother/infant attunement and relationship (Kestenberg Amighi, Loman, Lewis & Sossin, 1999). The dance/movement therapist, who is educated to be aware of nonverbal behavior, can detect and respond if a potential crisis is apparent in the movement of a group participant (Davis, 1970).

In the course of a session, movement experiences may elicit symbolic images (Sandel, 1993a; Schmais, 1985) and associations to relevant themes from the lives of the participants. Feelings may also emerge from the movement associations. The therapist helps the participants integrate these responses by developing them nonverbally in the dance or exploring them further verbally. This gives participants the opportunity to be recognized, communicate, and give meaning to their expression during a time in which their sense of self may be fragmented, their relationship to others disturbed, and their connection to reality tenuous. The participants engage together in a creative process that supports human dignity and affirms each person's need for and right to self-expression. Through dance/movement techniques the leader supports the participant's strengths as resources in recovery. In the same way, the well person's participation in creative or improvisational dance can be a creative, health supporting, and validating endeavor.

Dance/Movement and Anxiety

Dance/movement is suited to the treatment of anxiety. Anxiety involves physical and psychological discomfort that is common in everyday living, change and growth. However, in an anxiety disorder, distressing physical symptoms are intensified and can result in paralyzing self-restriction and avoidance accompanied by a psychological sense of danger, apprehension of the future, and often a fear of losing control. The leader, working with a client who has anxiety as a primary complaint, may first intervene by using movement to enhance a sense of control on a body level. Sessions might initially consist of structured exercises, designed to decrease tension and support physical mastery- exercises that the client can learn to use to lessen physical symptoms when they recur. Once some sense of control is established at the body level, the leader will work to address psychological issues and avoidant behaviors related to the anxiety. In an expressive movement process, the leader helps the anxious client attend to and tolerate physical sensations, understand the meaning he or she assigns to triggering physical and interpersonal experiences, and through dance engage in exploratory and expressive behaviors that have previously been curtailed by anxiety. Erwin-Grabner completed a pilot study in which dance/movement therapy provided an intervention to alleviate test taking anxiety in a group of university students (Erwin-Grabner, Goodill, Schelly Hill, & Von Neida, 1999). Leste and Ruste (1990) found a significant reduction in anxiety through participation in a modern dance class alone. In normal anxiety, engaging in dance may help the person, literally and psychologically, "move through" the temporary immobilization or physical agitation of the anxiety experience.

Trauma involves a particular anxiety experience. Often the site of trauma is the body itself as in sexual abuse or assault, many cases of survival of war or disaster, and accidental physical injury. Traumatic body-memories and anxiety may inhibit and fragment body awareness, "prohibiting spontaneous and integrated action" (Casey in Pylvanainen, 2003, p. 51). Movement attends to the linked physical and psychological sequelae of trauma. Dance/movement techniques can experientially access and address traumatic memories in the movement process. The leader can also facilitate movement that supports a sense of body integrity and coherence. It is especially important in the case of trauma to establish a sense of safety, both on the body level through titration of arousal and through a trusting relationship with a skilled leader (Gray, 2001). Resolution of trauma is a process that requires patience. Dance/movement techniques are in use in therapeutic work with survivors of physical torture at the Rocky Mountain Survivor's Center in Boulder, Colorado, in London with Amnesty International, and in Haiti at the Restorative resources Training Center. Dance/movement therapists also oftentimes work with survivors of sexual abuse (Ambra, 1995; Bernstein, 1995) and those recovering from traumatic physical injury.

Dance/Movement and Depression

Dance/movement therapy can be helpful to those experiencing depression. Again dance/movement effectively works on two levels: movement assists in alleviating the vegetative or agitated symptoms of depression, while the expressive aspect of a dance/movement process attends to the underlying psychological or emotional issues and responses which compromise coping. Beggs (2005) describes a 10-week dance/movement module to support women coping with depression. The design includes a three-phase process: Meeting in Movement, Exploring Meaning in Movement, and Moving Forward. Each session utilizes a dance experience relevant to the phase and responsive to the participants, followed by an opportunity to express the dance experience in art, a debriefing and a closing reflection.

An outstanding research project in Iran studied the effect of dance/movement techniques on depression of elderly women (Sayadi, Nazer, Ansary, & Khaleghi, 2004). Thirty women 60 to 75 years old were involved in the study which examined the affects of 30 dance/movement sessions. Mean scores on a depression scale dropped from a pretreatment score of 20.87 to postdance/movement sessions scores of 16.40.

Brooks and Stark (1989) investigated the effects of dance/movement therapy on affect. They suggested that through dance/movement therapy individuals can "discover how they change, alter, direct, destroy, or control (these) subtle muscular sensations which affect the experience or expression of feelings" (p. 103). Depression and anxiety scores on the Multiple Affect Check List were significantly reduced postdance/movement therapy.

Movement for Eating Disorders and Body Image Issues

Dance/movement is often used with women who have eating disorders or who are in other ways conflicted in relationship with their bodies. Our bodies naturally provide us with sensory feedback about needs, feelings, and relationships with others. In eating disorders, awareness of the sensations involved in the body's communications may be suppressed and experience may become "disembodied." Susan Kleinman and Terry Hall have developed particularly suitable dance/movement techniques for women in outpatient and residential programs at the Renfrew Foundation sites in Florida and Philadelphia and in private practice. They found that dance/movement techniques serve as a powerful means for women with eating disorders to explore their relationship to their bodies (Kleinman & Hall, 2004). Movement awakens physical sensation that leads to self and interpersonal connection. As a psychotherapeutic method, Kleinman and Hall state "dance/movement therapy reveals and articulates the body's expressiveness as participants explore and examine behavioral patterns, feelings, and memories hidden in the body" within the safety of the therapeutic relationship (p. 4). Participants may in time replace habitual patterns of compulsive exercise, body numbness, disconnection, tension, rigidity, or passivity with a renewed body relationship in which the body is valued as a source of information, vehicle for self-expression, and relationship to others.

A woman does not need to suffer an eating disorder to struggle with acceptance of her body and herself. "From an early age, the way females feel about their bodies correlates strongly with the way they feel about themselves, consequently, for most women, the ability to differentiate who they are from how they experience their appearance is extremely difficult" (Ressler & Kleinman, 2004, p. 3). Dance/movement therapists have refined skills for working with body-image issues. However, participation in expressive dance or another dance form may in itself facilitate a healthier relationship to one's body. Dance sets the body in motion, effecting a shift from the body as a one-dimensional object of appearance to a dynamic "body-self" (Dosamantes-Alperson, 1981), "a core self that experiences and interacts" (Pylvanainen, 2003, p. 50), is expressive, and serves one's ability to function. Experiencing oneself through movement offers a vital experience of the body-self that can support psychological and physical health.

Movement Therapy in Wellness and Growth

Individuals may seek the support of dance/movement therapy to enhance wellness. Many persons today are aware of the interrelationship of body and mind, and seek movement approaches for an integrated experience of mental, emotional, and physical well being and personal growth. This represents an apparent rediscovery of old truths. In several publications, anthropologist and movement research scholar Judith Lynne Hanna has addressed the relationship of dance to stress reduction and healing in previous eras and cultures (Hanna, 1988, 2006).

Coccari and Weiler (2004) examined the impact of dance/movement techniques in enhancing the personal vitality in eleven wellness-seeking individuals. Results showed increases in energy and stamina for accomplishing goals each day. Coccari and Weiler also found that work with breathing relieved tension, facilitated relaxation, and increased overall cognitive ability.

Attention to breath is central to many body-mind disciplines. The respiratory process is vital in physical functioning. Breath is also significant in that it relates to the inner space of the body (Bartenieff & Lewis, 1980, p. 232; Hackney, 2002, p. 41), is an indicator of emotional states (Chang, 2004), and represents an interaction between the self and the environment. It is perhaps remarkable that something as natural and essential to life as breathing is also a process of frequent disturbance. In *Making Connections: Total Body Integration through the Bartenieff Fundamentals*, Peggy Hackney

(Hackney, 2002) offers simple movement explorations, initiated in Breath Patterns, in which anyone can engage to enhance awareness and connectivity The dance/movement leader works with the breath in support of movement expression. Breath support is at the heart of "Bartenieff Fundamentals." The Bartenieff Fundamentals are a series of six fundamental exercises and elaborations developed by physical therapist and dance/movement therapy pioneer Irmgard Bartenieff within the framework of Laban Movement Analysis (LMA) (Bartenieff & Lewis, 1980). The developmentally informed movement sequences incorporate LMA principles to enhance both expressivity and functioning. The requisites of effective physical movement clearly have correlates in psychology and behavior and are a basis for effective movement through life. Practice of the Bartenieff fundamentals may be an integral part of a holistic dance/movement wellness approach.

In wellness applications it is not unusual for the dance/movement leader to have a practice foundation in a second body-mind discipline, combining dance/movement therapy skills with the methods of Yoga, Tai Chi or other practices. Dance/movement therapist Meg Chang has presented widely on Mindfulness-Based Stress Reduction (MBSR), as developed at Massachusetts Medical Center by Jon Kabat Zinn, and its potential for practice integration with dance/movement techniques (Chang, 2004). Chang respects the individual integrity of each approach and explores the possible integration of the two. She has found that dance/movement techniques fostered self-esteem in participants and contributed group cohesiveness to mindfulness practice sessions.

Authentic Movement is a dance/movement technique that may be practiced as a movement discipline. Authentic Movement originated with Mary Starks Whitehouse as Movement in Depth, an integration of Jungian depth analysis and creative dance (Whitehouse, 1979). In practice, participants in Authentic Movement seek personal truth through the wisdom of the body. This self-discovery process is suited for psychologically healthy persons or "normal neurotic" persons with stable ego functioning. The Authentic Movement process involves both a Mover and an observing Witness. In the basic structure of the practice, the Mover begins in a receptive stillness, often with eyes closed. The Mover attends deeply to physical sensations from which may arise an awareness of an inner impulse to move. The Mover allows the impulse to take form in physical action, sometimes as a very small movement that repeats and is developed over time. Whitehouse describes the mover's experience as one of "both moving and being moved," an expression "authentic" to the self. The Mover and Witness meet following the movement process. Each describes the movement sequence as well as awareness of inner experiences (images, thoughts, and feelings) that arose in the course of the movement. The theory is that through this discipline a space is provided for listening to the unconscious. Themes emerge that can be further explored both in words and movement. Sometimes the witness will suggest a simple exploratory movement structure relevant to these themes. The structure often takes the form of exploring an image or a conceptual "polarity" such as yielding and resistance, stillness and activity. In a world full of multi-tasking and external performance demands, taking time to move from within may be deeply self-restorative.

Joan Chodorow and Janet Adler, have developed this work with varied emphasis. Joan Chodorow (1997) emphasizes "active imagination" and the inclusion of other creative arts in the expressive process. Adler (2002) has developed the spiritual aspect of the work and initiated training groups that have served as labs for exploration of Authentic Movement as a group as well as an individual discipline. The former Authentic Movement Institute in San Francisco, the Authentic Movement Program at Naropa Institute, and the C.J. Jung Center in Houston, Texas have been institutional centers for the development of Authentic Movement practice in this country. Authentic Movement is practiced as "Contemplative Movement" at an annual summer institute at Hampshire College. Many others throughout the country practice Authentic Movement in therapy and studio settings.

Many of life's developmental milestones and transitions are expressed in cooccurring changes in psyche, social role, self-image, and body. Movement can embody personal history as well as emerging change. Ott (2003) demonstrated in a research project with pregnant and postpartum women that dance/movement techniques can support the body in transition and the psychological process of birth, offering the women a preventive therapeutic intervention to help reduce the risk of potentially traumatic postnatal adjustment. Often dance/movement methods effective in supporting life passages have an element of creative ritual and ceremony. Dance/movement techniques provide support in times of life transition in support groups for pregnancy, parenting, midlife transition, aging (Fersh, 1980; Sandel, 1978, 2004a), and for those facing end of life issues in hospice care (Deihl, 1992; O'Maille, 2005).

Medical Dance/Movement Therapy

The act of moving is in itself health enhancing. Dance/movement techniques used for support of those with medical conditions is a developing arena of dance/movement practice. Sharon Goodill, who is the Director of Drexel University's Hahnemann Creative Arts in Therapy Program, published the first full text of Medical Dance/Movement Therapy (Goodill, 2004). Penny Lewis addressed the ADTA membership in 2003 at the Thirty Eighth Annual Conference in Boulder, Colorado on themes of health and healing through movement. Berrol (1992, 2006) has described the neurophysiological mechanisms which underpin the body-mind connection and the movement relationship in dance/movement therapy practice.

Much of the work with adult medical illness and dance/movement involves contributions to psychosocial support in illness, often within a support group setting. In a recent article, Goodill makes the point that "It is logical to surmise that if phenomena and changes in the physical body are a source of pain, distress, anger, or isolation, then a somatically oriented method of psychosocial support and intervention will have meaningful impact" (Goodill, 2006, p. 52). The group movement process and dance expression provide psychological and social support in a process which fosters positive attention to the self, mediation of the physical effects of illness, and at times provides a medium for exploring the spiritual and existential questions that arise when one faces life threatening illness. There are a number of dance/movement therapists who have been working with women who are breast cancer survivors, each with a slightly varied focus (Dibbel-Hope, 2000; Sandel, 2004b; Serlin, Classen, Francis, & Angell, 2000). Other areas of medicine in which dance/movement therapists have specialized include neurological insult

(Berrol, Ooi & Katz, 1985; Berrol et al., 1997), chronic pain, and pediatric medical care (Cohen, 2005; Cohen & Walco, 1999; Tortora, 2005). Goodill, citing a review of cost offset data (Friedman, Sobel, Meyers, Caudill, & Benson, 1995) asserts that there can be cost savings in the healthcare system when psychological issues are addressed (Goodill, 2004, p. 33).

An interesting study conducted at the Department of Public Health and Caring Sciences within Uppsala University and Hospital, Uppsala, Sweden examined changes in stress-related hormones with fibromyalgia participants before and after dance/movement intervention (Bojner-Horowitz, Theorell, & Anderberg, 2003). The differences in hormone levels for participants in the treatment group and the controls did not reach a significance threshold. However, a 14-month follow-up showed increased cortisol levels both in plasma and in the saliva for the dance/movement therapy treatment group. And there were significant changes in the D/MT treatment group on all three variables studied in a video interpretation of movement patterns: movement pain, mobility, and life energy. This debilitating disease causes generalized pain and other physical and psychological symptoms and significantly limits quality of life. A reduction in symptoms through dance/movement techniques is a significant contribution to well-being.

The meeting of arts and medicine has occurred through the work of dance artists as well as dance/movement therapists. Dancer and community dance artist Anna Halprin (2000) tells a personal tale of recovery from cancer which she attributes to her experience with the self-healing qualities of dance. For decades Halprin brought communities of people together to address social issues through dance. After wrestling with and creating from her own illness, she extended her dancemaking into dance creation with cancer survivors and those diagnosed with AIDS. The Tamalpa Institute in Northern California, founded with her daughter, is a center for healing through dance and community dance ritual. Bill T. Jones is another dance artist whose experience of his partner's death to AIDS, in addition to a personal experience with HIV, led to performance themes of life and illness in *Still/Here* and dance workshops with persons with terminal illness (Moyers, 1997). Movement, which is an expression of life itself, lends itself as a medium for self-exploration and expression in illness and in the face of the specter of death.

Dance/Movement for Children

The language of infancy is a movement language, so it is not surprising that dance/movement therapists have had a historical presence in early childhood intervention. Movement researcher and child psychiatrist Judith Kestenberg, M.D. developed the Kestenberg Movement Profile (KMP) (Kestenberg, 1967) through which she charted the rhythms of this language, and the interactional rhythms within the caregiver-child relationship. In Germany a researcher used the Kestenberg-Movement-Profile to observe mothers and infants at play (Lier-Schehl, 2004). Results found significant differences in shape flow between mothers and their infants depending on the psychological diagnosis of the mother. Depressed mothers were often under involved in movement while mothers with psychosis were often over involved or disorganized. Birklein and Sossin (2006) examined "correspondences between specific patterns of parent and child nonverbal behaviors and indices of parental stress" (p. 128). Susan

Loman, a Kestenberg protege and Director of Dance/Movement Therapy Education at Antioch New England Graduate School (Loman, 1994, 1998), and Suzi Tortora in New York City (Tortora, 1994, 2004, 2005) are leaders in work with caregiver-infant pairs. In her recent book, *The Dancing Dialogue: Using the Communicative Power of Movement with Young Children*, Tortora (2005) talks about the process of entering the child's world and creating a social-emotional bond through movement attunement and mirroring, then creating a "dancing dialogue", and "exploring and expanding the child's vocabulary" (pp. 259–263), in a developing dance of interaction. Her work involves parents in a progressive series of observational exercises that develop awareness of "their child's unique personal styles of communicating, interacting, and self-expressing through body postures and actions" (p. 339), while reflecting on their own responses. In time, the exercises engage the parent in the dance of parent-child movement relatedness.

At the 2002 American Dance Therapy Conference, Claire LeMessurier (2002) reported on the role of dance/movement therapy in a federal grant initiative in Vermont (CUPS), designed to foster collaborative relationships among agencies and personnel serving children and designed to bring mental health services to the field of early childhood. LeMessurier spoke to how infants learn to cope with emotions and learn self-regulation through back and forth nonverbal communication with their caregivers, whereby negative states are diminished and positive states are amplified. Israeli dance/movement therapist Nava Lotan has been studying the movement elements of "secure attachment" in mother infant pairs. Lotan's study of children's body movement patterns and parent presence in the falling asleep process of toddlers suggest some practical applications (Lotan & Yirimya, 2002). Dance/movement techniques can effect change by helping parents observe nonverbal expression and attune to children on a body level through movement and touch.

Using a systems model for work with families, Dulicai (1977) developed an assessment instrument that added to the tools that can be used to identify consistent patterns of interaction within families and to guide family interventions more precisely. Adapting the work of Scheflen (1972) and adding the dynamic qualities of Laban (1971) allows the researcher to notate nonverbal behavior and the accompanying emotional expression within the context of themes discussed during interviews. Subsequently, the study has been replicated numerous times with a wide variety of problems in diverse types of families.

Some of the earliest dance/movement therapy work with children involved treatment for those with autism disorders. Thirty years ago, many in a generation of prospective dance/movement therapists were drawn to the profession of dance/movement therapy as they watched a young therapist, Janet Adler, enter the nonverbal world of an autistic child and engage in a movement relationship in a classic film "Looking for Me" (Bartlett & Brock, 1970).

In recent years, Autism Spectrum Disorders have been an increasingly prevalent diagnostic category. Dance/movement is a natural treatment modality for disorders that involve developmental deficits in relationship and communication. Using mirroring techniques such as those pioneered by Marian Chace with psychiatrically hospitalized adults, the leader nonverbally attunes to and gradually develops a relationship with the autistic children with whom they work; joining, responding to, communicating with, and shaping behavior and relationships through movement. As mentioned earlier, Kalish (1976) developed the first movement assessment of autistic children in her dissertation at Bryn Mawr College. Later her work was included in the broad assessment device, Behavior Rating Instrument for Autistic and Other Atypical Children (Ruttenberg et al., 1978). At the Center for Autism in Philadelphia, formerly the Developmental Center for Autistic Children, dance/movement has been integral to treatment of children with autism spectrum disorders for more than 25 years. The dance/movement therapy program at this center began under Kalish, and continued on through Gayle Gates (2005), Elise Tropea and Particia Miron (2005) who continue to actively contribute to work in this area.

Federal bills insuring services to children with special needs, No Child Left Behind (NCLB) and the Individuals with Disability Act (IDEA), include dance/movement therapy under related services personnel. Children may be eligible for these services at their school upon request. In some states children are served within their schools. In others, school districts contract with children's community mental health centers for these services.

A pilot study conducted in Stockholm paired two boys diagnosed with Attention Deficit Hyperactivity Disorder (ADHD) in short-term dance/movement therapy treatment which included creative dance and improvisational movement play. Results found that the dance/movement therapy treatment course partly reduced the behavioral and emotional symptoms of the participants and had a positive effect on their motor function (Gronlund, Reneck, & Weibul, 2005). ADHD is a common disorder presented in the school population that is distressing and highly disruptive to the learning and functioning of the child involved as well as others in the classroom. This pilot study points to the treatment potential of dance/movement therapy with this population and the need for larger studies that include dance/movement therapy over an extended period of time.

The dance/movement therapy work of Tina Erfer in New York City public schools helps students with autism take advantage of learning opportunities within the classroom. Dance/movement therapist William Freeman has designed, developed and implemented innovative programs in movement and expressive arts education and therapy for children and youth for 25 years. He conducts a movement program in the school district of southern Vermont that includes movement assessments at the beginning of movement intervention and at six month intervals, measuring the progress of children. An outstanding component of the program is the inclusion of the movement report with other modes of assessment as part of a battery of testing. *You're Okay Right Where You Are: Expressive Movement in Education*, is a videotape that demonstrates his innovative work and identifies his philosophy of working with and expanding the child's strength and enhancing self-confidence (Freeman, 1998). The American Dance Therapy Association web site listed in the appendix at the close of the chapter allows the reader to click on contacts for programs in specific states.

Arts Programs Serving Children

There are a number of arts programs for children that warrant mention here:

- The Very Special Arts (VSA) is an international nonprofit organization founded in 1974 by Ambassador Jean Kennedy Smith. VSA is creating a society where people with disabilities can learn through, participate in, and enjoy the arts. Five million people participate in VSA arts programs every year through a network of affiliates in every state and over 60 countries worldwide (wwww.vsaarts.org).
- Mark DeGarmo & Dancers has researched a dance program in PS 142 in New York City. The pilot program offered third grade students a curriculum in which the arts were integrated with all other subjects. In a three-year partnership the New York Department of Education offered classroom teacher professional development through DeGarmo & Dancers. The program involved research-grounded and arts-based teaching, interdisciplinary practice, and qualitative artistic assessment and evaluation methods. Parents participated in the program through a Parents As Arts Partners sponsored by the Center for Arts Education and the New York State Council on the Arts.
- Arts & Science for the Disabled, Inc. is a successful program in Long Beach, California that offers Therapeutic Arts Program I & II and Therapeutic Arts and the EPI center. This is a successful private center staffed by volunteers and actively supported by the community.
- The state of Texas recently completed a research project funded by the Ford Foundation which involved fourth graders at James S. Hogg Elementary school in Dallas. With the support of the project thousands of elementary school teachers integrated field trips and artist residencies in their lesson plans for such core subjects as reading, math, science and social studies. Since 1998 all but a few of the city's 157 public elementary schools have worked with arts groups with the purpose of boosting students' academic achievement.

Dance/Movement in Prevention Programs

A current surge in the development of dance/movement work with children is in the arena of prevention and support for at-risk children in educational and community settings. Various dance/movement based violence prevention programs are in place across the country. Dance/Movement Therapist Sue Ellen Fried, founder of Bully Safe USA and her daughter Paula Fried cowrote one of the early books addressing the phenomena of "bullying" in childhood (1996). A number of dance/movement therapists have since designed and successfully piloted movement based prevention programs in educational settings. All of the following programs have utilized movement to address the problem of youth violence: The PEACE program designed by Lynn Koshland in Salt Lake City (Koshland, 2003; Koshland, Wilson & Wittaker, 2004), Nancy Beardall's *Creating a Peaceable School: Confronting Intolerance and Bullying* curriculum in Massachusetts (1998), and Rena Kornblum's curriculum guide *Disarming the Playground: Violence Prevention through Movement* developed at the Hancock Center of Arts and Therapies in Madison, Wisconsin (Kornblum & McCutchan, 2002). Kornblum makes the point that since violence is often a physical response to emotional arousal, it is in the body that awareness must be developed and responses learned anew. In all of these programs, experientially based movement activity that is enjoyable and in some cases combined with story and other arts experiences, help the child develop self-awareness, self-regulation, and a positive relationship to self and others.

Dance/movement techniques in the field of dance/movement therapy, have often addressed symptoms in participants with diagnosed psychosocial disorders. A few pioneers introduced application of the techniques to provide support to participants without clinical disorders. They provided assistance with everyday problems of living. North (1972) applied her movement skills to enhance the individual strengths and remediate weaknesses in all children, not only those who were identified with clinical and learning problems. Kestenberg's innovative work with mothers and children at the Children's Development Research Center she founded in Sand's Point, New York supported parents so they could develop responses that increased positive bonding within parent-child dyads and suggested alternatives for those behaviors that diminished positive bonding.

Dance/movement therapy in mainstream educational settings is developing. Karen Kohn Bradley, movement educator and Laban practitioner was invited to visit a fourth grade classroom in a large urban center to advise the teacher on dance/movement techniques that might be helpful in her struggles with a chaotic classroom. Kohn visited during a day in which the Stanford-9 tests were to be administered. She introduced the children to growing and shrinking movements based on breath rhythms with music. The students then immediately responded to a waltz rhythm and continued to enthusiastically engage in dance/movement techniques for the next twenty minutes. Following this movement session, the students were able to return to their desks and begin their tests quietly. **Thus**, dance/movement therapists can provide consultation to teachers about useful dance/movement techniques in the classroom as well as provide direct intervention.

As dance/movement therapy expands its scope of practice, it is wise to remember that preventative research is difficult due to the multiple variants that contribute to an identified problem. However, it is clear that movement provides a useful way of looking at and understanding an individual. Dance/movement mobilizes the mind and body and can bolster coping mechanisms that help mediate life conflicts. Participants in dance/movement sessions leave with a sense of responsiveness to their body messages and with movement techniques they can practice. The process of achieving self-understanding takes time. However, dance/movement therapy is often time and cost efficient as it addresses both body and mind; attending to the physical expression of psychological issues in movement patterns and symptoms. Qualified dance/movement therapy practitioners (ADTR), work from a position of a person's strengths which can preclude serious difficulty or reduce the incidence of recurring difficulties whether emotional, physical, psychosocial or cognitive.

Appendix A

American Dance Therapy Association, www.adta.org 2000 Century Plaza, Suite 108, 10632 Little Patuxent Parkway, Columbia, Md. 21044–3263

Arts & Services for Disabled, Inc., 3962 Studebaker Road, Suite 206, Long Beach, CA 90808
The Center for Arts Education, www.cae-nyc.org
Center for Autistic Children, www.autismhelp.com
Contemplative Dance, www.contemplativedance.org
The Hancock Center for Arts and Therapy, Madison WI, www.hancockcenter.net
Laban Bartenieff Institute of Movement Studies, www.limsonline.org
Laban Centre, Creekside, London, SE8 3DZ, UK, www.Laban.org
Laban Movement Analysis Database, www.laban-analyses.org/index.html
Mark DeGarmo & Dancers, MARKDEGARMODANCE@AOL.COM
National Dance Educators Organizations www.ndeo.org
Renfrew Center Foundation, www.renfrew.org
Tamalpa Institute, www.tamalpa.org
VSA Arts, www.vsarts.org 1300 Connecticut Avenue, NW, Suite 700, Washington, DC 20036

References

Adler, J. (2002). *Offering from the conscious body: The discipline of authentic movement*. Rochester, VT: Inner Traditions.

Allport, G. W. & Vernon, P. E. (1933). *Studies in expressive movement*. New York: The Macmillan Co.

Ambra, L. N. (1995). Approaches used in dance/movement therapy with adult women incest survivors. *American Journal of Dance Therapy, 17*(1), 15–24.

American Dance Therapy Association (2006). Fact sheet www.adta.org/about/factsheet.cfm

Amighi, J., Loman, S., Lewis, P. & Sossis, M. (1999). The meaning of movement: Developmental, multicultural, and clinical perspectives as seen through the Kestenberg Movement Profile. Newark, N. J. Charles C. Thomas.

Bartenieff, I., & Lewis, D. (1980). *Body movement: Coping with the environment*. New York: Gordon and Breach Science Publishers.

Bartlett, V. (Director), & Brock, N. (Producer) (1970). *Looking for me* [Motion Picture]. United States.

Bates, J. A., & Malhotra, A. (2002). Genetic factors and neurocognitive traits. CNS Spectrums, *7*, 4.

Beardall, N. G. (1998). *Creating a peaceable school: Confronting intolerance and bullying*. MA: Newton Public Schools.

Beggs, S. (2005). Looking back and moving forward: Dance/movement therapy in the treatment of women with depression. *Proceedings of the Fortieth Annual Conference of the American Dance Therapy Association*.

Bernstein, B. (1995). Dancing beyond trauma: Women survivors of sexual abuse. In F. J. Levy (ed.), *Dance and other expressive art therapies*. New York: Routledge.

Berrol, C. F. (1978). The effects of two movement remediation programs on selected measurers of perceptual-motor ability, academic achievement and behavior on first-grade children manifesting learning and perceptual-motor problems. Unpublished doctoral dissertation, University of California, Berkeley.

Berrol, C. F. (1992). The neurophysiologic basis of the mind-body connection in dance/movement therapy. *American Journal of Dance Therapy, 14*(1), 19–29.

Berrol, C. F. (2006). Neuroscience meets dance/movement therapy: Mirror neurons and the therapeutic process and empathy. *The Arts in Psychotherapy* (in press).

Berrol, C. F., & Katz, S. S. (1985). Dance/movement therapy in the rehabilitation of individuals surviving severe head injuries. *American Journal of Dance Therapy, 8*, 46–66.

Berrol, C. F., Ooi, W. L., & Katz, S. S. (1997). Dance/movement therapy with older adults who have sustained neurological insult: A demonstration project. *American Journal of Dance Therapy, 19*(2), 135–160.

Birdwhistell, R. L. (1963). The kinesic level in the investigation of the emotions. In P. H. Knapp (Ed.), *Expressions of the emotions in man*. New York: International Universities Press.

Birklein, S., & Sossin, M. K. (2006). Nonverbal indices of stress in parent-child dyads: Implications for individual and interpersonal affect regulation and intergenerational transmission. In S. C. Koch, & I. Brauninger (Eds.), *Advances in dance/movement therapy: Theoretical perspectives and empirical findings* (pp.128–139). Berlin: Los Verlag.

Bojner-Horowitz, E., Theorell, T., & Anderberg, U. M. (2003). Dance-movement therapy and changes in stress related hormones. A study of fibromyalgia patients with video interpretation. *Arts in Psychotherapy: An International Journal, 30*, 255–264.

Brooks, D., & Stark, A. (1989). The effects of dance/movement therapy on affect: A pilot study. *American Journal of Dance Therapy, 11*(2), 101–111.

Chaiklin, S., & Schmais, C. (1979). The Chace approach to dance therapy. In P. Lewis (Ed.), *Eight theoretical approaches in dance/movement therapy* (p. 16). Dubuque, IA: Kendall Hunt.

Chang, M. (2004). Mindfulness-based stress reduction & dance-movement therapy. Theory and practice: Potentials or pitfalls? *Proceedings of the Thirty-Ninth Annual Conference of the American Dance Therapy Association*, 24–26.

Chodorow, J. (1991). *Dance therapy and depth: The moving imagination*. London: Routledge.

Cigaran, S. R. (2004). *The effect of Dance Movement Therapy work on patients with fybromyalgia in 1st International Research Colloquium in Dance/Movement Therapy* (p. 6). Germany: German Dance Therapy Association.

Coccari, G., & Weiler, M. (2004). Exploring the impact of dance/movement therapy on personal vitality in wellness-seeking individuals. *American Journal of Dance Therapy, 26*(1), 53–54.

Cohen, S. (2005). Holistic management of symptoms. *Palliative care for infants, children, and adolescents*. Baltimore: The Johns Hopkins University Press.

Cohen, S., & Walco, G. (1999). Dance/movement therapy for children and adolescents with cancer. *Cancer Practice, 7*(1).

Condon, W. S. (1968.) Linguistic-Kinesic research and dance therapy. *Proceedings of the Third Annual Conference of the American Dance Therapy Association*, 21–44.

Darwin, C. (1872). *The expression of the emotions in man and animals*. New York: Philosophical Library.

Davis, M. (1970). Movement characteristics of hospitalized psychiatric patients. *Proceedings of the Fifth Annual Conference of the American Dance Therapy Association*.

Davis, M. (1975). *Towards understanding the intrinsic in body movement*. New York: Arno Press.

Davis, M. (1977). Methods of perceiving patterns of small-group behavior: Effort-Shape analysis. New York, N. Y. Dance Notation Bureau.

Davis, M. (1991). *Guide to movement analysis methods part 2: Movement Psychodiagnostic Inventory*. (available from [Martha Davis, 1 West 85th Street, New York, NY 10024]).

Deihl, L. (1992, October). The dying process eased through body empathy. Paper presented at the American Dance Therapy Association 27th Annual Conference, Columbia, MD.

Deutsch, F. (1947). Analysis of postural behavior. *Psychoanalytic Quarterly, 16*, 195–213.

Dibbel-Hope, S. (2000). The use of dance/movement therapy in psychological adaptation to breast cancer. *The Arts in Psychotherapy: An International Journal, 27*(1), 51–68.
Dosamantes-Alperson, E. D. (1981). Experiencing in movement psychotherapy. *American Journal of Dance Therapy, 14*(2), 33–44.
Dulicai, D. (1977). Nonverbal assessment of family systems: A preliminary study. *The Arts in Psychotherapy: An International Journal, 6*(2), 55–62.
Dulicai, D., & Berger, M. R. (2005). Global dance/movement therapy growth and development. *Arts in Psychotherapy, 32*(3), 205–216.
Erwin-Grabner, T., Goodill, S., Schelly Hill, E., & Von Neida, K. (1999). Effectiveness of dance/movement therapy on reducing test anxiety. *American Journal of Dance Therapy, 21*(1), 19–33.
Fersh, I. (1980). Dance/movement therapy: A holistic approach to working with the elderly. *American Journal of Dance Therapy, 3*(2), 33–43.
Ford Foundation Report, www.fordfound.org/publications
Freeman, W. (Producer) (1998). *You're okay right where you are: Expressive movement in education* [videofilm]. United States.
Freud, S. (1938). Symptomatic and chance actions. In A. A. Brill (Translator), *The basic writings of Sigmund Freud.* New York: Random House.
Fried, S., & Fried, P. (1996). *Bullies & victims: Helping your child through the schoolyard battlefields.* New York: Evans & Company.
Friedman, R., Sobel, D. S., Meyers, P., Caudill, M., & Benson, H. (1995). Behavioral medicine, Clinical health psychology, and cost offset. *Health Psychology, 14*(6), 509–518.
Gallese, V., Keysers, C., & Rizzolatti, G. (2004). A unifying view of the basis of social cognition. TRENDS in cognitive sciences, *8*, 9.
Gates, G. (2005). Moving to the heart of the matter. In C. N. Ariel, & R. A. Naseef (Eds.), *Voices from the spectrum: Parents, grandparents, siblings, people with autism, and professionals share their wisdom.* Philadelphia: Jessica Kingsley.
Goodill, S. W. (2004). An *introduction to medical dance/movement therapy: Health care in motion.* New York: Jessica Kingsley Press.
Goodill, S. W. (2006). Dance/movement therapy for populations living with medical illness. In S. C. Koch, & I. Brauninger (Eds.), *Advances in dance/movement therapy: Theoretical perspectives and empirical findings.* Berlin: Logos Verlag.
Gray, A. (2001) The body remembers: Dance/movement therapy with an adult survivor of torture. *The American Journal of Dance Therapy, 23*(1), 29–43.
Gronlund, E., Reneck, B., & Weibull, J. (2005). Dance/movement therapy as an alternative treatment for young boys diagnosed as ADHD: A pilot study. *American Journal of Dance Therapy, 27*(2), 63–85.
Hackney, P. (2002). *Making connections: Total body integration through Bartenieff Fundamentals.* The Netherlands: Gordon and Breach.
Halprin, A. (2000). *Dance as a healing art: Returning to health with movement and imagery.* Mendocino, CA: Life Rhythm.
Hanna, J. (1988). *Dance and Stress: Resistance, reduction, and euphoria: Stress and modern society.* New York: AMS Press.
Hanna, J. (2006). *Dancing for health: Conquering and preventing stress.* Lanham, MD: Alta Mira Press.
Kalish, B. (1976). Body movement scale for autistic and other atypical children: An exploratory study using a normal group and atypical group. (Doctoral Dissertation, Bryn Mawr College, 1977). *Dissertation Abstracts International*, 37, 12. (UMI no. 77–06524) Bryn Mawr College.
Kestenberg, J. (1965a). The role of movement patterns in development I. Rhythms of movement. *Psychoanalytic Quarterly, 34*, 1–26.
Kestenberg, J. (1965b). The role of movement patterns in development II. Flow of tension and effort. *Psychoanalytic Quarterly, 34*, 517–563.

Kestenberg, J. (1967). The role of movement patterns in development III. The control of shape. *Psychoanalytic Quarterly, 36*, 356–409.

Kestenberg Amighi, J., Loman, S., Lewis, P., & Sossin, K. M. (1999). *The meaning of movement: Developmental and clinical perspectives of the Kestenberg Movement Profile*. The Netherlands: Gordon and Breach.

Kleinman, S., & Hall, T. (2004). Dance/movement therapy: A method for embodying emotions. In B. Davis, & S. Kleinman (Eds.), *Healing through relationship: Working with eating disorders. The Renfrew working papers* (p. 1). The Renfrew Center Foundation. Philadelphia, PA.

Kornblum, R., & McCutchan, C. T. (2002). *Disarming the playground: Violence prevention through movement and pro-social skills*. Oklahoma City, OK: Wood & Barnes Publishing.

Koshland, L. (2003). Testing the effectiveness of a dance/movement therapy violence prevention program with a multicultural school population. In R. Cruz (Ed.), *Research poster session abstracts, American Dance Therapy Association Conference, 2001–2002*.

Koshland, L., Wilson, J., & Wittaker, B. (2004). PEACE through dance/movement: Evaluating a violence prevention program. *American Journal of Dance Therapy, 26*(2), 69–89.

Laban, R. (1971). *The mastery of movement*, Boston: Plays, Inc.

Lambert, M. J. (1992). Implications of outcome research for psychotherapy integration. In J. C. Norcross, & M. R. Goldfried (eds.), *Handbook of psychotherapy integration* (pp. 94–129). New York: Basic Books.

LeMessurier, C. (2002). Integrating a movement perspective with early childhood mental health services. *Proceedings of the Thirty Seventh Annual American Dance Therapy Association Conference*.

Leste, A., & Ruste, J. (1990). Effects of dance on anxiety. *American Journal of Dance Therapy, 12*(1), 19–25.

Levy, F. (2005). *Dance/movement therapy: A healing art*. Reston, VA: American Alliance for Health, Physical Education, Recreation and Dance.

Lewis, P. (2003). Marian Chace Foundation Annual Lecture. Dancing with the Movement of the River. *American Journal of Dance Therapy, 25*(1), 17–37.

Lier-Schehl, H. (2004). Identification of early relationship from the analysis of movement patterns in mother-infant interaction. In 1st International Research Colloquim in Dance/Movement Therapy, February 2004, Germany.

Loman, S. (1994). Attuning to the fetus and young child: Approaches from dance/movement therapy. *Zero to Three: Dance/Movement and Expressive Arts Therapy with Very Young Children, 1*, 20.

Loman, S. (1998). Employing a developmental model of movement patterns in dance/movement therapy with children and their families. *American Journal of Dance Therapy, 20*(2), 101–115.

Lomax, A., Bartenieff, I., & Paulay, F. (1968). Dance style and culture. In *Folk Song Style and Culture*. Washington, D.C., American Association for the Advancement of Science, 88.

Lotan, N., & Yirimya, N. (2002). Body movement, presence of parents, and the process of falling asleep in toddlers. *International Journal of Behavioral Development, 26*(1), 81–88.

Miron, T. (2005). Circle of devotion. In C. N. Ariel, & R. A. Naseef (Eds.), *Voices from the spectrum: Parents, grandparents, siblings, people with autism, and professionals share their wisdom*. Philadelphia: Jessica Kingsley.

Moyers, B. (1997). *Bill T. Jones: Still/Here with Bill Moyers*. Princeton: Films for the Humanities and Sciences.

National Dance Educators Organization (2001). Mission statement. To move forward: An affirmation of continuing commitment to arts education. http://www.ndeo.org/ToMove.pdf

North, M. (1972). *Personality assessment through movement.* London: UK Macdonald and Evans Limited.
O'Maill, T. (2005). PASSAGEDANCE©: Dance/Movement therapy for aging and dying. *Proceedings of the Fortieth Annual American Dance Therapy Conference.*
Plomin, R. & DeFries, J. C. (1998). The genetics of cognitive abilities and disabilities. Scientific American, May.
Pylvanainen, P. (2003). Body image: A tripartite model for use in dance/movement therapy. *American Journal of Dance Therapy, 25*(1), 39–55.
Reich, W. (1949). *Character-Analysis* (3rd ed.). New York: Farrar, Straus & Giroux, Noonday Press.
Ressler, A., & Kleinman, S. (2004). Reframing body image identity in the treatment of eating disorders. In B. Davis, & S. Keinman (Eds.), *Healing through relationship: Working with eating disorders. The Renfrew working papers* (Vol. 1). The Renfrew Center Foundation. Philadelphia, PA.
Ruttenberg, B. A., Kalish, B., Wenar, C., & Wolf, E. G. (1978). *Behavior rating instrument for autistic and other atypical children (BRIAAC).* Chicago, Illinois: Stoelting Co.
Sandel, S. L. (1978). Resminiscence in movement therapy with the aged. *Arts in Psychotheraphy, 5*(4), 217–221.
Sandel, S. L. (1993a). Imagery in dance therapy groups: A developmental approach. In S. L. Sandel, S. Chaklin, & A. Lohn (Eds.), *Foundations of dance/movement therapy: The life and work of Marian Chace.* Columbia: MD: The Marian Chace Memorial Fund of the American Dance Therapy Association.
Sandel, S. L. (1993b). The process of empathic reflection in dance/movement therapy. In S. L. Sandel, S. Chaklin, & A. Lohn (Eds.), *Foundations of dance/movement therapy: The life and work of Marian Chace.* Columbia: MD: The Marian Chace Memorial Fund of the American Dance Therapy Association.
Sandel, S. L. (2004a). Moving into meaning. *Proceedings of the Thirty Ninth Annual American Dance Therapy Association Conference*, 79–83.
Sandel, S. L. (2004b). Dance and movement program improves quality of life measure in breast cancer survivors. *Proceedings from the Thirty Ninth Annual Dance Therapy Association Conference*, 105–108.
Sandel, S. L., Chaiklin, S., & Lohn, A. (Eds.). (1993). *Foundations of dance/movement therapy: The life and work of Marian Chace.* Columbia, Maryland: The Marian Chace Memorial Fund of the American Dance Therapy Association.
Sayadi, A. R., Nazer, M., Ansary, A., & Khaleghi, A. (2004). *Effect of movement therapy on depression of elderly women in 1st International Research Colloquium in Dance/Movement Therapy* (p. 25). Germany: Germany Dance Therapy Association.
Schappin, N. (2003) A movement-based assessment tool and outcome monitor of creative arts therapy treatment responses. In R. Cruz (Ed.), Research poster session abstracts American Dance Therapy Association Conferences 2001–2002. *American Journal of Dance Therapy, 25*(1).
Scheflen, A. (1972). *Body language and social order.* Englewood Cliffs, NJ: Prentice-Hall, Inc.
Schmais, C. (1974). Dance therapy in perspective. In K. C. Mason (Ed.), *Dance therapy: Focus on Dance VII.* Reston, VA: American Alliance for Health, Physical Education, Recreation and Dance.
Schmais, C. (1985). Healing processes in group dance therapy. *American Journal of Dance Therapy, 8*, 17–36.
Schoop, T., & Mitchell, P. (1974). *Won't you join the dance: A dancer's essay into the treatment of psychosis.* USA: Mayfield Publishing Co.
Serlin, I. A., Classen, C., Francis, C., & Angell, K. (2000). Symposium: Support groups for women with breast cancer: Traditional and alternative expressive approaches. *The Arts in Psychotherapy: An International Journal, 27*, 123–128.

Tortora, S. (1994). Join my dance: The unique movement style of each infant and toddler can invite communication, expression, and intervention. *Zero to Three, 15*(1), 1.

Tortora, S. (2004). Our moving bodies tell stories that speak of our experience. *Zero to Three, 24*(5).

Tortora, S. (2005). *The dancing dialogue: Using the communicative power of movement with young children*. Baltimore: Brookes Publishing.

Whitehouse, M. (1979). C. G. Jung and dance therapy: Two principles. In P. L. Bernstein (Ed.), *Eight Theoretical Approaches in Dance/Movement Therapy*. Dubuque, IA: Kendall Hunt.

10

Pleasant, Pleasurable, and Positive Activities

Joan S. Anderson

The intention of the author of this chapter is to lead the reader through a series of steps so that, at the end, a desire for engaging in pleasant activities will be compelling. This chapter will explore differences between leisure and recreation and between pleasure and enjoyment. The effects of leisure on mood, a discussion of play and games, and the spiritual, ethical, psychological and physiological issues behind the benefits of leisure will bear scrutiny. Because balance in life is so important and there is no yin without yang, there will be some notations on boredom. Finally, there is a list of some kinds of activities to consider, most of which cost little and many of which have major benefits.

A Bit of History

To the ancient Greeks, one's health and happiness were paramount. Perfection of the body was a goal and sports were the ideal showcase, which attitude led to the origin of the Olympics. Pastimes were designed to reflect Hellenic philosophy and attitudes. The word for leisure was *skole*, from which our word 'school' evolved. The word illustrated that time was to be used wisely and not frivolously. To the ancient Romans, leisure was enmeshed with the need for social order and the latter took precedence over an individual's personal freedom. Later, as the Roman conquests brought more wealth, free time increased and the people began to indulge in more gaudy pastimes. The *lud*i or public games began and, by the end of the Roman Empire, the carnal leisure activities had degraded the Roman people and their culture. There were 175 holidays in a year!. Possibly reflecting leisure as involving nature, fifteenth-to seventeenth-century China focused on gardening as a fine art. The impressionists in the nineteenth century reflected in their art upper class interests and activities such as the races, grand strolls in fashionable clothing, and balls. Leisure was paramount (Russell, 1996). Early Muslims followed Muhammad's philosophy found in the HADITH, "Recreate your hearts hour after hour for the tired hearts go blind." (Ibirham, 1991). For the Mayan's, around 300 AD, the predominant leisure was in religious festivals. For the Aztec, much later, around 1400 AD, religion was also important and their leisure activities differed within the social classes. In Medieval Europe, the Catholic Church was the main civilizing force and taught abstinence from worldly pleasures. Feudalism was established with wealthy nobleman, whose lives and leisure centered around fighting, drinking, games, and passive entertainment such as minstrels. (Russell, 1996). The clergy, also part of the feudal system, devoted their lives almost entirely to church. The more beleaguered peasants typically worked six days a week from dawn to dusk and used their free time for dancing, sacrilegious or vulgar songs, and general partying. Around 1300 AD, medieval Europe moved into the early Renaissance and changes in leisure occurred. The church influence was weakened and great achievements were seen in scholarship and art. It was an age of adventure and curiosity. Travel increased as did exploration. Music and ballet flourished. Dances, exhibitions, hunts, and theater activities abounded. Children, however, were still dressed and treated like miniature adults who only engaged in adult entertainment and were to be seen and not heard or considered (Russell, 1996).

In late eighteenth-century America, leisure was constrained by hard work and a Puritan ethic. In 1791, Philadelphia carpenters went on strike for the 10 hour day! Throughout the nineteenth and the twentieth centuries, reduction of work time was one of our nation's most pressing social issues. Work time steadily decreased until around 1970 when, for the first time by choice, Americans began to *increase* their workload. By 1997, it was estimated that, after work, sleep, and home chore hours were counted, there were only 16 ½ hours a week of free time. In contrast, Western Europe had about 320 more leisure hours per year than we did. Americans may think they have more free time now but that is a false perception because, in reality, they are only spending less time sleeping and tending to family (Harris, 1998). Women who have worked outside of the home in increasing numbers since World War II have spent 20% more of their time in work than before they entered the workforce. They have jobs *and* households to run. While labor saving devices have increased, norms for cleanliness and standards of mothering have also been on the rise (Schor, 1993). The Martha Stewart mentality prevails. The average American vacation is two weeks in length while Western Europeans enjoy up to five weeks as a norm.

Problems come with lack of leisure time and include an increase in stress related diseases, more workman's compensation claims, sleep disorders and a constant feeling of being rushed and/or unable to complete one's work. Marriages and families suffer from lack of time and children are not receiving the quality of care it takes to reach their potential. Physical and psychological problems increase dramatically as stress increases. The argument here is for more leisure time; for the option of Americans to move from a work/spend mentality, where material objects are most important, to a family/community model where relationships come first. Time is the commodity and it is only our free time which, when used wisely, can afford satisfaction, self-actualization, family connection and community spirit.

Leisure

Life is a great big canvas; throw all the paint on it you can. (Danny Kaye)

Leisure, in its basic definition, is the opposite of work and evolves from the Latin *licere* which translates into "to be permitted." Americans spend billions of dollars each year on leisure activities and jealously guard their discretionary time. Leisure can engender feelings of freedom, a positive mental state, and intrinsic motivation. It affords people the opportunity to explore the limits of their potential and to expand the range of mental, physical, social or spiritual growth. It is free activity that aims one toward self-actualization. (Eysenck, 1982). In the 1960s, Wolpe postulated his Systematic Desensitization theory around the hypothesis that one cannot be tense and relaxed at the same time and that, therefore, relaxation is an automatic antidote for anxiety. In people's activities, the more freedom of choice, the more attitude change would occur. Most people have bosses and, in working for someone else, have rules, time clocks, and many fewer choices than during their leisure time. Control of one's time is limited in the work environment but, within ethical constraints, is fully available during respite. In selecting a leisure event, one confirms what is "me" and "not me", a step toward identity and individuation. Leisure activity can be self-affirming as in "I can do well" at this or that. It can be a distraction from the troubled world and a mental and physical rest. The internal locus of control inherent in leisure is a reinforcement to freedom, defines us as separate from others, and moves us toward our desired view of ourselves (Bem, 1972).

If we also see ourselves as part of a community, we can commit to goals that aim us toward an even higher self-fulfillment. Leisure is borne in the mind and must be taught (Sylvester, 1987). Yet, individualism can become self-indulgence and we can better define our ideal selves if we see ourselves as part of a larger community and ultimately of the world. Tinsley and Kass (1979) described eight primary areas which seemed to benefit from positive leisure activities, including: (1) self-expression (fulfilling the need to express one's self and enjoy recognition); (2) companionship (fulfilling the need to engage in playful and supportive relationships); (3) personal power (fulfilling the need to be in control of one's situation and enjoy the center of attention); (4) compensation (fulfilling the need to experience something new or unusual); (5) security (fulfilling the need to make a commitment and be rewarded for one's efforts); (6) service (fulfilling the need to help others); (7) intellectual aestheticism (fulfilling the need for intellectual stimulation); (8) solitude (fulfilling the need to do things alone without feeling threatened).

Mood Effects of Leisure

I have found that if you love life, life will love you back. (Arthur Rubinstein)

Mood can be explained as the subtle, subjective state of a person at any given time; the affect or feelings. Mood can have many components: (a) communication such as facial expression, motor responses, and interactions with others, (b) physiological responses such as arousal, and digestion and (c) cognitive responses such as awareness of mood and of the precursors and reactions to mood. Tompkins (1981) identified nine fundamental moods (fear, anger, enjoyment, disgust, interest, surprise, contempt, shame, and distress) and hypothesized that all others were combination of those moods. Other authors agree with the concept but delineate different fundamental moods. This author includes only happy, mad, sad and scared as the basic moods.

One means of describing, predicting, and explaining mood had its roots in the works of Berlyne (1960) who posited a PAD explanation based on Pleasure, Arousal, and Dominance which he called the three major dimensions of mood. Each of the dimensions is bipolar and can be described as more or less pleasurable, more or less arousal causing, and as being more or less dominant or submissive. Arousal plus pleasure equal excitement; pleasure without arousal equal relaxing; lack of pleasure coupled with lack of arousal equal boredom; displeasure plus arousal equal chaotic, etc. Mood has strong effects on our immune system, attention, cognitive behavior and affiliation. Common sense and anecdotal reports tell us that good leisure induces good mood. There is also empirical evidence of the same. Stone (1987) found that leisure events were significantly associated with positive moods, more so than almost all other daily events. Mannell, Zuzanek, and Larson (1988) found the same results. Driver, Brown, and Peterson (1991 p. 254) identifies four factors likely to influence mood in recreational activities: (a) alertness (the rock climber or channel swimmer must be more alert than the reader or the sunbather), (b) activity-environment fit (swimming in the muddy Mississippi is not as satisfying as it would be in the crystal waters of the Caribbean), (c) other people (there may be commitments to or judgments by others. People are often unpredictable and crowding can cause aggressive responses) and (d) environment itself (a beautiful view can be pleasure on its own).

Mood can influence our relationships, our future goals and our mental health. Persons experiencing positive moods during activities are more likely to have positive self-concepts (Graef, Czikszentmihalyi, & Ginaninno, 1983). One aspect of mental health is the ability to let go of negative moods and to work through or at least compartmentalize negativity. Leisure activities are an enormous opportunity to accomplish those goals.

Prosocial behavior increases with good mood, creativity is enhanced by a positive outlook, performance is better when one has perceived control. Physiological responses such as heart rate, respiration, blood pressure, gastrointestinal functioning and hormonal changes are all affected by mood. There are many environmental influences of mood some of which we wish to avoid, such as carbon monoxide, negative ions and other chemicals leading to fatigue, anxiety, and sometimes death. There are those we seek such as nature or concert halls. Light, sound, smell, taste, temperature, vibration and other conditions influence mood, however subtly (Hull, 1981).

Czikszentmihalyi (1990) postulated the concept of "Flow," a state of being in which one becomes so involved in an activity or thing that nothing else seems to matter. He describes Flow as an experience so compelling, so gripping, so absorbing, so satisfying that it is done for the pure value of itself. In all of the activities reported by people in Czikszentmihalyi's research, the optimum enjoyment occurred when the opportunities for action perceived by the individual were equal to his or her capability and when challenge and skill matched, whether very simple or very hard. Another important aspect of Flow was the merging of action and awareness. When concentration is so fully on the task at hand that only a select range of information is allowed into awareness, when there is a loss of self-consciousness, when there is a clear goal and immediate feedback, when there is a sense of control and no worry about losing control, when time is encapsulated such as the sense of it is lost, and especially when the activity is auto-telic, an end in itself, then Flow occurs and is immensely satisfying (Czikszentmihalyi, 1990). He postulated that certain activities can become out of control and be destructive. Hazing might be an example. Those antisocial activities may be "play-like" and even enjoyable to some but do not typically produce feelings of Flow and are personally destructive and disintegrating. They cannot be self-actualizing except in a distorted way. On the other hand, solitary, nonsocial, activities can contribute to flow, actions such as meditation, yoga, intensely interesting hobbies and even some intellectual endeavors. Schools which present active, engaging programs that produce Flow experiences maximize children's attention, foster their reflection, and lead to creativity. The perfect experience is one which simultaneously includes the best of all three of Freud's Elements of the Mind: Id (pure wild pleasure), ego (regulation and organization) and superego (the conscience). Flow appears to be an Id experience with the protection of Ego boundaries within the framework of Superego acceptance. Research in Flow theory shows that blue collar women feel work to be a situation of anti-flow with only home activities possibly producing such good feelings. On the other hand, professional women experience their greater sense of flow both at home and at work. The major source of anti-flow for *both* groups in nonwork settings occurred while doing housework. Evidently repetition leads to antiflow feelings (Allison & Duncan, 1987).

One neglected aspect of mood enhancement is the memorializing of good leisure activities which later produces concomitant good moods. How often do people come home from vacations armed with movies and still pictures of their happy adventures? Maintaining films and picture albums allows good moods again to be evoked. Writing a diary of events to go along with the pictures is even more evocative of the original pleasure. The more senses we can involve in our memories, the more they will mimic the original event (Rumelheart, 1977); (Czikszentmihalyi & Rockbird-Halton, 1981).

Recreation

Follow the grain in your own wood. (Howard Thurman)

Recreation, derived from the Latin *recreare* meaning to create anew, is the word applied to the accomplishing of activities one takes part in during leisure. Recreation means to refresh after toil. It is usually engaged in actively and always takes place during leisure time. It affords freedom of choice and is as purposeful and necessary for sustaining the best of the human body and psyche as is food or water. There are many kinds of recreation including:

Spiritual leisure – Experiencing things and activities spiritually can be a significant part of a person's sense of control over life and can provide a sense of connectedness with other people who are alive or who have departed this life. Adding a spiritual dimension can provide a potential for personal development, may be a means for greater understanding and is often a source of comfort for the future. Spirituality may or may not be the same as religion. Spiritual activities include such things as integration of public and private domains and intensely private and personal communion, the most intimate of activities. At the same time, spirituality provides an opportunity, if one wishes, to share a perceptual process while still maintaining one's own interpretation. Introspection, humility, a sense of belonging, peace, comfort and endurance in hard times are states of mind that have been described as 'spiritual.' One can have a spiritual experience, a sudden epiphany, a mystical happening or a gradual spiritual growth. Any one of those events impacts the individual with new awareness and moves one to new insights and understanding (James, 1936). Ragheb (1989) identified Spiritual wellness as one of the six wellness measures correlated with leisure satisfaction, most strongly with aesthetic/environmental leisure. Maslow's "Peak Experience", Czikszentmihalyi "Flow Experience" and Glasser's "Transcendental State" are very similar to one another and seem to occur in many religious and spiritual rituals when the person is receptive.

One's spirituality may be fed by the environs of a particular place. To some, nature is conducive to being in touch with a higher being; to others, the place may be a building such as a church or a synagogue. One has only to think of Thoreau's Walden Pond or the Sistine Chapel to understand the 'sacredness' of a setting. Mountains and seashore are notoriously relaxing and conducive to spiritual experiences. Some have said that being able to view a horizon captures the wonder and the vastness of the universe.

Shared spirituality can be affirming or stifling depending upon how important it is to 'do the right thing.' Some individuals equate peak experiences with mental illness or loss of control. The possibility of a spiritual experience being judged is increased in group activity. At best, spiritual experiences can bring one to introspection, feelings of belonging, peace, opportunity to help others, and a deeper meaning to life. Beneficial to one's well being are a potential for greater understanding of and acceptance of others and one's self, and a sense of connectedness with others in the world (Driver et al., 1991).

Solitary Leisure – The Self as Entertainment (Mannell, 1984) describes a match between the free time available and the capacity to meaningfully fill it with a solitary activity. People high on the SAE scale do not experience boredom or loneliness and do not find time hanging heavily on their hands. They are engaged and involved during their free time. Mannell says that they have a more developed ability to engage in fantasizing and make believe and for using knowledge based in memory. They rely less heavily on social and physical opportunities or on other people's assessment of them than do people who need company to relax. High SAE scale people truly enjoy their own company and typically have a variety of activities that can be enjoyed alone as well as with others. With the mind unsullied by external stimuli, there is more chance of one being able to focus on the activity at hand and to benefit from it in a different way than one would gain from more public activities.

Play Play has typically been thought of as an activity for children. It is usually motivated by the enjoyment of living with no outside judgment or solutions, and is characterized by relaxed and free activity. Play is crucial for our mental creativity and for our health and happiness. It lifts stress, restores optimism, and appears to enhance our brain's ability to exercise flexibility and to renew neural connections that allow us to adapt and meet even difficult environmental conditions. Play can protect us and improve our memory and cognitive abilities (Marano, 1999). The exploration and manipulation of objects enables children to learn about specific characteristics of those objects and, more important, to relate interactively with the outer world. Play has been linked theoretically and through research with the development of convergent and divergent problem solving ability. In convergent thinking, there is one correct solution; in divergent thinking, there may be multiple solutions. Experimentation with new behaviors is typical of play as is using objects for purposes not meant in the context of their original use (Bruner, 1972). Give a child a large brown box and observe the phenomenon. Children who were given the opportunity, in varying conditions, to play with objects on their own, objects that would later be used to solve a specific task, performed better on that task than same age/stage children who had not had the opportunity to do so (Sylva, 1974). Later research clarified that it was not the specific play that allowed success on the subsequent task, but more likely that play provides the child with a more flexible approach to problem solving and contributes to the development of a generalized mode of cognitive approach (Driver et al., 1991). Play has been found to contribute to creativity and has been correlated positively with three aspects of divergent thinking: ideational fluency, originality, and spontaneous flexibility (Torrance, 1961). Children, in play, distort reality to fit their fantasies and that activity results in novel associations, unusual connections, increase in thought flexibility, and creativity (Lieberman, 1965). It appears that make-believe play is most likely to have such effects. Play that is imitative, intellectually based or adult directed apparently does not produce the same results.

As we can see in other leisure activities, it is the *active* and *self-directed* participation in an activity that leads to changes in awareness, self-satisfaction and self-actualization. In the social development area the importance of interpersonal interaction and play is documented in Harlow's studies with young monkeys. Even brief daily play between infant monkeys raised by wire mothers compensated to some degree for the lack of real mothering (Harlow, 1969). Play facilitates an individual's integration into its group and even affects eventual reproductive success and ability to enjoy sexuality. If children lack the opportunity to enjoy interactive play, they can be either maladjusted or excluded from their social group or both (Altmann, 1965). Altmann showed that it is the development of a system of meta- communication learned in play that allows the animals to participate fully and successfully in adult behavior. Learning social cues, communication subtleties, and certain communication sequences depends upon experience and allows for the prediction of others' behaviors. Play enhances development and can provide an avenue for reducing anxiety. Freud argued that play allowed the mastery of anxiety producing events. NeoFreudians conceive of play as having a cathartic affect more than emphasizing mastery. Play can mitigate tensions, anxieties and aggressive tendencies thereby freeing energy for cognitive tasks (Erikson, 1963; Singer, 1973).

Adults also play. Usually their play is motivated simply by the enjoyment of living and no other ulterior motive. Look at karaoke participants, sports enthusiasts and people on a dance floor and you typically see great joy and abandon. We use play in our vernacular as we play on words, play the horses, play the stock market, play dumb, play up to somebody, play along with somebody, make a play for somebody, etc. Futurists predict that people will spend up to 50% of their time in recreating and note that the leisure, entertainment and hospitality industries will be the next economic wave by 2015. People who want to play will buy experiences, not things (Wetzstein, 2000). Adams (2000) calls for "a right to play," for a play ethic to balance the work ethic.

Games, both passive and active, both indoors and out, consume a large amount of play time for adults. Game is a word derived from the German *gaman* meaning glee. Today, many games are highly structured, organized, regulated by the kind of activity and almost always have a win-lose aspect. Most have rules, often require a particular place or specialized equipment, often take place in a particular time span, are artificial, and mimic reality, e.g. Monopoly mimicking business. Callois (1961) distinguishes four types of games: agon – competitive games; alea – games based on luck; mimicry – games involving role playing like children's make believe; and ilinx – games involving vertigo or sensory stimulation such as hang-gliding or drug use. Humor is a form of play. While it may be only a venting of nervous energy, it can also be an intellectual reaction to something unexpected or a self-congratulatory derogation of someone else. We know that laughter can stimulate endorphins in the brain which are natural pain killers and people including Norman Cousins have written about the curative effects of laughter (Cousins, 1979). We read more and more about making sure that our days contain events that make us dissolve into guffaws and belly laughs. Even without the documented positive health effects, laughter is just plain fun.

Play can be destructive. There are many pastimes forbidden by law, custom, or belief such as substance abuse, vandalism, and activities that are inherently harmful to self or others. Deviant behavior is learned through others and through desensitization to the harmful effects on one's behavior. For example, video games involving hurting or killing others have been shown to add to delinquency of those playing the games. (www.killology.com). Most of the children who have been responsible for killing in the schools have been teased and hazed by their peer mates.

Ethics

Character is doing what is right when no one is looking. (J.C. Watts, Jr.).

In the same manner that any other activity involves ethical or nonethical behavior, so does recreation. Ethical pastimes are not self indulgent, they enhance connectedness to others, do not hurt others or the environment, and are typically part of the human community. Bellah, Madsen, and Sullivan (1985) cite*s* family as the clearest example of a sense of community and speaks of family as "a context in which identity is formed in part through identifying with and incorporating aspects of other members." They say that commitment is not the same as conformity and that different isn't wrong. In fact, utter conformity may be a sign of anxiety and not of commitment, and individuality and community are two halves of a whole which make up what is called the "Ensembled Self." There may be a need to formulate a code of environmental ethics, including protection and preservation of nature, and a need to differentiate activities on the basic of morality in that sense (Dustin, 1989). The "me" generation has fostered unbridled self-fulfillment instead of adhering to the Aristotelian concept of "combining reflection and action with deeply routed attachment to one's community," the cultivation of civil character and the capacity for shared existence, the ability to be open toward truth so as to "come together in pursuit of themselves and the world around them." (Hemingway, 1998) Charles Ketering of General Motors stated sometime back that business needed to create a dissatisfied customer and proceeded to make annual changes in GM cars thus forwarding a consumption ethic that still prevails today. As in any other activity in our lives, we must consider who or what our decisions benefit and who or what they hurt.

Boredom

Be kind, for everyone you meet is fighting a hard battle. (Plato)

According to Bertrand Russell (1968) "Boredom is essentially a thwarted desire for events, not necessarily pleasant ones, but just occurrences such as will enable the victim of ennui to know one day from another. The opposite of boredom is not pleasure, but excitement." (p. 36). As participation in satisfying leisure activities increases, boredom decreases. Those activities most likely to reduce boredom are social activities, sports participation, outdoor recreation and reading. Cultural activities, hobbies, and passive media experiences are less likely to reduce boredom (Ragheb, 1989). Boredom is basically under-stimulation and disconnection. It is not intrinsic to the object or event but is a product of how those objects or events are experienced by the individual. Factors contributing to boredom include repetition, lack of interaction, and minimal variation (Isohola 1990; Selb, 1998). Those authors showed how boredom increased with reduction in perceived social competence, and also reduction in chosen entertainment, intrinsic leisure motivation, self-esteem, leisure ethics, and either mental or physical health. In most of the research we learn that the process of engaging meaningfully in leisure is learned early in life and that there is a continuum of boredom – passivity on one end and action – pleasure/enjoyment on the other.

Pleasure has been described as the satisfaction of a desire, a state which does not require skill or drive to reach its potential. Examples would be drinking when thirsty, petting a dog, winning the lottery, or sex. Activities contributing to pleasure can be repeated and still not be boring. There are various kinds of pleasure such as sensory, expressive, and intellectual (Smith, 1991). Smith et al. also say that the pleasure center of the brain is in the limbic system and is basic to most warm blooded animals who are neurologically intact. Enjoyment, on the other hand, requires activity and ability, and will drive us to new heights and potentials. One drifts into boredom without new challenges and when one loses the capacity to make the more mundane events of everyday life enjoyable. It is pointed out in the literature over and over again that it is *activity*, not passivity that provides leisure activity with its potential to enhance growth in the participant.

Activity, in this sense of the word, is not synonymous with aerobics but with active participation, interest, involvement, and choice. It is perfectly fine to fill one's time partially with activities that do not require any effort and do not produce any reward but one must realize there will be none but the present pleasure from such time spent, no seeds of self-actualization planted and no hope of future gain. Pleasure for itself? Of course. There are times when we can bask in the sensory joys, especially as our work lives are reduced. In an aging population, there is more free time expected for America's seniors and an opportunity to fill time with pleasure and enjoyment. At a stage of life characterized by social losses, leisure activities can create new social ties and literally sustain life. (Kelly, Steinkamp, & Kelly, 1986).

Benefits of Leisure

While we have the gift of life, it seems to me the only tragedy is to allow part of us to die – whether it is our spirit, our creativity or our glorious uniqueness. (Gilda Radner)

Brightbill (1961) made some points that seem pertinent even today: Were people trying to find appreciations, interests and skills that would help them use leisure all through their lives in personally satisfying, decent and wholesome ways, he would set them down as follows:

1. Those that aid body development, movement and motor coordination; such activities would include many sports and athletic endeavors. Most cities have municipal parks and running tracks, tennis courts, golf courses, etc. There are also inexpensive ways of being active without leaving one's neighborhood such as bike riding, skating, dancing, and back yard games like Frisbee and various ball play. Children can play hopscotch, jump rope, kick the can and hide and seek while, at the same time, meeting and enjoying the neighbors. Playgrounds with swings and slides and seesaws provide a safe place for children to play and for parents to chat. Most YMCA's have small monthly dues but part of their philosophy is not to turn families away if they are truly needy. Little League play is a grand opportunity for children to learn athletic skills and for parents to coach, work out with them or simply provide refreshments and support.
2. Those that contribute to safety and survival; such activities would include things like swimming, learning to drive various vehicles and perhaps martial arts. Most cities have pools; some have usable ponds and lakes. For children, there are summer day and sleep-away camps often sponsored by inner city groups or entities such as Boy and Girl Scouts or churches, places where skills such as water safety, survival, and camping are taught.
3. Those that help make the individual an interesting and articulate conversationalist and reflect social graces; such activities would include cooking skills, fashion design and hosting/hostessing. Many stores give free or low cost seminars lasting from an hour to a day. The Internet is a ready resource for increasing one's knowledge of cooking, flower arranging, housekeeping and interior design. In this area, it is practice that makes perfect just as in the development of athletic or intellectual skills. What could be more fun for a parent and child than planning, preparing for, and having a party? Parlor games are a good way for children to learn to be comfortable performing in front of others. Table games and cards can help teach sportsmanship and 'charm under fire.'
4. Those that make use of creative hands in shaping materials; such activities would include things like drawing, painting, tying flies, sewing, knitting and many crafts. All ages can enjoy hand work and the products which result. Making a photo album for the hostess of a party or the bride or one's family brings pleasure to the maker and the recipient. Things that produce a product are most satisfactory to one's inner sense of accomplishment.

5. Those that bring good literature into minds and lives; this category would include reading, some public television, tapes, CD's, and attendance at plays and movies. Public libraries are a source for most of the above. Many cities have 'dollar movies' with films that are a few months old instead of brand new. Instead of the path of entertainment described above, local drama groups and many religious groups offer opportunities for citizens to participate in shows, either on or backstage. Scrabble and crossword puzzles increase vocabulary and are joyful activities themselves.

6. Those that bring appreciation and enjoyment of the outdoors and that bring us close to the natural world around us; such activities would include use of parks and public outdoor facilities. Join your local Parks and Recreation Department. There are year-round events listed with nominal or no charges. Many outdoor amusement parks have year-round passes which may appear expensive at first but which, when amortized over a season, end up being inexpensive (Beam, 2004). Visit a lighthouse or a port, go to the fire station, or find a very dark place from which to look at the stars. Hike on a trail or go to the zoo or have a picnic. Walk through an arboretum, do some bird watching, take pictures of your loved ones amidst wild flowers in the spring. Plant a garden.

7. Those that make it possible to create vocal and instrumental music or at least make it possible to enjoy listening to it; such activities would include listening to radio, tapes, CD's and especially live performances. Again, many cities provide free concerts, both pop and classical, as do schools and churches. Form a family band with inexpensive instruments. Barter for lessons. Most people have a talent or product that can be swapped for music lessons. Find a needy choir and enjoy the camaraderie as well as the lessons and the productions. Christmas carol groups are wonderful fun for children and adults alike. Sing in the shower to start your day.

8. Those that allow us to express ourselves through drama, even though in elementary form, and certainly those that help us appreciate it; the activities in this group would be passive and active. Live dramatic performances can be found at little or no cost through most schools and colleges and at some municipal facilities or drama clubs. Expressive dance might be a subcategory here. One could form a group and, in that way, a teacher's shared payment would be small. Book signings at libraries or local book stores are fun and often include the authors reading of a passage or two. Join or, better yet, start a book club or a current events discussion group.

9. Those that encourage us and provide satisfaction in being service to others. Volunteer work would be a perfect example of this kind of activity. One can accomplish that by giving time to an already organized entity or by choosing one's own way to serve others such as driving an elderly neighbor to the doctor. Read the local newspaper for listings of groups who need volunteer services. Fostering one's favorite cause is a good way to find inner-satisfaction. One way of helping a child understand good fortune is to have him give to someone less fortunate. The earlier the concept of sharing one's time and money with the community is instilled, the better it is learned and the more it is enjoyed.

Brightbill (1961) commented that there was not a Neuropsychiatric hospital with a credible record in the United States that did not include recreation in its program for participants. The latter is still true today. The benefits of leisure include physical and mental health, social skill development, and community growth. A recent review of the literature confirmed that physical inactivity carries a far higher risk of coronary heart disease and some forms of cancer than smoking, drinking, and poor diet (Carney, 2001). Driver et al. (1991) identified 43 specific types of benefits of leisure in general, 18 physiological benefits, 24 social benefits, and 11 categories of environmental benefits. The grand total was 105 benefits all supported by research.

Regular physical activity is associated not only with increased life expectancy, but with reduced incidence of coronary heart disease, diabetes, colon cancer, hypertension, obesity and osteoporosis. An active lifestyle extends independent living in older adults and interacts positively with strategies to improve diet and reduce the use of alcohol, tobacco, and drugs (Knowler et al., 1996; (Department of Health and Human Services, 1996). Inactivity is the most significant risk for coronary heart disease and that physical activity can increase the average age expectancy by as much as two years (Paffenbarger, Hyde, & Wing, 1986; U.S. Centers for Disease Control). Many health insurance companies are recognizing the benefits of staying physically fit and are offering, especially to seniors, financial assistance in obtaining fitness and health education through community centers, senior centers and recreational parks and pools (Stahl, 2003). Senior Dimension is a federally funded Medicare and Choice program in Nevada, a prototype which will hopefully spread as its successes are documented. Public and private partnerships for community or corporate health initiatives are fairly common as many medical centers and businesses have workout facilities and incentive programs. Health plans in your area can be found through the American Association of Health Plans website at www.aahp.org.

The study of benefits is a complex process of observing and measuring variables and a simplistic approach to the study cannot be made. Benefits rarely stand alone as a measurable outcome nor are they easy to identify. For example, if physical health is a benefit to be measured, there are considerable confounding variables that contribute to this measurement. Also, one benefit can overlap with other benefits and build upon benefits until an ultimate perceived benefit is achieved (Driver et al., 1991, p. 483). "Recreation-related mental or physical relaxation might promote higher productivity at work, which could lead to increased economic security, which has been identified as an important contributor to life satisfaction." (p. 9) One of the better books on recreation, a catalog published by the Parks and Recreation Federation of Ontario, focused heavily on recreation providers and public decision makers as an audience rather than on the general public (Parks and Recreation Federation of Ontario, 1992).

Health is much more than physical and includes mental health, emotional health, social health and spiritual health (Williams & Knight, 1995). Psychological measures are more common among leisure researchers and more complex to understand than the physiological measures. Research results on physiological benefits are clear and, in summary, show that mortality from all causes and longevity are influenced by exercise, fitness and other considerations of lifestyle (Paffenbarger et al., 1986). Psychological benefits of leisure activities included intellectual stimulation, catharsis, expressive compensation, hedonistic companionship, supportive companionship, secure solitude, routine, temporary indulgence, moderate security, and expressive asceticism (Tinsley, 1979; Tinsley & Tinsley, 1986). Self-identity becomes a potentially important benefit of leisure participation and the perception of internal locus of control is an important contributor to positive attitude change (Haggard & Williams, 1991).

The contribution to mental and emotional health is evidently quite dependent upon whether the individual perceives the activity as freely chosen and an end in itself or as an activity chosen by someone else. Those who are in control of their leisure time and experiences feel engaged, are healthier than those not in control, and feel less detached (Iso-Ahola & Weissinger, 1984). Recreational activities can play an important role in helping people to manage stress and to interpret stressful situations in a less negative way. Certain types of physical activity, running in particular, can target some forms of mild depression. A New York study involving older men and women showed that those with high participation in leisure activities such as walking, playing cards, and listening to music, were 38% less likely than controls in the study to develop dementia (Scarmeas et al., 2001). Verghese et al. (2003) found the same results. Large muscle activities help ease frustration, anger and hostility (Sullivan, 2001). Several studies have shown that people engage in recreational activities specifically for social reasons and that friendships generated through these recreations are closer than those generated in other life situations such as work (Coleman & Iso-Ahola, 1993). Mortality is three times higher in individuals with few close relationships (Anspaugh, Hamrick, & Rosato, 1991). Several studies have shown that recreation has a positive impact on quality of family life and on marital satisfaction. Spiritual health extends beyond commitment to a religious organization. Recreation's contribution to spiritual health is best exemplified in the development and provision of parks and open spaces (Kanters, 1996).

The relationship between leisure activities and social benefits are multidirectional and the most difficult of all potential benefits to measure. When families participated together in leisure activities, family bonding occurred and the related benefits included family satisfaction, family interaction, and family stability. Husbands and wives who shared joint recreational activities together tended to be much more satisfied in their marriages (Orthner & Mancini, 1991).

If leisure is the mirror of the personality which tells us what kind of person we are, we must not ignore it. We must be prepared for nonwork time and *ready* for free time. So much of our lives is regulated and routinized by someone or something else that, when we have great blocks of free time, we are much like the dog who had been chained for years to the house and, when the chain is removed, never leaves his place.

"When we empty or free our minds from distracting thoughts, we are more receptive to our surroundings and the options presented. If your mental cup is full, then how can you receive more information? By emptying the cup, you actually become more capable of receiving....Our belief starts to affect external factors. Experience shows that, as soon as you decide to make a change, you have already begun this process. It's like telling a child he can have ice cream. The moment the words spill out of your mouth, the ice cream is already happening in his mind. By focusing attention on your positive intentions, constructive improvement and change greets you at every turn."
(Stewart & Stewart, 2005)

We must make a commitment to leisure.

Summary

Leisure is the time when we are most free to make choices that can renew or recreate us and lead to higher self-esteem and community spirit. Pleasure and enjoyment typically result in renewed vigor, and we go back to the chores of life refueled and often with new ideas to apply to old problems. Our health is changed in a positive way with constructive, and especially active, participation in enjoyable events which result in stress reduction, skill enhancement, and immunological boosts. Psychological effects include self-affirmation, self-actualization, development of leadership skills, cognitive and social development in children, skill and knowledge acquisition, mood enhancement, and an increase in life satisfaction. Spiritual leisure activities lead to increases in feelings of affiliation, better appreciation for others, opportunities to apply ethics and values to real-life situations through ministry, and feelings of belonging (Mannell, 1988). Family leisure activities can lead to more authenticity in relationships, better bonding, and just plain fun. Couples who play together stay together. Enjoying activities together builds memories, creates stories and histories, and can increase adolescents' feelings of belonging to a significant group. As we grow within ourselves, grow within our family and grow within our community, it is very easy to slip into becoming a world citizen, one who sees the value in all others, who can extend a helping hand when appropriate and who can sleep at night knowing that the peace is well deserved.

With my loved ones around me, I will always choose my home
Over the glory that was Greece and the grandeur that was Rome (Anon).

References

Adams, R. (2000). Let's all go out to play. *New Statesman, 129*(4512), 36.

Allison, M. T., & Duncan, M. C. (1987). Women, work and flow. *Leisure Sciences, 9*, 143–161.

Altmann, S. A. (1965) Sociobiology of rhesus monkeys. II. stochastics of social communication. *Journal of Theoretical Biology, 8*, 490–522.

Anspaugh, D. J., Hamrick, M. H., & Rosato, F. D. (1991). *Concepts and applications of wellness*. St. Louis, MO: Mosby Year Book.

Beam, J. (2004). 'Cheap Thrills'. *Doll – The Dollaar Stretcher*. www.stretcher.com/stories.

Bellah, R. N., Madsen, R., & Sullivan, W. M. (1985) *Habits of the heart: Individualism and commitment in American life* (p. 298). Berkley, CA: University of California Press.

Bem, D. (1972). Self-perception theory. In L. Berkowitz (Ed.), *Advances in experimental social psychology* (p. 6). New York, NY: Academic Press.

Berlyne, D. (1960) *Conflict, arousal, and curiosity* (p. 48). New York, NY: McGraw Hill.

Brightbill, C. K. (1961). *Man and leisure, a philosophy of recreation* (pp. 232–233). Englewood Cliffs, NJ: Prentice-Hall, Inc.

Bruner, J. S. (1972). Nature and uses of immaturity. *American Psychologist, 27*, 687–708.

Callois, R. (1961). *Man, play and games*. Glenco, IL: Free Press of Glenco.

Carney, C. (2001). *Health benefits of physical activity; a literature review*. Edinburgh: Report for Scottish Natural Heritage.

Coleman, D., & Iso-Ahola, S. E. (1993). Leisure and health: The role of social support and self determination. *Journal of Leisure Research, 25*(2): 111–128.

Cousins, N. (1979). *Anatomy of an illness as perceived by the patient.* New York: W. W. Norton and Company, Inc.

Czikszentmihalyi, M. (1990). *Flow: the psychology of optimal experience.* New York: Harper and Row.

Czikszentmihalyi, M., & Rockbird-Halton, E. (1981). *The meaning of things: domestic symbols and the self.* Cambridge: Cambridge University Press.

Department of Health and Human Services (Vs) (1996). *Physical activity and health: A report of the surgeon general.* Atlanta: Department of Health and Human Services, Centers for Disease Control and Prevention, National Center for Chronic Disease Prevention and Health Promotion.

Driver, B. L., Brown, P. J., & Peterson, G. L. (Eds.). (1991). *Benefits of leisure* (pp. 218–219). State College, PA: Venture Publishing, Inc.

Dustin, D. L. (1989). Recreation rightly understood. In T. Goodale, & P. Witt (Eds.), *Recreation and leisure: issues in an era of change* (3rd ed.). State College, PA: Venture Publishing, Inc.

Erikson, E. H. (1963). *Childhood and society* (p. 445). New York, NY: W. W. Norton.

Eysenck, M. W. (1982). *Attention and arousal.* Berlin: Springer Verlag. In *Benefits of leisure*. State College, PA: Venture Publishing, Inc.

Graef, R., Czikszentmihalyi, M., & Ginaninno, S. M. (1983). Measuring intrinsic motivation in everyday life. *Leisure Studies, 2*, 155–168.

Haggard, M., & Williams, D. R. (1991). Self-identity benefits of leisure activity. In B. L. Driver, P. J. Brown, & G. I. Peterson (Eds.), *Benefits of leisure* (pp. 103–119). State College, PA: Venture Publishing, Inc.

Harlow, H. F. (1969). Age mate or peer affectional systems. In D. S. Lehrman, R. A. Hinde, E. Shaw (Eds.), *Advances in the study of behavior* (Vol. II, pp. 334–384). New York, NY: Academic Press.

Harris, L. (1998). *Americans and the arts* (p. 60, Table 1). New York: Louis Harris and Associates.

Hemingway, J. L. (1998). Leisure and civility: Reflections on a Greek Ideal. *Leisure Sciences, 10*(3), 179–191.

Hull, R. B. (1981). Mood as a product of leisure: Causes and consequences. In Driver et al. (Eds.), *Benefits of leisure* (p. 253). State College, PA: Venture Publishing, Inc.

Ibirham, H. (1991). *Leisure and society: A comparative approach.* Dubuque, IA: W. C. Brown.

Iso-Ahola, S. E. (1990). Perceptions of boredom in leisure. *Journal of Leisure Research, 22*(1), 1–17.

Iso-Ahola, S. E., & Weissinger, E. (1984). Leisure and well-being: is there a connection. *Parks and Recreation, 19*(6), 40–44.

James, W. (1936). *The varieties of religious experience.* New York, NY: The Modern Library in Benefits of Leisure; State College, PA: Venture Publishing, Inc.

Kanters, M. A. (1996). The health benefits of parks and recreation. *Illinois Parks and Recreation*, January/February.

Kelly, J., Steinkamp, M., & Kelly, J. (1986). Later life leisure: how they play in Peoria. *The Gerontologist, 26*(5), 531–537.

Knowler, W. C., Barrett-Conner, E., Fowler, S. E., Hamman, R. F., Lachin, J. M., Walker, E. A., et al. (1996). Diabetes prevention program research group. Reduction in the incidence of type 2 diabetes with lifestyle intervention or metformin. *New England Journal of Medicine, 346*: 393–403.

Lieberman, J. N. (1965). Playfulness and divergent thinking. *Journal of Genetic Psychology, 107*: 219–224.

Mannell, R. C. (1984). Personality in leisure theory: The self as entertainment. *Society and Leisure, 7*, 229–242.

Mannell, R. C., Zuzanek, J., & Larson, R. (1988) Leisure states and "flow" experiences: Testing perceived freedom and intrinsic motivation hypothesis. *Journal of Leisure Research, 20*, 289–304.

Marano, H. E. (1999). The power of play. *Psychology Today, 32*(4), 36. Sussix Publishers.

National Institutes of Health (NIH) (1996). Physical activity and health. NIH consensus development panel on physical activity and cardiovascular health. *Journal of the American Medical Association, 276*, 227.

Orthner, D. K., & Mancini, J. A. (1991). Benefits of leisure for family bonding. In B. L. Driver, P. J. Brown, & G. L. Peterson (Eds.), *Benefits of leisure* (pp. 289–301). State College, PA: Venture Publishing, Inc.

O'Sullivan, E. (2001). Repositioning: parks and recreation as essential to well-being – national programs: fitness and active lifestyles, *Parks and Recreation*, October 2008, Wholistic Health Promotion (p. 88).

Paffenbarger, R. S., Hyde, M. A., & Wing, A. L. (1986). Physical activity: All cause mortality, and longevity of college alumni. *New England Journal of Medicine, 314*, 605–613.

Parks and Recreation Federation of Ontario (1992). *The benefits of parks and recreation: A catalog* (p. 98). Ontario, Canada: Parks and Recreation Federation of Ontario.

Ragheb, M. (1989). In a paper entitled Leisure and Wellness, presented at the Southeastern Recreational Research Conference; Ashville, NC, February.

Rumelheart, D. E. (1977). *Introduction to human information processing* (p. 306). New York, NY: Wiley.

Russell, B. (1968). *The conquest of happiness* (p. 36). New York: Bantam.

Russell, R. V. (1996). *Past times: the context of contemporary leisure* (pp. 8–13). Chicago, IL: Brown and Benchmark.

Scarmeas, N., Levy, G., Tang, M-X., et al. (2001). Influence of leisure activity on the incidence of Alzheimer's disease. *Neurology, 57*, 2236–2242.

Schor, J. B. (1993). NY: Basic Books. (pp. 1–15)

Selb, H. M. (1998). Cognitive correlates of boredom proneness. *Journal of Psychology: Interdisciplinary and Applied, 132*(6), 642–652.

Singer, J. L. (1973). *The child's world of make believe: experimental studies of imaginative play* (p. 294). New York, NY: Academic Press.

Smith, S. L. J. (1991). On the biological basis of pleasure. In T. L. Goodale, & P. A. Witt (Eds.), *Recreation and leisure: issues in an era of change*. State College, PA: Venture.

Stahl, J. (2003). Prescription for senior health: recreation. Looksmart. http: www.looksmart.com/ParksandRecreation. June 2003.

Stewart, B. K., & Stewart, L. D. (2005). *Your way home: the psychology of place inside and out*. Charleston, SC: Inner Arts Press.

Stone, A. A. (1987). Event content in a daily survey is differentially associated with concurrent mood. *Journal of Personality and Social Psychology, 52*, 56–58.

Sylva, K. (1974). *The relationship between play and problem solving in children 3–5 years old* (p. 144). PhD Dissertation. Cambridge, MA: Howard University.

Sylvester, C. D. (1987). The ethics of play, leisure and recreation in the 20th century, 1900–1983. *Leisure Sciences, 9*(3), 173–188.

Tinsley, H. E. A., & Kass, R. A. (1979). The latent structure of the need satisfying properties of leisure activities. *Journal of Leisure Research, 11*, 278–291.

Tinsley, H. E. A., & Tinsley, D. J. (1986). A theory of the attributes, benefits, and causes of leisure experienced. *Leisure Sciences, 8*(1), 1–45.

Tompkins, S. S. (1981). The quest for primary motives. *Journal of Personality and Social Psychology, 41*, 306–329.

Torrance, E. P. (1961). Priming creative thinking in the primary grades. *Elementary School Journal, 62*, 139–145.

Verghese, J., Lipton, R. B., Katz, M. J., Hall, C. B., Derby, C. A., Kuslansky, G., Ambrose, A. F., Sliwinski, M., & Buschke, H. (2003). Leisure activities and the risk of dementia in the elderly. *New England Journal of Medicine, 348*, 2508–2516.

Wetzstein, C. (2000). More play, less work foreseen for Americans. *Insight on the News, 16*(6), 32.

Wolpe, J. (1958). *Psychology by reciprocal inhibition.* Palo Alto, CA: Stanford University Press.

Section IV

Secondary Writing Approaches

The writing medium has come into its own only recently. Its resurgence has taken place in spite of a long history of applications that in many instances preceded the use of talking for preventive and psychotherapeutic purposes (Esterling, L'Abate, Murray, & Pennebaker, 1999; Lepore & Smyth, 2002). Recent considerations about the expensive nature and relative inefficiency of the verbal medium (L'Abate, 1999, 2005) have brought into the fore the importance of expanding mental health practices of adding the nonverbal (Section 3 this volume) and writing media to traditionally verbally based preventive and psychotherapeutic armamentaria. Perhaps through this expansion it may be possible to reach the goal of matching a method of intervention with a particular problem. For instance, one could argue that given the well-known resistance and poor results of treating externalizing personality disorders and criminals when the verbal medium is used, it would seem that group nonverbal methods might offer a more cost-effective approach to help increase self-awareness. One time only offenders might profit by writing rather than by talking (McMahan & Arias, 2004; Reed, McMahan, & L'Abate, 2001). With internalizing disorders, where the motivation to change seems somewhat higher and there is greater amenability to collaborate than in externalizing disorders (L'Abate, 2005), writing, as a more cost-effective approach, may be coupled with the verbal modality for greater synergistic effectiveness.

The spoken medium, talk, although necessary for communication, is not the only medium of communication available to promote physical and mental health. Both nonverbal and writing media are available even though they have not been used in preventive and psychotherapeutic practices as widely as the spoken medium. Rather than wonder why that lopsided emphasis has occurred, we need to look at the characteristics of these media to understand why talk has been used exclusively at the expense of the other two. Words allow us to communicate easily for most of the information needed. However, both the verbal and nonverbal media are infinite in their manifestations. There are no limits to what one can say or do. They are both infinite domains, in the sense that their manifestations are limitless in their expression. Although one could use the same argument for the written medium, one would argue that while the spoken and nonverbal media are not controllable, the written medium is relatively more controllable than the other two media, once a specific topic is assigned to participants. We cannot control what participants (individuals, couples, and families) will say to therapists any more than we can control what therapists will say to participants, no matter how many therapy manuals we may use to decrease a therapist's variability (L'Abate, 2005). Furthermore, as long as we rely solely on the verbal medium, we cannot control what participants will say and do outside the therapy office, unless we administer between-sessions homework assignments (Kazantzis, Deane, Ronan, & L'Abate, 2005; Kazantzis & L'Abate, 2007). If and when we give participants instructions or suggestions verbally, we can predict that many participants will tend either to forget or to distort them, especially if no written contract or Informed Consent Form was signed from the very outset of the relationship. If something is important, it needs to be put in writing. This is how societies move forward.

Talk requires personal, f2f contact, unless one uses the phone, while the written medium does not require it. Through writing, a relationship can take place at a distance, through the mail, fax, or Internet, and does not require personal, f2f contact. Writing, therefore, is a cheaper and, perhaps more cost-effective medium of communication than talking. The written medium is controllable to the extent that written instructions and written homework assignments can be administered, where distortions, generalization, and deletions, will be minimized.

As long as the verbal medium is used as the major or only source of information about the process of psychotherapy, it will be difficult if not impossible to learn more about psychotherapy and answer the question about which method of treatment is better than the others. As long as treatment takes place verbally, one needs to record and transcribe what is going on and then code it in order to reduce it to manageable units of research. However, as long as we rely on the spoken word, the costs of studying therapist-participant interactions, process and outcome, are going to be expensive if not prohibitive. Research will be limited to those few who are able to marshal grant support for this type of research. Early estimates indicated that it might take at least 28 hours of clerical and technical time to reduce verbal therapist-participant interactions to manageable units of research. Perhaps, through new technological advances in voice and writing reproductions, it is possible to cut down on the time and clerical help it takes to transform spoken records or recordings to the written form. Nonetheless, using the written modality, either as an alternative medium of therapeutic interaction or as a paratherapeutic addition to the verbal medium, may allow us to learn more (and faster) about various methods of treatment than would be possible through an analysis of verbal interactions. The verbal modality is very expensive in terms of professional time, while writing, in its proper use, might be cost-effective, but under certain conditions, as discussed in Chapter 14.

Consequently, through written records it is possible to advance the field of mental health, among many other technological advances of the last century, including TV, broadband, fax, telephone, mail, CD-Roms, etc. As long as f2f talk is used solely in the delivery of mental health services, research and practice in f2f psychological interventions will remain, and are destined to remain, separate fields of endeavor, with no hope of being united and integrated for the betterment of humanity's ills. Through writing it will be possible to keep records of what professionals and participants feel, think, and do, with a minimum of professional time and effort.

Writing may fulfill quite a few functions, many already elaborated in previous publications cited in Chapter 14 in this volume. Briefly, writing can be used as an alternative to or as an aid and adjutant to prevention and psychotherapy, provided that a written contract about its use is made from the very outset of professional contacts. Writing can be used as a method to assess motivation for change by increasing the active involvement of participants in the process of change. In this fashion, writing puts greater responsibility for change on participants rather than on therapists. By possibly shortening the process and length of prevention and therapy, an area that is crying out for empirical evidence, writing may also become a cost-effective parapreventive and paratherapeutic approach as well as a easier method for research in mental health. By tapping in the cognitive coping realm, writing would fit into the cognitive therapies field, even though it can be oriented to tap into the affective and behavioral realms as well.

As a means of self-growth, writing can be individualized to run a parallel, synergistic process with or without f2f, talk-based (tb) prevention or therapy sessions. It can be used before, in parallel, or in tandem with preventive and therapeutic efforts. It can also be used by itself, especially if, as shown in the chapters of this section, there are so many ways of intervening with writing to promote physical as well as mental health. By giving participants something concrete to do about their problem above and beyond the 50-minute f2f session, it provides an impetus for carrying relevant themes further and deeper than a costly f2f tb session would allow. Providing a structure and focus by breaking down relevant problems into more manageable parts will be illustrated by chapters in this section. By increasing the sense of direction, writing also increases participants' sense of responsibility for their own progress. The use of writing increases options available to professional helpers as well as participants. At a minimum, it may increase awareness and critical evaluation of set beliefs, cognitions, and behavioral patterns with a greater sense of choice about them. Rehearsal and practice of certain behavior patterns can be administered and monitored through written instructions just as well as verbally. In fact, one could argue that certain routine instructions, administered in writing, decrease the chances of deletions, distortions, and unwarranted generalizations in participants.

Not completing written homework assignments can become as lucrative "grist for the helping mill" as completing them, because sources of resistance to change can be brought out through writing assignments that would not be brought out otherwise. Tangential or parallel practices after the assignment of writing assignments to participants may consist of confronting reasons for either not completing an assignment or not completing it well. Questions raised by this practice would focus on: (1) "What worked or didn't work for you?" (not all assignments work well for all participants); (2) "Where might this practice be or not be helpful to you?" As will be seen in the chapters in this section, writing can be as individualized and tailor-made just as well and perhaps even better than talking, by writing *ad hoc* assignments for specific patterns not covered elsewhere. Thus, writing increases the preventive and therapeutic repertoires and gives more options to participants by opening doors that may stay closed otherwise, by using verbal or nonverbal therapies alone.

Of course, writing cannot be used for illiterates or unmotivated individuals, even though audiotapes and volunteer intermediaries could be used to mediate its use with these populations. Ultimately, though, the most important function of writing is to link evaluation with treatment in ways that are impossible or very expensive to achieve through either the verbal or the nonverbal media. This last point will be elaborated on in the various chapters of this section.

Stress on the written medium does not mean that reliance on speaking should be down played or eliminated. On the contrary, all three media should be used synergistically rather than exclusively, if not, in some instances, antagonistically. The written medium fulfills functions that do not overlap with the spoken one. For instance, writing can be used primarily to increase generalization from the professional's office to the home. Thus, the spoken word could be used to establish rapport and trust between professionals and participants, which includes contracts about the use of regular appointments and homework assignments to be completed at home by participants to parallel whatever is going on in the professional's office (Kazantzis et al., 2005; Kazantzis & L'Abate, 2007). However, treatment or generalization outside the therapist's office needs to take place through the written medium, including instructions about interventions covered in Sections II, III and V of this volume.

Why is writing a secondary intervention that promotes physical and mental health? There are at least four lines of thinking that lead toward including writing not only to promote physical and mental health, but also to prevent illness (Lepore & Smyth, 2002), and make preventive and psychotherapeutic processes more effective and possibly more efficient (Esterling et al., 1999).

In the first place, writing is learned through training, while talking is learned automatically, earlier than talk, which is learned spontaneously, mostly without training. Consequently, one can assume that talk and writing may affect and may be affected by different parts of the brain (Hugdahl & Davidson, 2004). Whether they are and how they are affected needs to be ascertained further. Nonetheless, there is no question that there are at least two different intellectual processes, and, very likely, two different neurological processes underlying them. Simplistically, to begin with, writing involves eyes and hands. Talk involves ears and mouths. As Denes-Ray and Epstein (1994), supported by more recent work (Dawes, 2001; Savitsky and Gilovich, 2003; Savitsky et al., 2001), found, one intellectual process is deliberate and the other is intuitive. The latter is based on personal experience, is influenced quickly by emotions, and is involved in the here and now. The former process is based more on logic and deduction, consideration of the pros and cons of a situation, and follows more rational pathways.

L'Abate (L'Abate & Hecker, 2004; McMahan & L'Abate, 2001) suggested that the emotional process is related "relatively more" to the right hemisphere of the brain, while the rational process necessary for writing is related "relatively more" to the brain's left hemisphere. Whether this symmetry is valid remains to be seen, because the issue is much more complex than an either-or position (Hugdahl & Davidson, 2004). Is is possible, however, that talk-based psychotherapy, in its immediacy, may relate "relatively more" to the right hemisphere, while writing, in its necessary delay, may relate "relatively more" to the left hemisphere.

In the second place, talk and writing may possess different functions. Talk is based on communicating immediately, with little if any thinking. Writing, on the other hand, requires a modicum of thinking if nothing else, to connect from thinking to writing. Of course, there are many examples of abusive and thoughtless writing, just as much or worse than talk. The immediacy of talk makes it possible to use it therapeutically, while the relative delay of writing makes it possible to use it not only therapeutically but also promotionally and preventively. As the chapters in this section demonstrate, writing in its various structures can be used synergistically as an approach with functional participants, and as an additional medium of help for dysfunctional individuals and their relationships.

The fields of psychotherapy and prevention, however, have been slow in acknowledging the importance of writing as an additional medium of intervention besides just talk and medication. Among the many available examples of this limited dichotomous view, a recent source (Beitman, Nair, & Viamontes, 2004), for instance, commented that: "No one clinician has found the ideal formula for treating medications and psychotherapy to achieve this condition," that is, "...creating a therapeutic environment in which the patient can feel safe..." (p. 23). This thinking, either talk-based psychotherapy or medication, or both, fails to acknowledge Bloom's (1992) findings that even psychotic participants can use and profit by using (and writing into) computers. Those original results seem supported by the possibility that psychotic participants in remission do respond to objective written tests, a process that seems to increase rapport with the examiner (Cusinato, 2005). Hospitalized schizophrenic participants do seem to improve when responding to written assignments from a workbook which deals with severe psychopathology (Tarquinio et al., 2005). Whether this is indeed the case, needs to be demonstrated further.

Indeed, writing may possibly help initiate a process of self-awareness that is not present in severe psychopathology when talk is involved (Beitman, Nair & Viamontes, 2004). Programmed, emotionally neutral written questions or tasks may allow schizophrenics to answer through writing in ways that are not possible in the talk-based, inevitably emotionally charged, contact with another human being, professional or otherwise. By the same token, writing charged with emotionality, as in the case of expressive writing (Chapter 13 this volume), may be counterproductive with schizophrenic participants. This is an important area to study. It may open up new possibilities for the treatment of severe psychopathology (James Pennebaker, personal communication, May 10, 2005).

In the third place, as argued elsewhere (L'Abate, 1999, 2005), words are infinite and uncontrollable while writing is finite and controllable in its *specificity and explicitness*. Writing by its very nature is replicable. Words are difficult to record and score because they are neither specific nor explicit. Because of the expenses needed to convert them into a written format, overall, especially in private practice, they are not replicable. If recorded through audio or videotapes, as noted earlier, words are very expensive to code. There are many different scoring systems and there is no agreement on which system to use.

In the fourth place, writing can be classified according to: (a) its degree of structure – which varies from least structured or open-ended, to focused, guided, to the most structured extreme, i.e., programmed, and (b) its content – from traumatic to trivial or from abstract to concrete. Focused writing essentially suggests one specific topic that should be the major focus of concern for writing, as for instance, one's journaling (Chapter 11 this volume), autobiography (Chapter 12 this volume), and expressive writing (Chapter 13 this volume). From reading the outcome of this assignment, professional helpers may progress to the next step of guided writing by asking specific questions to be answered also in writing. For instance, they can ask for elaboration of unclear passages in one's journal, autobiography, or focused writing. After guided writing helpers may progress to programmed writing, a planned, already prepared approach based on a previously designed series of assignments around a specific topic, which form a program, or workbook (Chapter 14 this volume). This sequence does not need to occur through f2f tb interventions. It already occurs every day on the Internet (Chapter 15 this volume).

Even though there are various classifications of talk, there have been relatively few heuristic classifications of writing. Among others, writing can be classified according to four levels of structure. The first level, at the extreme of little if any structure, is found in *open-ended* diaries and journals (Chapter 11), even though they are no longer as open-ended as in the past. The second, more *focused*, level of structure, is found in autobiographies (Chapter 12) and expressive writing (Chapter 13). The third level, *guided* writing, includes responding in writing to written questions. This level, however, is not included here for lack of available and reliable information about its use. The fourth level, highly structured, is found in *programmed* writing or workbooks (Chapter 14). All these approaches can be implemented fully and extended to various populations, clinical and nonclinical on the Internet (Chapter 15 this volume).

The foregoing classification may be outdated in the sense that diaries (Chapter 11 this volume) and autobiographies (Chapter 12 this volume) are now highly structured. Hence, degree of structure may no longer be a valid basis for classification. A different classification based on more valid criteria may be needed. For instance, an intervention that might qualify as a relational approaches but that is difficult to classify either in this section or in any other sections of this volume is bibliotherapy (Minna Levine, personal communication, August 10, 2005; Santrock, Minnett, & Campbell, 1994; Norcross et al., 2000). As the evidence (Ackerson, Scogin, McKendree-Smith, & Lyman, 1998) and a three-year follow-up study (Smith, Floyd, Jamison, & Scogin, 1997) indicates, bibliotherapy is self-administered, very economical, and lasts a long time. Hence, it possesses eminently all the qualities of a promotional approach. Why then not include it in this book?

It could be included in this section, even though it is sometimes based on a passive reading of the written word and relies, albeit minimally in the research, and on someone checking on whether readings have occurred on a regular basis. The relationship is usually with a lower level professional (mostly graduate students) who administers pre-post tests and checks weekly on the regular progress of reading. How can one justify not including bibliography in this volume? One could claim an oversight. Another could claim a bias toward bibliotherapy. One could claim an oversight due to a bias against bibliotherapy. Admittedly, bibliotherapy, when used solely in research seems like a passive endeavor, reading and nothing else. At least in the sources that have been researched, there is no discussion of the contents of the information read with anyone. Apparently, whatever is learned remains passively "inside" the reader and no information seems available about the process of understanding and accommodating to the information acquired.

In most cases (not covered by the research cited here) in the real world of clinical practice, usually bibliotherapy is part of the psychotherapeutic process. Assigned readings are actively discussed with a therapist. The process is based then on a prolonged f2f relationship with a therapist based on talk, making it difficult to classify bibliotherapy as an approach in and by itself. When bibliotherapy is part of this prolonged and expensive process, it ceases to act as an approach. One would be hard put to disentangle the outcome of this process between the effects of the approach and the effects of the therapeutic relationship. On the other hand, when administered solely by itself, without a prolonged relationship with a monitor, bibliotherapy may indeed act as an approach. When bibliotherapy readings consist also of writing exercises (assignments, exercises, handouts, or worksheets) and various types of interactive tasks (Minna Levine, personal communication, April 12, 2005), then bibliotherapy may be considered, at least in part, as an approach to be contained with the writing classification. However, not knowing how much of the outcome in using writing exercises is due to their effects or to other variables, makes it difficult, at this time, to include bibliotherapy as a writing approach. Perhaps, in the future, bibliotherapy, by any other name, except "therapy", may become an approach in its own right.

References

Ackerson, J., Scogin, F., McKendree-Smith, N., & Lyman, R. D. (1998). Cognitive bibliotherapy for mild and moderate adolescent depressive symptomatology. *Journal of Consulting and Clinical Psychology, 66*, 685–690.

Beitman, B. D., Nair, J., & Viamontes, G. I. (2004). Why self-awareness? In B. D. Beltman, & J. Nair (Eds.), *Self-awareness deficits in psychiatric participants: Neurobiology, assessment, and treatment* (pp. 3–23). New York: W. W. Norton.

Bloom, B. L. (1992). Computer-assisted psychological intervention: A review and commentary. *Clinical Psychology Review, 12*, 169–197.

Cusinato, M. *Valutare per intervenire: Misure di competenza relazionale in pazienti psichiatrici* (Evaluate to intervene: Measures of relational competence in psychiatric participants). Submitted for publication.

Dawes, R. M. (2001). *Everyday irrationality: How pseudoscientists, lunatics, and the rest of us fail to think*. Boulder, CO: Westview Press.

Denes-Raj, V., & Epstein, S. (1994). Conflict between intuitive and rational processing: When people behave against their better judgment. *Journal of Personality and Social Psychology, 66*, 819–829.

Esterling, B. A., L'Abate, L., Murray, E., & Pennebaker, J. M. (1999). Empirical foundations for writing in prevention and psychotherapy: Mental and physical outcomes. *Clinical Psychology Review, 19*, 79–96.

Hugdahl, K., & Davidson, R. J. (Eds.). (2004). *The asymmetrical brain*. Cambridge, MA: MIT Press.

Kazantzis, N., Deane, F. P., Ronan, K. R., & L'Abate, L. (Eds.). (2005). *Homework assignments in cognitive-behavioral therapy*. New York: Routledge.

Kazantzis, N., & L'Abate, L. (Eds.). (2007). *Handbook of homework assignments in psychotherapy: Theory, research, and prevention*. New York: Springer-Verlag.

L'Abate, L. (1999). Taking the bull by the horns: Beyond talk in psychological interventions. *The Family Journal: Therapy and Counseling for Couples and Families, 7*, 206–220.

L'Abate, L. (2005). *Personality in intimate relationships: Socialization and psychopathology*. New York: Springer-Verlag.

L'Abate, L., & Hecker, L. L. (2004). The status and future of workbooks in mental health: Concluding commentary. In: L. L'Abate (Ed.), *Using workbooks in mental health: Resources in prevention, psychotherapy, and rehabilitation for clinicians and researchers* (pp. 351–373). Binghamton, NY: Haworth.

Lepore, S., & Smyth, J. M. (2002). *The writing cure*. Washington, DC: American Psychological Association.

McMahan, O., & Arias, J. (2004). Workbooks and psychotherapy with incarcerated felons: Replication of research in progress. In L. L'Abate (Ed.), *Using workbooks in mental health: Resources in prevention, psychotherapy, and rehabilitation for clinicians and researchers* (pp. 205–213). Binghamton, NY: Haworth.

Norcross, J. C., Santrock, J. W., Campbell, L. F., Smith, T. P., Sommer, R., & Zuckerman, E. L. (2000). *Authoritative guide to self-help resources in mental health*. New York: Guilford.

Reed, R., McMahan, O., & L'Abate, L. (2001). Workbooks and psychotherapy with incarcerated felons. In L. L'Abate (Ed.), *Distance writing and computer-assisted interventions in psychiatry and mental health* (pp. 157–167). Westport, CT: Ablex.

Santrock, J. W., Minnett, A. M., & Campbell, B. D. (1994). *The authoritative guide to self-help books*. New York: Guilford.

Savitsky, K., Epley, N., & Gilovich, T. (2001). Do others judge us as harshly as we think? Overestimating the impact of our failures, shortcomings, and mishaps. *Journal of Personality and Social Psychology, 81*, 44–56.

Savitsky, K., & Gilovich, T. (2003). The illusion of transparency and the alleviation of speech anxiety. *Journal of Experimental Social Psychology, 39*, 618–625.

Smith, N. M., Floyd, M. R., Jamison, C., & Scogin, F. (1997). Three-year follow-up of bibliotherapy for depression. *Journal of Consulting and Clinical Psychology, 65*, 324–327.

Tarquinio, C., Santamato, W., Sgobbio, A., Cialdella, C., Storelli, M., & De Giacomo, P. (2005). Integrazione tra farmacoterapia ed interventi psicologici manualizzati (Integration of Pharmaco-therapy and manualized psychological interventions). Department of Neurological and Psychiatric Sciences, University of Bari (Italy). Paper read at the Second Thematic National Conference on the origin of psychopathological disturbances. Rome, Italy, 22–24 June 2005.

11

The Recording of Personal Information as an Intervention and as an Electronic Health Support

Minna Levine and Ronald Calvanio

Freud & Breuer (1976) were likely the first to advocate the recording of dreams and memories. Recently, this recording has ramified into a variety of practices. It has expanded to include the recording of current experiences, and the recording of thoughts about the future. This growth continues unabated in response to multiple influences: ideas from cognitive psychology (Clark, Beck, & Alford, 1999), better research methodology (Barlow & Hersen, 1984), the availability of personal technology (Appendix) and the need to contain care costs. We will review current recording practices and those on the horizon. To do so, we will distinguish practices in terms of recording format and purpose.

There are two basic recording formats: journal and diary. Others are a hybrid of these two. Journal formats entail a prose response. Journal subtypes involve differences in topic choice, prose formats, time schedules, and social context. Journal hybrids contain a few diary features. The diary format replaces prose with quantitative responses: rating scales, counts, magnitude estimates and checklists. The topics are assigned by a counselor, with input from the client. Recording takes a few minutes one or more times per day. Recording can be done quickly on a handheld computer, and then uploaded to the Internet where the recordings are automatically graphed to show symptom trends (Appendix). This practice is a form of electronic health support.

There are two recording purposes: recording as an intervention, and recording as a support to intervention. Intervention recording is a procedure for promoting positive personal change. That is, the act of recording is viewed as having a restorative or habilitative agency. Supportive recording has a different purpose. It is a procedure that enhances the impact of an intervention such as using a workbook, engaging in psychotherapy, or using a psychotropic medication, etc. Supportive recording provides feedback. For example, if indices of distress are recorded, the response of these indices to an intervention can be used to guide decisions about modulating, reconfiguring, or redirecting the intervention for maximum benefit.

Table 11.1. Journal and diary formats and purposes.

Recording purpose	Recording format: Journal	Recording format: Diary
Intervention	1. Intervention Journals Free-form writing Expressive writing Prescriptive writing	2. Intervention Diaries Recording for mindfulness Re-minding through When-To and How-To Reminders
Intervention Support	4. Intervention Support Journals Analysis of journal contents to adjust treatment dosage	3. Intervention Support Diaries ESM/EMA paradigms Electronic disease management

Recording's two formats (journal and diary) and two purposes (intervention and intervention support) join to define four recording practices as depicted in a two by two table (Table 11.1). We will describe these recording practices subject to the following qualifications and clarifications.

First, our use of the terms "journal" and "diary" can accord roughly with professional usage of these terms. A closer correspondence is not possible since there are no established conventions. Second, supportive journals (cell 4) are used almost exclusively in research, not in clinical practice. For example, they are used to record side-effects in order to determine optimum drug dosages in a Phase-2 drug trial. Since our focus is on counseling and self-help, we will not discuss this cell. Third, the recording distinctions in Table 11.1 not only distinguish helping practices, they also coincide with two cost control strategies: containing psychological care costs through lower-cost interventions versus, containing total service costs through intervention supports. These distinctions, qualifications, and clarifications may be difficult to keep in mind especially as more are added. To reduce confusion, we offer Table 11.2 as a reference.

Journal and Diary Subtypes

Free-Form Journals

In a free-form journal method, the journal writer chooses the topics, the length of passages, and the frequency of entry. Freud encouraged participants to use free association and to write down distressing memories (Kern, 1995). Jung (1989) emphasized the importance of recording dreams and inner imagery. Today, journal writers are encouraged: to vent frustrations, find solutions to problems, admit to fears and emotions that can't be discussed with others, or fantasize about a different life.

Expressive Writing Journals

The expressive writing journal places a single restriction on the free-form method. The counselor asks the writer to focus on a single topic, and to bring out deepest thoughts and feelings. In the Pennebaker (1990) version of expressive writing, the writing is done over 3 to 5 consecutive days, for 15 to 30 minutes. The Pennebaker method, the most researched and validated form of journaling, has its own chapter in this book (Chapter 13).

Table 11.2. Characteristics of intervention journals and diaries.

	Intervention journals	Intervention diaries
Response Type	Prose Free-form Assigned topic Specified structure	Pre-formatted short answers Scales Magnitude judgments Checklists
Length	Medium to long	Short
Entry schedule	As requested by treater As thoughts come to mind	Daily Multiple times/day Event-driven
Representation	Can be summarized	Quantifiable and graphable
Temporal reference	Retrospective	Current/Prospective
Intervention Mechanism	Bringing distressing memories to greater awareness nullifies them through: Objective discrediting Emotional release Narrative closure	Successful coping counteracts distressing memories via a cascade of mechanism starting with: A coping response yields a positive outcome, Which enhances self-esteem, Which boosts the likelihood of a more coping responses, Which boosts coping skill, Which creates a history of successful coping, Which interferes with the activation of negative memories, Which weakens then extinguishes them.
Examples	CBT homework, bibliotherapy, workbooks, self-instruction, expressive writing	Paper and electronic diaries online or on handheld computers, used as part of research or interventions

Prescriptive Journals

In prescriptive journals the author/counselor not only assigns topics, he/she also specifies the prose response formats. For example, there may be time lines for life cycle events, traumatic experiences, and accomplishments. Other formats include pro versus con lists, annotated steppingstone diagrams, decision trees, etc. Hybrid prescriptive journals often include a diary method feature: rating scales for tracking symptoms. Workbooks (L'Abate, 2001, 2004) and self-help books (Burns, 1999), which are available for consumer purchase, as well as Cognitive Behavior Therapy (CBT) homework, are typically hybrid journals.

Diary Variations

The questions in a diary change, of course, to correspond with the nature of the health challenge or educational challenge that is addressed. Besides question content, diaries also vary in the medium used: traditional paper and contemporary electronics. Electronic diaries, unlike paper ones, are actually diary systems with multiple components. Besides a component for recording data, there are also components for reminding to record, and reminding to perform other self-help activities. Some systems also contain a component for charting the impact of the interventions on the indices that are monitored in the recording component.

Paper diaries have been used more extensively than the newer electronic systems. They have been used for both intervention and intervention support purposes. They are used to develop insight, to monitor symptoms, and to guide the use of coping strategies in response to problems. Their use is an integral part of several high profile Cognitive Behavioral Programs: Borderline Personality Disorder (Linehan, 1999), Depression (Beck, 1995) and Anxiety (Barlow, 1988).

A major limitation of paper diary use is user unreliability, which likely occurs for a variety of reasons. The data collected with paper diaries is hard to interpret because the data are not routinely charted; some charting would take considerable time and effort. As a result, caregivers do not review diary contents with participants on a routine basis. This lack of interest in the diary content, sends a message to the client that diary use isn't a high priority, thereby reducing recording reliability. Other sources of unreliability may be user forgetting, inconvenient portability, and unfriendly response formats. Electronic diary systems have overcome the limitations of paper diaries through electronics. Consequently, our review will focus largely on electronic diary use. Our review of diaries will focus on the information processing power. The virtues of electronic diary system power make it a lower cost (i.e., less than $200/year) option for intervention and support.

Journals and Diaries: Mechanisms of Intervention

Four hypotheses have been advanced to explain why the recording of personal information has therapeutic agency. We have titled these hypotheses: (1) Objective Discrediting, (2) Emotional Release, (3) Narrative Closure, and (4) Evidence-based Coping.[1] All four rationales begin with a common starting point, the recall of disturbing memories. They differ in terms of the role they assign this recall starting point. One rationale, Evidence-Based Coping, assigns a prospective role. The evidence base includes both disturbing memories and performance ratings. This information is used for a prospective purpose. It is used to formulate coping techniques to meet *future* challenges particularly those influenced by the disturbing memories. In contrast, the three other rationales all posit a more retrospective role for recalling disturbing memories. That role is to use the restorative agency of recall to repair the past. That is, the recall process, by digging deeper into the disturbing memory corpus, can change the "encoding" of the past, and thereby reduce or eradicate its harm. The three rationales differ regarding how the recall, restorative encoding works. Capsule descriptions of the differences among the four rationales appear below.

[1] The reader should note that the phrase "evidence-based" is used here differently than it is usually used. It most often refers to empirical findings published in refereed journals, as in "evidence-based medicine."

Objective Discrediting

The act of free-form writing is said to enable the writer to not only bring to mind negative experiences, thoughts, and feelings, but also to bring them to mind with a diminution of the negative affect that had blocked their recall. The memories come to mind with a diminished negative affect because the act of free-form writing enables the writer to come at the memory from a variety of perspectives. This varied access is the key to fostering a more objective, less emotionally charged memory encoding. Once the excavated memories come to light in a more objective status, the writer can then see how absurd they are and can discredit them (Robson, 2003).

Emotional Release (Catharsis)

A second viewpoint is the classical Freudian thesis with a twist: memories come to light in the *unguarded* moments of intense writing with *full* negative emotional release. Freud and Breuer posited a disinhibitory process with four re-encoding steps: "We found . . .that each . . .symptom immediately and permanently disappeared when we had succeeded in [1] bringing clearly to light the memory of the event by which it was provoked and [2] in arousing the accompanying affect, and [3] when the patient had described that event in the greatest possible detail and [4] had put the affect into words." (Freud & Breuer, 1976)

Narrative Closure

A third view emphasizes the restorative power of the main product of writing: a personal narrative. This view (see Pennebaker, 2001) posits that what makes the negative psychic residue so disabling is its disorganized, unresolved, negatively valenced encoding. Painful experiences that remain encoded in this fashion will continue to remain open: they will draw attention or will otherwise influence thinking, feeling, and action. Pennebaker hypothesizes that a narrative that organizes negative memories into a coherent, settling story, will close the memories, and enable a psychological moving on in a positive direction. Recording works when this narrativization is accomplished.

Evidence-Based Coping

Evidence-based coping is the use of personal data to inform the selection, formulation, use and evaluation of coping techniques. As indicated, the coping techniques are based in part on the recall of disturbing memories and other functional information. A person learns and uses these techniques to cope with a debilitating functional challenge (e.g., having panic attacks in large public venues, such as a shopping mall). Successful coping works through a series of mechanisms. An instance of successful coping produces a more positive outcome in the situation in which it is used. This positive outcome boosts self-esteem, and also strengthens the likelihood that the coping technique will be used again. Each repetition of this success scenario will increase coping expertise. Each repetition will also diminish the likelihood that negative influences will come into play. The eventual impact of this repetition is the eradication or dissolution of the memorial substrate, or a weakening of its negative influence.

Journal Research

The body of journal intervention research is small and is dwarfed by the large variety of practices. Consequently, we will only be able to address a single broad issue: How does journaling work to produce a benefit according to available evidence.

We will begin our account of the action mechanism from the vantage point of phenomena involving recall and negative emotion. This is an appropriate starting perspective for two reasons. First, it is after all, the disabling impact of emotional pain that is associated with an experience(s) that draws interest in promoting further recall of the experience(s). Second, how negative emotion is managed during recall turns out to have important implications for its therapeutic utility, efficacy and safety.

Emotional factors in recall were considered in our account of the Objective Discrediting and the Emotional Release hypotheses. Both hypotheses posit that in unguarded moments during writing, previously repressed or inhibited information comes forth. These hypotheses as they stand, however, leave unaddressed the best way to foster unguarded moments. Are some recording formats better at an early stage in intervention to get things going, and others at a later stage to keep them going? If so, Emotional Release or Objective Discrediting may be the mechanism of either early or later stage intervention efficacy. Similar questions about intervention format and efficacy can be framed in terms of emotion related individual differences (e.g., personality, coping style, etc.). Fortunately, this potentially large set of questions can be reduced to one: Is it necessary to structure recording assignments differently for different persons and purposes? The literature's answer to this question is yes, as follows.

Ira Progoff (1992) cautioned that free-form writing can engender wandering "around in circles", rather than positive change. Getting nowhere might not just be ineffectual, however; it may be detrimental. The writer may interpret the wandering as failure, and feel increased despair. Additionally, because writers are free to frame experiences negatively or positively, a negative choice would feed rumination and depression. Several studies imply that these concerns are warranted.

First, two studies combine to suggest that depressed persons require different writing formats. One recording study (Campbell, Chew, & Scratchley, 1991) described the many differences that distinguish depressed individuals, and those with reduced self-esteem, from healthier minded peers. They are more likely: (1) to report that negative events affect their mood, (2) to take responsibility for negative events, (3) to express self-doubts, (4) to respond retroactively, not proactively to negative events, and 5) to appraise an event *more negatively* as time goes by. A second study (Cameron & Nicholls, 1998) reported that pessimists, unlike optimists, did not show a positive response to an expressive writing exercise, whereas pessimists like optimists responded positively when a coping plan exercise was added to the writing assignment. Together these two studies imply that persons who are depressed, who have low self-esteem or who are pessimistic (1) have a number of distinctive issues to address, and that (2) chances of addressing an issue successfully is enhanced when the issue is addressed with the right recording task.

Second, a study involving college students who kept daily journals (Nolen-Hoeksema, Morrow, & Fredrickson, 1993) indicates that ruminative thinking is another feature of depression that must be addressed. Students differed in terms of the type of journal entry they made in response to events that provoked sadness or depression. Some made a ruminative writing response, while others made a distracting writing response. What is more, those who had a ruminative style had significantly longer episodes of depressed mood. This study implies that the coping assignments should contain exercises that can interfere with, and extinguish, ruminative responding. Another set of studies, however, sharply qualifies this statement.

Schacter (2001), citing the work of others (Foa & Meadows, 1997; Keane, Fairbank, Caddell, & Zimering, 1989), has pointed out that soon after a traumatic event people benefit from telling and retelling their story, using pictures and visualization, while in a safe environment. This exposure intervention yielded the greatest reduction in symptoms of PTSD. He also indicated (Wegner, 1994; Wegner & Gold, 1995) that persons who soon after a trauma are inhibited from expressing unwanted thoughts (thought suppression) show a rebound effect: "They later think about the forbidden subjects more often and intensely than they would have if they had never attempted to suppress thinking about it in the first place." Schacter's commentary implies that the earlier recommendation to employ exercises to suppress rumination requires amendment as follows. Early after a trauma, focusing on the trauma and responding to it in appropriate ways leads to habituation (the emotional content is drained through repeated exposure (Schacter, 2001)) and should be encouraged. Some time after the trauma – when after trauma is not clear – ruminative thoughts suppression should be undertaken. Note that this early-later distinction runs parallel with the early-late Emotional Release-Objective Discrediting hypothesis advanced above.

Third, and finally, Stanton and her colleagues (Stanton & Danoff-Burg 2002; Stanton et al., 2002; Stanton, 2005) produced results that imply that format must be structured in a way that is consonant with coping "orientation". They found that women being treated for breast cancer, who were also depressed and/or anxious, showed a mood elevation immediately after engaging in a "benefit finding" writing exercise. In contrast, women with an avoidant coping style became more upset after an expressive writing exercise, whereas nonavoidant women did not. The authors concluded that the expressive writing task that asked participants to explore their deepest thoughts and feelings about cancer was threatening to the avoidant women who had devoted considerable effort to not confronting these themes. Later, Stanton (2005) concluded that the utility of psychological intervention depends on the match up between attributes of the method and participants.

Stanton's conclusion reinforces our earlier claim that Objective Discrediting and Emotional Release hypotheses are inadequate as stated. Neither specifies the retrieval strategies for initiating or sustaining recall, and how these strategies are related to individual differences. Perhaps the recall process, and its memory nullification sequel, require more guidance: recording formats should have specifications that give, or yield, retrieval hooks to enhance recall. Recently Pennebaker has proposed a hypothesis which may bear fruit in this direction.

Pennebaker has dropped his initial Emotional Release hypothesis in favor of a narrativization hypothesis. He now hypothesizes that expressive writing is effective when participants compose narratives that settle disturbing issues and permit a psychological moving on. In support of this narrativization hypothesis, Pennebaker has offered three post hoc findings from his studies (2001). First, during debriefings, participants explained their success in cognitive terms suggestive of their having engaged in a successful storytelling enterprise. Phrases such as "understanding", "realize", "come to terms" and "getting past" appeared frequently. Second, post hoc tests did not support an emotional release hypothesis. Third, post hoc tests correlating healthier outcomes with writing indices that reflect storytelling effort (e.g., more positive than negative words) were significant. These findings are suggestive; they await a definitive test that is yet forthcoming. There are, however, several lines of evidence from cognitive psychology that lend support to Pennebaker's narrativization hypothesis.

Unresolved memories do call a person's attention until closure is reached. This Pennebaker claim is not only true, it is a principle called the Zeigarnik Effect (Bruner, 1966, p. 119): "tasks that are interrupted are much more likely to be returned to, and completed, and much more likely to be remembered, than comparable tasks that one has completed without interruption." To interpret new or "unclosed" experiences, people routinely use a preferred set of story schemata. That is, each of us has particular kinds of stories ready and waiting to interpret events, particularly novel, ambiguous, or dangerous ones (Schank, 1990). What is more, the motivation to tell stories is a driving force behind the child's acquisition of language (Bruner, 1990). Finally, stories are preferred because they provide a convenient structure (who, what, where, when, which, why, how) for organizing, and simplifying, event processing (Bartlett, 1932).

These findings indicate the centrality of narrative structure in human thought. They thus indirectly support the Pennebaker hypothesis. What is more, other bodies of evidence identify useful story criteria (Bruner, 1990), and sources of story distortion (Schacter, 2001). These latter findings suggest possible retrieval hooks that can aid intervention recall.

CBT combines hybrid journal homework with face-to-face counseling. This intervention structure can be viewed as a response to Stanton's recommendation to more closely link treatment methods with personal attributes. In particular, its prospective coping exercises, and its diary based progress tracking, bring treatment into closer connection with day-to-day functioning. Several studies of the CBT method have reported a significant reduction in DSM IV diagnosed depression (Burns & Nolen Hoeksema, 1991, Burns & Spangler, 2000). Other studies using the same recording materials in a bibliotherapy context (no face-to-face counseling, only phone calls to promote adherence) found similar benefits (Jamison & Scogin, 1995; Smith, Floyd, Scoggin, & Jamison, 1997) or reported mixed results (Ackerson, Scogin, McKendree-Smith, & Lyman, 1998). These studies imply that prospective recording, used with CBT counseling or administered as bibliotherapy, can yield a statistically significant reduction in DSM IV level depression.

Two aspects of these methodologically important depression studies remain unclear. First, the CBT depression studies reported that depression reduction was significantly correlated with CBT coping exercise compliance. There was no data, however, about what aspects of coping exercises were most important and emphasized. What is also not clear is why outcomes become mixed when social support was reduced. The answers to these questions are important not only because they help to identify action mechanisms, but also because by identifying essential intervention ingredients, caregivers can contain the risk of treatment failure. We pursue these questions further in the Diary Research section.

Journal Product Availability

This section lists intervention recording instruments that are, or may become, available to professionals for use with their participants. This listing is designed to aid the reader in selecting journal products. A diary listing appears in a later section.

Free-Form Journals

Clear evidence of free-form journal popularity was the recent publication of a *Complete Idiot's Guide to Journaling* (Neubauer, 2001). Both the *Idiot's Guide* and *The New Diary* (Rainer, 1978), describe how to use four modes of expression: catharsis (releases and expresses the emotions), description (conveys perceptual information), free-intuitive writing (releases writing from the conscious control), and reflection (developing connections from a broader perspective). Dozens of websites offer low-cost computer software (under $75), storage for private journal entry (Appendix), and journaling via blogs and personal websites. None of these sources provides efficacy data beyond anecdotes and testimonials.

Expressive Writing

Pennebaker (1990, 2001, 2002, 2004) has pioneered a version of the expressive writing paradigm, which he and his colleagues have studied extensively. The typical, expressive writing (or "emotional disclosure" writing) protocol requires participants to write about a major, negative, emotionally charged topic of their choosing. Participants are encouraged to describe their deepest thoughts and feelings about a stressor. In some protocols the stressor is ongoing (e.g., recent job loss), in others the stressor occurred in the more distant past (abuse, illness). See Pennebaker's coauthored chapter in this volume (Chapter 13) to learn more about the possibilities and the demonstrated effectiveness of this approach.

Prescriptive Journals

The distinctive feature of prescriptive journals is the varied formats imposed on the form of written expression. We identify particular authors and their formats below. We then refer you to Table 11.3 for a list of structured formats. Treaters may assign the prescriptive journal as homework, or direct it in one-to-one treatment, or in a group setting. Consumers also purchase these journals and use them in a self-help context.

Two popular CBT self-help books (Burns, 1999; Greenberger & Padesky, 1995) provide structured exercises to teach users to identify thoughts, moods, behaviors and physical reactions. They are used as homework in a CBT therapeutic program. They can also be purchased as self-help books at low cost.

Table 11.3. Prescriptive journal format options.

Narratives

Writing about Past Traumas

1. Describe a stressful situation or a time when you were angry (or anxious or worried). Describe what actually happened and the thoughts and feelings experienced then. (1, 2)
2. List the individuals with whom you feel your relationship, past, present, and future warrants further exploration. Write a brief and direct statement describing the essence of the whole relationship (reflecting thoughts and feelings) and where it is now. (3)
3. Topics: positive/negative instances/experiences.
4. Write an unsent letter – a letter to someone expressing feelings that might be inappropriate or damaging if it was sent.

Writing Perspectives

1. Catharsis: feelings toward
2. Description: just facts: what heard, saw
3. Reflection: apparent reasons why
4. Intuitive: hidden reasons why
5. Futuristic: where from here

Time Lines

Steppingstones™(3)

1. Writing about the course one's life has taken from its beginning to the current moment.
2. Create the time line (with in terms of eight or ten key steps) from different vantage points: spiritual journeys from doubt to conversion, education-related events, events in a relationship, professional steps, steps in your health/with your body changes.
3. Write similar time lines of other important people in your life to understand your relationship.

Assessing Progress with Daily/Weekly Logs

1. Daily ratings of moods/feelings (select the ones you want to examine), from 0 to 100 (1, 2) or multiple times/day (2)
2. Recapitulation: recall and recreate events of the day (3)
3. Current Recording: as things happen, record thoughts, feelings, situations that are stressful (2, 3, 4)
4. Complete an anxiety or depression inventory weekly and chart progress. (1)

Reflecting about Past, Current & Future Choices

1. List all the "Intersections" – all the "Roads Taken" and "Not Taken" that you can think of in your life. (3)
2. Consider the choices not taken, but avoid self recrimination. Evaluate if there are unlived possibilities that still hold potential for your life.

Two-Sided Dialogues with Oneself

Each of the examples below is two-column point-counterpoint type format for journals. For each example, the writer adds information to the left column and then comments on or evaluates that information in the right column. Each format has a sample input inserted in the table. Some authors recommend additional columns for writing substitute more realistic thoughts or for ratings of the likelihood/of the left column occurring.

Evaluating Thoughts for Distortions (1)	
Negative Thought	*Identify Distortion in Thought*
"I can't write papers."	Overgeneralization from this instance. Discounting the positives.
Support for Thoughts (2)	
Thoughts	*Support/Lack of Support*
"I'll never understand this chapter."	"The girl in my study group said she'd explain things to me."
Finding The Meaning of Thoughts/Feelings (4)	
Thoughts, Feelings	*Meaning, Perspective*
"I have been a mother, an attendant, a cook...All these made me more depressed."	"The jobs make me tired, being tired makes me depressed..."
Pros/Cons of Change (1)	
Advantages to Change	*Disadvantages to Change*
"If I change my belief that I have to be perfect, I will feel better about myself when I make an occasional mistake."	"If I don't change my belief, I will always worry people will know I am a fraud."
Evaluation of Fears (1, 2)	
Imagined Events & Actions	*Perceived Likely Scenario*
"When I give my presentation, I will say stupid things."	Probability of that happening = 20%

[1] Burns, 1999
[2] Greenberger and Padesky, 1995
[3] Progoff, 1992
[4] Durgahee, 2002

Their effectiveness with and without much professional support was described in the Research section of this chapter. An advantage of some self-help books is that they contain educational materials as well as exercises. Readers can refer back to them as reference books, well after therapy is completed, and many do (Smith et al., 1997). When used in bibliotherapy, the bibliotherapy procedure entails very brief weekly calls to encourage compliance and to answer questions.

Another type of prescriptive journaling is a therapeutic workbook. In contrast to self-help books that contain educational material and are written for broader application, workbooks have a narrower content. They contain exercises for more specifically defined disorders. Workbooks too can be used on their own or in conjunction with face-to-face talk-based psychotherapy. See L'Abate and Goldstein's chapter of this volume (Chapter 14) to learn more about the possibilities and effectiveness of this approach.

An early example of a prescriptive type of journal, Ira Progoff's Intensive Journal tools (1992), illustrates the great variety of writing formats that can be used (See Table 11.3). Participants learn to use these tools in an Intensive Journal workshop. A typical workshop may cost as much as $875 per person for a five-day session, including three meals a day. While this is not a low-cost intervention available for mass-dissemination, Dialogue House (Appendix), which runs the workshops, has run sessions in prisons and is looking for opportunities to make its methodology available for broader use. More recently, Durgahee (2002) described a prescriptive journaling method, which unlike Progoff's multiple writing formats method, uses a single versatile format. The journal writer's task is to examine thoughts, feelings, beliefs and ideas from many angles. Duragahee provides a compare and contrast format (a dialogic journal) to facilitate this process (Table 11.3). The author described his journal tool as a way to improve quality of care at low cost. The cost containment comes from enabling caregivers to understand participants with fewer contact hours.

Diary Research

As indicated earlier, the benefits to be derived from diaries are tied to the components available in the diary system.

The Benefits of Recording

Diary recording can provide an intervention benefit that comes from repetitive and reflective responding. This benefit is comparable to the benefit of prescriptive journal writing that brings information to consciousness (Ollendick & Ollendick, 1990; Peterson & Tremblay, 1999). In both practices the act of recording, combined with reflection, should lead to awareness of important stimulus-response patterns. For example, an unrecognized source of arguments between two people might be revealed through recording (See Case Anecdote at the end of this chapter, for example). An interesting, but to our knowledge untried practice would be to combine electronic diary recording with journal writing. In this combination, the stimulus-response patterns discovered through electronic diary recording, can be used as diary data. These data also could be used as memory retrieval cues to enhance the benefits of journaling: emotional release, narrativization, and object discrediting.

The Benefits of Recording and Reminding

e-Diaries plus CBT. The value of recording plus reminding with an electronic diary system should support CBT. Together they should prompt action and outcome evaluation. Newman et al. conducted two studies that investigated the impact of different CBT configurations on panic disorder (Kenardy et al., 2003; Newman, Kenardy, Herman, & Taylor, 1997). They offered participants different amounts of manualized face-to-face CBT therapy: 6 sessions or 12 sessions administered about once per week. They also offered participants different amounts of paper-based coping exercise homework: 6 weeks or 12 weeks. This homework incorporated such methods as imagined exposure to provocative stimuli; guided use of coping methods such as deep breathing; the guided discrediting of fearful predictions regarding the consequences of exposure, the careful recording of symptomatology and coping success. Their Group 1 provided participants 12 weeks of both face-to-face treatment and coping exercise homework. Their Group 2 received the same contents as Group 1, but condensed into 6 weeks. Group 3 had the same number of interventions as Group 2. Group 3 differed from 2, however, in the medium used to implement homework. They used handheld computers rather than paper. In practice this added two features to homework implementation. Group 3 participants received computer delivered reminders five times a day to do homework. In addition, computer use enabled participants to practice coping in response to actual panic situations encountered in the community rather than in response to imagined situations. One additional distinguishing feature for Group 3 versus 2 was that participants continued to carry the handheld computer for six additional weeks, thereby permitting continued self-help.

All three groups showed significant improvement posttreatment, over untreated participants on a waiting list. There was no statistically significant difference between the treatment benefits obtained with the standard 12-hour protocol and the 6-hour plus computer use protocol (Group 3). The 6-hour protocol without computer support (Group 2) came in third. Kenardy et al.'s posttreatment results indicate that adding computer supported homework tends to compensate for a reduction in weeks in the standard 12-week protocol thereby replicating equivalent earlier findings by Newman et al. (1997). These findings from the Newman group when combined with the CBT depression findings reported earlier (journal research section) justify four conclusions. First, computer supported community coping exercise is more effective than coping exercises supported by reflective homework. Second, the greater the compliance in performing the CBT exercises the greater the therapeutic benefit. Third, given the importance of community situated homework compliance, methods that enhance this compliance should be emphasized. Fourth, since the use of handheld computers supports this compliance and is less expensive ($1,200 for standard therapy, $680 for computer-assisted brief therapy and $600 for brief therapy), briefer computer assisted protocols should be advocated over longer, non-computerized standard protocols.

e- Diary Applications Without CBT Counseling. We will describe two other examples of diary-based intervention. These interventions were not performed in conjunction with CBT. They illustrate the potential e-diary systems have for tackling a broad range of disability problems.

The first example is a study in which the authors and colleagues provided diary reminders on handheld computers to students with Asperger's Disorder (O'Callaghan, Fishbein, Calvanio, Grant, & Levine, 2004). The reminders were designed to heighten student awareness of classroom social behavior: cooperation with teachers, interactions with peers, self-expression of needs, and self-control when distressed. The reminders guided students by having them periodically review, and rate, their feelings and social behavior. Teachers simultaneously reviewed student social behavior and affect as well Figure 11.1.

The simultaneous electronic monitoring by teachers and students produced two insights. It enabled teachers to detect possible disorders comorbid with the Asperger's disorder. Eleven of 20 students were found to have multiple feelings deviations involving sadness, anger, sleepiness, tension or boredom. These deviations were of sufficient magnitude to merit either continued monitoring, or in two instances, referral to a physician for drug toxicity and covert depression. Figure 11.2

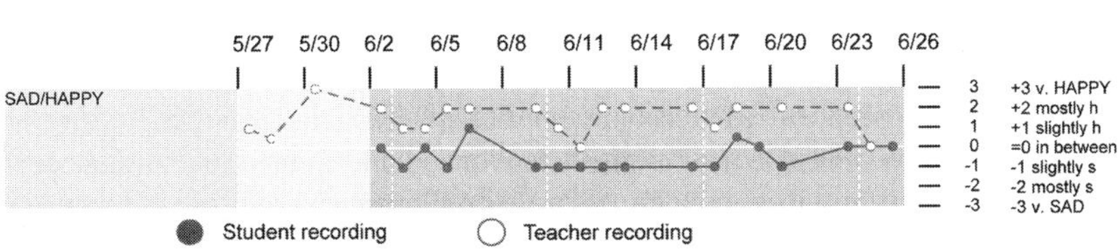

Figure 11.1. Recordings consistent with covert depression. This student was chronically sad on a day-to-day basis, which he hid from teachers. Similar findings were obtained for Peaceful/Angry and Calm/Nervous Ratings.

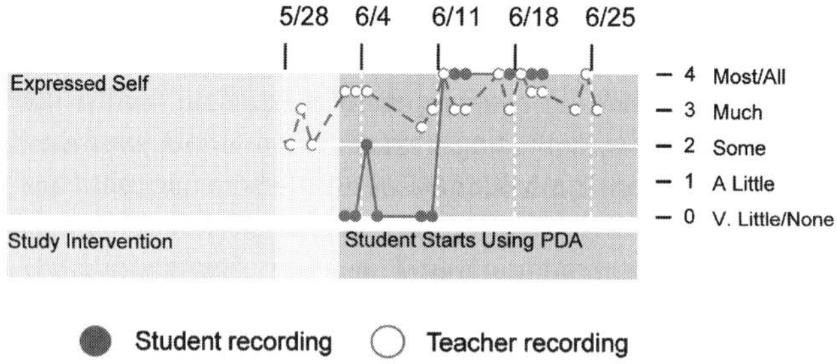

Figure 11.2. Impact of reminders on student's self-expression. Change from light gray to dark gray indicates the beginning of reminding via handheld computer. This student improved her self-expression in the estimation of teachers as well as, subsequently, from her own perspective.

Second, the insight produced by our study was the identification of students who could improve their social behavior through social mindfulness reminding. Nine of twenty students showed significant social behavior improvement from routine mindfulness reminding. That is, routine (3 times per day) recording and reflecting about feelings and social behavior improved social behavior without the need for additional interventions. It was instructive that 8 of 9 of these students had medically well-managed, comorbid disorders. In contrast, ten of 11 students who did not benefit from mindfulness reminding did not have properly identified, or well managed, comorbid disorders. Given the high rate of comorbidity in Asperger students, these findings imply that a combination of pharmacotherapy and electronic diary supported mindfulness will be needed to promote better social functioning in this population.

Our second example of a diary-based intervention is a case anecdote. We offer this case anecdote because it conveys a picture of real personal change that can't be captured in a graph. The first patient to use the SymTrend prototype was RD, a 25-year old woman who suffered a brain injury as the result of a motor vehicle accident. RD developed attention, memory and executive functioning problems as a result. As part of treatment prescribed by her psychiatrist, RD used a treatment diary on a handheld computer for a year. She received hourly reminders on her handheld, which were announced by a ring. She then checked off activities undertaken or completed in the previous hour. At these times RD also recorded symptom levels on rating scales and checklists. Because of RD's reduced awareness of the passage of time, she had prospective memory difficulties: she forgot to do things she was supposed to do. She also often got "lost" in time – for example, she would go grocery shopping for a half hour, not to emerge until after an hour or more – forgetting that she had appointments. This forgetting led to numerous arguments with RD's mother who minded RD's dog when RD went shopping. RD's tardiness increased her mother's tardiness at work, to her mother's great displeasure.

The hourly beep of RD's handheld helped RD manage her tardiness problem in several ways. One of these was quite unexpected. First, the beep enabled RD to check the time. This time checking made some inroads on the tardiness problem. Second, RD's recording of events at the beep, generated an awareness that many of her arguments with her mother were related to her tardiness. This increased awareness enabled her ability to apologize to her mother. Both of these changes pleased RD's mother. Third, the hourly beeps unexpectedly did more: they provided structure to RD's day. That is RD, after a while, learned to anticipate the alarm's ring minutes before the alarm rang. RD used this renewed ability to appreciate an hour's duration to break up her day into hour-long time periods. These periods became a temporal scaffolding by which she could manage her affairs. In particular, she planned activities in terms of what she might accomplish in an hour. Finally her greater punctuality and efficiency made her look more responsible to those around her. This newfound responsibility enabled her to take a teacher's assistant position in a local grammar school.

The Benefits of Recording and Charting

A major benefit of electronic diary systems is derived from the combination of recording and charting. Charts based on daily diary entries, made before and after an intervention, constitute a superior database for promoting positive functional change at a relatively low cost. One element of the superiority is the quality of the data in the database. Recording of psychological indices of functioning on a daily basis, or in closer temporal proximity to significant events, tends to reduce memory bias that develops in the days after an event has occurred (Schacter, 2001). A second source of superiority is the versatility of the database. The electronic diary database can be easily charted and routinely checked for various data patterns that can inform life change decision-making. The availability of symptom charts can be used in a number of ways to support treatments. We present here idealized charts in order to make points clearly, given limitations of space and reader time. In all instances, the chart uses are based upon actual clinical data.

Diary Charts: Uses

Example 1: To See If Treatment is Working. A diary chart can reveal intervention impact in detail. For example, Figure 11.3 depicts how mood

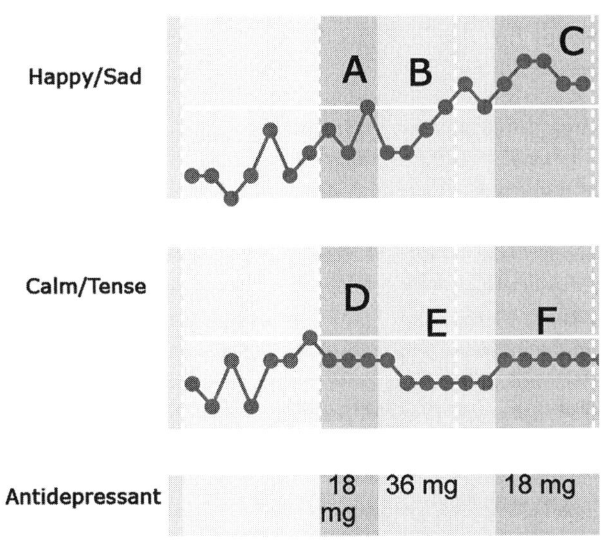

Figure 11.3. How is the Treatment Working? The antidepressant worked differently for different symptoms.

(Happy/Sad in A, B, C) and tension (Calm/Tense in D, E, F) responded to an intervention. In A, the start of a medication brought a small mood improvement. It was so small that it might escape notice for report in a follow-up visit. In B, a dosage increase boosted mood further. In C, a slight dosage decrease, to reduce side-effects (not shown), leveled off the mood improvement. In D, tension became less variable with the start of medication. No symptom improvement occurred in E, however, as occurred in B.

Example 2: To Check for Side-Effects. A diary chart can be used to check for side-effects. Side-effects may occur immediately with a dose increase, or after a few days at a new dose. In Figure 11.4, a dosage increase of an antidepressant (line 4) increased sleep disturbance and jitteriness (lines 2 and 3). A sleeping pill improved sleep (line 2), but appeared to bring on headaches (line 1).

Example 3: Risk Factors. A symptom can be influenced by a body state change, by exposure to a substance, by a frightening experience, etc. Small influences can add up slowly over time, or can suddenly start multiplying and rapidly escalate. Clinicians can use diary charts to identify negative influences (risk factors) and positive influences (palliatives). Figure 11.5 illustrates a subtle risk factor in operation. It depicts how an as-needed medication (line 3), over time, produced stomach distress (line 2), which then exacerbated irritability (line 1). A similar diary chart pattern might illustrate the link between drinking alcohol, hangovers, irritability, and violence.

Example 4: Triggers. Some events are so powerful that only one or two occurrences are needed to produce either a negative or positive impact. You can use diary charts to identify these "triggers". Figure 11.6 illustrates how the start of an antidepressant was undermined by a trigger event. In the example, the symptom improvement depicted in the line chart at A was reversed at B by a trigger onset, depicted in the event chart below the line chart (at C). The negative trigger could have been physiological (menstruation, asthma attack) or personal (argument, bad grade).

Example 5: Warning Signs. Symptoms can increase insidiously to dangerous levels. With diary charts, a clinician can identify reliable warning

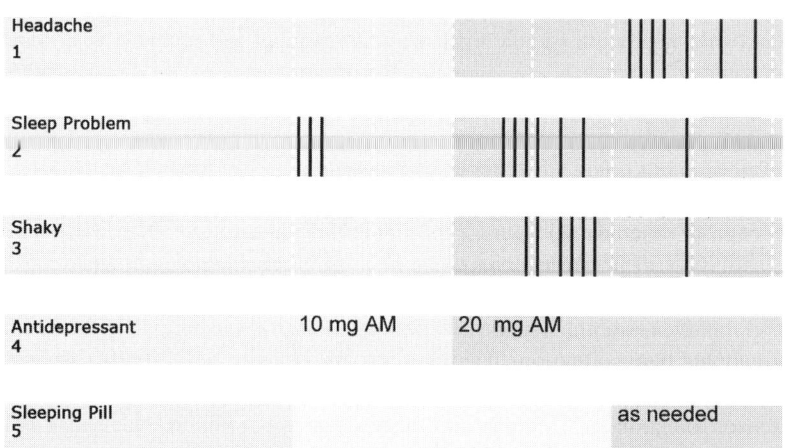

Figure 11.4. Are There Any Side Effects? Different side effects appeared for different medications at different dosages.

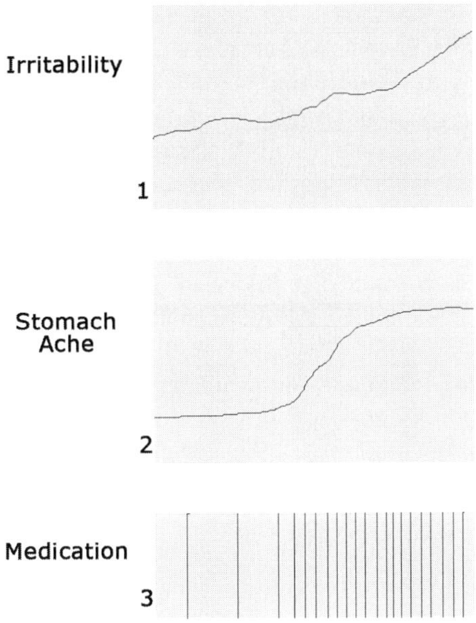

Figure 11.5. Can risk factors be identified? There is a gradually developing linkage between increased mediation use, stomachache, and irritability.

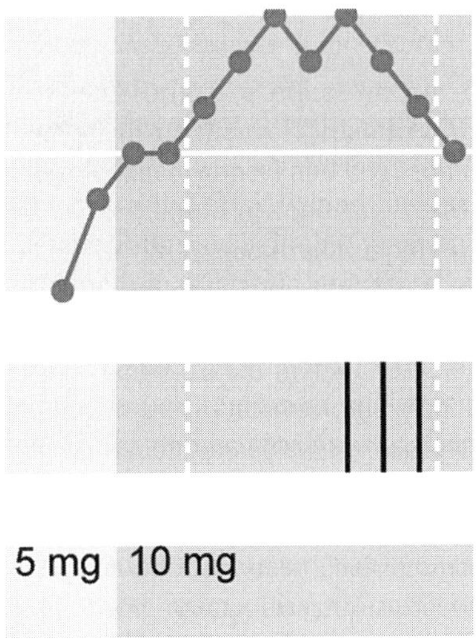

Figure 11.6. Did a trigger undermine drug action? The growing drug benefit at A was undermined at B.

signs as alerts to take preventative action. A warning sign may be something that is not inherently an indication of something wrong, but for a particular person, it may be a signal that something unpleasant or harmful is brewing. Figure 11.7 identifies a warning sign relationship. It shows a relationship between the occurrence of teary outbursts (line 1) and cumulative, antecedent fatigue (line 2). The fatigue was brought on by: lost sleep (line 3), work

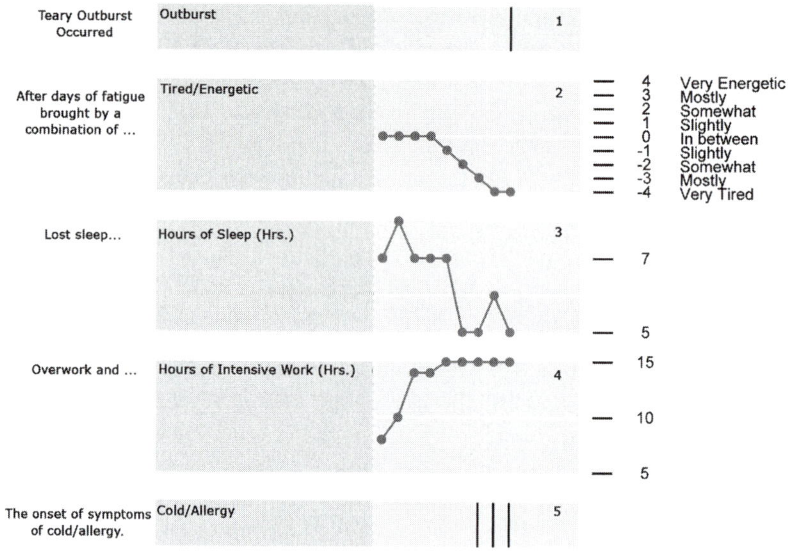

Figure 11.7. Is there a warning sign that has a subtle etiology? The development of fatigue was multi-factorial and was a harbinger of tearful outbursts.

stress (line 4), and by a cold or allergy (line 5). Thus, the frequency of teary outbursts illustrated here was more due to multiple increasing stresses. It was not due to a worsening of a biological depression that required an antidepressant dosage increase. Making an unnecessary dose increase can bring on side effects that can reduce treatment adherence. It can also more quickly bring on the time when first drug "poop-out" occurs, and requires augmentation with a second one.

Instead of fatigue and teary outbursts, the above data patterns in Figure 11.7 might illustrate the links among self-harm, negative thoughts, and repeated bad days. In either case, to be forewarned is to be alerted to take appropriate preventive or reactive measures. Being able to identify risk factors, triggers, and warning signs are important for understanding failures to thrive in response to treatment. Once one of these signals is identified, it can become the target for further exploration, and its source may become the target for cognitive behavioral management in conjunction with medical treatment. Understanding the etiology of symptom increase also leads to more efficient and less costly care.

Electronic Diary Product Availability

We begin this section with a description of those e-diary systems currently in use, together with comments about availability and suitability as a low-cost intervention. As for research findings, besides Newman et al.'s work, we could find no electronic diary method data that has been published in English language peer reviewed journals. Instead, we wrap up with an anecdotal case of our own plus data we presented in poster format at an NIH-sponsored Complexities of Cooccurring Conditions conference in June, 2004. The poster data indicates how diary data can be used to detect inadequately identified, or inadequately treated comorbid disorders in Autism. In addition, we illustrate the data of one student who, among a total of 9 out of 20, was able to use reminders to improve social behavior in a classroom.

Recording Methods

The history of electronic diary recording methods is quite short. The use of programmable watches is about 20 years old; the use of handheld computers is about 15 years old, and the use of the Internet about 5 years old. Three practices have emerged that use these media with different formats and for different purposes (Bolger, Davis, & Rafaeli, 2003). These practices differ in format, purpose, and electronic media. The Experience Sampling Methodology (ESM; Csikszentmihalyi & Larson, 1987; deVries, 1992) employs a watch that signals when to record. The recording is done at multiple random times during the day. When the watch rings, paper forms are filled out that include both quantitative and prose responses. The purpose of this method is primarily intervention support in a research context. The random sampling enables participants to record information in different circumstances, so as to assess symptom change as a function of intervention and circumstance. Delespaul, one of the early ESM developers indicated that he uses ESM in clinical practice as a repeated assessment tool that generates daily life data, which can be used in personalized interventions and cognitive behavioral therapy (personal communication).

The Ecological Momentary Assessment paradigm (EMA; Stone & Shiffman, 1994) is primarily used in an intervention research context. It also uses a random sampling of symptoms to check for the impact of circumstances. EMA uses handheld computer signaling and recording, however. Consequently, its recording data capture is in the form of rating scales and short-answer questions. EMA has made a major contribution to the research technology used to study addictions (e.g., recording the immediate antecedents of cigarette smoking – Shiffman et al., 2002; studying the impact of stress on cardiovascular activity – Kamarck et al., 1998). EMA comes closer to what we have characterized as electronic diary support recording.

The third method is our own SymTrend method (SymTrend, 2005). Like EMA, it uses handheld computer technology, but it also incorporates the Internet. SymTrend expands on EMA in several ways. It is designed for both individual case intervention use and research applications. It incorporates a more extensive reminding capability, and it incorporates a symptom graphing capability for individual patient/self/client intervention. The reminding capability includes How-To Reminders (how to perform a task), which expand the diary's treatment capability and emulates Newman et al.'s work described earlier in this chapter. It also has two forms of When-To Reminders: (1) fixed schedule reminders and (2) the random time When-To Reminders of EMA and ESM. Charting is included for two reasons: (1) to provide feedback about intervention progress, and (2) to support intervention decision-making. Finally, SymTrend has both standard and customizable features. It has standard disease and disorder specific recording and graphing protocols. It also has customizable options to enable a professional to tailor a protocol to meet client needs as well as to accommodate a professional's ideas about recording, reminding, feedback, and decision-making.

Diary methods are no cost or low cost for a variety of common problems (seizures, headaches, pain, depression, anxiety, and ADHD, among others. See Appendix for a listing). Several paper diaries for clinical and research applications are available online and through the professional literature. Behavioral Tech, LLC publishes its DBT diary online (Behavioral Tech, 1999–2003; Linehan, 1999). The NIMH Bipolar Lifechart is available online (Leverich & Post, 1997). These diaries are a one-size-fits-all product. Using the diaries as supportive recording usually requires the assistance of a professional for interpreting findings, modifying treatment, and evaluating treatment efficacy. Individuals, however, can use the paper diaries and SymTrend.com on their own. EMA and ESM technologies or multiple symptom recorders like the Health Buddy are also used to record physical health related data that is uploaded to a server for monitoring by a clinical or research staff.

Reactivity of Diaries and Journals

Recording in a diary (or in a journal) requires attention. While attention can improve accuracy during recording, it can also, some have argued, heighten awareness of what is being recorded. This heightened awareness may produce an exaggerated, more intense rating response (this systematic bias is called reactivity). Current research findings, however, minimize this concern. Cruise, Broderick, Porter, Kaell, & Stone (1996) studied chronic pain in a study and found no bias. Ruble's (1977) survey of menstrual-related symptoms found that other biases were of far greater concern. In particular, belief-based bias affects symptom reports and requires counteractive practices. Our own data suggest that electronic self-reporting reduces rather than creates error. For example, we found that students were more willing to reveal distress levels, of which teachers were unaware, to a computer, and that these revelations had clinical validity.

Summary

This review has found that intervention recording methods should use:

1. Workbooks that more closely correspond with participants' diagnoses and personal status (L'Abate, Chapter 14 this volume).
2. Expressive writing techniques that encourage successful narrativization of negative experiences. A successful narrative brings a form of closure that leads in a more positive direction (Pennebaker, Chapter 13 this volume).
3. Procedures that enhance learning, and use, of coping techniques (Burns, 1999).
4. Electronic or other means to support a) community based coping exercises and b) close to real time self-evaluation (Kenardy et al., 2003; Newman et al., 1997).
5. All three components of an electronic diary system (this chapter).

Appendix: Treatment Diary and Journal Websites

Journaling Sites	
http://www.journalingtools.com.	Prescriptive and free-form journaling tools
http://www.mindsview.com/	Journaling software
http://www.lifejournal.com/	Journaling software
http://www.higherawareness.com/index.shtml	Journaling tools and articles
http://www.bgsu.edu/cconline/Scenters-Zapico/background/two.htm	Information about dialogic journals.
http://www.intensivejournal.org/	Progoff's site
Disease Specific Treatment Support Diaries	
http://www.symtrend.com	Diaries for ADHD, Anxiety, Asperger's Disorder, Autism, Cancer, Depression, Neurological Disorders & Women's Health.
http://www.myadhd.com	ADHD
http://www.stoppulling.com	Trichotillomania
http://www.stoppicking.com	Skin picking
http://www.depnet.com.au/	Depression diary/ journal site
http://www.paniccenter.net	Panic center diaries and information about anxiety
http://www.imetrikus.com/prod_MC.asp	Diabetes and asthma
http://www.achenet.org/your/diary2.php	Headache diary
http://www.migrainehelp.com/pdf/MigraineDiary.pdf	Paper headache diary
Resources for Creating Diaries for Research & Treatment (e.g., ESM)	
http://www.invivodata.com	Custom handheld applications for research
http://www.psychiatry.uchc.edu/faculty/files/conner/ESM.htm	ESM overview and links to software for researchers
http://www.phtcorp.com	Commercial electronic diaries for clinical trials
http://www.symtrend.com	Authoring tool for custom handheld applications for research or individual use by participants, families, educators, and clinicians.

References

Ackerson, J., Scogin, F., McKendree-Smith, N., & Lyman, R. D. (1998). Cognitive bibliotherapy for mild and moderate adolescent depressive symptomatology. *Journal of Consulting and Clinical Psychology, 66*, 685–690.

Barlow, D. H. (1988). *Anxiety and its disorders: The nature and treatment of anxiety and panic*. New York: The Guilford Press.

Barlow, D. H., & Hersen, M. (1984). *Single case experimental designs: Strategies for studying behavior change* (Pergamon General Psychology Series, Vol. 56). Boston: Allyn & Bacon.

Bartlett, F. C. (1932). *Remembering*. Cambridge, MA: Cambridge University Press.

Beck, J. S. (1995). *Cognitive therapy*. New York: The Guilford Press.

Behavioral Tech (1999–2003). *Dairy Card Instructions*. Retrieved November 1, 2005 from: http://www.behavioraltech.com/downloads/diarycrdinstructions.pdf.

Bolger, N., Davis, A., & Rafaeli, E. (2003). Diary methods: Capturing life as it is lived. *Annual Review of Psychology, 54*, 579–616.

Bruner, J. S. (1966). *Toward a theory of instruction*. Cambridge, MA: The Belknap Press of Harvard University Press.

Bruner, J. S. (1990). *Acts of meaning*. Cambridge, MA: Harvard University Press.

Burns, D. D. (1999). *The feeling good handbook*. New York: Plume.

Burns, D. D., & Nolen-Hoeksema, S. (1991). Coping styles, homework assignments and effectiveness of cognitive-behavioral therapy. *Journal of Consulting and Clinical Psychology, 59*, 35–311.

Burns, D. D., & Spangler, D. L. (2000). Does psychotherapy homework lead to improvements in depression in cognitive-behavioral therapy or does improvement lead to increased homework compliancc. *Journal of Consulting and Clinical Psychology, 68*, 46–56.

Cameron, L. D., & Nicholls, G. (1998). Expression of stressful experiences through writing: Effects of a self-regulation manipulation for pessimists and optimists. *Health Psychology, 17*, 84–92.

Campbell, J. D., Chew, B., & Scratchley, L. S. (1991). Cognitive and emotional reactions to daily events: The effects of self-esteem and self-complexity. *Journal of Personality, 59*, 473–505.

Clark, D. A., Beck, A. T., & Alford, B. A. (1999). *Scientific foundations of cognitive theory and therapy of depression*. New York: John Wiley & Sons, Inc.

Cruise, E. D., Broderick, J., Porter, L., Kaell, A., & Stone, A. A. (1996). Reactive effects of diary self-assessment in chronic pain participants. *Pain, 67*, 253–258.

Csikszentmihalyi, M., & Larson, R. (1987). Validity and reliability of the Experience Sampling Method. *Journal of Nervous and Mental Disease, 175*, 526–536.

deVries, M. (Ed.). (1992). *The experience of psychopathology: Investigating mental disorders in their natural settings*. Cambridge, England: Cambridge University Press.

Durgahee, T. (2002). Dialogism in action: talking fact and fiction. *Journal of Psychiatric and Mental Health Nursing, 9*, 419–425.

Foa, E. B., & Meadows, E. A. (1997). Psychosocial treatments for posttraumatic stress disorder: A critical review. *Annual Review of Psychology, 48*, 449–480.

Freud, S., & Breuer, J. (1976). Studies on hysteria. In J. Strachey (Ed.), *The Standard Edition of the Complete Psychological Works of Sigmund Freud* (Vol. 11, p. 6). New York: Norton & Co. (Original work published in 1895).

Greenberger, D., & Padesky, C. A. (1995). *Mind over mood*. New York: Guilford Press.

Jamison, C., & Scogin, F. (1995). Outcome of cognitive bibliotherapy with depressed adults. *Journal of Consulting & Clinical Psychology, 63*, 644–650.

Jung, C. G., & Jaffe, A. (Editor), Winston, R., & Winston, C. (Translators) (1989). *Memories, Dreams, Reflections*. New York: Vintage.

Kamarack, T. W., Shiffman, S. M., Smithline, L., Goodie, J. L., Paty, J. A., Gnys, M., & Jong, J. Y. (1998). Effects of task strain. Social conflict, and emotional activation on ambulatory cardiovascular activity: daily life consequences of recurring stress in a multiethnic adult sample. *Health Psychology, 17*, 17–29.

Keane, T. M., Fairbank, J. A., Caddell, J. M., & Zimering, R. T. (1989). Implosive (flooding) therapy reduces symptoms of PTSD in Vietnam combat veterans. *Behavior Therapy, 20*, 245–260.

Kenardy, J. A., Dow, M. G. T., Johnston, D. W., Newman, M. G., Thomson, A., & Taylor, C. B. (2003). A comparison of delivery methods of cognitive-behavior therapy for panic disorder: an international multicenter trial. *Journal of Consulting and Clinical Psychology, 71*, 1068–1075.

Kern, J. W. (1995). On focused association and the analytic surface: clinical opportunities in resolving analytic stalemate. *Journal of the American Psychoanalytic Association, 43*, 393–422.

L'Abate, L. (2001). Distance writing and computer-assisted interventions in psychiatry and mental health. In L. L'Abate (Ed.), *Distance writing and computer-assisted interventions in psychiatry and mental health*. Connecticut: Ablex Publishing.

L'Abate, L. (2004). The role of workbooks in the delivery of mental health services in prevention, psychotherapy, and rehabilitation. In L. L'Abate (Ed.) *Using workbooks in mental health: Resources in prevention, psychotherapy, and rehabilitation for clinicians and researchers*. Binghamton, NY: Haworth Press.

Leverich, G. S., & Post, R. M. (1997). *The LCM– S/P*™. Washington, DC: NIMH Biological Psychiatry Branch. Retrieved November 1, 2005 from: http://www.bipolarnews.org/pdfs/Patient%20Prospective%20Manual.pdf.

Linehan, M. M. (1999). *BRTC Diary Card*. Retrieved November 1, 2005 from: http://www.behavioraltech.com/downloads/diarycrdexamples.pdf.

Neubauer, J. R. (2001). *The complete idiot's guide to journaling*. Indianapolis, Indiana: Alpha Books.

Newman, M. G., Kenardy, J., Herman, S., & Taylor, C. B. (1997). Comparison of palm-top-computer-assisted brief cognitive-behavioral treatment to cognitive-behavioral treatment for panic disorder. *Journal of Consulting & Clinical Psychology, 65*, 178–183.

Nolen-Hoeksema, S., Morrow, J., & Fredrickson, B. L. (1993). Response styles and the duration of episodes of depressed mood. *Journal of Abnormal Psychology, 102*, 20–28.

O'Callaghan, C., Fishbein, H., Calvanio, R. J., Grant, C., & Levine, M. (June, 2004). *Electronic monitoring of co-morbidity in Asperger's students*. Poster presented at Complexities of Co-Occurring Conditions conference, Washington, DC.

Ollendick, T. H., & Ollendick, D. G. (1990). Tics and tourette syndrome. In A. M. Gross, & R. S. Drabman (Eds.), *Handbook of clinical behavioral pediatrics* (pp. 243–252). New York: Plenum.

Pennebaker, J. W. (1990). *Opening up: The healing power of expressing emotions*. New York: Guilford Press.

Pennebaker, J. W. (2001). Explorations into the health benefits of disclosure: inhibitory, cognitive, and social processes. In L. L'Abate (Ed.), *Distance writing and computer-assisted interventions in psychiatry and mental health*. Conneticut: Ablex Publishing.

Pennebaker, J. W. (2002). Writing, social processes, and psychotherapy: From past to future. In S. J. Lepore, & J. M. Smyth (Eds.), *The writing cure: How expressive writing promotes health and emotional well-being*. Washington, DC: American Psychological Association.

Pennebaker, J. W. (2004). Theories, therapies, and taxpayers: On the complexities of the expressive writing paradigm. *Clinical Psychology: Science and Practice, 11*, 138–142.

Peterson, L., & Tremblay, G. (1999). Self-monitoring in behavioral medicine: Children. *Psychological Assessment, 11*, 458–465.

Progoff, I. (1992). *At a Journal Workshop* (Rev. ed.). Los Angeles: Jeremy P. Tarcher, Inc.

Rainer, T. (1978). *The new diary*. Los Angeles: J. P. Tarcher, Inc.

Robson, J. (2003). Go deeper…reach higher…Journaling for self-empowerment. Retrieved November 1, 2005 from: http://www.journalingtools.com.

Ruble, D. N. (1977). Premenstrual symptoms: A reinterpretation. *Science, 197*, 291–292.

Schacter, D. L. (2001) *The seven sins of memory: How the mind forgets and remembers*. Boston, MA: Houghton Mifflin Company.

Schank, R. C. (1990). *Tell me a story: A new look at real and artificial memory*. New York: Charles Scribner's Sons.

Shiffman, S., Gwaltney, C. J., Balabanis, M. H., Liu, K. S., Paty, J. A., Kassel, J. D., Hickox, M., & Gnys, M. (2002). Immediate antecedents of cigarette smoking: An analysis from Ecological Momentary Assessment. *J. Abn Psychology, 111*, 531–545.

Smith, N. M., Floyd, M. R., Scoggin, F., & Jamison, C. S. (1997). Three-year follow-up of bibliotherapy for depression. *Journal of Consulting and Clinical Psychology, 65*, 324–327.

Stanton, A. L. (2005). How and for whom? Asking questions about the utility of psychosocial interventions for individuals diagnosed with cancer. *Journal of Clinical Oncology, 23*, 1–2.

Stanton, A. L., & Danoff-Burg, S. (2002). Emotional expression, expressive writing, and cancer. In S. J. Lepore, & J. M. Smyth (eds) *The writing cure: How expressive writing promotes health and emotional well-being*. Washington, DC: American Psychological Association.

Stanton, A. L., Danoff-Berg, S., Sworowski, L. A., Collins, C. A., Branstetter, A. D., Rodriguez-Hanley, A., et al., (2002). Randomized controlled trial of written emotional expression and benefit finding in breast cancer participants. *Journal of Clinical Oncology, 20*, 4160–4168.

Stone, A. A., & Shiffman, S. (1994). Ecological momentary assessment (EMA) in behavioral medicine. *Annals of Behavioral Medicine, 16*, 199–202.

SymTrend, Inc. (2005). Retrieved from http://www.symtrend.com on November 1, 2005.

Wegner, D. M. (1994). Ironic processes of mental control. *Psychological Review, 101*, 34–52.

Wegner, D. M., & Gold, D. B. (1995). Fanning old flames: Emotional and cognitive effects of suppressing thoughts of a past relationship. *Journal of Personality and Social Psychology, 68*, 782–792.

12

Teaching to Remember Ourselves: The Autobiographical Methodology

Duccio Demetrio
With contribution by Chiara Borgonovi

Inspired by philosophical thought, almost a century ago the human sciences discovered that collecting life stories was necessary for shedding light on circumstances, for penetrating more deeply into the explanations of events, which, when observed solely from the outside – even thoroughly and systematically – certainly could not reveal the whole of what they have to tell us. Written and oral stories (autobiographies) narrated by people can instead disclose what they feel inside. They communicate the experiences of narrators and their subjective points of view (Polkinghorne, 1983). Therefore, no one should claim the right to speak for someone else without first listening to him or her.

But knowledge of life stories is a means of self-analysis first and foremost for the one who writes about him or herself: every man and woman mindfully grows in relation to his or her ability to reprocess the past as a resource for the present (Demetrio, 1992, 1995a, b, 1998, 2003; Mayo, 2004; Polster, 1987; Progoff, 1975), and being in the present means also knowing how to think, write, and communicate better. Written autobiography may stimulate self-knowledge. The autobiography, a spoken tale told to others who collect the stories and reconstruct them into a written narrative text, also invites the illiterate to better understand themselves.

Tales can never be anything but unique: two identical (cloned) tales cancel each other, since their distinguishing feature is their absolute originality and uniqueness. Millions of tales have been produced and are continuously produced every day, and their uniqueness can be used to trace the uniqueness of the writer or narrator. While we can gather tales into types and typologies, nevertheless each of them has an individual character that stands out because of its unique author (Bruner, 1990). Therefore, for clinical research and autobiographical approach in educational theory the individual, not considered a "sample of a series", is addressed and listened to, invited to write and speak of himself or herself simply as a unique individual in history, in the culture, in his or her genetic and physical structure.

Theory: Written Autobiographical Memories

Writing about oneself includes a great variety of narrative forms. Besides *greater* forms (the actual autobiography, memoirs, the systematic epistolary, the systematically kept journal), *lesser* forms, should not be overlooked, such as personal notes, graffiti, letters and today e-mail messages stating private feelings and thoughts about oneself.

Autobiography represents a unique example, with implications not present in the other cited forms. It is not, in fact, a spontaneous narration: it requires effort, patience, diligence, a willingness to go back over an existential path whose tracks have been lost. Supposedly, the autobiographical method soothes and creates self-esteem (Birren and Deutchman, 1991; Polster, 1987; Progoff, 1975), which helps the writer to overcome problems of self-confidence especially in illness, in long-sought oblivion, in the inevitable law of forgetting in order to survive. Realizing that we can write as well as we can speak of ourselves, when everything is collapsing within and around us, certainly does not solve problems, but at least it strengthens our defenses and makes us feel alive with everything necessary to contemplate and continue explaining the world.

Autobiographies and journals are therefore the primary means through which writing about oneself achieves its most sought-after and profound formative results, both visible and invisible. Certain studies, in fact, have shown that autobiographical writing might improve relationships through empathy and better understanding of others (Howard, 2000). Besides, people who regularly put down their own experiences, emotions and thoughts, on paper, and acquire a habit of self-reflection, can act with greater deliberation and self-control and pay more attention to the needs of others. Writing about oneself can in fact help to avoid transferring one's affliction elsewhere, since it teaches one to coexist both with pain and life's most secretive and intense moments (Foucault, 1988). A relationship with suffering, as with beauty, explored through writing about oneself, is a source of maturity and improvement.

On the other hand, beyond observable manifestations of their "diversity," writers who write about themselves know very well how this work improves self-awareness (Baldwin, 1977) and produces changes and the discovery of new dimensions of thought and sensitivity (Progoff, 1975).

Although autobiographies and journals are at the core of writing about oneself, we trace all types of narrator focused writing – short, epigrammatic, formal, in prose or poetic – to the "autobiographical genre". This leads us to specify that, pedagogically, what interests us is the attention to the ego, that is to say, according to psychoanalysis, to the conscious dimension of thinking activities (Wilson, 2005). In fact, without neglecting that every personal writing always conceals unconscious, symbolic and hidden dimensions under its immediate semantics, in the autobiographical genre we search for forms that express awareness of one's self and of the world. Even spattered graffiti on walls shouts something to our conscience of annoyed city dwellers and, beyond the cultural, instinctive, and desiderative implications, it is in any case a sign of an anonymous self that wants to send messages to others.

Today, every expression presented orally or even through nonverbal codes, based on the principle of a recognizable ego-narrator, is included in the autobiographical genre. Self-portrait, dance, mime, even personal ways of organizing one's own space and living environment, are considered autobiographical since their "languages" reconstruct an idea about oneself, allowing us to get to know an author, his or her feelings and story. In short, we are "in autobiography" and we are dealing with autobiography whenever attention is dedicated to our own ego-narrator (or that of others). It tries to explain actions, reasons for living, relationships with others and, first and foremost, relationships with ourselves. In this broad sense of autobiography, therefore, we do not limit ourselves to telling a story, we also reflect, sometimes in writing, but also through all those forms of intelligence and art that are unequivocal signs of our conscious being.

When faced with any explicit reference to the first person singular (I am, I was, I will be, I did, I am doing, etc.), we catch sight of autobiographical evidence, that is often waiting for someone to help it find the theme of a possible tale, its absolutely unique story. The autobiography therefore becomes an invitation to acknowledge one's self, free to autonomously articulate it (Bruner, 1990).

All of the above, however, should be understood in a broad epistemological sense. Here, rather, we will mainly deal with autobiography in the strict sense: in its original reference to writing. So, we will look to the autobiographical self that comes to life the moment it becomes a sentence, a period, a work readable by the author and by others, recognized as a self that wants to be recognized and desires something more, personal development, larger self-knowledge and wisdom, in a fertile transition from the roots of memory to the autobiographical imagination (Eakin, 1985). Creating an autobiography, in this sense, means not only leaving a written evidence of our story, but also asking others to become interested in what we have experienced through the exercise of writing, and dealing with the writings of others as if they were one's own.

Research

Research in the field of autobiography has usually meant anecdotal rather than controlled evidence. Hence, in this section, we shall consider anecdotal/clinical first, phenomenological research second, and controlled evidence third. The latter means any findings that result from research using experimental and control groups with pre and postmeasures to evaluate any possible change that may have occurred from the experimental intervention.

Clinical and Autobiographical Viewpoints

When it was realized that every single story should not be merged with others into typologies, but rather valued for its uniqueness, a style of anecdotal research, born in the field of medicine, presented itself: the "clinical" research. According to this kind of research, each "case" is a story in and of itself before being traced to categories. As a result, every personal story, collected as a spoken tale from someone or provided through writings, not just regarding suffering and illness, can do nothing but arouse our clinical attention. Openmindedly and broadly speaking – even when not dealing with a pathology – it means not dispelling the tales of the individual narrator, his or her opinions and viewpoints (Demetrio, 1992, 1995a, b, 1998, 2003).

If the clinical viewpoint, later established in psychology thanks to the psychoanalytical revolution, represented and continues to represent an epistemological change in scientific research of primary importance, nevertheless here we prefer to call it "autobiographical," for at least three reasons. First, because the word "clinical" is now commonly used to refer to situations of malaise, illness, and abnormality. Secondly, because the clinical approach implies a repertory of knowledge going back to multiple movements and schools of thought. Finally, because, for the first reason, the clinical study of anyone, if announced as such, is frightening to the participant; it isolates and separates him or her from everyday life and relationships making him or her different.

The autobiographical viewpoint is, rather, conceptually more fluid, and it cannot be traced back to a certain school of thought that competes with others, but it is present transversely in all sciences that deal with uniqueness, not to mention literature and the figurative arts, since autobiography is a self-portrait, a novel or a poem. In fact:

(a) In its truest etymological idiom (*autos-bios-graphein*: to write about one's own life), this practice is present whenever anyone writes about him or herself, leaving us his or her vision as well as feelings, actions, loves, desires, etc.;
(b) In a broadest sense, an autobiography is anything we tell about ourselves to a real or imaginary person through words, during a spoken conversation, in a monologue, and await the reaction or otherwise of the other person;
(c) As a result, an autobiographical tale is also what is thought by someone in the secrecy of his or her own inner vicissitudes, whose profound consideration is invisible to others.

Furthermore, we do not expect autobiographies or biographies to provide us with ideas for general social or individual principles.

Memory: Establishing Responsibility and Awareness

One doesn't need to stress that memory constantly allows us to avoid errors and all kinds of trouble. It even suggests to us how to act. Nevertheless it must be pointed out that habitually recalling memories lets us, even in the irregularity of life, hold on to Ariadne's thread, which we all need so that we don't become totally confused and bewildered. Personal identity and the conception of our own existence as a whole are acquired through inserting our lived experience into a narrative structure that leads us to gain an understanding of our life as expression of a unique story in process, in a dynamic outlook which includes also the potential outlines of our evolution (Polkinghorne, 1988).

This makes memory the inner place of responsibility toward ourselves and others. It doesn't let us forget how much we were able to give and receive, how much we have done and attained compared to our starting point, how much progress we have made. Excessive attention to the present, dominant everywhere today, leads us to forget and continuously start over as if we weren't something before (Polster, 1987). Loss of memory leads us to be "transformist" people for personal advantage, and in this case an autobiography written in old age, only aimed at exonerating ourselves, is of no use.

Therefore, we should never forget that, if our memories were suddenly taken away, we would no longer be able:

- To think, since we would no longer have the raw material of thought;
- To find our direction, since memories teach and advise on what or what not to do, or, in any case, put us in a dilemmatic situation that increases cognitive activities;
- To dream or plan, since the desire for change and looking toward the future originates from memories;
- To recognize people, their faces, the role they played and play in our life.

Memory's worth is, however, both individual and collective (Ricoeur, 2000). In this case, the role of educating ourselves to remember the most terrible, cruelest errors and awful things committed by humanity is symbolic. As regards the value of remembering all of this, the educational theory of memory sets aside reference to our individual stories, psychological problems, and issues of success, for a broader and freer view. The result is that remembering is a right as well as a social and political duty. This concerns retrospective solidarity with those who went before us and intergenerational alliance.

Memory Training through Autobiography in Education

Memory in education has long been an object of suspicion and prejudice. It has been stated that memory is not considerable in children because they haven't had experiences, so adults have the job of transmitting their knowledge, without questioning too much what happened before in their histories. This complies with a vision of an all-absorbing performative pedagogy, which can be found in famous metaphors like those of *filling the empty vase* or *the soft wax to be molded*, as the educator desires.

Attention to memory and experiences that each person has in an educational context responds, rather, to what belongs to a tradition of activism, which never considers the individual as a blank sheet on which to record knowledge (Dewey, 1938). Certainly educating is also transmitting rules, instructions, ways of being and doing. But educating cannot be reduced to this, since each of us has a story, a tangled web of stories that precede that moment. These must be kept in mind, so that educating means developing natural potential, encouraging and discovering one's own resources (Ruth, 1987). We must even start from what was learned during the very first moments of life. Intentionally prepared educational time, as an opportunity not just for instruction but also for experiencing emotions, encounters, new experiences, is a large playground for human growth founded on remembering.

Existential Memories

We call "existential" memories those recollections that build our Self and make each of us who we are. They are present even in those who, according to a very scholastic definition, "can't remember" or "can't memorize," but, when faced with very personal questions, demonstrate they can remember more than those students who never forget anything or almost anything that is explained to them, or that they read or learn elsewhere.

Existential memories can cover at least four operational areas, in the sense that, by evoking them – spontaneously or planned, through writing or other expressive forms – the mind works in different ways (Nelson, 1993, 2003):

1. *Sensory* memories concern moments of perceptual and sensory intensity absolutely an end unto themselves, connected with the mental area of pleasure and pain (for example: *My memories often take me back to the warm smell of carrot cake just out of the oven*).
2. *Procedural* memories surface when we remember events connected with sequences of experiences, when we use "before" and "after" categories, managing to remember something that happened according to an actual narrative sequence (for example: *I remember when I learned how to tie my shoes by myself, how to move my fingers*).
3. *Pre-semantic* memories appear as very vivid memories, mental scenes connected especially with places or strong emotional events, but not connected with evaluations or instructive, moral messages, etc. (for example: *I remember when I lived in a trailer. I went with my brother, Jonah, to a place where there were lots of toys*).
4. *Semantic* memories are complex memories – that also include the previous types – to which the person assigns a personal meaning, which therefore attest to a judgment or assessment of what was witnessed or done. The episode remembered is reconstructed in a narrative synthesis and inserted into an interpretative map that testifies as to its pedagogic value (since it holds an admonition, a lesson, an understanding...). It also bears witness to the presence of someone else, a mirror figure, that induced a line of reasoning, forbade something or simply interacted.

This shows that semantic memory is always relational and allows us to think back to the people who were the source of the mnestic fixation, accompanied by considerations and stories that were probably added afterwards or whose recollection by others was so frequent that it was impressed on one's memory. For example, a woman remembered an episode that occurred when she was two-and-a-half years old:

> My mom told me [...] she was going to the dry-cleaner's. I asked her why she was going and she told me she needed to have some clothes cleaned. When she went out, I left my room and went into the bathroom, took off my pants and put them in the toilet. Then my mom returned and she asked why I put them there and I told her that I wanted to help her by washing them myself. She said that was very nice of me but it would probably be better if she washed the clothes.

Therefore, semantic memories are "indirect", or have narrative mediation, because they are tied to events that probably would have vanished into oblivion if they hadn't had spectator-narrators that confirmed or judged (Ricoeur, 2000). Like in this other example: *They told me that the first word I said was "alone" because I wanted to do everything by myself.*

In short: memory is not just "memorizing." First of all, as to what was stated, we must explain to students, whatever their ages, that memory cannot be reduced to the fateful "memorizing" of factual knowledge (poetry, dates, names, statements, etc.), which has caused such anguish and suffering in scholastic teaching. It is undoubtedly indispensable that all of this be remembered. The problem, however, is to do it in such a way that those quickly defined as children or young people that "can't memorize" are not considered inferior to others. Although it is true that genetics play a role in the greater or weaker ability to remember, in education it must be kept in mind that:

(a) We remember better what has impressed us and stirred our emotions. So, the more pupils who are involved in a didactic experience, the more it can be expected they will retain the information longer. In fact, it will be located in what we call semantic memory. The knowledge will be difficult to forget if it is associated with relational situations, reasons, and natural as well as sparked interest;
(b) Even purely factual recollections stick and remain engraved if we can "work on them," apply them as quickly as possible to verify their usefulness within a system of integrated learning that allows complex neuronic networks to be constructed;
(c) Information is registered in the mind the more it is associated with pleasant or unpleasant, motivating or depressing events.

Autobiographies of Children

Both autobiography and journal can help us to hold ourselves together existentially and psychologically. Even when we accept that living means getting through endless transformation, we need to give ourselves a direction, to find an orchestration, an organized concept of self as a scenery with figures in the limelight and backgrounds. Living, we need to connect, and interconnection produces synthesis, cognitive patterns, forms of interpretation. If identity is a tale, it's a tale in progress, and we have to perform and carry out it as well as to interpret it on the way: it's telling or writing about ourselves that we become really subjects in the full sense of the word (Bruner, 1990; Ricoeur, 1990). Therefore, directing precocious children to the habit of writing, we can help them to feel more themselves as subjects, as autonomous persons. With the youngest, recalling and narrating the most significant experiences of life helps the process of self-construction, offering them the feeling of being owners of something absolutely original that they can share with others. "Remember to narrate, narrate to exist" it is not a play on words. It is an activity that has to come to life, one that teachers can suggest through experiences centered on listening to others.

A recent research project which used fifth-grade students of elementary schools in the north of Italy, allowed us to present some examples of autobiographical practice in education. It was aimed to help the growth of a more and more mature self awareness and to stimulate sensory and cognitive self perception. The autobiographic laboratory that took place in a school of Lissone (Milano), was particularly directed to the study of the role played by narrative thought and autobiographical memory in the process of the construction of identity. The purpose was to investigate how one tells stories about one's self in infancy, brings back to life and reconstructs the past experiences through language, takes part in the elaboration of a concept of self, of one's own identity and position in the world. Narrations were stimulated by using a version adapted to children of the "Life's Game," that assumes the structure of a traditional table game, transforming it into an autobiographical instrument through which the players are invited to talk about themselves to others, starting from the themes suggested in the squares on which they must stop before arriving at the final goal. The choice of the topics has privileged daily experiences, and therefore the dimension of present time, although in the participants were sped up also memories about past time and, on the other side, hopes, desires and plans for the future.

Among the more significant aspects that come to light thanks to these suggestions, it must be considered the fundamental role that, in the identity construction, assumes the development of self perception. Special relevance has perception of one's own body and, above all, of specific characteristics and tastes which distinguish each person from the others. Collected stories, in fact, show children's desire to manifest their preferences in every field, through the definition of what they like or dislike, and emphasizing their own peculiarity regarding the other known persons. It is evident, for example, when children, invited to tell about food, describe their tastes:

> I don't like meat very much, because it is hard, but I eat fish. My grandmother cooks always roast meat, but I don't like it. So, she cooks also meatballs for me, and I eat them with potatoes, while all they [sic] eat roast meat. (Sara, 10 years old)
>
> I like stew, that mummy cooks with white rise [sic], and my sister and I always stir them in the same dish, while daddy eats the rise [sic] before and after the meat. (Yuri, 10 years old)

The starting points for autobiographical work can be, already during the kindergarten, the evoking of the "earliest" memory, of pleasant or frightening episodes, or of recollections closely connected to the sensory dimension (smells, tastes, sounds, materials one liked to touch, etc). Initial work on memory should also be carried out with the help of journals, freely writing about growing up. In any case, it should be well understood that memory, from an autobiographical point of view, is the product of a poetic-literary vision of experiences. For example, stories like this can be found when children are asked to mention stories about their first experiences:

> I remember that as soon as I was born, to celebrate my dad shot a gun into the woods with his friends. It was so dry that the forest caught on fire. The firemen and police came. I was just born. I'm still afraid of gunshots now.
>
> When I was born I sneezed and scared the nurse, the doctor, and all the doctors that were there. I remember everything.

With children of elementary school grades, however, ways of memory can follow more complex progressions, which can give rise to narrative moments based, for example, on the comparison between past and present time. This is what happened in a school in Bologna. Here, the topic of overcoming one's own weaknesses and limits – looking ahead and behind in life, telling about memories and about plans for the future – has lead up to their writing short narrations in which the theme of difference emerges, as well as the relations between desires and reality, hopes and errors or behaviors to avoid. For example:

> Ahead. To be able to go alone to school. To be able to cook meat in the oven. To have understood that horror films are made thanks to special effects. To be able to run alone with my bicycle to cool down my anger. To be happy when my parents are not at home, while before I always cried. Behind. To need the lamp lighted to fall asleep. To moan and cry when my older brother does something to spite me. To cry when my parents are away. *(Lorenzo, 10 years old)*

> Ahead To read quite big books. To ignite the oven or the gas cooker. To begin listening to television news and to the adult's speeches. To begin to do my homework by myself. To dress myself as I want. To think to[sic] the boys. To confide secrets to my mother. To see films with red stamp [sic]. To telephone secretly. Behind To need that mammy kiss me goodnight and tuck in my bed-sheets. To have my dress prepared. To be fear[sic] to sleep alone. To sleep sometimes in my parents bed. *(Cristina, 9 years old)*

The suggestion of this topic is particularly interesting because it gives rise to writings that show us the exercise of a memory we could define "auto-pedagogical" already in pre-adolescents. In their writings – and through them – children manifest and exercise their ability to feel themselves growing up, to describe their own transformation, evidencing what they were a short time before and comparing it with what they would want to become.

Phenomenological Research on Autobiographies

Memory qualities for positive, negative, and neutral autobiographical events, were investigated in 101 participants aged 18 to 32 years. Participants were asked to recall two personal experiences of each type and then rated their memories on several characteristics (e.g., sensorial and contextual details). They were also asked to report on whether they "saw" these events in their memories from their own perspective (field memories), or whether they "saw" the self engaged in the event as an observer would ("observer" memories). Positive memories contained more sensorial (vision, smell, taste) and contextual (location, time) details than both negative and neutral events, whereas negative and neutral memories did not differ on most dimensions. Positive and negative events were more often recollected with a field perspective than neutral events (D'Argembeau, Comblain, & Van der Linden, 2003).

Furthermore, there may be age-related differences in phenomenal characteristics of autobiographical memories for positive, negative, and neutral events. Emotional (both positive and negative) memories may contain more sensorial and contextual details than neutral memories in both young and old adults. Negative memories were associated with a higher intensity of positive feelings and a reduced complexity of story line in older as compared to younger adults (Comblain, D'Argembeau, & Van der Linden, 2005).

Autobiographical accounts of traumatic and stressful events may reveal how we understand and organize personally meaningful experiences. This analysis of traumatic and emotional narratives focuses on the ways in which a person's event memory predicts the impact of trauma and emotional experiences on psychological well-being (e.g. depression or positive morale). Analyses of narratives by adolescents experiencing trauma and by male caregivers to a partner with AIDS, showed that four factors account for the relationship between memory and psychological well-being: (1) Beliefs (evaluation) about the experience of trauma; (2) Specific emotions expressed in reaction to the events; (3) Beliefs about one's competence at coping with and overcoming adversity; and (4) Generation of new goals formulated to replace those lost.

The organization and narration of emotional understanding, while diverse and complex in content, is highly constrained as to the number and kind of emotions expressed. The relationship among specific emotions, antecedents, beliefs, and plans of action also are constrained. These constraints, as well as the use of a causal theory of emotion and goal-directed action, allow us to make predictions about psychological well-being and memory for emotional events (Stein, Trabasso, & Albro, 2001).

The emotional determinants of the phenomenal characteristics of autobiographical memories were examined in 84 participants who completed the Memory Characteristics Questionnaire (MCQ), after retrieving and orally describing a negative, a positive, and a neutral autobiographical memory. In addition, self-reports and physiological measures of emotional states at retrieval were recorded. Recall of perceptual, sensory, and semantic elements is better for emotional memories than for neutral ones. Emotional memories may be even more vivid but no more specific than are neutral ones. Positive memories yielded higher MCQ ratings than did negative memories for sensory, temporal, and contextual aspects. Positive correlations suggested possible relations between emotional states at retrieval and levels of phenomenal details of retrieved memories (Schaefer & Philippot, 2005).

Empirical Research about the Autobiographical Method

In this section, we shall report on research that used controlled conditions or conditions that could be repeated from one laboratory to another. For instance, 49 undergraduates were randomly asked to write autobiographically about profound topics (e.g., highly traumatic, traumatic, or guilty experiences) versus a control group that wrote about trivial topics (e.g., describing in great detail their bedroom or dormitory room) for 15 minutes per day for 4 consecutive days, during a two-week period. Both groups completed pre-post- and 6-week follow-up measures of suicidal thinking and mood, and self-reported health-center visits on pretest and follow-up, the experimental group tended to report ($p = .06$) a reduction in the number of health center visits from pretest to follow-up. There were no changes in measures of suicidal ideation or mood. These findings support those obtained from expressive writing discussed in Chapter 13 (this volume).

Childhood Amnesia

When undergraduates labeled childhood events (e.g., when your first permanent tooth came in) as known or recollected memories and estimated their age at the event's occurrence, the estimated transition from mostly known memories was roughly 4.7 years. This transitional estimate was replicated in a sample of adults aged 25 to 65 years. Undergraduates' memories of public events (e.g., the Challenger explosion) was roughly 6 years. Therefore, the wane of childhood amnesia appears to occur around 4.7 years (Multhaup, Johnson, & Tetirick, 2005).

Childhood Memories

Two seemingly separate but related factors may account for autobiographical memory in children: (1) Theory of mind or the ability to know what another can and cannot know, and (2) Narrative skill, or the ability to tell a coherently structured story. In the autobiographies of 22 preschoolers, theory of mind predicted the "how" or structure of the children's fictional story narratives, whereas narrative skills predicted the "how much" or content of the children's memory (Kleinknecht & Belke, 2004). Content analyses of elderly individuals' recollections about three points in family life focused on episodes that illustrated the initial occurrence of family themes and values. In contrast, recollections of their families when they were middle-aged and their families of today showed a tendency to identify continuing themes and trends from the early episodes of their families' lives. These findings may indicate that reminiscences of family lives change as the relative importance of family developmental tasks changes (Byrd, 2001).

Emotional remembering in functional populations of children depends on the attributes of memories other than their historical accuracy. The structure and content of young children's emotional memories is coconstructed by the children and their parents, a process that varies from culture to culture and also depends on the child's gender. This coconstruction is important for many reasons, among them, it is one of the essential means through which children gain a foundation for understanding themselves and their autobiographies. Also crucial here are the ways in which parent-child reminiscing about stressful experiences can guide the child's understanding of and coping with aversive events (Fivush & Sales, 2004).

The Nun Study

The now historical Nun Study (Snowdon, 2001) consisted of examining autobiographies of nuns in a convent. This study has been a fruitful source of continued analyses and breakthrough knowledge about the long-time effects of autobiographical writings. Handwritten autobiographies from 180 nuns, composed when they were on the average 22 years of age, were scored for emotional content and related to survival rates during ages 75 to 95. A strong inverse relationship existed between positive emotional content and risk of mortality in late life ($p < .001$). As the quartile ranking of positive emotions in early life increased, there was a stepwise decrease in risk of mortality resulting in a 2.5 fold difference between lowest and highest quartiles. Positive emotional content in early life autobiographies was strongly associated with longevity 6 decades later (Denner, Snowden, & Friesen, 2001).

Relationships between early life variables, cognitive function, and neuropathology were examined in the same participants. An early life variable was idea density, which is a measure of linguistic ability, derived from the same autobiographies. Six discrete categories of cognitive function, including mild cognitive impairment, were evaluated using the battery of cognitive tests developed by Consortium to Establish a Registry for Alzheimer Disease (CERAD). Early-life idea density was significantly related to the categories of late-life cognitive function, including mild cognitive impairments. Low idea density was associated with lower brain weight, greater impairment, higher degree of cerebral atrophy, more severe neurofibrillary pathology, and the likelihood of meeting neuropathologic criteria for Alzheimer's disease (Riley, Snowden, Desrosiers, & Markesbery, 2005). These findings would support the importance of early, structured training to become aware of emotional feelings and how to express them positively (Chapters 15 and 16 this volume).

Gender Differences

Adult women and men may differ in the affective qualities of their autobiographical reports. If that is the case, gender differences in emotional content should appear in autobiographical memories of both remote and recent past and whether these memories extend to internal states other than emotions. Forty-eight women (aged 19 to 47 years) and 30 men (aged 19 to 31 years) provided written accounts of four events from early in life (before age 7) and four events from age 7 or later. Narratives were coded for mention of emotions, cognitions, perceptions, and physiological states. Coding showed that women used more emotion terms in their descriptions of events from later in life, relative to men. Across life phases, similar trends were observed for cognition and perception terms, but not for physiological states. Internal states were more coherent for women than for men. These results support the possibility that women and men experience different socialization practices regarding expression of internal states (Bauer, Stennes, & Haight, 2003).

Autobiographies of Deviant Populations

It is important to see how autobiographies can give us important information about the genesis and development of deviant behaviors.

Incarcerated Offenders: Autobiographies of 48 incarcerated adult male sexual offenders were used to generate retrospective self-report measures of childhood maternal and paternal attachment, sexual abuse experiences, and onset of masturbation. Contrary to expectations, all offenders more often reported secure than insecure maternal and paternal attachment. However, rapists and intrafamilial child molesters were more likely to report insecure paternal attachment than were extrafamilial child molesters. Offenders with insecure paternal attachment were more likely to report having been sexually abused than were those with secure paternal attachment. Sexually abused offenders in turn reported earlier onset of masturbation than did those who were not sexually abused (Smallbone & McCabe, 2003).

Addictions and Intoxications: An analysis of three autobiographies of two drug-addicted physicians and one recovering alcoholic mother raises questions about traditional notions of addictions being rooted in the self (Keane & Wales, 2001).

The sharing of life stories is the most important social practice among members of Alcoholic Anonymous (AA). Close attention to autobiographic story-telling provides clues as to how AA works to heal alcoholism by creating a community of recovering alcoholics. There are at least three major ways that AA stories create community. First, in the course of performance of autobiographic narratives, expert AA speakers create social structures between themselves and their audience. Second, proper AA stories are the means by which AA members acquire and maintain their identities as recovering alcoholics. In this manner, story-listening is just as important as story-telling. Third, through the invocation of strong feelings, both tragic and humorous, AA story-tellers create a kind of intimacy based on shared emotions (Swora, 2001).

Autism Spectrum Disorder: Children may develop a succession of theories of mind that, like scientific theories, postulate abstract coherent mental entities and laws, and provide predictions, interpretations, and explanations. These processes, in turn, enable children to interact successfully with other people. Individuals with autism or Asperger's syndrome are said to be unable to theorize about other minds, and this results in difficulties in relating to people around them. It could be argued also that typical children do not have to theorize that there are minds as they can immediately experience other people's intentions and feelings within their affective, coregulated interactions with others. High-functioning individuals with autism, on the other hand, do need to engage in theorizing about minds if they are to bridge the gap between themselves and other people. An interpretative phenomenological analysis of ten published autobiographical accounts written by individuals diagnosed with either high-functioning autism or Asperger's syndrome seems to support the latter argument (Williams, 2004).

Computerized Content Analyses of Autobiographies

The computer has opened new vistas in the promotion of health and prevention of mental illness (Chapter 16 this volume) (Chapter TK). For instance, the computer can be used for content analyses of autobiographical writings (Gottschalk & Bechtel, 2005; Gottschalk, Defrancisco, & Bechtel, 2002).

To assist older participants in the telling of their life stories, a digital recorder and voice-to-text software were administered to ten older participants. These machines would free participants from the labor of creating a formal record of their life stories, either through typing, writing, or manual transcription of audio tapes. On a hand-held recorder, and in a one-to-one interview format, each participant's voice was converted to digital form as the narration proceeded. The digital recording was then transcribed electronically into a computer, which subsequently converted the digital voice record into text. The resultant text was corrected to mirror the audible story, and a printed copy was given to each participant. Adapting this emerging technology to a one-on-one interview process presented many challenges, the most significant of which was correcting the machine-generated text to mirror the audio recording. The technique of assisted life stories has potential for more widespread usage when software programs are developed that more adequately address the unique requirement of an interview format and require a shorter training period (Harlow, Boulmetis, Clark, & Willis, 2003).

Practice

One of the advantages of the autobiographical method lies in its being used to help couples in therapy, benefitting by adding it to on-going group, face-to-face talk therapy, thus saving time (Hoang, 2005), for school counselors in training (Holcomb-McCoy, 2004), student teachers (Estola, 2003), teacher education (Bushnell & Henry, 2003). Indeed, teachers' autobiographies may influence their responses to children's behaviors in the classroom (Weiss, 2002a, b).

Existential Teaching Methodologies

We can outline three means for making the above an educational project, regardless of the ages of those participating in activities like courses, labs or seminars, within or outside scholastic and instructional settings. We are writing about ourselves, telling our own stories, and self-reflections.

The first methodology favors the task – infinitely superior to others – that writing carries out. Nothing else can accentuate the ability of ingraining memories in the mind and transforming them into a myriad of possibilities and combinations. When we write about ourselves, we teach ourselves to concentrate. Concentrating is not so much using an hypothetical focal point around which every other thought gravitates, but rather a cognitive ability based on the emotional pleasure of peacefully being alone, taking time for ourselves, a moment of retreat in which attention is centered on our inner world (Metzger, 1992; Progoff, 1975). In religious cultures, prayer, contemplation and meditation have always carried out this role, necessary for the well-being of the psyche. St. Augustine, by no accident a convert, was the first to remind us that secular writing about what we've experienced (and therefore about ourselves) means carrying out a special mental exercise, a combination of abstract thought (because memories become abstract concepts) and concrete thought (because memories are experiences).

The second, rather, encourages public speaking, the self-presentation of who we are, talking about ourselves freely and no longer being afraid to talk, getting used to being narrators, creating atmospheres and captivating the attention of others.

The last means develops speculative thought, both about personal decisions that must be made for the present and for the future, and for the pure pleasure of freely philosophizing and wandering, beginning with the experiences that life inevitably introduces along each of our paths of existence. We think about ourselves when emotional and professional decisions must be made, when we evaluate our resources, when we question our values and principles and when suffering, mourning or love inevitably suggests that we separate ourselves from others and ponder the meaning of life.

We define these three teaching methodologies as "existential" because, although during scholastic time and continuing education they have special moments related to different ages of life, they crisscross our existence, creating a sort of *curriculum* for learning how to live with a greater awareness of ourselves and of the world, while being independent and autonomous. They continuously strengthen us morally and internally to face the unease and adversities that life entails. It also means we have confidence and hope, both consequentially dependent upon the sense of self, the awareness of existing, gained through the understanding that we have a story, we can tell a story about ourselves that organizes all the events of our lives into a meaningful whole (Metzger, 1992).

As teachers and educators of young people and adults (and as therapists, and those in educational fields interested in these methodologies), we must consequently act so that the story we want to listen to and assemble brings past experiences back to life. Anyone not suffering from serious mental problems, in fact, even if there may be some initial difficulties, can draw on his or her personal history as a wealth of knowledge, also called self-knowledge, of which we are not always aware. This is how we discover that we are never empty: we always have something to narrate, since each of us has lived and our mind biologically and culturally possesses a tendency to think without being obliged to answer to anyone else.

Scholastic Education for Young People and Autobiographical Suggestions

If in extra-scholastic contexts autobiographical methodologies are used by specialized figures of educators, in scholastics education work on memory can be carried out – with children and young people – thanks to the work of teachers who have been trained to the autobiographical approach, acquiring the instruments to introduce narrative and autobiographical moments into scholastic activities.

Memory and autobiographical writing represent a special way among all that practices that have always nourished inner and, therefore, mental life. We can induce young people to cultivate inner life encouraging any activity that stimulates introspection and leads to experiences that do not involve immediate socialization, dependence on others or the media. Among these: reading, activities that develop thought and questioning, activities that encourage concentration and observation (like various forms of expressive creativity), experiences in which silence is important (meditation, solitary sports, etc.), creative narrative writing. And, obviously, autobiographical writing, as a diary or retrospectively, where memory turns out to be invisible knowledge that we gradually accumulate, consciously or without realizing it, which writing brings back to our attention and that of others, if we desire.

The narrative teaching methodology, which focuses on writing about oneself, has evident educational objectives of a cognitive nature. Dealing with autobiography in strict sense, in fact, doesn't mean only dealing with memory; it involves the activation and integrated exercise of several cognitive abilities and forms of thought – retrospective and introspective, logical and metaphorical, reflective and explorative, etc. – as well as the development of self-reflective or meta-cognitive abilities, related to reflection on the work of one's own mind (Foucault, 1988; Lejeune, 1975; Olney, 1972).

Writing, erasing and rewriting is the true initiatory road to mental work because the burden, requested of the writer, to keep watch over his or her words and states of consciousness is more direct. In many it triggers inner work fed from desire, that will be endless, and that will sanction the beginning of the adult psychological condition, since it is primarily a time for reflection, of transitioning from the youthful age of unease to the mature age of unquiet consideration.

The spontaneity of young people's writing is therefore not a certainty or even enough for a school whose core is education. Consequently, adults who operate in school, educators, teachers, tutors and coaches, have a large responsibility in this respect: they can stimulate (without being intrusive). They can request more precise and effective thinking, that tries to be less anonymous (without being pedantic). They can become mentors of narration, dwelling on life's main themes, that young people are beginning to experience: on love and pain, on effort and on the conquest of one's own place in the world (without being importunate).

Therefore, school should be able to offer a variety of opportunities aimed at increasing narrative skills, setting up autobiographical labs dedicated both to journal and retrospective writing. The purpose is to create a special space at school for young people and to promote actual pedagogic projects aimed at allowing them to live through a time of reflection on themselves, and also to "narrate themselves" in public, to share their own stories with others, and experience various narrative genres, from poetry to theater. In such a way a private question is transformed into education to communication and social interaction: especially inspiring habits that defend and respect one's own inner life, contributing to make them able to manifest their own affection and feelings, well over scholastic learning time. Teaching how to cultivate writing about oneself in this case means to provide young people with a method for learning how to look within themselves and understand others (Calkins, 1983). All of this can spawn behavior aimed at transitioning into adulthood and new awareness.

The didactic and educational objectives can therefore be summed up as:

1. Legitimize the role that personal literature has for centuries played as a lesser literary genre (journals, memoirs, autobiographies, etc.) in art, film, television and music;
2. Demonstrate how the school, just as it can withdraw from young people's free desire to talk about themselves, can also help them narrate, inquire into the life stories of peers, and much more: it can itself learn from the individual memories that populate it and from local ones in much hoped-for and experienced intergenerational meetings.

Some Guiding Principles

The following principles must be kept in mind to realize effective autobiographical teaching and didactics.

Memory is a cognitive activity. Using memory means cultivating one's mind, beginning with whether we can or cannot remember, discovering that this originates within ourselves, giving us the sensation of being the builders and first interpreters of our life, the sensation of having more autonomy and a sense of freedom.

Cultivating memory is the basis of all education. Memory controls the ways of access to knowledge and how abilities are returned.

Cultivating memory favors the exercise of various kinds of expressive languages (technical-procedural, descriptive, but also the language of novels and poetry).

Cultivating memory stimulates cognitive activity as a whole. It teaches how to: choose between memories, contextualize memories, interpret memories using analogies, comparisons.

Cultivating memory stimulates identification of its cognitive processes, as shown below, where we have included sentences stated by students during experiential workshops and activities that we organized:

– reminiscence *(I have a story if I can remember something)*
– recognizability *(I have had many features)*
– fulfillment *(I'm not so empty)*

– reassociation *(I have more memories than I thought I had)*
– reorganization *(I don't have just scattered memories, I can link them to create scenes, descriptions of life, etc.)*
– relation *(I can't forget who was next to me that day, that time).*

Cultivating memory invites us to think about other people's memories, it generates curiosity about other people's stories. Stories tell us about who we are and who we were. If we don't listen to the story of another person, we can't get to know each other.

Cultivating memory means growing emotionally, since remembering is also a feeling. We continuously nourish ourselves with stories; we are born within the stories of others and we are partially guided by them our entire lives. Some impact us deeply, indelibly and then we need to talk about them in an appropriate clinical setting or at least write about them.

We borrow other people's stories: they help us, they prop us up and support us during difficult times. They give us direction when we don't have one or when we've lost it. We can feel healing when we are bewildered and assimilate other people's stories, make them ours, invent others. We tell stories to find connections and significant explanations.

Conclusions

In spite of its widespread use and enthusiastic endorsements of its advocates, the evidence for the use of autobiography as a vaccine relies mostly on the results of the Nun Study. In addition to being easy to administer to large masses of people, that study, fortunately for its advocates, is one of the best pieces of evidence to demonstrate the long-term outcome of writing autobiographies at an early age. However, by the same token, one needs to look at *the kind of writing* before making a pall-mall declaration of universal applications for autobiographies as vaccines. The evidence from that study shows how autobiographies can be used diagnostically to predict how long and how well one will live, on the basis of idea density and use of positive emotion words, as supported by other research (see Chapter 14 this volume) (Chapter TK).

Consequently, on the basis of the definition of a vaccine as an easy to administer, low-cost intervention to large groups of people, with some benefits for a certain few, the use of autobiographies will benefit from research on individual differences on how and why some individuals benefit by it and why some will not.

References

Baldwin, C. (1977). *One to one: self-understanding through journal writing*. New York: M. Evans & C.

Bauer, P. J., Stennes, L., & Haight, J. C. (2003). Representations of the inner self in autobiography: Women's and men's use of internal states language in personal narratives. *Memory, 11*, 27–42.

Birren, J. E., & Deutchman, D. (1991). *Guiding autobiography groups for older adults. Exploring the fabric of life*. Baltimore, MD: John Hopkins University Press.

Bruner, J. (1990). *Acts of meaning*. Cambridge, MA: Harvard University Press.

Bushnell, M., & Henry, S. E. (2003). The role of reflection in epistemological change: Autobiography in teacher education. *Educational Studies: Journal of the American Educational Studies Association, 34*, 38–41.

Byrd, M. (2001). Elderly individuals' reminiscences about the life-span development of their family. *International Journal of Aging & Human Development, 52*, 253–263.
Calkins, L. (1983). *The art of teaching writing*. Portsmouth. NH: Heinemann.
Comblain, C., D'Argembeau, A., & Van der Linden, M. (2005). Phenomenal characteristics of autobiographical memories for emotional and neutral events in older and younger adults. *Experimental Aging Research, 31*, 173–189.
Danner, D. D., Snowden, D. A., & Friesen, W. V. (2001). Positive emotions in early life and longevity: Findings from the nun study. *Journal of Personality and Social Psychology, 80*, 804–813.
D'Argembeau, A., Comblain, C., & Van der Linden, M. (2003). Phenomenal characteristics of autobiographical memories for positive, negative, and neutral events. *Applied Cognitive Psychology, 17*, 281–294.
Demetrio, D. (1992). *Micropedagogia. La ricerca qualitativa in educazione*. Firenze: La Nuova Italia.
Demetrio, D. (1995a). *Raccontarsi. L'autobiografia come cura di sé*. Milano: Raffaello Cortina.
Demetrio, D. (1995b). *Per una didattica dell'intelligenza. Il metodo autobiografico nello sviluppo cognitivo*. Milano: Franco Angeli.
Demetrio, D. (1998). *Pedagogia della memoria. Per se stessi, con gli altri*, Roma: Meltemi.
Demetrio, D. (2003). *Ricordare a scuola. Fare memoria e didattica autobiografica*. Roma-Bari: Laterza.
Dewey, J. (1938, 1997). *Experience and education*. New York: Touchstone.
Eakin, P. J. (1985). *Fictions in autobiography: Studies in the art of self-invention*. Princeton, NJ: Princeton University Press.
Eakin, P. J. (1999). *How our lives become stories: Making selves*. Ithaca, NY: Cornell University Press.
Estola, E. (2003). Hope at work-Student teachers constructing their narrative identities. *Scandinavian Journal of Educational Research, 47*, 181–203.
Fivush, T., & Sales, J. M. (2004). Children's memories of emotional events. In D. Reisberg (Ed.), *Memory and emotion* (pp. 242–271). New York: Oxford University Press.
Foucault, M. (1988). Technologies of the self. In Martin, L. H., Gutman, H., and Hutton, P. (Eds.), (1988) *Technologies of the self: A seminar with Michel Foucault* (pp. 16–49). Amherst, MA: University of Massachusetts Press.
Gottschalk, L. A., & Bechtel, R. J. (2005). Computerized content analysis of writings of Mahatma Gandhi, *Journal of Nervous and Mental Disease, 193*, 210–216.
Gottschalk, L. A., Defrancisco, D., & Bechtel, R. J. (2002). Computerized content analysis of some adolescent writings of Napoleon Bonaparte. A test of the validity of the method. *Journal of Nervous and Mental Disease, 190*, 542–548.
Gunn, J. V. (1982). *Autobiography: Toward a poetics of experience*. Philadelphia: University of Pennsylvania Press.
Harlow, G., Boulmetis, J., Clark, P. G., & Willis, G. H. (2003). Computer-assisted life stories. *Computers in Human Behavior, 19*, 391–406.
Hillman, J. (1983). *Healing fictions*. Dallas: Spring Publications.
Hoang, L. (2005). "I thought we came for therapy": Autobiography sessions in couple work. *Australian and New Zealand Journal of Family Therapy, 26*, 65–72.
Holcomb-McCoy, C. (2004). Using the family autobiography in school counselor preparation: An introduction to a systemic perspective. *Family Journal: Counseling and Therapy for Couples and Families, 21*, 21–25.
Howard, D. E. (2000). *Autobiographical writing and performing: An introductory, contemporary guide to process and research in speech performance*. New York: McGraw-Hill.
Keane, H., & Wales, R. W. (2001). Public and private practices: Addiction autobiographies and its contradictions. *Contemporary Drug Problems, 28*, 567–595.

Kleinknecht, E., & Belke, D. R. (2004). How knowing and doing inform an autobiography: Relations among pre-schoolers' theory of mind, narrative, and event memory skills. *Applied Cognitive Psychology, 18*, 745–764.
Lejeune, P. (1975). *Le Pacte autobiographique*. Paris: Seuil [Transl. (1989) On *autobiography*. Minneapolis, MN: University of Minnesota Press]
Lepore, S. J., & Smyth, J. M. (Eds.) (2002). *The writing cure: How expressive writing promotes health and emotional well-being*. Washington, DC: APA Books.
Mayo, J. A. (2004). Using mini-autobiographical narration in applied psychology to personalize course content and improve conceptual application. *Journal of Constructivist Psychology, 17*, 237–246.
Metzger, D. (1992). *Writing for your life. A guide and companion for the inner worlds*. San Francisco: Harper.
Multhaup, K. S., Johnson, M. D., & Tetirick, J. C. (2005). The vane of childhood amnesia for autobiographical and public event memories. *Memory, 13*, 161–173.
Nelson, K. (1993). The psychological and social origins of autobiographical memory. *Psychological Science, 4*, 7–14.
Nelson, K. (2003). Self and social functions: individual autobiographical memory and collective narrative. *Memory, 11*, 125–136.
Newkirk, T. (1997). *The performance of self in student writing*. Portsmouth, NH: Heinemann/Boynton-Cook.
Olney, J. (1972). *Metaphors of self: The meaning of autobiography*. Princeton, NJ: Princeton University Press.
Polkinghorne, D. (1983). *Methodology for the human sciences: Systems of inquiry*. Albany, NY: State University of New York Press.
Polkinghorne, D. (1988). *Narrative knowing and the human sciences*. Albany NY: State University of New York Press.
Polster, E. (1987). *Every person's life is worth a novel*. New York: Norton.
Progoff, I. (1975). *At a journal workshop, The basic text and guide for using the intensive journal*. New York: Dialogue House Library.
Progoff, I. (1983). *Life study: Experiencing creative lives by the intensive journal method*. New York: Dialogue House Library.
Ricoeur, P. (1990). *Soi-mème comme un autre*. Paris: Seuil [Transl. (1992) *One self as another*. Chicago, IL: University of Chicago Press].
Ricoeur, P. (2000). *La mémoire, l'histoire, l'oubli*. Paris: Seuil [Transl. (2004) *Memory, history, forgetting*. Chicago, IL: University of Chicago Press].
Riley, K. P., Snowden, D.A., Desrosiers, M. F., & Markesbery, W. R. (2005). Early life linguistic ability, late life cognitive function, and neuropathology: Findings from the nun study. *Neurobiology of Aging, 26*, 341–347.
Ruth, L. (1987). Reading children's writing. *The Reading Teacher, 40*, 756–760.
Schaefer, A., & Philippot, P. (2005). Selective effects of emotion on the phenomenal characteristics of autobiographical memories. *Memory, 13*, 148–160.
Smallbone, S. W., & McCabe, B. A. (2003). Childhood attachment, childhood sexual abuse, and onset of masturbation among adult sexual offenders. *Sexual Abuse: Journal of Research and Treatment, 15*, 1–10.
Snowdon, D. (2001). *Aging with grace: What the nun study teaches us about living longer, healthier, and more meaningful lives*. New York: Bantam Books.
Stein, N. L., Trabasso, T., & Albro, E. R. (2001). Understanding and organizing emotional experience: Autobiographical accounts of traumatic events. *Empirical Studies of the Arts, 19*, 111–130.
Swora, M. G. (2001). Narrating community: The creation of social structure in Alcoholic Anonymous through the performance of autobiography. *Narrative Inquiry, 11*, 363–384.
Valverde, M. (2002). Experience and truth-telling: Intoxicated autobiography and ethical subjectivity. *Outlines: Critical Social Studies, 4*, 3–18.

Weiss, S. (2002a). How teachers' autobiographies influence their responses to children's behaviors: The psychodynamic concept of transference in classroom life. Part I. *Emotional & Behavioral Difficulties, 7*, 9–18.

Weiss, S. (2002b). How teachers' autobiographies influence their responses to children's behaviors: The psychodynamic concept of transference in classroom life. Part II. *Emotional & Behavioral Difficulties, 7*, 109–127.

Williams, E. (2004). Who really needs a "Theory" of mind? An interpretative phenomenological analysis of the autobiographical writings of ten high-functioning individuals with an autism spectrum disorder. *Theory & Psychology, 14*, 704–724.

Wilson, L. (2005). Biography, autobiography and history. *International Journal of Psychoanalysis, 86*, 155–158.

13

Expressive Writing: An Alternative to Traditional Methods*

Ewa Kacewicz, Richard B. Slatcher, and James W. Pennebaker#

Researchers and clinicians have begun to search for alternative treatments that are lower in cost and easier to implement than traditional treatment methods. One promising alternative is expressive writing. When people transform their feelings and thoughts about emotional experiences into language, their physical and mental health often improves. An increasing number of studies indicate that having people write about their deeply felt emotions and thoughts can result in healthy improvements in social, psychological, behavioral, and biological measures. Expressive writing offers an alternative to traditional therapies with the advantage of lower cost and greater accessibility. This chapter will begin with an overview of the writing paradigm followed by evidence supporting the efficacy of expressive writing, as well as its potential limitations. The more compelling reasons for why expressive writing works will be presented next. The chapter will conclude with possible real-world applications and future directions.

The Expressive Writing Paradigm

In the first expressive writing study, people were asked to write about a trauma or about superficial topics for 4 days, 15 minutes per day. We found that confronting the emotions and thoughts surrounding deeply personal issues promoted physical health, as measured by reductions in physician visits in the months following the study, fewer reports of aspirin usage, and overall more positive long-term evaluations of the effect of the experiment (Pennebaker & Beall, 1986). The results of that initial study led to a number of subsequent investigations, in our laboratory and by others, with a wide array of intriguing results. We briefly review the writing paradigm and basic findings below.

The standard laboratory writing technique involves randomly assigning participants to one of two or more groups. All writing groups are asked to

*Preparation of this paper was aided by a grant from the National Institutes of Health (MH52391).
Correspondence: James W. Pennebaker, Department of Psychology A8000, University of Texas, Austin, TX 78712 (e-mail: Pennebaker@psy.utexas.edu).

write about assigned topics for one to five consecutive days, for 15–30 minutes each day. Writing is generally done in the laboratory with no feedback given. Those assigned to the control conditions are typically asked to write about superficial topics, such as how they use their time. The standard instructions for those assigned to the experimental group are a variation on the following:

> For the next three days, I would like for you to write about your very deepest thoughts and feelings about the most traumatic experience of your entire life. In your writing, I'd like you to really let go and explore your very deepest emotions and thoughts. You might tie this trauma to your childhood, your relationships with others, including parents, lovers, friends, or relatives. You may also link this event to your past, your present, or your future, or to who you have been, who you would like to be, or who you are now. You may write about the same general issues or experiences on all days of writing or on different topics each day. Not everyone has had a single trauma but all of us have had major conflicts or stressors – and you can write about these as well. All of your writing will be completely confidential. Don't worry about spelling, sentence structure, or grammar. The only rule is that once you begin writing, continue to do so until your time is up.

Whereas the original writing studies asked people to write about traumatic experiences, later studies expanded the scope of writing topics to general emotional events or to specific experiences shared by other participants (e.g., diagnosis of cancer, losing a job, coming to college). The amount of time people have been asked to write has also varied tremendously from 10 to 30 minutes for 3, 4, or 5 days – sometimes within the same day to once per week for up to 4 weeks.

The writing paradigm can be powerful. If nothing else, the technique demonstrates that when individuals are given the opportunity to disclose deeply personal aspects of their lives, they readily do so. Even though a large number of participants report crying or being deeply upset by the experience, the overwhelming majority report that the writing experience was valuable and meaningful in their lives. Interest in the method has grown since the original expressive writing study, and by 2006 well over 150 studies have been published in English language journals. Below, we briefly summarize some of the more promising findings. For a more detailed and technical summary, also see a recent paper by Pennebaker and Chung (2006).

Effects of Expressive Writing

Researchers have relied on a variety of physical and mental health measures to evaluate the effects of writing. Writing or talking about emotional experiences relative to writing about superficial control topics is associated with significant drops in physician visits from before to after writing among relatively healthy samples. Over the last decade, as the number of expressive writing studies has increased, several meta-analyses either have been conducted or are currently being conducted.

Meta-Analysis Findings

The original expressive writing meta-analysis was published by Smyth (1998). It was based on 14 studies using healthy participants. The primary conclusions were that the writing paradigm is associated with positive outcomes with a weighted mean effect size of d = 0.47, and noted that this effect size is similar to or larger than those produced by other psychological interventions. The strongest effect sizes were for psychological (d = 0.66) and physiological outcomes (d = 0.68), which were greater than those for health (d = 0.42) and general functioning outcomes (d = 0.33).

Almost seven years after the Smyth article was published, another meta-analysis by Meads, Lyons, and Carroll (2003) was released by the Cochran Commission. In an analysis of dozens of studies, the author concluded that there wasn't sufficient evidence to warrant adopting the writing method as part of clinical practice. One problem that the report underscored was the lack of any large randomized clinical trials (RCTs) that were based on large, clearly identified samples. Coming from a medical background, Meads was befuddled by the fact that most of the experimental studies of expressive writing were more theory-oriented and not aimed at clinical application. Since the release of the Meads paper, a new wave of RCTs are now being conducted with a diverse group of patient populations.

Most recently, Frisina, Borod, and Lepore (2004) performed a similar meta-analysis on 9 writing studies using clinical populations. They found that expressive writing significantly improved health outcomes (d = 0.19). However, the effect was stronger for physical (d = .21) than for psychological (d = .07) health outcomes. The authors suggested that a possible reason for these small effect sizes were due to the heterogeneity of the samples. Writing was less effective for psychiatric than physically ill populations. Indeed, health improvements were exhibited by participants with a chronic illness (asthma or rheumatoid arthritis) after writing, relative to participants with chronic illness writing about neutral topics (Smyth, Stone, Hurewitz, & Kaell, 1999). Health improvements gauged by reduction in physician assessed disease severity provided evidence for the effectiveness of writing.

Immune System and Hormonal Effects

Writing and/or talking about emotional topics also influences immune functioning in beneficial ways, including t-helper cell levels as well as growth, antibody response to Epstein-Barr virus, and antibody response to hepatitis B vaccinations. Other studies are finding effects on wound healing, changes in objective symptoms associated with arthritis and asthma. Yet other projects report faster healing following surgery among participants with cystic fibrosis. It is beyond the scope of this paper to summarize these many effects. Interested readers are encouraged to read recent reviews by Lepore and Smyth (2002), Pennebaker and Chung (2006), and Sloan and Marx (2004a).

Autonomic and Cardiovascular Effects

Activity of the autonomic nervous system is also influenced by expressive writing. Among those participants who disclose their thoughts and emotions to a particularly high degree, skin conductance levels are significantly lower during the trauma disclosures than when they are describing superficial topics. Systolic blood pressure and heart rate drops to levels below baseline following the disclosure of traumatic topics but not superficial ones (Pennebaker, Hughes, & O'Heeron, 1987). In short, when individuals talk or write about deeply personal topics, their immediate biological responses are congruent with those seen among people attempting to relax. McGuire, Greenberg, and Gevirtz (2005) have shown that these effects can carry over to the long term in participants with elevated blood pressure. One month after writing, those who participated in the emotional disclosure condition exhibited lower systolic and diastolic blood pressure (DBP) than before writing. Four months after writing, DBP remained lower than baseline levels.

Objective Behavioral Effects

Behavioral changes have also been found. Students who write about emotional topics evidence improvements in grades in the months following the study (e.g., Lumley & Provenzano, 2003). Senior professionals who have been laid off from their jobs get new jobs more quickly after writing (Spera, Buhrfeind, & Pennebaker, 1994). Writing about intimate relationships is associated with the relationships lasting longer (Slatcher & Pennebaker, in press). Interestingly, relatively few reliable changes emerge using self-reports of health-related or social behaviors.

Self-Reports of Depression and Distress

Self-reports also suggest that writing about upsetting experiences, although painful in the days of writing, produces long-term improvements in mood and indicators of well-being compared to controls. Although expressive writing is a decidedly psychological intervention, it rarely has been applied to psychiatric populations. One reason for the hesitancy was a brief report by Gidron, Peri, Connolly, and Shalev (1996) that indicated that Israeli PTSD individuals who wrote about traumas reported increases in symptoms five weeks later. The Gidron procedure, however, required participants to read and openly discuss their writing with others in the group. Since then, several researchers (including Gidron) have reported positive effects with people reporting PTSD symptoms without the public reading of stories (e.g., Gidron, Gal, & Freedman, 2001; Nishith, Resick, & Griffin, 2002).

As of this writing, there are virtually no expressive writing studies with clinically depressed samples. However, several studies have found drops in self-reported depression or distress among people who have been classified as formerly depressed, or who initially reported elevated depression symptoms among mixed psychiatric, medical and community samples. Although most bereavement studies have not found expressive writing benefits among people with uncomplicated grief reactions, writing appears to be potentially beneficial for more traumatic grief experiences, such as suicide or murder (e.g., Stroebe, Stroebe, Schut, Zech, & van den Bout, 2002).

Procedural Differences in Expressive Writing Studies

Writing about emotional experiences clearly influences measures of physical and mental health. In recent years, several investigators have attempted to define the boundary conditions of the disclosure effect. Some of the most important findings are as follows.

Topic of Disclosure

Although some studies have found that health effects only occur among individuals who write about particularly traumatic experiences, most have found that disclosure is more broadly beneficial. Choice of topic, however, may selectively influence outcomes. Although virtually all studies find that writing about emotional topics has positive effects on physical health, only certain assigned topics appear to be related to changes in behaviors in other domains. For beginning college students, for example, when asked to write specifically about emotional issues related to coming to college, both health and college grades improve. However, when other students are asked to write about emotional issues related to traumatic experiences in general, no improvements in academic performance are found.

Over the last decade, an increasing number of studies have experimented with more focused writing topics. Individuals diagnosed with breast cancer, lung cancer, or HIV, have been asked to write specifically about their living with the particular disease. Similarly, people who have lost their job have been asked to write about that experience. In each case, however, participants are asked to write about this topic in a very broad way and are encouraged to write about other topics that may be only remotely related. For example, in the job layoff project, participants in the experimental conditions were asked to explore their thoughts and feelings about losing their jobs. Fewer than half of the essays dealt directly with the layoff. Others dealt with marital problems, issues with children, money, and health.

It has been our experience that emotional upheavals often bring to the fore other important issues in people's lives. We recommend that writing researchers and practitioners provide sufficiently open instructions to allow people to deal with whatever important topics they want to write about. As described in greater detail below, the more that the topic or writing assignment is constrained, the less successful it usually is.

Topic Orientation: Focusing on the Good, the Bad, or the Benefits

There are a number of theoretical and practical reasons to assume that some strategies for approaching emotional upheavals might be better than others. With the growth of the field of Positive Psychology, several researchers have reported on the benefits of having a positive or optimistic approach to life. A handful of studies were conducted to examine whether the effects of expressive writing differed for optimists versus pessimists. For example, in one study which examined adjustment to college among previously classified optimists and pessimists, Cameron and Nicholls (1998) demonstrated that overall, only participants in the disclosure condition (writing about thoughts and feelings only) had higher GPA scores at follow-up. However, they did find that only participants in the self-regulation condition (writing about thoughts and feelings towards coming to college and then formulating coping strategies) experienced less negative affect and better college adjustment to college over controls. Interestingly, optimists visited their doctors less in the following month if they had participated in either the self-regulation or disclosure condition, whereas pessimists only reaped these benefits if they had participated in the disclosure condition.

Along similar lines, Laura King and her colleagues have demonstrated that when instructed to write about intensely positive experiences, participants reported significantly better mood, and fewer illness-related health center visits than did those who wrote about trivial topics (Burton & King, 2004). In another study, students were asked to write about traumas in the standard way, a benefit-finding way, or a mixed condition in which participants were first asked to write about the trauma, and then switch to the perceived benefits of the trauma (King & Miner, 2000). Counter to predictions, the trauma only and benefits only participants evidenced health improvements whereas the mixed group did not. It could be that writing about the perceived benefits is enough to organize thoughts and feelings about a trauma, and to cope effectively. However, as evidenced from the mixed condition, if people aren't able to integrate their perceived benefits into their trauma story in their own way, writing may be ineffective.

Although several variations on the expressive writing method have been tested, none have been found to be consistently superior to the original method that encourages participants to freely choose their writing topic. Forcing individuals to write about a particular topic or in a particular way may cause them to focus on the writing itself rather than the topic and the role of their emotions in the overall story.

Actual or Implied Social Factors

Unlike psychotherapy and everyday discussions about traumas, the writing paradigm does not employ feedback to the participant. Rather, after individuals write about their own experiences, they are asked to place their essays into an anonymous-looking box with the promise that their writing will not be linked to their name. In one study comparing the effects of having students either write on paper that would be handed in to the experimenter or on a magic pad (wherein the writing disappears when the person lifts the plastic writing cover), no autonomic or self-report differences were found. The benefits of writing, then, occur without explicit social feedback.

Typing, Handwriting, and Finger-Writing

Although no studies have compared ways of writing on health outcomes, a few have explored if the mode of writing can influence people's ratings of the expressive writing procedure itself. Brewin and Lennard (1999), for example, reported that writing by hand produced more negative affect, and led to more self-rated disclosure than did typing. One possibility is that writing by hand is slower and encourages individuals to process their thoughts and feelings more deeply.

Recently, we have begun to test the idea of finger writing. In finger writing exercises, people are asked to use their finger and to "write" about a trauma as if they were holding a pen. Over the last 2 years, six expressive writing workshops have been given (see Pennebaker & Chung, 2006) in which participants have been asked to write for 5–10 minutes about an emotional topic on at least two occasions. People are typically asked to write using a pen; however, one time they are asked to write only with their finger. At the conclusion of each workshop, when asked to rate how valuable and meaningful each of the writing exercises was, individuals rate writing using a pen versus using a finger as equally valuable. Interestingly, women significantly prefer the finger writing to men because many felt freer to express some of their most secret thoughts. Indeed, in every workshop, several people reported that they used more swear words when finger writing compared to writing with a pen.

Timing: How Long After a Trauma

Is there an optimal time after a trauma that expressive writing would most likely work? Unfortunately, no parametric studies have been conducted on this. Over the years, we have been involved in several projects that have attempted to tap people's natural disclosure patterns in the days and weeks after upheavals. For example, using a random digit dialing in the weeks and months after the 1989 Loma Prieta Earthquake in the San Francisco Bay area, we asked different groups of people the number of times that they had thought about and talked about the earthquake in the previous 24 hours. We used a similar method a year later to tap people's responses to the declaration of war with Iraq during the first Persian Gulf War. In both cases, we found that people talked with one another at very high rates in the first 2–3 weeks. By the 4th week, however, talking rates were extremely low. Rates of thinking about the earthquake and war showed a different pattern: it took considerably longer (about 8 weeks) before people reported thinking about them at low rates (from Pennebaker & Harber, 1993).

More recently, we have analyzed the blogs of almost 1,100 frequent users of an internet site in the 2 months before and 2 months after the September 11 attacks. Rates of writing increased dramatically for about 2 weeks after the attacks. More striking was the analysis of word usage. Use of 1st person singular (I, me, and my), dropped almost 15% within 24 hours of the attacks and remained low for about a week. However, over the next 2 months, I-word usage remained below baseline (Cohn, Mehl, & Pennebaker, 2004). Usage of 1st person singular is significant because it correlates with depression (see Pennebaker, Mehl, & Niederhoffer, 2003 for review). What was striking was that these bloggers – who expressed an elevated rate of negative moods in the days after 9/11 – were generally quite healthy. They were psychologically distancing themselves from the emotional turmoil of the event.

Considering the current evidence, it is likely that defenses such as denial, detachment, distraction, and distancing may, in fact, be quite healthy in the hours and days after an upheaval. A technique such as expressive writing may be inappropriate until several weeks or months later. Indeed, we now encourage clinicians to delay their use of expressive writing until at least 1–2 months after an upheaval or until they think their patient is thinking "too much" about the event. Obsessing and ruminating about a trauma a few weeks after it has occurred is probably not too much; thinking about it at the same high rate six months later might in fact signal that expressive writing may be beneficial.

Timing Between Writing Sessions

Different experiments have variously asked participants to write for one to five days, ranging from consecutive days to sessions separated by a week, ranging from 10 to 45 minutes for each writing session, for anywhere from

1 to 7 sessions. In Smyth's (1998) meta-analysis, he found a trend suggesting that the more days over which the experiment takes place, the stronger the impact on outcomes.

Two subsequent studies that actually manipulated the times between writing failed to support Smyth's findings. The first, by Sheese, Brown, and Graziano (2004), asked students to write either once per week for 3 weeks or for 3 continuous days about traumatic experiences or superficial topics. Although the experimental-control difference was significant for health center differences, no trend emerged concerning the relative benefits of once a week versus daily writing. More recently, we had 100 students randomly assigned to write either about major life transitions or about superficial topics. Participants wrote three times, 15 minutes each time, either once a day for 3 days, once an hour for 3 hours, or three times in a little more than an hour. Immediately after the last writing session and again at one-month follow-up, no differences were found between the daily versus 3-times-in-one-hour condition. Indeed, at follow-up, the three experimental groups evidenced lower symptom reports than the controls after controlling for the prewriting symptom levels.

Time Until Benefits Are Seen

Expressive writing outcomes have been measured up to about 6 months after the writing sessions are completed. While some psychological and physical health changes may be immediately apparent, they may be fleeting. On the other hand, some effects may take days, weeks, months, or even years to emerge as significant changes on various measures, if at all.

Considering all the other variants on the writing method already mentioned, it would be difficult to come up with some standard time for follow-up. Instead, knowing the general time-course of proposed underlying mechanisms, and providing multiple convergent measures to validate specific outcomes may be a more practical approach in thinking about follow-up assessments.

Why Does Expressive Writing Work?

Over the last two decades, a daunting number of explanations have been put forward and many are partially correct. Ultimately, there may not be a single cause for a phenomenon as complex as expressive writing. The reason is twofold. First, any causal explanation can be dissected at multiple levels of analysis ranging from social explanations to changes in neurotransmitter levels. Second, an event that takes weeks or even months to unfold will necessarily have multiple determinants that can inhibit or facilitate the process over time.

This section will briefly summarize some of the more compelling explanations for the expressive writing-health relationship. Keep in mind that many of these processes occur simultaneously or may influence one another.

Individual and Social Inhibition

The first expressive writing projects were guided by a general theory of inhibition. These studies showed that people who had experienced one or more traumas in their lives were more likely to report health problems if they did not confide in others about their traumas than if they had done so (e.g., Pennebaker & Susman, 1988). The inhibition idea was that the act of inhibiting or in some way holding back thoughts, emotions, or behaviors is associated with low level physiological work. Further, people were especially likely to inhibit their thoughts and feelings about traumatic experiences that were socially threatening. Hence, individuals who had experienced a sexual trauma would be far less likely to talk about it with others than if they had experienced the death of a grandparent.

Emotions and Emotional Expression

Emotional reactions are part of all important psychological experiences. From the time of Breuer and Freud (1957/1895), most therapists have explicitly or tacitly believed that the activation of emotion is necessary for therapeutic change. The very first expressive writing study found that if people just wrote about the facts of a trauma, they did not evidence any improvement. Consistent with an experiential approach to psychotherapeutic change, emotional acknowledgement ultimately fosters important cognitive changes (Ullrich & Lutgendorf, 2002).

A variation on the emotional expression idea is that the benefits of writing accrue because individuals habituate to the aversive emotions associated with the trauma they are confronting. A test of a habituation model would be to see if people who wrote about the same topic in the same general way from essay to essay would benefit more than people who changed topics. Research on changes in autonomic reactions to distressing topics over the writing days tends to support features of this argument (e.g., Sloan & Marx, 2004b).

An alternative approach looks specifically at the topics on which participants write. If habituation is a strong argument, one would assume that the more you write about the same thing, the more you would habituate to it. If people wrote about different emotional upheavals, rather than a single topic, one could argue that they would have less opportunity to habituate. Empirical tests of this idea are mixed. In earlier studies, judges evaluated the number of different topics people wrote about across a 3-day writing study. Number of topics was unrelated to health improvements. Using a more mathematically sophisticated strategy, we attempted to learn if the content similarity of essays written by people in the experimental conditions in three previous writing studies was related to health improvements (Campbell & Pennebaker, 2003). The answer is no. If anything, the more similar the writing content was from day to day, the less likely people's health improved.

The Construction of a Story

One of the basic functions of language and conversation is to communicate coherently and understandably. By extension, writing about an emotional experience in an organized way is healthier than writing about it in a chaotic way. Indeed, growing evidence from several labs suggests that people are most likely to benefit if they can write a coherent story (e.g., Smyth, True, & Souto, 2001). Any technique that disrupts the telling of the story or the organization of the story is undoubtedly detrimental.

Although talking about the upsetting experience will help to organize and give it structure, talking about such a monumental experience may not always be possible. Others may not want to or even be able to hear about it. Within the discourse literature, particular attention has been paid to the role of written language in demanding more integration and structure than spoken language (Redeker, 1984; see also Brewin & Lennard, 1999). It would follow that writing – and to a lesser degree talking – about traumatic experiences would require a structure that would become apparent in the ways people wrote or talked about the events.

The Components of a Story: The Analysis of Cognitive Words

The degree to which individuals are able to cognitively organize the event into a coherent narrative is a marker that the event has achieved knowledge status and can be determined through the language people use. Words or phrases such as, "I now realize that..." or "I understand why..." suggest that people are able to identify when they have achieved a knowing state about an event. Consistent with this, linguistic analyses find promising effects for changes in insight and causal words over the course of emotional writing (see also Klein and Boals, 2001; Petrie, Booth, & Pennebaker, 1998). Specifically, people whose health improves, who get higher grades, who find jobs after writing go from using relatively few causal and insight words to using a high rate of them by the last day of writing. In reading the essays of people who show this pattern of language use, judges often perceive the construction of a story over time. Building a narrative, then, may be critical in reaching understanding or knowledge. Interestingly, those people who start the study with a coherent story that explained some past experience generally do not benefit from writing.

Writing as a Way to Change Perspective

A central tenet of all insight-oriented therapies is that through psychotherapy people are able to develop a better understanding of their problems and reactions to them. Inherent in this understanding is the ability to stand back and look at oneself from different perspectives.

Using a variety of computerized text analysis methods, we are discovering that people's linguistic styles can predict who benefits from writing. Linguistic style is reflected in function words, which include pronouns, prepositions, conjunctions, articles, and auxiliary verbs (Pennebaker et al., 2003). Analyzing three previous expressive writing studies, we found that the more that people oscillated in their use of 1st-person singular pronouns (I, me, my) and all other personal pronouns (e.g., we, you, she, they) from day to day in their writing, the more their health improved (Campbell & Pennebaker, 2003). If individuals wrote about emotional upheavals across the 3–4 days of writing but they approached the topic in a consistent way – as measured by pronoun use, they were least likely to show health improvements. The findings suggest that the switching of pronouns reflects a change in perspective from one writing day to the next. Interestingly, it doesn't matter if people oscillate between an I-focus to a we- or them-focus or vice versa. Rather, health improvements merely reflect a change in the orientation and personal attention of the writer.

Implications for Treatment

The purpose of this chapter has been to present expressive writing as an alternate low-cost intervention strategy for improving mental health. Evidence for the efficacy of expressive writing, its boundary conditions, as well as possible reasons for why it works were offered in an effort to gain a better idea of practical limitations in the real world. For this chapter and certainly for this book, the most important aspects of expressive writing include low cost, ease of implementation, and its proven efficaciousness in improving mental health.

Writing forces people to stop and reevaluate their life circumstance, which is especially relevant for people suffering from mental illness. The mere act of writing also demands a certain degree of structure as well as the basic labeling or acknowledging of their emotions. All of these cognitive changes have the potential for people to come to a different understanding of their circumstances without the restrictions of expensive therapy. This provides compelling evidence for the potential use of expressive writing as a low-cost alternative to traditional methods.

Despite the large number of promising studies, expressive writing is not a panacea. The overall effect size of writing is modest at best. It is still uncertain for whom it works best, when it should be used, or when other techniques should be used in its place. Despite these shortcomings, it is reasonable to assume that expressive writing methods have the potential to be used on a large-scale basis. Given the current status of the discipline, some recommendations for treatment may be of value.

- *Anonymity and confidentiality*. In the treatment world, there is often a sense that the therapist always knows best. Many therapists, then, feel as though they need to read whatever writing samples that their participants produce. Our research suggests otherwise. If finger writing is potentially beneficial, there may not be a need for participants to read their writings to others or to give them to a therapist.
- *Diaries, journaling, and number of writing sessions*. In some quarters, there is a belief that the more that people write, the better their health. Again, expressive writing research does not support this idea. It may be that a fixed number of writing sessions – perhaps only 3–5 – may be sufficient to optimize improvement. Too much writing, in fact, may simply begin to reflect the processes of rumination or obsession.
- *Flexibility in topic, timing, and genre*. It is often helpful for participants and therapists to have a structured treatment method. Although structure and organization may be manna to practitioners of CBT, all evidence suggests that too much structure in the writing world is not beneficial. Some people may not want to write about something. This may be a healthy defense for them at the time. Others may want to write in verse rather than prose. Encourage it. Some may want to write for an hour a day; others for 5 minute sessions at different times of the day. Why not? There is no good evidence that one type of writing is necessarily better than others.
- *Flipping out, cracking up, and going insane*. Some ethics or IRB committees (especially in medical schools – ironically) have raised concerns that if people confront upsetting issues, they may regress into serious mental

decline. This "flip out" hypothesis has never been observed in our lab. To bypass this remote possibility, however, we often tell our participants about the *Flip Out Rule*. Prior to participation, we simply explain the flip out issue. We then note that if they feel as though they might flip out to simply stop writing or to write about another topic. The *Flip Out Rule* has been effective for many years (Pennebaker, 2004).

- *When writing fails*. Expressive writing is much like every other intervention: it works for some people and not for others. Despite a great deal of research, we still can't predict exactly who will benefit. We have had people who have been in psychotherapy for years who immediately benefited from writing. We've had many people who found the expressive writing boring and irrelevant. Others have fallen into a trap of writing more and more without ever getting any sort of closure. Our recommendation is to encourage people to try the method for perhaps 4 days, 20 minutes a day. If they find the method unhelpful or aversive, then try something else. If it is beneficial, it might be wise to try something else as well.
- *Workbooks, manuals, workshops, retreats, and therapy*. Effective therapy often requires a therapist who is a strong believer in the methods he or she is using. There is also an occasional feeling of territoriality among believers in different treatment methods. "My treatment is better than yours because I have had the certified training and am using the certified materials from the Certified Institute." As should be apparent, the expressive writing method is not certified, licensed, trademarked, or copyrighted. A feature that may work well with one therapist may not be effective for another. At the end of the day, we encourage practitioners to experiment with expressive writing. See what works and reject what doesn't.

Conclusion

Our understanding of expressive writing and, indeed, all psychotherapy is in the very early stages of knowledge. When expressive writing works, it is probably due to a variety of causes and contexts. In the years to come, we welcome comments and suggestions of therapists and participants about expressive writing. Together, we can begin to build a better understanding of the power of writing among people in the real world.

References

Breuer, J., & Freud, S. (1957). *Studies on hysteria* (J. Strachey, Trans.). New York: Basic Books. (Original work published 1895.)

Brewin, C. R., & Lennard, H. (1999). Effects of mode of writing on emotional narratives. *Journal of Traumatic Stress, 12*, 355–361.

Burton, C. M., & King, L. A. (2004). The health benefits of writing about intensely positive experiences. *Journal of Research in Personality, 38*, 150–163.

Cameron, L. D., & Nicholls, G. (1998). Expression of stressful experiences through writing: Effects of a self-regulation manipulation for pessimists and optimists. *Health Psychology, 17*, 84–92.

Campbell, R. S., & Pennebaker, J. W. (2003). The secret life of pronouns: Flexibility in writing style and physical health. *Psychological Science, 14*, 60–65.

Cohn, M. A., Mehl, M. R., & Pennebaker, J. W. (2004). Linguistic markers of psychological change surrounding September 11, 2001. *Psychological Science, 15*, 687–693.

Frisina, P. G., Borod, J. C., & Lepore, S. J. (2004). A meta-analysis of the effects of written emotional disclosure on the health outcomes of clinical populations. *The Journal of Nervous and Mental Disease, 192*, 629–634.

Gidron, Y., Gal, R., & Freedman, S. (2001). Translating research findings to PTSD prevention: Results of a randomized-controlled pilot study. *Journal of Traumatic Stress, 14*, 773–780.

Gidron, Y., Peri, T., Connolly, J. F., & Shalev, A. Y. (1996). Written disclosure in posttraumatic stress disorder: Is it beneficial for the patient? *Journal of Nervous & Mental Disease, 184*, 505–507.

King, L. A., & Miner, K. N. (2000). Writing about the perceived benefits of traumatic events: Implications for physical health. *Personality & Social Psychology Bulletin, 26*, 220–230.

Klein, K., & Boals, A. (2001). Expressive writing can increase working memory capacity. *Journal of Experimental Psychology: General, 130*, 520–533.

Lepore, S. J., & Smyth, J. M. (2002). *Writing cure: How expressive writing promotes health and emotional well-being*. Washington, DC, US: American Psychological Association.

Lumley, M. A., & Provenzano, K. M. (2003). Stress management through written emotional disclosure improves academic performance among college students with physical symptoms. *Journal of Educational Psychology, 95*, 641–649.

McGuire, K. M. B., Greenberg, M. A., & Gevirtz, R. (2005). Autonomic effects of expressive writing in individuals with elevated blood pressure. *Journal of Health Psychology, 10*, 197–207.

Meads, C., Lyons, A., & Carroll, D. (2003). *The impact of the emotional disclosure intervention on physical and psychological health – a systematic review*. Technical Report 43 (ISBN 07044 24347), West Midlands Health Technology Assessment Collaboration, University of Birmingham, UK.

Nishith, P., Resick, P. A., & Griffin, M. G. (2002). Pattern of change in prolonged exposure and cognitive-processing therapy for female rape victims with posttraumatic stress disorder. *Journal of Consulting and Clinical Psychology, 70*, 880–886.

Pennebaker, J. W. (2004). *Writing to heal: A guided journal for recovering from trauma and emotional upheaval*. Oakland, CA: New Harbinger Press.

Pennebaker, J. W., & Beall, S. (1986). Confronting a traumatic event: Toward an understanding of inhibition and disease. *Journal of Abnormal Psychology, 95*, 274–281.

Pennebaker, J. W., & Chung, C. K. (2006). Expressive writing, emotional upheavals, and health. In H. Friedman and R. Silver (Eds.), *Foundations of Health Psychology*. New York: Oxford University Press.

Pennebaker, J. W., & Harber, K. D. (1993). A social stage model of collective coping: The Loma Prieta earthquake and the Persian Gulf War. *Journal of Social Issues, 49*, 125–145.

Pennebaker, J. W., Hughes, C. F., & O'Heeron, R. C. (1987). The psychophysiology of confession: Linking inhibitory and psychosomatic processes. *Journal of Personality & Social Psychology, 52*, 781–793.

Pennebaker, J. W., Mehl, M. R., & Niederhoffer, K. G. (2003). Psychological aspects of natural language use: Our words, our selves. *Annual Review of Psychology, 54*, 547–577.

Pennebaker, J. W., & Susman, J. R. (1988). Disclosure of traumas and psychosomatic processes. *Social Science & Medicine, 26*, 327–332.

Petrie, K. P., Booth, R. J., & Pennebaker, J. W. (1998). The immunological effects of thought suppression. *Journal of Personality and Social Psychology, 75*, 1264–1272.

Redeker, G. (1984). On differences between spoken and written language. *Discourse Processes, 7*, 43–55.
Sheese, B. E., Brown, E. L., & Graziano, W. G. (2004). Emotional expression in cyberspace: Searching for moderators of the Pennebaker disclosure effect via email. *Health Psychology, 23*, 457–464.
Slatcher, R. B., & Pennebaker, J. W. (2006). How do I love thee? Let me count the words: The social effects of expressive writing. *Psychological Science, 17*(8), 660–664.
Sloan, D. M., & Marx, B. P. (2004a). Taking pen to hand: Evaluating theories underlying the written disclosure paradigm. *Clinical Psychology: Science & Practice, 11*, 121–137.
Sloan, D. M., & Marx, B. P. (2004b). A closer examination of the structured written disclosure procedure. *Journal of Consulting & Clinical Psychology, 72*, 165–175.
Smyth, J. M. (1998). Written emotional expression: Effect sizes, outcome types, and moderating variables. *Journal of Consulting and Clinical Psychology, 66*, 174–184.
Smyth, J. M., Stone, A. A., Hurewitz, A., & Kaell, A. (1999). Effects of writing about stressful experiences on symptom reduction in patients with asthma or rheumatoid arthritis: A randomized trial. *Journal of the American Medical Association, 281*, 1304–1309.
Smyth, J. M., True, N., & Souto, J. (2001). Effects of writing about traumatic experiences: The necessity for narrative structuring. *Journal of Social and Clinical Psychology, 20*, 161–172.
Spera, S. P., Buhrfeind, E. D., & Pennebaker, J. W. (1994). Expressive writing and coping with job loss. *Academy of Management Journal, 37*, 722–733.
Stroebe, M., Stroebe, W., Schut, H., Zech, E., & van den Bout, J. (2002). Does disclosure of emotions facilitate recovery from bereavement? Evidence from two prospective studes. *Journal of Consulting & Clinical Psychology, 70*, 168–178.
Ullrich, P. A., & Lutgendorf, S. L. (2002). Journaling about stressful events: Effects of cognitive processing and emotional expression. *Annals of Behavioral Medicine, 24*, 244–250.

14

Workbooks for the Promotion of Mental Health and Life-Long Learning

Luciano L'Abate and Demián Goldstein

The purpose of this chapter is to provide a rationale and background for using self-administered, self-help workbooks to promote mental health in functional rather than dysfunctional individuals, couples, and families. If the goal of any science is to understand, predict, and control, then one needs to know how progress in science, law, industry, and medicine occurs. The first writer has maintained that understanding, predicting, and controlling deviant or dysfunctional relationships is not going to occur as long as face-to-face (f2f) talk remains the major if not the only medium of communication between participants (clients, patients, or subjects) and professional helpers. Progress takes place more efficiently, through writing rather than through talk. Consequently, if progress is to occur in the delivery of physical and mental health services, it will occur through writing and not through f2f talk. Current preventive and psychotherapeutic practices, based on the f2f talk-based paradigm, are not going to meet the mental health ills and needs of this or any other nation (L'Abate, 1999; L'Abate & De Giacomo, 2003). An evolutionary shift from talking to writing media will allow expansions to populations that were heretofore unreachable through f2f talk. These populations become reachable once writing, computers, and the Internet become the vehicles of service delivery and possible healing (L'Abate, 1992, 2001, 2002, 2003a, 2005a, b).

Understanding, Predicting, and Controlling Relationships through Prescriptive Writing

Control of deviant and troubled relationships was partially established in the last century through psychotherapy, while prevention of deviant and troubled behavior was established through a variety of structured programs, as already discussed in Chapter 1. However, both psychotherapy and prevention will not advance as long as they rely solely on f2f talk between professionals and participants. Why? Because both f2f talk is difficult and expensive to record and replicate. Talk is nonspecific, extremely variable, and uncontrollable (L'Abate, 1999, 2005a, b). Hence, attempts to make psychotherapy and prevention into separate sciences are bound to take time and expense. Furthermore, research about psychotherapy and its process, as well as prevention, as already argued in Chapter 1, will remain in the hands of few North American researchers who qualify for grants. Research will be out of reach from Main Street professionals. Recording, transcribing, and classifying psychotherapy or prevention audio-recordings is a very time-consuming job left for a handful of grant-supported researchers, not for professional helpers in private practice. Hence, the often-commented on gap between researchers and practitioners will only widen.

Advances can and will take place unless the processes of promotion, prevention, and psychotherapy occur through the writing medium between professionals and participants (Esterling, L'Abate, Murray, & Pennebaker, 1999; L'Abate, 2003a, 2004a, b). Why? Through writing one can keep records of the process, about what is occurring between professionals and participants. Instead of talk, participants should be required to rely as much as possible on writing rather than on just talk. Written protocols can be completed at home and sent back to professionals through the mail, Internet, or fax (Lepore & Smyth, 2002). This approach requires making homework assignments an integral part of preventive and psychotherapeutic approaches (Kazantzis, Deane, Ronan, & L'Abate, 2005; Kazantzis & L'Abate, 2007; L'Abate, 2005a, c). Through homework assignments one can actively and interactively intervene in helping participants become responsive and responsible for any positive changes in their lives, taking away the burden of responsibility off the shoulders of professional helpers. To attempt to help and heal all the people who are hurt through f2f talk is simply impossible. Psychotherapy and prevention are the last remaining fields of endeavor (in addition to preaching) where only f2f talk is required. The outcome is a veritable Tower of Babel, where extreme, unproven, sometimes harmful, and even ridiculous gimmicks and remedies are administered by duly licensed professionals who, for whatever reason, have forgotten and left behind their scientific heritages.

As a result, the only record of what has occurred between professionals and participants is found in the notes of professionals. These notes are kept private and there is no way one can find how accurate or complete they are. They cannot be used to prove whether improvement in participants has occurred. They are kept in the professional's private office. Those notes are not going to be used to improve one's professional practices. Furthermore, there is no way to find out how self-serving those notes are, even if they supposedly document process and progress in psychotherapy or in prevention.

This conclusion does not mean that f2f talk should be eliminated from the process of healing. On the contrary, it means that the written medium needs to be added to f2f talk in ways that will increase synergistically not only the power of both media, f2f talk and distance writing, but will also include nonverbal interventions (see Section III this volume. In most cases, however, in the not-too-distant future, distance writing, instead of just supplementing f2f talk, will most likely supplant it, especially in preventive and promotional interventions, as shown by the work of Seligman, Steen, Park, and Peterson, 2005). Greater control is established through writing than through talk (L'Abate, 1999, 2005a, b, c).

A Mental Health Technology for the 21st Century: Self-Administered Programmed Workbooks

The last quarter of a century has seen the rise of a completely American technology, the production of countless self-administered, self-help mental health workbooks to deal with just about any known clinical and nonclinical human condition for children, youth, adults, couples, and families (L'Abate, 1996, 2004a, b). A workbook consists of a series of written homework assignments around a specific topic to be answered in writing by participants. Workbooks supposedly are cost-effective, mass-producible, versatile, and specific enough to allow evaluation of the theory or model from which workbooks were derived (L'Abate, 2005a). However, recent results raise serious questions about the cost-effectiveness of workbooks in outpatient psychotherapy (L'Abate, L'Abate, & Maino, 2005). Instead of shortening the number of psychotherapy sessions with individuals, couples, and families, workbooks were found to lengthen it significantly, apparently increasing the involvement of participants in the process. Hence, one cannot longer claim, as the first writer has done repeatedly in the past, that workbooks are cost-effective, even though more research will be needed to reach a definite conclusion on this matter, as shown below. Whether the increased number of psychotherapy sessions would lead to greater efficacy is an open question that could not be answered in that research. However, this is the reason for including Goldstein's work below. Even though his workbook was administered to clinical inpatients, the important dependent variable to evaluate was the number of days in the hospital. This variable is needed to check on whether the results of L'Abate, L'Abate, and Maino's (2005) are a single time occurrence or are replicated by Goldstein's results. Consequently, if cost-effectiveness cannot longer be claimed for workbooks, perhaps other advantages may still justify their administration.

Workbooks and Their Advantages

Workbooks fulfill a variety of advantages while their disadvantages are yet to be discovered fully.

Mass-Orientation

Mass-orientation for workbooks is a given, because questions asked on a piece of paper or on a computer through the Internet are a much cheaper approach than if the same questions were asked verbally f2f by a professional helper. Professional time and expertise are a hundred times more expensive and less replicable than one or two pages of questions that can be administered before-consultation, between-sessions homework assignments, or after therapy-termination, through mail, faxes, and the Internet. Hence, the f2f talk paradigm of the last century is giving way to distance writing approaches reaching populations that cannot and will not be reached solely by f2f talk and helping to change troubled people's behaviors and relationships for the better. This potential is realized in the work by Seligman et al. (2005) using the Internet to reach a vast range of willing participants.

Versatility

This advantage means that a workbook can be administered under different conditions in different settings. For instance, workbooks can be administered f2f as structured interviews between professionals-in-training and participant, in spite of their cost. They can be used at a distance from participants when assigned as homework in addition to f2f talk-based sessions. They can be used in prevention and rehabilitation where mass-orientation and cost-effectiveness are important criteria to consider. They can be used solely or in conjunction with preventive or psychotherapeutic practices or medication (L'Abate, 2004a, b).

Specificity

The specificity of workbooks is achieved by their matching a referral question, a test profile, or a test score with a diagnostic label or a reason for referral. Given the diagnosis of depression, for instance, there are at least a half a dozen workbooks designed to deal with such a diagnosis. This specificity allows the fulfillment of a major desideratum of mental health practices: matching treatment with diagnosis in a way that cannot be reached and will not be reached when f2f talk is the sole medium of exchange between professionals and participants. If and when the match between evaluation and treatments is claimed to exist verbally (Beutler, 1989), it cannot be proven that it produced results.

Matching Diagnosis with Treatment

The goal of linking evaluation with treatment can be accomplished through the creation of *prescriptive* rather than solely *descriptive* or, at best, *predictive* diagnostic instruments (L'Abate, 1990, 1992). In addition to the *descriptive-predictive-prescriptive* distinction, we need to consider two other distinctions of relevance to evaluation using workbooks, and that is, the *nomothetic-idiographic* and the *direct-indirect* ones. Through workbooks we can use what is essentially a nomothetic approach and apply it in an idiographic manner, as discussed below. Furthermore, evaluation can be direct, as, for instance, a semantic differential, or indirect, as in the instrument to be described in the Problems In Relationships Scale (PIRS).

Through workbooks, the link between evaluation and intervention is straightforward and direct, in a way that would be difficult if not impossible to achieve verbally. If a workbook is derived from a validated list of items defining depression, as in the case of the Beck Depression Inventory or Hamilton Depression Scale, for instance, workbooks derived from both tests, as described below, are now directly linked to the diagnostic label of depression. Therapists would not need to demonstrate that, verbally or through therapy notes, they have followed a treatment plan that derives from the original diagnosis. The workbook itself will fulfill this function, allowing direct demonstration and documentation that there is indeed a direct link between evaluation and intervention. No wonder that the market for self-help programmed workbooks has increased exponentially in the last decade (L'Abate, 1996, 2004a, c).

Furthermore, as long as talk is used, it will be very difficult, if not impossible, to link evaluation with a specific form of treatment, as attempted conceptually in many instances but never substantiated empirically (Beutler, 1989; Hurt, Reznikoff, & Clarkin, 1991; Perry, Frances, & Clarkin, 1985). One could argue that as long as treatment relies mainly or solely on talk such a link or match will remain virtually impossible for the large majority of psychotherapists, or certainly difficult and expensive to accomplish even for those few who can do it. The use of treatment manuals has been one way of decreasing therapist variability. However, thus far no one has won any prizes through the use of manuals (Bleuter, 1991; L'Abate, 2005b). Again, research will be limited to those few, very skilled, specialized researchers who are able to obtain research grants. However, the majority of psychotherapists will be unable to participate in research activities because of the time and energy required to find such a link through the verbal medium. Publication trends in psychotherapy outcome research show a continuing failure to replicate crucial studies, plus a few other disadvantages that are peculiar to the nature of the spoken word. Writing, on the other hand, has the qualities of explicitness and specificity that cannot be found in the spoken word. Consequently, replication would take place at a much cheaper cost than would be the case with the spoken word. Writing can be replicated easily. The spoken word cannot. One advantage of programmed writing, among others, lies in its potential to solve the long-standing problem of linking evaluation with treatment in a more specific way than it can be accomplished through talk (L'Abate, 1992).

Test-Derivation and Theory-Testing

One way in which workbooks become interactive instruments of theory testing is through the construction of workbooks directly from test instruments. Among them, one can find workbooks on juvenile anxiety and depression and on adult anxiety, or on depression from Beck's Depression Inventory as well as Hamilton's Depression Scale. This link is achieved through a very simple, easy device. One can take all the items from any test or from any factorially or research-derived list of behaviors, signs, and even symptoms, and transform them into a workbook. This transformation is obtained simply by asking participants to define (in writing, of course!) each item in the list and give also two examples for each item. After completing this task, participants are asked to rank-order the items according to how much each item applies to them, from a great deal to nonapplicable. The rank-order is then used to administer all the subsequent assignments according to a standard format. This format is the same from one assignment to another, but with a different title for each assignment that follows the original sequence of rank-ordered items. Since almost all tests used in this fashion were copy-written, special permission was required to convert them into workbooks (L'Abate, 1996, 2002).

Using this simple device, therefore, workbooks can become nomothetic as well as idiographic. They can fulfill research functions in the sense that all participants can answer the same number of assignments, usually no more than six. They are also idiographic, in the sense that the sequence of homework assignments follows specifically what individual, couple, or family participants have deemed as applying uniquely to them.

Consequently, one can then transform most tests into active and interactive vehicles of theory-testing from a relatively inert, static, and passive collection of paper-and-pencil, self- or other-report instruments. This process has already taken place for both single or multiple score tests (L'Abate, 1996, 2002). Once a workbook has been derived from a theoretical or empirical model, it becomes a direct instrument of theory- or model-testing. This advantage adds to the versatility of workbooks. In addition to being mass-oriented and versatile, workbooks become another interactive way to verify the validity of theoretical models.

Levels of Theoretical Connectedness

Evidence to support or invalidate models of a theory can be broken down into three possible levels between evidence and theory. Workbooks have been developed from: (1) constructs, concepts, tests, or evaluative instruments that are conceptually similar but completely independent from theoretical models, strictly created from professional experience or clinical predilection, as found, for instance, in a workbook about arguing and fighting in couples (L'Abate, 1996, 2002), (2) constructs or concepts that are conceptually similar and somewhat related to theoretical models, as found, for instance, in different depression workbooks developed from different tests, like Beck's or Hamilton's, and (3) constructs or concepts that are completely and directly derived, i.e., driven from models of a theory itself, as in the case of many workbooks derived from models in a relational competence theory (L'Abate, 2005a). Consequently, there are workbooks that are *independent* of a theory but that are deemed to be conceptually similar to some of its models, as described below. There are workbooks that are in some way *related* to the models of a theory. There are workbooks that are completely and directly *derived* or driven from models of a theory.

In the case of relational competence theory (L'Abate, 2005a), there are workbooks that are independent from models of this theory but derived from models that are similar but independent from the theory. For instance, a model-derived workbook about depression may relate to a depression workbook developed from Beck's model of depression, as well as an empirically derived model of depression based on the MMPI-1 Content Scale (L'Abate, Boyce, Fraizer & Russ, 1992). An example of a theory-related workbook may be found in assignments in the Negotiation workbook derived from social exchange theory (L'Abate, 1996). Additionally, examples of theory-derived workbooks are: Intimacy, Planned Parenting,Who am I? Priorities, and Self-Other from the Selfhood model of personality propensities (L'Abate, 2003, 2005b; L'Abate & De Giacomo, 2003). Therefore, within these three levels, workbooks can be and are active and interactive vehicles of validation for models of a theory, relational or otherwise.

Bridging the Semantic Gap

There is another clinical advantage implicit into this transformation from statically inert tests into interactive workbooks. By administering a list of items defining any psychological construct or symptom, and asking participant to define them and give two examples, as discussed above, one is able to bridge the considerable semantic gap between professionals and participants (L'Abate, 2004b). Instead of giving a diagnostic label with serious and likely threateningly stigmatizing connotations, i. e., "depression," "anxiety," "severe psychopathology," or even "bipolar" or "schizophrenic disorder," the administration of a workbook constructed from test items or any other list of items, allows participants to learn exactly what is meant by labels or diagnoses assigned to them by professionals. This process would demythologize a great deal of the professional jargon that keeps participants distant from professionals in a one-down positions, because the use of the diagnostic label attributes the professional powers that participants likely have not acquired yet (L'Abate, 2004b).

Increase in Feedback Loops

Furthermore, instead of one feedback change loop from professionals to participants through f2f talk, which is essentially a nonspecific and relatively expensive medium of communication, workbooks increase the number of feedback change loops available to participants. For instance, participants now have to answer questions that they may have never been asked before. This process could be conceived as a form of self-monitoring, especially if it takes place at specific, predetermined times and places. Participants now have to think on their own about how to answer each question, rather than talking to a professional. If they have a partner or family members who are answering the same set of questions separately, they can set appointment times to exchange, compare, contrast, and discuss their answers with those of others. Even if participants have no one to discuss their answers with, like single adults or single parents, their completed assignments become grist for discussion with the professionals who administered the workbook, as would be the case with couples and parents.

Disadvantages of Workbooks

Research about possible disadvantages of workbooks is still lacking. Resistance to their use in clinical practice comes from deeply and rigidly entrenched professional helpers who still believe in the power of personal f2f contact and talk and are unwilling to change their practices, while paradoxically claiming to help others change (L'Abate, 1997, 1999). Possible disadvantages derive from a mismatch between the reason for referral or condition and the chosen workbook. In the case of workbooks presented at the end of this chapter, their aim is to help improve mostly those with nonclinical conditions or clinical conditions who have improved after therapy is terminated and who need "booster-shots" toward normalization. Hence, there should be little danger of a mismatch. Failing to evaluate objectively any condition might also lead to a mismatch that would be perilous for participants who take it upon themselves to self-administer workbooks without professional consultation.

There is no question that future applications of workbooks will bring to light more objectively their advantages and disadvantages.

Research on the Clinical Usefulness of Workbooks

Research advantages of workbooks will be illustrated through summaries of a few exemplary research projects. For a more extensive review of past research, the reader can consult an entire chapter devoted to a detailed description of research studies performed years ago in the first author's laboratory (L'Abate, 2004b).

Evaluation of Workbooks with Individuals

Three research projects will be summarized here to illustrate how programmed writing can help us perform research functions at a cheaper and faster rate than the verbal modality (L'Abate et al., 1992). In the first study, undergraduates were selected for scoring on the upper third or half of the distribution on two paper-and-pencil tests for depression, the Center for Epidemiological Studies Depression scale (CES-D) and the Beck Depression Inventory (BDI). In a pilot study, participants were divided into four groups. A control group (N = 16) received nothing and was retested at the same time as the other three experimental groups. A second group (N = 13) received a workbook developed from this author's model of depression (L'Abate, 1986). A third group (N = 10) was administered a workbook developed from Beck's cognitive theory and treatment of depression (Beck, 1976). A fourth group (N = 11) received a depression book patterned after the Minnesota Multiphasic Personality Inventory-2 Content Scale of depression (Butcher, Graham, Williams, & Ben-Porath, 1990). This workbook is available in L'Abate et al. (1992). None of these participants was ever seen f2f. The whole treatment was performed entirely through the mail. The average depression scores for all four groups before treatment were 25.83 (S.D. = 7.88) for the BDI and 34.95 (S.D. = 10.14) for the CES-D. On posttest after treatment (about 7–8 weeks), the control group means were 19.94 (S.D. = 7.54) on the BDI and 30.12 (S.D. = 8.91) on the CES-D. The means for the three treatment groups were 10.26 (S.D. = 11.34) on the BDI and 28.37 (S.D. = 13.09) for the CES-D.

These results failed to reach statistical significance, but were suggestive and encouraging enough to repeat and replicate the same procedure with another sample of undergraduates. In this sample, the control group (N = 14) scored 22.79 (S.D. = 4.66) on the BDI and 34.21 (S.D. = 8.83) on the CES-D on pretest and 19.17 (S.D. = 8.82) on the BDI and 30.00 (S.D. = 8.55) on the CES-D on posttest. The three experimental groups scored means of 23.37 (S.D. = 7.42) on the BDI and of 33.28 (S.D. = 8.12) on the CES-D on pretest. On posttest these groups scored means of 12.52 (S.D. = 8.13) on the BDI and 10.68 (S.D. = 10.23) on the CES-D. An ANCOVA for repeated measures (4 × 2 × 2) yielded a $F = 5.91$ (df, 3, 63), $p < .001$ for the BDI. The same level of significance resulted for the CES-D ($F = 7.18$, df, 3, 63), $p < .001$).

A second study explored the effectiveness of using programmed and open-ended writing as treatment for generalized anxiety in undergraduates. They were selected on the basis of their T-scores above 65 on the Anxiety Content Scale of the MMPI-2 (ACS). From a pool of volunteers there were 35 males and 37 females who were randomly assigned to one of three treatment groups. In the programmed writing group there were 13 males and 13 females. In the open-ended writing group there were 11 males and 12 females. In the comparison, control group there were 11 males and 12 females. From the original group of 72 participants, 71.4% of the males and

81.1% of the females completed the study. They were administered Spielberger's State Trait Anxiety Inventory (STAI) as well as the ACS before and after completion of all written assignments. The programmed writing group received six homework assignments designed to treat anxiety on the basis of the DSM-III definition of generalized anxiety disorder. The open-ended group was asked to write about anything that came to mind for about 30 minutes once a week for 6 weeks, just as the first treatment group. The control group were tested before and after without any treatment. A factorial ANCOVA yielded significant treatment effects (p. $< .05$), that is, significant mean scores reduction, on the ACS and on the state Anxiety scale of the STAI with no significant interactions or gender effects. Trait anxiety scores remained unchanged. There were no significant differences between programmed and open-ended homework assignments, a finding that substantiates Pennebaker's work (2001), as well as the replications of his work by Murray and his associates (Murray, Lamnin, & Carver 1989). An examination of the open-ended writings indicated that most of them were focused on anxiety related topics, since this was the initial set for the study.

This approach can be accomplished with individuals using an objective test like the MMPI-2. To determine the effectiveness of programmed writing in lowering the peak scores on the MMPI-2 Content scales (Butcher et al., 1990), 54 undergraduate participants were administered this test on a before-after basis. They were randomly assigned to one of three groups, a control group without homework assignments, a group with workbooks designed to match each of the 15 Content Scales (L'Abate, 1992), and another experimental group that in addition to programmed writing received written feedback about and after each assignment was turned in. As in all the previous studies, personal contact between participants and experimenters was either nonexistent or minimized. One-way MANOVA was used to examine mean differences in peak scores subtracted from average profile elevation of the remaining 14 scores on the Content Scales on a pre-post treatment basis. Although between-groups effects yielded no significant difference ($F = 2.03$; df[.]2,5, $p > .14$) among the three groups, the within-effect yielded a significant difference among these same groups ($F = 24.12$; df[.]2,51, $p < .001$). Although the mean peak scores decreased significantly, in this study, the control group's mean peak scores went down as well as those of the two control groups, decreasing the validity of the results. Some additional findings concerned the validity of the Content Scales, as related by the students' behavior during the study. For instance, students scoring highest on the Type A Personality Scale were the most prompt in returning assignments, while those scoring highest on the Antisocial Practices Scale handed in incomplete assignments, made the most excuses, were often late, and dropped out the most from the study. Nonetheless, in spite of the questionable statistical significance of the results, where control groups decreased their mean scores as well as those of the experimental group, this study supported the thesis that programmed writing can be linked to evaluation on a prescriptive-idiographic basis (L'Abate, 2002, 2003a, 2005a).

The proposed classification of workbooks shown in Table 14.1 illustrates how it is possible to make systematic sense of an otherwise unyielding mass of information (L'Abate, 2004c).

Table 14.1. Toward a Classification of Workbooks.*

Participants Composition: Children, Adolescents, Single Adults, Couples, Families
Theoretical Orientation: Theory-derived or driven versus theory-free directly or indirectly, and based solely on clinical experience or on research data.
Format: Fixed-nomothetic versus Flexible-idiographic or both
Derivation: From referral question versus single score tests (e.g., BDI) or from multi-dimensional test profiles (e.g., MMPI-2).
Style: Linear-straightforward versus circular-paradoxical
Level of Functionality:Normalization, Externalization, Internalization, Severe Psychopathology.
Content: addictions, affective disorders, acting-out disorders, intimacy, etc. (L'Abate, 1996, 2004a)

* Adapted from L'Abate, 2004c.

A Problem Solving "Problem-Solving Workbook"

This workbook (Goldstein, 2002, 2004) was administered at the SOE (Observation and Evaluation Service) which is part of the Acute Inpatient Emergency Unit (AIEU) of the Hospital de Salud Mental Dr. Braulio Moyano of Buenos Aires, Argentina. This Hospital serves female inpatients between the ages of 18 and 65. The SOE has been established to seek faster and accurate discharge of acute inpatients, thus avoiding a long-term hospitalization. Treatment modality is chosen according to the degree of decompensation present (psychosis, impulsivity, depression, etc.). Subsequent planning is based on whether the participant may be discharged within a 4-day period, or else be admitted to a longer-term service. In this hospital, there are insufficient professional resources available because most of the professionals serve *pro bono*. They do so because of the large amount of easily available participants who provide a solid learning experience, and who otherwise would not receive any treatment. The two major avenues of treatment are medication and very short-term crisis psychotherapy. Many cases consist of decompensated Axis II personality disorders who have undergone some form of crisis or trauma.

Within the context of a public charity hospital, a workbook may reduce the number of f2f sessions by training participants in problem solving, decision making, and greater assertiveness through homework assignments. The theoretical basis of this workbook derives from the work of D'Zurilla and Nezu (1982, 1999). The frame in which this workbook was formatted relied heavily on Cognitive Behavioral Therapy (Beck, 1976). It follows the principles of programmed writing (L'Abate, 1992). Assignments follow a logical sequence with each assignment stating its specific purpose, separating diagnostic from problem-solving questions. Participants are asked to: (1) define terms, (2) describe the possible benefits of proposed changes, and (3) elaborate on ways each topic is relevant to its specific condition. To produce change at the cognitive level, each assignment contains specific sub-assignments for certain relevant behaviors. Participants in this hospital have plenty of time to complete assignments, since they do not receive a great deal of attention from the meager number of staff members. For a more detailed explanation of this workbook, the reader may consult Goldstein (2004).

The workbook was administered to 40 Participants picked at random, diagnosed with DSM-IV criteria for Axis I and Axis II disorders. This sample included 12 Personality Disorders (PD), 12 Borderline, 8 Histrionic,

8 Dependent, and 2 Narcissistic. Workbooks were not administered to participants with Axis II Cluster A disorders, Avoidant, Obsessive Compulsive, and Antisocial Personality Disorders. Some comorbidity occurred with Axis I disorders, such as Bipolar II, Major Depressive Episodes, Dysthimic Disorder, and Substance Dependency (the most prominent were alcohol, pychopharmacological agents, and illegal drugs). The average age for participants with Histrionic PD was 40 years, Borderline participants ranged between 20 and 35 years, and Dependent PD participants between 40 and 50 years (Goldstein & Molina, 2004). A control group of 20 participants with similar characteristics as those described above was selected. These participants were treated by the same team, with the same pharmacological guidelines, but no workbook was administered. In many cases it was possible to discharge participants much faster when the workbook was completed. The main conflict promoting the decompensatory crisis was circumscribed, which made it easier to work directly with the most relevant issues. Length of stay was reduced from 8+/−1 day without workbook, to 4+/−1 day with workbook. Workbook administration, therefore, helped reduce the length of stay by 50%. This significant outcome has a direct impact on per-patient costs and other administrative issues, such as a higher bed rotation.

This workbook was provided as a donation from Janssen-Cilag Pharmaceutical Company. They printed a total of 800 copies at a cost of US $0.35 each. The average cost of full hospital stay and treatment at the AIEU per day per participant is about US $25. If the workbook helped reduce the length of stay in participants with PD by 50%, the cost per participant was reduced by US $100. Since 40% of the participants coming to this hospital are diagnosed with PD with an average of 1,000 hospital participant a year with 400 with PD diagnoses, the savings could reach up to US $40,000 a year! This savings could cover approximately 7 yearly salaries for psychiatrists or psychologists. This in turn could improve the provision of inpatient care and further outpatient services. It is noteworthy that the average readmission rate of Participants who used the workbook was 10%, after 4 months of discharge. Participants who were not administered the workbook showed a readmission rate of 20% after 4 months of discharge. Results from this pilot study are summarized in Table 14.2. They need replication from other inpatient and outpatient settings.

Finally, there was an increase in the DSM-IV's Global Assessment of Functioning (GAF) scores. Participants who were administered the workbook showed an increment of 30% in the posttreatment GAF score after one month of discharge, compared to baseline. Participants who did not receive the workbook showed no change in their GAF scores, or else they showed an average 10% increase compared to baseline. These results tend to disagree with those found in L'Abate et al. (2005) study with an outpatient rather than

Table 14.2. Results for two samples of participants with or without workbook administration.

	Average length of stay	N° of. Sessions	GAF range Pre Treat.	GAF range Post Treat.	Readmissions after 4 months
Workbook $n = 30$	4+/−1	3–5	50–70	65–75	10%
No Workbook $n = 20$	8+/−1	6–9	50–70	55–70	20%

with an inpatient population mentioned earlier. Hence, the jury is still out on the issue of costs. The question, then, remains: "Under what conditions will workbooks decrease or increase the number of therapy sessions in an outpatient or length of stay in an inpatient population?" Even more specifically, which workbooks foster dependency and which ones foster greater autonomy? However, the intriguing hypothesis raised by Goldstein's results suggests that workbooks may increase involvement and hence a greater number of outpatient sessions, while workbooks in a hospital setting may shorten the length of stay for inpatients.

Evaluation of Workbooks with Couples

We can obtain the same link between evaluation and treatment with couples using two different instruments to measure the same dimensions from two different vantage points, the direct and the indirect, using a nomothetic approach in an idiographic manner. A program in this context means the combination of two tests with an isomorphic series of programmed assignments that can be prescribed on the basis of agreements among scores on the two test profiles. For instance, to test a theory-derived model for intimate relationships, a prescriptive instrument and a workbook linked to it were constructed – the Problems in Relationships Scale and program (PIRS, L'Abate, 1992). Most marital problems and polarizations were summarized in 20 conflictual and polarized dimensions (dominant-submissive, weak-strong, oversensitive-undersensitive) that are the bases for the creation of the PIRS. This test consists of 240 items answered on a 5-point Likert scale.

The creation of this paper-and-pencil, self-report test took place in parallel with the development of an isomorphic workbook, whose assignments correspond to the 20 dimensions measured by the test, plus four personality propensities derived from a theoretical selfhood model: Selful, Selfish, Selfless, and No-self (L'Abate, 2005a). It became possible, therefore, to identify which of the 20 dimensions were the most conflictual in a couple and to rank them from the most to the least conflictual. Each couple, therefore, can then be administered only the assignments that correspond to their most conflictual dimensions. In this fashion, we have a nomothetic method in the test and in the workbook. The administration of specific assignments for each couple, however, is idiographic to fit the specific dimensions reported by each couple. The validity of a total discrepancy score was substantiated by its negative correlation with the Spanier Dyadic Adjustment Scale (McMahan & L'Abate, 2001).

Using the same rationale, a simpler instrument to parallel the one just presented was created. This Semantic Differential (SD) instrument consists of 7-points ratings for each of the 20 dimensions of polarization; the participant rates self and partner. The PIRS is an *indirect* (supposedly subtle!) way to assess couples and assign specific written homework assignments matching most conflictual dimensions. The SD format, on the other hand, is a more *direct* way to measure the validity of these rankings and of their more indirect counterparts on the PIRS. In addition, it gives a more straightforward view of how each partner perceives the other, which is not given by the PIRS, because of its indirection. Ideally, the administration and sequencing of assignments should be based on the convergent agreement concerning the most conflictful dimensions between the direct (SD) and the indirect test (PIRS), as well as discussions with each couple's consent (L'Abate, 1992).

In preliminary, informal, and unpublished research to evaluate the reliability of the PIRS, 18 couples drawn from the undergraduate volunteer pool at a large urban university were administered the PIRS twice, at the beginning and at the end of the quarter, with a minimum interval of about 4–6 weeks. A Pearson r was used to assess this test's reliability. The Selful and No-self scales for women were stable, while the Selfish and the Selfless scales were not. For men, only the Selfless scale was significantly stable. Some of these nonsignificant correlations were due to the effects of single, very deviant scores from one or two couples.

More relevant was the difference between means for men and women. On pretest, undergraduate women tended to score higher on Selflessness than men ($df = 32$, $t = 2.50$, $p < .05$), while clinical women seemed to reverse this trend in comparison to men. The No-self dimension was also significantly higher for women than for men ($t = 6.45$, $p < .01$). On posttest, differences between men and women on Selflessness ($t = 3.79$, $p < .01$) and in No-self personality propensities ($t = 4.82$, $p < .01$) persisted. To evaluate the concurrent validity of the Selfishness scale it was correlated with the Narcissism Personality Inventory (NPI) using another group of undergraduate participants. No correlation between these two scales was found, which suggested that Selfishness in the intimate realm may be quite different from narcissism as an intrapsychic dimension void of an intimate context. Of course, these suggestive data thus far gathered are based on too small samples to arrive at meaningful conclusions.

This approach, however, does indicate that diagnostic tests can be transformed into prescriptive workbooks, thus linking evaluation with treatment in a way that cannot be accomplished through talk.

Practice

Most of the research studies summarized above were conducted with functional populations of undergraduates, supporting the notion that workbooks can and should be used to promote mental health especially in populations that can use them the most, namely, functional ones. While most workbooks produced by the first writer (L'Abate, 1996) deal with symptoms and clinical conditions which place them outside the province of this chapter and this Handbook, there are, however, workbooks developed to normalize individuals, couples, and families who have successfully completed a preventive or psychotherapeutic program, or who, being without any specific symptom or reason for referral, could use help in becoming more "normal," or "functional," if that is humanly possible.

Consequently, this section summarizes workbooks that promoted mental health rather than prevented mental illness. By necessity, longer descriptions of most workbooks are found in L'Abate (2002, pp. 116–120).

Normative Workbooks for Individuals

Development of Emotional Competence

Emotionality is by now on the forefront of current hot topics in psychology. We realize as professionals and as humans that we need to "get in touch with our feelings." However, how is this process to occur? Certainly not through talk. It would take a great deal of professional time and energy to teach people how to achieve greater awareness of their feelings (as accomplished in Chapter 25 this volume, on emotional intelligence). Hence, the eleven assignments of this workbook condense the work of quite a few "emotion" theorists.

Emotional Expression (EE)

The previous workbook was produced according to a fixed sequence of assignments, this EE workbook, instead, consisted of 3+ assignments, and is based on a list of feelings that are to be defined first with two additional examples. Once this nomothetic task is accomplished, these feelings need to be ranked according to how they apply to the single participant. This idiographic ranking is used to administer assignments that will follow from the feeling that applies the most to the feeling that applies less frequently.

Self-Awareness

This workbook was developed by Piero De Giacomo (L'Abate & De Giacomo, 2003). It was expanded and translated into English by L'Abate. It consists of 12 assignments that can be administered either in a fixed or in a flexible format. Self-awareness is not only lacking in psychiatric participants (Beitman & Nair, 2004), but to some degree in functional individuals as well. Consequently, this workbook may be useful along the whole range of awareness, from too little to too much.

Emotional Intelligence

This workbook is based on the manual developed by Bar-On (1997). As in the case of the two preceding workbooks, the first assignment is prescriptive in the sense that all subsequent assignments follow from scores either from the original test and/or from the subjective rank-order given by participants.

Multiple Abilities

This workbook consists of 15 assignments that include a combination of most "intelligence" theorists as well as an extra one not contained in the work of those theorists, and that is: sex and sexuality.

Normative Experiences

Three different workbooks were developed from Goldberg's (1999) research. They are generic and neutral enough to be administered to relatively well-functioning individuals. All three are based on a beginning prescriptive assignment, a standard assignment to be assigned in subsequent sessions, and a concluding, follow-up assignment.

Social Skills

This workbook is based on an inventory by the same name, using the same flexible (3+) format available in some of the workbooks listed above.

Who Am I?

This workbook was developed from a model of developmental differentiation which is part of a relational theory of personality socialization in intimate relationships that is isomorphic with the DSM-IV (L'Abate, 2005a).

Priorities Workbooks

These workbooks were developed from a model of priorities that is part of a relational personality theory isomorphic with the DSM-IV (L'Abate, 2005a). There are workbooks for various stages of the life cycle: elementary, middle, and high school, college, and adulthood (3+ assignments).

Workbooks for Couple Normalization

Premarital Preparation

This workbook is designed to help couples prepare for marriage in better ways than they would without any direction or support (3+ assignments).

Relational Quality

Three workbooks (3+ assignments each) were developed from the work of Hassenbrauk and Fehr (2002). The workbooks listed all the possible features of couple relationships.

Workbooks for Family Normalization

Family Profile Form

The purpose of this workbook is to help families learn to communicate better than they have done in the past. It consists of defining and ranking various dimensions of family functioning with 11 assignments in a *fixed* format, introduction, 9 dimensions, and final follow-up.

Family Functioning

This workbook consists of defining and ranking various dimensions of family functioning developed by Bloom (1985) in ways that are complementary to the Family Profile Form (3+ assignments).

Planned Parenting

This workbook is based on various models included in a relational personality theory (L'Abate, 2005) isomorphic with the DSM-IV (10 assignments).

Relationship Styles

This workbook was developed by Piero De Giacomo and his collaborators (L'Abate & De Giacomo, 2003) from his Elementary Pragmatic Model of relationships (12 assignments).

Conclusions

How much evidence will be necessary to change traditional therapeutic practices based on f2f talk to include also both nonverbal and writing modalities? No matter how much research evidence one may muster, it is doubtful whether any amount of evidence will hold sway on traditionally current verbally-mediated preventive and psychotherapeutic practices. Ultimately, the decision to change and to incorporate new or perhaps more cost-effective practices may need to be mandated by third parties. Resistance to the use of writing in psychotherapy or preventive practices and research, either by itself or in conjoint with the verbal modality, is inevitable. As long as psychotherapy or prevention are based mainly on talk, progress in both fields will be slow and difficult, limited mostly to those few who can receive research grants.

Research with workbooks shows how it is possible to: (1) study comparatively different therapeutic models in the treatment of depression and reduce, at least temporarily, state anxiety through the use of programmed workbooks in student populations, (2) possibly increase coping skills in former participants, and (3) link and match evaluation with treatment through test scores or link specific symptomatologies with specifically matched workbooks. More relevant to the purposes of this Volume and this chapter, there are workbooks that can be administered to functional individuals, couples, and families when no symptoms or reasons for referral are present.

The advent of the new workbook technology will speed up progress in making mental health services more available to larger segments of the population that could not receive these services because of their cost. The future for their applications is wide open. Mental health professionals have nothing to fear about their applications decreasing their income. Workbooks, thus far, on an outpatient basis may prolong rather than decrease the number of therapy sessions. On an inpatient basis, they may shorten the length of hospital stays. Whether this length is associated with greater involvement and lasting improvement remains to be seen.

References

Bar-On, R. (1997). *Bar-On Emotional Quotient Inventory: User's Manual.* Toronto, ON: Multi-Health Systems.

Beck, A. (1976). *Cognitive therapy and the emotional disorders.* New York: Meridian Press.

Beitman, B. D., & Nair, J. (2004). *Self-awareness deficits in psychiatric participant: Neuro-biology, assessment, and treatment.* New York: W. W. Norton.

Beutler, L. E. (1989). Differential treatment selection: The role of diagnosis in psychotherapy. *Psychotherapy, 26*, 271–281.

Beutler, L. E. (1991). Have all won and must all have prizes? Revisiting Luborsky et al.'s verdict. *Journal of Consulting and Clinical Psychology, 59*, 1–7.

Bloom, B. L. (1985). A factor analysis of self-report measures of family functioning. *Family Process, 24*, 225–239.

Butcher, J. M., Graham, J. R., Williams, C. L., & Ben-Porath, Y. S. (1990). *Development and use of the MMPI-2 content scales*. Minneapolis: University of Minnesota Press.

D'Zurilla, T. J., & Nezu, A.M. (1982). Social problem solving in adults. In P. C. Kendall (Ed.), *Advances in cognitive-behavioral research and therapy*, vol 1. New York: Academic Press, pp. 202–274.

D'Zurilla, T. J., & Nezu, A. M. (1999). *Problem-solving therapy: A social competence approach to clinical intervention* (2nd edn). New York: Springer Publishing Co.

Esterling, B. A., L'Abate, L., Murray, E. J., & Pennebaker, J. W. (1999). Empirical foundations for writing in prevention and psychotherapy. *Clinical Psychology Review, 19*, 79–96.

Goldberg, L. R. (1999). The Curious Experiences Survey: A revised version of the Dissociative Experiences Scale: Factor structure, reliability, and relations to demographic and personality variables. *Psychological Assessment, 11*, 134–145.

Goldstein, D. F. (2002). *Cuaderno de resolución de conflictos, (Problem Solving Workbook.)* Printed and distributed by Laboratorio Janssen-Cilag of Argentina. e-mail: cognitas@fibertel.com.ar

Goldstein, D. F. (2004). Schema focused cognitive therapy: A stage specific schema workbook approach. In L. L'Abate (Ed.), *Using workbooks in mental health: Resources in prevention, psychotherapy, and rehabilitation for clinicians and researchers*. Haworth Clinical Practice Press, New York, pp. 129–139.

Goldstein, D. F., & Molina, F. A. (2004). *Crisis descompensatoria de los trastornos de personalidad* (Decompensatory Crises of Personality Disorders). Buenos Aires, Argentina; Bleu Editora.

Hassenbrauck, M., & Fehr, B. (2002). Dimensions of relationship quality. *Personal Relationships, 9*, 253–270.

Hurt, S. W., Reznikoff, M., & Clarkin, J. F. (1991). *Psychological assessment, psychiatric diagnosis, treatment planning*. New York: Brunner/Mazel.

Kazantzis, N., Deane, F. P., Ronan, K. R., & L'Abate, L. (Eds.). (2005). *Homework assignments in cognitive-behavioral therapy*. New York: Routledge.

Kazantzis, N., & L'Abate, L. (Eds.). (2007). *Handbook of homework assignments in psychotherapy: Theory, research, and prevention*. New York: Springer-Verlag.

L'Abate, L. (1986). *Systematic family therapy*. New York: Brunner/Mazel.

L'Abate, L. (1990). *Building family competence: Primary and secondary prevention strategies*. Newbury Park, CA: Sage.

L'Abate, L. (1992). *Programmed writing: A self-administered approach for interventions with individuals, couples, and families*. Pacific Grove, CA: Brooks/Cole.

L'Abate, L. (1996). Workbooks for better living. < *mentalhealthhelp.com* >

L'Abate, L. (1999). Taking the bull by the horns: Beyond talk in psychological interventions. *The Family Journal: Therapy and Counseling for Couples and Families, 7*, 206–220.

L'Abate, L. (Ed.). (2001). *Distance writing and computer-assisted interventions in psychiatry and mentalhealth*. Westport, CT: Ablex.

L'Abate, L. (2002). *Beyond psychotherapy: Programmed writing and structured computer-assisted interventions*. Westport, CT: Ablex.

L'Abate, L. (2003). *Family psychology III: Theory building, theory testing, and psychological interventions*. Lanham, MD: University Press of America.

L'Abate, L. (2004a). *A guide to self-help workbooks for mental health clinicians and researchers*. Binghamton, NY: Haworth.

L'Abate, L. (2004b). Systematically written homework assignments: The case for homework based treatment. In L. L'Abate (Ed.), *Using workbooks in mental health: Resources in prevention, psychotherapy, and rehabilitation for clinicians and researchers*. Binghamton, NY: Haworth, pp. 65–102.

L'Abate, L. (Ed.). (2004c). *Using workbooks in mental health: Resources in prevention, psychotherapy, and rehabilitation for clinicians and researchers.* Binghamton, NY: Haworth.

L'Abate, L. (2005). *Personality in intimate relationships: Socialization and psychopathology.* New York: Springer-Verlag.

L'Abate, L. (in press) What I really believe about family psychotherapy. Journal of Family Psychotherapy.

L'Abate, L., & Baggett, M. S. (1997). *The self in the family: Toward a classification of personality, criminality, and psychopathology.* New York: Wiley.

L'Abate, L., Boyce, J., Fraizer, L., & Russ, D. (1992). Programmed writing: Research in progress. *Comprehensive Mental Health Care, 2*, 45–62

L'Abate, L., & De Giacomo, P. (2003). *Intimate relationships and how to improve them: Integrating theoretical models with preventive and psychotherapeutic applications.* Westport, CT: Praeger.

L'Abate, L., L. L'Abate, B. L., & Maino, E. (2005). A review of 25 years of part-time professional practice: Workbooks and length of psychotherapy. *American Journal of Family Therapy, 33*, 19–33.

Lepore, S. J., & Smyth, J. M. (Eds.). (2002). *The writing cure: How expressive writing promotes health and well-being.* Washington, DC: American Psychological Association.

McMahan, O., & L'Abate, L. (2001). Programmed distance writing with seminarian couples. In L. L'Abate (ed) *Distance writing and computer-assisted interventions in psychiatry and mental health.* Westport, CT: Ablex, pp. 137–156.

Murray, E. J., Lamnin, A., & Carver, C. (1989). Emotional expression in written essays and psychotherapy. *Journal of Social and Clinical Psychology, 8*, 414–429.

Pennebaker, J. W. (2001). Explorations into the health benefits of disclosure: Inhibitory, cognitive, and social processes. In L. L'Abate (ed), *Distance writing and computer-assisted interventions in psychiatry and mental health.* Westport, CT: Ablex, pp. 33–44.

Perry, S., Frances, A., & Clarkin, J. (1985). *A DSM-III casebook of differential therapeutics: A clinical guide to treatment selection.* New York: Brunner/Mazel.

Seligman, M. E. P., Steen, T. A., Park, N., & Peterson, C. (2005). Positive psychology progress: Empirical validation of interventions. *American Psychologist, 60*, 410–421.

15

Computers and the Internet

Myron L. Pulier, Timothy G. Mount, Joseph P. McMenamin, and Marlene M. Maheu

Delivery of low-cost interactive multimedia-enhanced behavioral interventions by computer and Internet can achieve unprecedented public health impact (Clarke et al., 2005). Computer technologies and Internet communication offer the practical advantages of availability, adaptability, attractiveness, anonymity, and affordability (Maheu, Pulier, Wilhelm, McMenamin, & Brown-Connolly, 2005). Combining images, video, sound, music, text, and automatically generated speech, as well as supplementary e-mail communication with experts and peers, boosts clinical efficacy. Early research suggests a promising future for the prescription of technologically mediated "behavioral vaccines."

This chapter begins by focusing on theory related to applying communication and information processing technology to behavioral vaccines. Next, research covering the effect of technology on behavioral vaccine effectiveness and cost reduction is reviewed. Finally, practical considerations for delivering behavioral vaccines are discussed, including the Online Clinical Practice Management Model (Maheu et al., 2005).

Theory

Availability can determine whether a person takes advantage of a behavioral intervention. Prompt intervention following a traumatic event may improve long-term prognosis (Lange et al., 1999). The effectiveness of a behavioral intervention may thus depend on intercepting a consumer at a "teachable moment" (Stevens, Severson, Lichtenstein, Little, & Leben, 1995). Technology can enable a healthcare provider to take advantage of an opportunity when it would not be feasible to clear time or assemble personnel to deliver the intervention without it (Maio et al., 2005).

The classes of technology most applicable to delivering low-cost behavioral interventions are hardware devices (such as the computer), software programs, and information transmission channels (such as the Internet).

Today's computerized devices are very different from their slow, room-sized ancestors. Although the basic body plan of the ancient computers of the 1940s (Goldstine & von Neumann, 1946) is still in use, the evolution of computer technology has brought miniaturization, enlarged capacity, portability, greater speed, lower cost, and sophisticated "peripheral" devices.

The central processing unit (CPU) has become the almost invisibly small microprocessor at the heart of desktop computers and other devices. The CPU can quickly send data to a unit that displays information (e.g., a monitor or screen) or to a printer or other peripheral device, and can receive data from input devices such as a keyboard, mouse or microphone. Today's video recorders, telephone answering machines, and cellular telephones are all controlled by microprocessors, a sign of how computers are converging with other forms of equipment. These devices are becoming ubiquitous and part of a general information network, and hence are losing their individual identities.

Computer software requires more attention when it comes to exploiting technology for behavioral interventions. It is largely the software that determines how a user will experience a technologically delivered behavioral vaccine, thereby limiting what a vaccine can accomplish. Early computer programs were procedural; that is, they proceeded step-by-step toward completion in a linear fashion until the desired output was achieved. Current computer operating systems (such as Linux or Microsoft Windows) are input-driven and support multitasking. Input-driven means that the device is always ready to accept a user's input (e.g., a mouse click or keystroke) after which it responds, then awaits further input. In other words, it is capable of conducting a sort of dialogue. Multitasking means that the computer does many tasks at once, such as maintain a dialogue with several application programs simultaneously. Actually, computers are still procedural, but clever programming allows both programmer and user to take it for granted that the machine is truly input-driven and engaged in multitasking.

The input-driven style of today's computers supports the "feedback" capability that confers a major advantage on technologically delivered behavioral vaccines. Curiously, the need for feedback is what led to the development of computers. During World War II, hand-operated antiaircraft guns were no match for approaching airplanes that would twist and turn before delivering their lethal munitions. Mathematician Norbert Wiener helped develop the theory necessary for automatic rangefinders that predicted where a shell would strike an attacking aircraft based on the plane's recent trajectory. Wiener was intrigued not only with how intelligently the machines seemed to "learn" from their "experience", but also how they developed pathological behaviors – uncontrolled oscillations – when internal friction was reduced. From Arturo Rosenbleuth, who had worked with Walter B. Cannon (the developer of the concept of homeostasis), Weiner learned that injury to the cerebellum could produce similar dysfunction in humans. Wiener and his young collaborator Julian H. Bigelow came up with the idea of the feedback loop, where information about the effect of an action immediately corrects further action. Joined by neurophysiologist Warren McCulloch and other scientists in a series of seminars, Wiener developed the theory he named "cybernetics" (Wiener, 1948), Claude Shannon and Warren Weaver founded information theory (Shannon, 1948) and John von Neumann laid the basis for the modern computer (Goldstine & von Neumann, 1946).

John von Neumann's architecture allowed the modern computer to switch rapidly from one program to another. It seems as if the computer is dealing with all the programs at once. At first, computer capability was exploited for "time sharing," where users at several terminals (keyboards and displays wired directly to the computer) could each feel they were continuously "on line". This capability is now essential for a computer's ability to interrupt whatever it is doing, such as showing a video clip that is streaming in from the Internet, to service the user's input. It is also the basis for the computer's ability to provide the immediate corrective "feedback" that gives a technology-enhanced behavioral vaccine an advantage over standard ones.

In a network where a computer has several attached terminals, each giving and receiving data, it is relatively straightforward to substitute another computer for one of the terminals. Likewise, it is relatively straightforward to connect several computers together to form a network. Once many such communication networks were established on the campuses of large corporations, universities, and military installations it became desirable to create a network of networks – the Internet. The first node on the forerunner of the Internet began operation in 1969 (Leiner et al., 2005).

One of the earliest applications of the Internet was e-mail. Another Internet service is the World Wide Web ("A little history of the World Wide Web", 2005). Essentially, a user's Web "browser" program sends out a request for a particular "Web page". A special computer on the Internet locates the computer hosting that page and forwards the request. The host computer sends the page to the requesting computer, which displays it on its monitor screen. A user's click on specially marked "hypertext" on a Web page causes the browser to request a particular new page. Such "hot spots" (which may be parts of images as well as text) link pages residing on computers all over the Internet, hence the name "World Wide Web."

In addition to hosting e-mail communications, today's World Wide Web conveys sound, pictures, animation, and continuously streaming video, as well as entire behavioral vaccine programs. The main bottleneck in using the Web is no longer within the Web but a matter of connecting to it – the transmission channel.

Most people in the US have access to the Internet at home or in public libraries, schools and workplaces. High-speed transmission channels, such as "DSL" telephone service, cable access or linkage through an overhead satellite are replacing slower conventional telephone connections to ISPs and enabling users to receive streaming video of a quality sufficient for many purposes. When it comes to behavioral vaccines, if a connection is too slow or high quality video is necessary, a video segment can be transmitted slowly, in advance of its use, and stored on the user's computer, then played at full speed when the behavioral intervention is activated. Where the bottleneck comes in is when a consumer is not "at" a computer. Communication companies are rapidly rolling out technologies permitting connection to the World Wide Web through cell phones or other portable devices. At the same time, computer-like devices are becoming ever smaller, more portable and more capable, with flexible electronic books likely to be standard consumer items before the decade is out. When this happens, behavioral intervention modules loaded from or operating on the World Wide Web will be unequivocally more accessible, convenient, and effective than printed versions. Already, even people without Internet experience can easily learn to handle automated patient education and decision-support tools. As this proportion increases, using technology for behavioral vaccines will become fully accepted and perhaps even expected.

Research

Among questions to be addressed by research are:

1. Where can technology provide behavioral interventions or enhance their effectiveness without requiring much professional involvement?
2. Where would adding some supplementary professional involvement be cost-effective for a behavioral intervention delivered primarily by computer or Internet?
3. How much can technology increase the cost-effectiveness of a behavioral intervention?
4. How can technology assist research into low-cost behavioral interventions?

Enhancement of Effectiveness

Interacting with an automated system can be crucial for behavioral vaccine efficacy. While printed self-help manuals seem ineffective for stopping a cigarette habit, feedback and outreach improve quitting rates. This suggests that hand-held computers and the Internet could be valuable in such efforts (Curry, Ludman, & McClure, 2003). Computer interaction enhanced women's realistic expectations about hormone replacement therapy (Rostom, O'Connor, Tugwell, & Wells, 2002). Introduction of computer technology increased the impact of an educational initiative for preventing sun-induced skin cancer (Hornung et al., 2000). HIV-infected participants who used the CHESS (Comprehensive Health Enhancement Support) system daily on their home computers experienced improved health and daily function (Gustafson et al., 1999). An 8-session self-administered cognitive-behavioral therapy CD-ROM program without added therapist input was associated with decreased eating disorder symptoms, particularly self-induced vomiting (Bara-Carril et al., 2004). Beating the Blues, an interactive multimedia cognitive-behavioral program, brought about improvements in depression and anxiety as well as in work and social adjustment when set up in a self-care center and operated under minimal supervision by a nurse (Proudfoot et al., 2004). Experience with self-help programs delivered to a home or library over the Web or by phone shows that many people suffering from various disorders can benefit significantly with little or no intervention by a clinician (Gega, Marks, & Mataix-Cols, 2004). The Fear Fighter program, transmitted to a patient's home through the Internet, produced satisfaction and significant improvement in a small open study (Kenwright, Marks, Gega, & Mataix-Cols, 2004). Self-treatment at home using a manual and a computer-driven telephone interview system (BT STEPS) enabled people with obsessive-compulsive disorder to reduce symptoms (Nakagawa et al., 2000).

Decision aids for participants are increasingly available over the Internet and may be judiciously prescribed by healthcare professionals. Taking advantage of the interactivity and adaptability of presentations delivered by computer and Internet, they differ from the usual patient education materials in being individualized and specific and in promoting decisions that are consistent with personal values. Many have been shown in controlled trials to improve knowledge and realistic expectations and to enhance participants' collaboration in decision making (O'Connor et al., 2005).

Adherence to treatment plans, particularly taking medication, is another area where computers and the Internet can supply effective intervention at low cost (Haynes, McDonald, Garg, & Montague, 2002). It can be difficult for the prescribing physician to assess compliance. A combined medication-dispensing device and electronic diary seemed to enable participants with schizophrenia to increase antipsychotic adherence from 50% to 94% of doses (Baker, 2005). The videocassette-sized Med-eMonitor http://www.informedix.com/med_emonitor.html records when the patient opens a compartment to obtain a dose of medicine. It also includes reminder and electronic diary functions and supports two-way communication with a clinician. The MEMS (Medication Event Monitoring System), a tiny microprocessor in the cap of a standard prescription bottle that records the time the container is opened (George, Peveler, Heiliger, & Thompson, 2000), can operate in concert with a computerized telephone system. The system can conduct an in-depth discussion with a patient about his or her reliability in taking medication, about "pocketing" medication "for later", and about how adherence might be enhanced (Farzanfar, Frishkopf, Friedman, & Ludena). Simply providing weekly graphic feedback reflecting a patient's pill-taking behavior enhanced compliance during a smoking cessation trial (Schmitz, Sayre, Stotts, Rothfleisch, & Mooney, 2005).

A less expensive "memory prosthetic" is a computer-generated telephone message or a beep on a pager to remind a patient or family to take a dose of medicine or to write down some observation (Milch, Ziv, Evans, & Hillebrand, 1996). Simplest and least costly of all is a computer program targeted at people who are already sitting at a computer. People experimentally advised to take stretch breaks while working at a computer actually obeyed (Monsey et al., 2003), and in one study suffered less skeletal discomfort (Fenety & Walker, 2002).

Benefit of Professional Supplementation

Some studies suggest that a small investment of time by a healthcare professional can boost a consumer's healthcare activity into being effective, and ultimately save professional time overall. Just the feeling that one is in contact with or watched by one's therapist or some knowledgeable and caring professional or authority may in itself be a powerful motivator, and reduce anxiety and enhance morale and patience. For example, daily home telehealth monitoring may have produced lower service utilization than more intensive weekly monitoring (Chumbler, Neugaard, Ryan, Qin, & Joo, 2005). A purely Internet-based intervention reduced self-reported depression in people also receiving standard treatment, provided that it was supplemented by e-mail and, if necessary, telephone reminders to continue participation (Clarke et al., 2005). In one lengthy 68-week clinical trial, regular contact with the research team maintained a remarkably high level of participation of families despite heavy demands of the study (Hellard, Sinclair, Forbes, & Fairley, 2001). Adding individual behavioral counseling through e-mail to a fully automated Web-based weight loss program enhanced success (Tate, Jackvony, & Wing, 2003). Subjects recruited by way of a Web site completed a highly structured series of writing assignments and received personalized feedback by e-mail from specially trained graduate students. The subjects reported marked relief of symptoms characteristic of posttraumatic stress disorder and fared significantly better than a randomized control group (Lange et al., 2003).

A technology-induced feeling of ongoing human contact might approach the impact of an in-person encounter in boosting the gain from bibliotherapy and other self-help and vaccine methods. Minimal-contact techniques for inducing such a feeling can range from a brief telephone interchange (Febbraro, 2005), through a system that allows a client to periodically transmit or record progress reports via a symptom diary that eventually will come to a clinician's attention, to having a client send e-mail messages (Tate & Zabinski, 2004). People who received professional feedback in the course of writing about their stress symptoms reported feeling close to therapists they never saw (Lange et al., 2003).

Just how much professional time, if any, is necessary to achieve the goals of a behavioral intervention is likely to vary with the characteristics of the participants and the problems being addressed (Tate et al., 2003). In one study an already effective eight-session CD-ROM based cognitive-behavioral intervention for bulimia nervosa was not further enhanced by three supplementary brief focused support sessions with a therapist (Murray et al., 2007). When it comes to weight loss, habit control and many other efforts, however, people by and large do not persist long on their own and soon are back in the "self-help" section of their bookstores seeking another approach, raising the question whether supplementing self-help with at least some oversight by a professional may be needed.

Cost Reduction

Technological enhancement of behavioral vaccine delivery seems to be highly cost-effective (McCrone et al., 2004) and to free clinicians for other tasks, but there are intrinsic barriers to developing sound scientific evidence for this impression (Monnier, Knapp, & Frueh, 2003). A quantifiable standardized assessment approach to evaluating any complex telehealth project may not do justice to its actual utility (Hailey, Bulger, Stayberg, & Urness, 2003) and may fail to take into account hidden costs in staff time, morale and effort or to factor in risks that happened not to materialize during the study period (Finch, May, Mair, Mort, & Gask, 2003). When it comes to services for a nonclinical population, standard mental health assessment instruments may be insensitive to attainment of humanistic goals, so that measurement of the value of some interventions may best involve client-defined outcomes (Boulton et al., 2001). Some guidance in designing research into cost reduction attributable to technology may be found in the report of a survey of 26 randomized controlled trials of multimedia computers for adult patient education in physicians' offices. The survey report concluded that computerized patient education can indeed save professional time (Wofford, Smith, & Miller, 2005). The authors applied outcome measures that addressed clinical indicators, knowledge retention, health attitudes, shared decision-making, health services utilization and costs.

Some expensive mass public education campaigns, such as for improved diet or encouraging a rapid and lifesaving response to symptoms of an acute myocardial infarction, failed to meet their goals (Atkinson & Nitzke, 2001). It may be inefficient to attempt to educate the population as a whole in risk avoidance, timely recognition of a need for treatment, and finding (and accepting) appropriate assistance. An indiscriminate blanket approach to a population through television or printed pamphlets may not capture the attention and recruit the participation of those people who would benefit from an intervention. Computers and the Internet bring a markedly different economic structure. It is hardly more costly to reach hundreds of thousands of people than to reach one, and the cost of a technology-driven behavioral vaccine is overwhelmingly in its creation, not in its delivery or operation. Since the World Wide Web abounds in advertisements and entertainment, however, simply posting a behavioral intervention program on the Web may recruit few users. If privacy concerns can be satisfactorily addressed, sending e-mail to people known to be at special risk may be a cost effective way to initiate contact and arouse interest. Of an entire class of students in a university solicited by e-mail, 44 percent participated in a study of drinking alcohol and driving (Bendtsen, Johansson, & Åkerlind, 2006). After responding to a quiz about their behavior on the study's website and being presented with individualized feedback about how their answers compared with those of a normative peer group, some participants indicated increased interest in improving how they handled drinking and driving.

Where an intervention entails significant cost it becomes desirable to restrict delivery to people at special risk so as to concentrate resources on discretely but effectively promoting the intervention to a selected subset (Paperny, 2004). For example, it was suggested that a computerized intervention for decreasing misuse of alcohol might best show efficacy if administered specifically to adolescents who have experienced drinking and driving (Maio et al., 2005). When only a small fraction of a population is at risk, as in postdisaster disorders, the cost of accurately identifying such people and specifically targeting them may be impractically high (Friedman, 2005). Advances in detection of vulnerability to stress-related disorders may change this (Kaufman et al., 2004). Even inexpensive screening, however, such as restricting intervention to reverse the reported increase in childhood obesity to obviously overweight children would be unacceptably stigmatizing, and indeed no such screening trials have been reported (Whitlock, Williams, Gold, Smith, & Shipman, 2005).

One way to avoid stigmatizing individuals yet hold down the incremental cost for a behavioral intervention is to piggy-back the intervention onto some already ongoing activity and perhaps to shift the focus away from at-risk individuals and onto the level of the family. For example, because food selection is strongly influenced by family practices and attitudes Nicklas et al., (2001) suggests providing schoolchildren with a CD-ROM they could all use to "teach" their families to increase their intake of fruits and vegetables. Younger children could compose a school report on a before-and-after family knowledge and attitude survey as a long-term homework assignment to be graded, of course, on quality of reporting rather than on success in effecting dietary change. For older students, software could help randomize the students' families so that the class as a whole could compare actual dietary outcomes of a purely informational/educational program versus one with a technology-supported stepwise goal-setting approach (Cullen, Baranowski, & Smith, 2001).

Advantages for Research

Automation of behavioral vaccines facilitates studying their impact. It can be easier to implement data-gathering features with an automated intervention than with one delivered by print. Turning to the World Wide Web to recruit participants can quickly bring a study population up to the size needed to test hypotheses. Recruitment bias inherent in this approach has not been systematically assessed, but a recent report suggests that salient characteristics of participants ascertained in this manner do not differ importantly from those engaged in conventional ways, so that results of such Internet-based studies can justifiably be generalized (Seligman, Steen, Park, & Peterson, 2005). Data acquired from an automated behavioral intervention is ready for electronic processing, avoiding transcription error and cost. Data can be accurately time-stamped. Detailed information can be acquired with relatively low demand on participants. Randomizing the order of presentation of answer choices in some modules can avoid a source of response bias. Even clinicians not ordinarily engaged in research can be induced to contribute to a study where the bulk of the data is supplied directly by their participants (March et al., 2005). Of course, a data set acquired from many professional practices, that involves numerous variables and that is "incomplete" because of the branching nature of an automated behavioral vaccine poses special problems for analysis.

Practice

One can acquire an automated behavioral vaccine as a CD or DVD data disk, download it from the Internet or interact over the World Wide Web with a vaccine running on a distant central computer. In this last method, a user can log on over a secure, encrypted connection using a familiar Web browser, have his or her identity authenticated and then interact with the remote computer, receive personalized feedback and optionally forward a summary of the session to the clinician who originally prescribed the intervention. Data lying outside predefined limits or meeting certain criteria can trigger sending a timely alert to a person's therapist or physician (Finkelstein, Khare, & Vora, 2003). Subsequent strategically timed "booster" interventions may enhance effectiveness (Walters, Hester, Chiauzzi, & Miller, 2005).

Medem (http://www.medem.com), a hybrid e-mail and Web service for medical practices, offers a treatment adherence system that, in the name of the prescribing physician, can e-mail to a patient a sequence of behavioral intervention modules, including reminders and boosters. With minimal investment of time the physician can register such modules into his or her online "library" from a general stock of behavioral interventions maintained by Medem, can fashion new modules or can obtain behavioral vaccines from a third party.

A computer can adjust its presentation to match the user's learning style or readiness to change, for example using conditional "skip logic" to "branch" past irrelevant content (Ellison, 2001). Another simple but probably effective way to tailor communication is to address the user by name and take into account the composition of the user's family: "What are you doing to keep little Jenny, your 3 year old daughter, from breathing-in the smoke from your cigarettes?" In one study those participants who expected personalized pamphlets to be helpful in quitting smoking responded better after reading printed booklets that seemed to have been tailored for them, even though the anti-smoking content was not actually altered; participants expressing indifference to personalization seemed better off with wholly standard pamphlets

(Webb, Simmons, & Brandon, 2005). This finding supports first assessing user preference and then providing true or apparent personalization only as indicated.

Individually targeted and personally tailored education for people at risk has been proposed to make interventions more effective (Moser, McKinley, Dracup, & Chung, 2005). Internet-delivered motivational programs, such as those counseling against tobacco use or excessive alcohol consumption, may be enhanced by including online assessment and individualized feedback (Walters et al., 2005). Even simple adaptability, such as a personalized graph showing that the user's drinking and driving put his or her chances of being jailed in the upper quartile of a comparison group may exert a more powerful influence than a "one size fits all" approach characteristic of print and broadcast presentations that may turn away users who are uncertain about what is applicable to them and what is generic (Kreuter, Strecher, & Glassman, 1999). Dijkstra and De Vries (1999) provided principles for implementing and evaluating personalized tailoring in automated behavioral intervention modules. Neala and Carey (2004) suggested that simple nonconfrontational but personalized normative feedback may dispel the myth that binge drinking is common and acceptable and thus nudge participants into taking part in a behavioral intervention. Indeed, after receiving automatically generated, individually tailored comparisons of their reported drinking patterns with national norms, college students indicated an increased willingness to change (Bendtsen et al., 2006).

Self-administered behavioral interventions must compete with a host of distractions for a consumer's time and attention. The multimedia and hypermedia features of computer presentations may be more compelling than print-based methods by appealing to users on many levels (Chambers, Connor, McGarvey, & Driver, 2001). The designer of a computer-based module has wide scope in setting such delivery and demand characteristics as pacing, presentation format and requests for user input. Furthermore, an automated intervention can continually adapt itself to a user's changing state as determined by the user's responses (Martindale & Ahern, 2002). Thus the intervention can shift between being challenging and reassuring. It can be rapid-fire and then allow the user to respond at leisure. Technology can quickly produce relevant content as well as adapt its format. An interactive "calculator" can instantly show how the expected number of healthy days remaining in the user's life varies as the user manipulates the various input parameters reflecting lifestyle changes. A spectacular version of a calculator artificially "aged" some children to depict how they will look and what they will be like if they don't improve their lifestyle ("Honey we're killing the kids!" 2005).

Immediate automated feedback and closely tailored, strategically timed reinforcement to shape behaviors in a way resembling standard psychotherapy (Claiborn & Goodyear, 2005) can be accomplished particularly well with miniature computers, called personal digital assistants (PDAs), that people carry throughout the day. A PDA can make vaccine programs available where and when a person might best interact with them. Late-model PDAs and cell phones can access sophisticated behavioral vaccines by connecting to the Internet's World Wide Web. In addition, portable computers can link to broadband "WiFi" wireless communications at many public locations.

Behavioral vaccination can be brought close to a user's daily life through mobile telephones, automated dialing, interactive voice response (IVR) and touch-tone sensitive systems to issue periodic reminders, provide immediate feedback to input from the consumer and support timely communication with peers in a support network. Just as telecommunication and computing instruments are converging into a compatible array of tabletop and wearable devices, communication services such as telephony, the World Wide Web and e-mail are converging into a seamless network able to locate an individual wherever he or she might be.

Some semblance of human contact or therapeutic alliance is important for efficacy of certain self-help modalities (Newman, Erickson, Przeworski, & Dzus, 2003). The Internet can leverage ongoing peer contact into a low-cost behavioral intervention. Technology can also foster a feeling of ongoing relatedness with a clinician even when little or no professional time is actually involved. Participants consider a good relationship with their physicians important for obtaining the best care (Towle, Godolphin, Manklow, & Wiesinger, 2003). Mutual trust and respect ordinarily rests on two-way communication, yet conveying psychological guidance and support by technology – even by telephone or videophone – may strike one as depersonalizing, a far cry from the traditional "laying-on of hands." Among available technologies, the Internet is especially able to let a therapist add a measure of interpersonal communication to a behavioral vaccine (Lange, van de Ven, Schrieken, & Emmelkamp, 2001). This can be effected at low cost and with little or no demand on the therapist's time through a combination of therapist-branded modules (e.g., the previously mentioned Medem treatment adherence system), automated feedback features, computer-generated personalized messages, returning to the therapist summaries of a consumer's interaction with a behavioral vaccine and limited supplementary e-mail communication.

An appropriate multimedia presentation can surpass the impact of verbal counseling, not just substitute for it. Among the therapeutic advantages of a purely written medium over face-to-face speech described by L'Abate (Introduction to Section IV this volume) is that writing entails less "immediacy" and greater opportunity for reflection and contemplation, thus recruiting different brain regions and different cognitive and perhaps emotional subsystems. A writing task may cause a person to reexperience and reassess feelings and ideas in a manner not possible during a face-to-face therapy session and to extend changes to otherwise unaffected parts of the brain. Beyond writing, incorporation of interactive multimedia adds tasks that demand interpreting graphics and images, listening and watching motion. Such active participation may produce even more widespread effects on the brain.

Reading the text of a behavioral vaccine can induce conscious "explicit" learning that supports deliberate behavior. Acquiring relatively automatic and "natural" behavior patterns may require actually enacting something or at least observing an enactment (Bird, Osman, Saggerson, & Heyes, 2005). Multimedia behavioral vaccines can not only provide explicit "book knowledge," but can also enable implicit learning by showing video segments of people performing a desirable behavior, by engaging the user in decision-making, and by simulating scenarios in which the user is invited to play out a role.

A properly designed website can adequately deliver behavioral vaccines with a rich array of multimedia features within the limits of technology readily available to most of the population of developed countries and without requiring high-speed Internet access.

The basic authoring tools for constructing interactive behavioral vaccines are nearly as simple and inexpensive as word processors. They are necessary because simply copying a printed module into an electronic file for online perusal or operation may not result in a satisfactory behavioral intervention. Not only may psychometric properties be degraded, but consumers may not tolerate long text passages or grainy and jerky images presented on a small "window" within a computer screen. There should be provision for a user to suspend participation in an intervention sequence and resume, perhaps a day or two later, without losing ground.

Home healthcare studies have found wireless networks and devices reliable for accurate transmission of medical data (Zhao, Fei, Doarn, Harnett, & Merrell, 2004). Sensitive communication should not be sent over dubiously secure systems, however. Many people would be surprised at the range of eavesdropping activities considered legal in the U.S. Encryption of data transferred to and from a website hosting a behavioral vaccine is imperative to keep private information from unauthorized third parties. Current widely available encryption can adequately conceal the content of transmissions but an electronic eavesdropper can readily ascertain the fact that a consumer is communicating with a particular website, such as one specializing in management of a stigmatized health condition. Using a neutral intermediary website that provides access to other websites is one way to hide the Web address one is accessing from a snooper. The Health Insurance Portability and Accountability Act (HIPAA) and in many instances state analogues require protected health information to be well guarded. While preventive behavioral vaccines may not be subject to the provisions of HIPAA it would be wise to contact legal advisors before electronically delivering behavioral vaccines that could be construed as treatment. Even where no statutory authorities are implicated, for example, a tort claim may lie at common law if appropriate precautions to protect privacy are not taken.

Such considerations led Maheu et al. (2005) to develop an "Online Clinical Practice Management" (OCPM) model to guide clinicians in the effective, safe, and ethical application of technology. Special professional training, the first of 7 steps in this model, will help the practitioner review the potential benefits and problems associated with various technologies and review federal, state, and local laws in order to decide which technology, if any, is best suited for a patient. Having chosen an appropriate technology the trained professionals will have the competence and skill to understand and correct any problems that may arise during treatment. In addition to sufficient expertise in the specific technology selected, practitioner competence should include a basic knowledge of the functioning of the computer system or communication channel being employed.

Making and accepting referrals, the second consideration of the OCPM, increasingly involves the World Wide Web. Websites may direct participants to a professional practice, may directly offer behavioral vaccines and may provide access to online support groups. Before signing up to accept referrals or otherwise associating with or recommending a website, a mental health professional should become familiar with the site's policies to ensure that sensitive data are kept secure and private, that information provided is trustworthy and that participants will not be misled or exploited for commercial purposes or to promote some nontherapeutic agenda of the website's sponsors. A clinician who offers behavioral vaccines on his or her own website should be aware of the professional implications of being involved with the entities supporting the website, of accepting advertising, of promoting particular vaccines and a host of other issues. For example, protection of sensitive personal information requires special measures even when an online user is supposedly "anonymous" and even when a home computer is used without connecting to the Internet. These considerations relate to steps 3 and 4 of the OCPM – patient education and informed consent (Maheu et al., 2005, pp. 331ff.). New technologies can cause participants to become anxious or feel incompetent. Depending on the technologies required for a specific vaccine professionals may need to provide a client with a full explanation and demonstration.

One self-guided Internet program for overcoming depression (Clarke et al., 2005) asks a user for a troublesome personal negative or irrational thought. It finds the closest matches to the keyed-in text in its library of negative statements, asks the user to select the one most similar to his or her idea, then offers several relevant counter-thoughts for the user to choose for behavior modification training and correlation with trigger events. Clearly, tailoring a presentation to an individual user in this way raises privacy issues. Sensitive personal information is particularly vulnerable to adverse exploitation or accidental embarrassing disclosure when transmitted over the Internet or when showing on an unguarded monitor screen. Users should be taught safeguards, but also be warned that no protection is foolproof. Those offering such services should document that these steps have been taken.

Mental health professionals who use technologies to deliver interventions may be working outside current standards of care. What seems absolutely safe can cause unexpected harm. Good intentions may offer little defense against claims for unintended consequences. It behooves both innovators and early adopters to keep abreast of the research on whatever technologies they propose to use. To be sure, a review of published and ongoing studies found no reports that engaging in a technology-mediated self-help treatment for psychological problems has resulted in harm or has rendered anyone more difficult to treat by conventional means (Andersson, Bergstrom, Carlbring, & Lindefors, 2005). The standard for judging the new technologies, however, will likely be the efficacy of existing, traditional therapies. As it stands, evidence for the efficacy of technology-based mental health treatment derives from a limited set of small-scale studies. A partial solution to this issue, beyond research designed to expand our understanding of the risks and benefits of use of the technology, is careful and carefully documented informed consent that addresses the additional vulnerabilities created by technology as such. Because efforts to enhance security can make a technology less convenient, a significant degree of vulnerability will probably always exist and an informed patient will have to make a reasonable decision about using it (Tjora, Trung, & Faxvaag, 2005).

The fifth step of the OCPM describes how clinical assessment, along with repeatedly reinforced education and frequently renegotiated consent, should continue throughout the therapeutic relationship. Ideally, behavioral vaccines will contribute valuable information towards understanding a client's problems and strengths and towards documenting progress in treatment.

Current practice standards, however, do not accommodate relying on behavioral vaccines for assessment to the exclusion of accepted methods.

Step 6 reviews the legal and ethical implications of psychotechnologies in direct care. The wide spectrum of psychotechnologies used for behavioral vaccines makes specific suggestions difficult, but the practitioner is advised to be fully informed about all standards and requirements before working with participants through psychotechnologies. Practitioners should also recognize that the standard of care is a moving target based on choice of prudent services at a given time. It is likely that eventually the standard of care may at times actually require the professional to use psychotechnologies with participants or, at least, that an advocate will be prepared to so claim.

The final step of OCPM is obtaining reimbursement. This area may be the greatest current stumbling block in the way of progress for low-cost behavioral interventions that by definition involve little or no professional time and thus cannot contribute directly to the financial "bottom line." If third party payers come to see behavioral vaccines as ways to reach objectives efficiently and to promote preventative measures that lower long-term health costs then clinicians may come under strong pressure to prescribe them appropriately. Clinicians may resist the prospect of "losing" participants to computers and the Internet until research demonstrates that prescribing behavioral vaccines can enhance clinical outcome, patient satisfaction and the reputation and even the financial success of a clinical practice.

Conclusions

Technology will have a transformative effect on low-cost behavioral interventions through enhancement of their affordability, dissemination, ease of access and use, personal relevance, appeal and engagement of multiple mental functions, as well as their facilitation of reporting results back to prescribers and researchers. Little special skill is required to apply many key technologies to behavioral vaccines. In the near future technology enhanced low-cost behavioral interventions will be available for self-help and prevention, but treatment applications will be restricted mainly to research settings. Current barriers to expanded clinical use of technologies for delivering behavioral vaccines are concern over privacy, uncertainty over integrating use of behavioral vaccines into existing clinical practice patterns, and the current paucity of prospects of immediate reimbursement for prescribing or developing technology enhanced behavioral vaccines. These impediments are likely to recede as the advantages of low-cost interventions become more obvious and widely known. Clinicians are well-advised to be familiar with how computers and the Internet will help make behavioral vaccines a valuable resource for mental health practice.

References

A little history of the World Wide Web (2005). World Wide Web Consortium. Accessed November 2, 2005 at http://www.w3.org/History.html.

Andersson, G., Bergstrom, J., Carlbring, P., & Lindefors, N. (2005). The use of the Internet in the treatment of anxiety disorders. *Current Opinion in Psychiatry, 18*(1), 73–77.

Atkinson, R. L., & Nitzke, S. A. (2001). School based programmes on obesity. *BMJ, 323*(7320), 1018–1019.

Baker, M. L. (2005). Electronic pill box proves to be good medicine. Retrieved March 24, 2005, from http://www.cioinsight.com/article2/0,1397,1778351,00.asp

Bara-Carril, N., Williams, C. J., Pombo-Carril, M. G., Reid, Y., Murray, K., Aubin, S., Harkin, P., Treasure, J., & Schmidt, U. (2004). A preliminary investigation into the feasibility and efficacy of a CD-ROM-based cognitive-behavioral self-help intervention for bulimia nervosa. *The International Journal of Eating Disorders, 35*(4), 538–548.

Bendtsen, P., Johansson, K., & Åkerlind, I. (2006). Feasibility of an email-based electronic screening and brief intervention (e-SBI) to college students in Sweden. *Addictive Behaviors, 31*(5), 777–787.

Bird, G., Osman, M., Saggerson, A., & Heyes, C. (2005). Sequence learning by action, observation and action observation. *British Journal of Psychology, 96*(3), 371–388.

Boulton, M., Boudioni, M., Mossman, J., Moynihan, C., Leydon, G., & Ramirez, A. (2001). 'Dividing the desolation': Clients views on the benefits of a cancer counselling service. *Psychooncology, 10*(2), 124–136.

Chambers, M., Connor, S. L., McGarvey, H., & Driver, M. (2001). User acceptance of a multi-media software application to increase preparedness for caring problems. *Health Informatics Journal, 7*(3–4), 152–157.

Chumbler, N. R., Neugaard, B., Ryan, P., Qin, H., & Joo, Y. (2005). An observational study of veterans with diabetes receiving weekly or daily home telehealth monitoring. *Journal of Telemedicine and Telecare, 11*(3), 150–156.

Claiborn, C. D., & Goodyear, R. K. (2005). Feedback in psychotherapy. *Journal of Clinical Psychology, 61*(2), 209–217.

Clarke, G., Eubanks, D., Reid, E., Kelleher, C., O'Connor, E., DeBar, L. L., Lynch, F., Nunley, S., & Gullion, C. (2005). Overcoming depression on the Internet (ODIN) (2): A randomized trial of a self-help depression skills program with reminders. *Journal of Medical Internet Research, 7*(2), e16.

Cullen, K. W., Baranowski, T., & Smith, S. P. (2001). Using goal setting as a strategy for dietary behavior change. *Journal of the American Dietetic Association, 101*(5), 562–566.

Curry, S. J., Ludman, E. J., & McClure, J. (2003). Self-administered treatment for smoking cessation. *Journal of Clinical Psychology, 59*(3), 305–319.

Dijkstra, A., & De Vries, H. (1999). The development of computer-generated tailored interventions. *Patient Education and Counseling, 36*(2), 193–203.

Ellison, J. (April 23, 2001). Computer-assisted instruction/ programmed instruction. Retrieved 24 September 2005, from http://www.informatics.buffalo.edu/faculty/ellison/Syllabi/519Complete/formats/programmedinstr/program.html

Farzanfar, R., Frishkopf, S., Friedman, R., & Ludena, K. (2006). Evaluating an automated mental health care system: Making meaning of human-computer interaction. *Computers in Human Behavior, 23*(3), 1167–1182.

Febbraro, G. A. R. (2005). An investigation into the effectiveness of bibliotherapy and minimal contact interventions in the treatment of panic attacks. *Journal of Clinical Psychology, 61*(6), 763–779.

Fenety, A., & Walker, J. M. (2002). Short-term effects of workstation exercises on musculoskeletal discomfort and postural changes in seated video display unit workers. *Physical Therapy, 82*(6), 578–589.

Finch, T., May, C., Mair, F., Mort, M., & Gask, L. (2003). Integrating service development with evaluation in telehealthcare: An ethnographic study. *British Medical Journal, 327*(7425), 1205–1209.

Finkelstein, J., Khare, R., & Vora, D. (2003). Home automated telemanagement (HAT) system to facilitate self-care of patients with chronic diseases. *Journal of Systematics, Cybernetics and Informatics, 1*, e5.

Friedman, M. J. (2005). Every crisis is an opportunity. *CNS Spectrums, 10*(2), 96–98.

Gega, L., Marks, I. M., & Mataix-Cols, D. (2004). Computer-aided CBT self-help for anxiety and depressive disorders: Experience of a London clinic and future directions. *Journal of Clinical Psychology, 60*(2), 147–157.

George, C. F., Peveler, R. C., Heiliger, S., & Thompson, C. (2000). Compliance with tricyclic antidepressants: The value of four different methods of assessment. *British Journal of Clinical Pharmacology, 50*(2), 166–171.

Goldstine, H. H., & von Neumann, J. (1946). On the principles of large scale computing machines. In A. H. Taub (1963), *John von Neumann Collected Works, Volume V, Design of Computers, Theory of Automata and Numerical Analysis*. New York: Pergamon Press, pp. 1–34.

Gustafson, D. H., Hawkins, R., Boberg, E., Pingree, S., Serlin, R. E., Graziano, F., & Chan, C. L. (1999). Impact of a patient-centered, computer-based health information/support system. *American Journal of Preventive Medicine, 16*(1), 1–9.

Hailey, D., Bulger, T., Stayberg, S., & Urness, D. (2003). The reality of applying an assessment guideline to a telemedicine mental health programme. *Journal of Telemedicine and Telecare, 9*(6), 344–348; discussion 348–349.

Haynes, R. B., McDonald, H., Garg, A. X., & Montague, P. (2002). Interventions for helping patients to follow prescriptions for medications. *Cochrane Database of Systematic Reviews, 2*, CD000011.

Hellard, M. E., Sinclair, M. I., Forbes, A. B., & Fairley, C. K. (2001). Methods used to maintain a high level of participant involvement in a clinical trial. *Journal of Epidemiology and Community Health, 55*(5), 348–351.

Honey we're killing the kids! (2005). [Broadcast Television]. United Kingdom: BBC Three.

Hornung, R. L., Lennon, P. A., Garrett, J. M., DeVellis, R. F., Weinberg, P. D., & Strecher, V. J. (2000). Interactive computer technology for skin cancer prevention targeting children. *American Journal of Preventive Medicine, 18*(1), 69–76.

Kaufman, J., Yang, B. Z., Douglas-Palumberi, H., Houshyar, S., Lipschitz, D., Krystal, J. H., & Gelernter, J. (2004). Social supports and serotonin transporter gene moderate depression in maltreated children. *Proceedings of the National Academy of Sciences, U S A, 101*(49), 17316–17321.

Kenwright, M., Marks, I. M., Gega, L., & Mataix-Cols, D. (2004). Computer-aided self-help for phobia/pamic via Internet at a home: a pilot study. *British Journal of Psychiatry,* 184(5), 448–449.

Kreuter, M. W., Strecher, V. J., & Glassman, B. (1999). One size does not fit all: The case for tailoring print materials. *Annals of Behavioral Medicine, 21*(4), 276–283.

Lange, A., de Beurs, E., Dolan, C., Lachnit, T., Sjollema, S., & Hanewald, G. (1999). Long-term effects of childhood sexual abuse: Objective and subjective characteristics of the abuse and psychopathology in later life. *The Journal of Nervous and Mental Disease, 187*(3), 150–158.

Lange, A., Rietdijk, D., Hudcovicova, M., van de Ven, J.-P., Schrieken, B., & Emmelkamp, P. M. G. (2003). Interapy: A controlled randomized trial of the standardized treatment of posttraumatic stress through the Internet. *Journal of Consulting and Clinical Psychology, 71*(5), 901–909.

Lange, A., van de Ven, J.-P., Schrieken, B., & Emmelkamp, P. M. G. (2001). Interapy, treatment of posttraumatic stress through the Internet: A controlled trial. *Journal of Behavior Therapy and Experimental Psychiatry, 32*(2), 73–90.

Leiner, B. M., Cerf, V. G., Clark, D. D., Kahn, R. E., Kleinrock, L., Lynch, D., C., Postel, J., Roberts, L. G., & Wolff, S. (2005). A brief history of the Internet [online document]. Internet Society. Accessed November 3, 2005 at http://www.isoc.org/internet/history/brief.shtml.

Maheu, M. M., Pulier, M. L., Wilhelm, F. H., McMenamin, J. P., & Brown-Connolly, N. E. (2005). *The mental health professional and the new technologies:*

A handbook for practice today. Mahwah, New Jersey: Lawrence Erlbaum Associates, Publishers.

Maio, R. F., Shope, J. T., Blow, F. C., Gregor, M. A., Zakrajsek, J. S., Weber, J. E., & Nypaver, M. M. (2005). A randomized controlled trial of an emergency department-based interactive computer program to prevent alcohol misuse among injured adolescents. *Annals of Emergency Medicine, 45*(4), 420–429.

March, J. S., Silva, S. G., Compton, S., Shapiro, M. A., Califf, R., & Krishnan, R. (2005). The case for practical clinical trials in psychiatry. *American Journal of Psychiatry, 162*(5), 836–846.

Martindale, T., & Ahern, T. C. (July 14–18, 2002). *Designing reusable learning objects: Matching delivery models to content.* Paper presented at the 6th World Multiconference on Systemics, Cybernetics, and Informatics, Orlando, Florida.

McCrone, P., Knapp, M., Proudfoot, J., Ryden, C., Cavanagh, K., Shapiro, D. A., Ilson, S., Gray, J. A., Goldberg, D., Mann, A., Marks, I., Everitt, B., & Tylee, A. (2004). Cost-effectiveness of computerised cognitive-behavioural therapy for anxiety and depression in primary care: Randomised controlled trial. *British Journal of Psychiatry, 185*, 55–62.

Milch, R. A., Ziv, L., Evans, V., & Hillebrand, M. (1996). The effect of an alphanumeric paging system on patient compliance with medicinal regimens. *American Journal of Hospital Palliative Care, 13*(3), 46–48.

Monnier, J., Knapp, R. G., & Frueh, B. C. (2003). Recent advances in telepsychiatry: An updated review. *Psychiatric Services, 54*(12), 1604–1609.

Monsey, M., Ioffe, I., Beatini, A., Lukey, B., Santiago, A., & James, A. B. (2003). Increasing compliance with stretch breaks in computer users through reminder software. *Work*, 21(2), 107–111.

Moser, D. K., McKinley, S., Dracup, K., & Chung, M. L. (2005). Gender differences in reasons patients delay in seeking treatment for acute myocardial infarction symptoms. *Patient Education and Counseling, 56*(1), 45–54.

Murray, K., Schmidt, U., Pombo-Carril, M.-G., Grover, M., Alenya, J., Treasure, J., & Williams, C. (2007). Does therapist guidance improve uptake, adherence and outcome from a CD-ROM based cognitive-behavioral intervention for the treatment of bulimia nervosa? *Computers in Human Behavior, 23(1), 850–859.*

Nakagawa, A., Marks, I. M., Park, J.-M., Bachofen, M., Baer, L., Dottl, S. L., & Greist, J. H. (2000). Self-treatment of obsessive-compulsive disorder guided by manual and computer-conducted telephone interview. *Journal of Telemedicine and Telecare, 6*(1), 22–26.

Neala, D. J., & Carey, K. B. (2004). Developing discrepancy within self-regulation theory: Use of personalized normative feedback and personal strivings with heavy-drinking college students. *Addictive Behaviors, 29*(2), 281–297.

Newman, M. G., Erickson, T., Przeworski, A., & Dzus, E. (2003). Self-help and minimal-contact therapies for anxiety disorders: Is human contact necessary for therapeutic efficacy? *Journal of Clinical Psychology, 59*(3), 251–274.

Nicklas, T. A., Baranowski, T., Baranowski, J. C., Cullen, K., Rittenberry, L., & Olvera, N. (2001). Family and child-care provider influences on preschool children's fruit, juice, and vegetable consumption. *Nutrition Reviews, 59*(7), 224–235.

O'Connor, A. M., Stacey, D., Entwistle, V., Llewellyn-Thomas, H., Rovner, D., Holmes-Rovner, M., Tait, V., Tetroe, J., Fiset, V., Barry, M., & Jones, J. (2005). Decision aids for people facing health treatment or screening decisions. *Cochrane Database of Systematic Reviews, 3.*

Paperny, D. M. N. (2004). A new model for adolescent preventive services. *The Permanente Journal, 8*(1), 74–79.

Proudfoot, J., Ryden, C., Everitt, B., Shapiro, D. A., Goldberg, D., Mann, A., Tylee, A., Marks, I., & Gray, J. A. (2004). Clinical efficacy of computerised cognitive-behavioural therapy for anxiety and depression in primary care: Randomised controlled trial. *British Journal of Psychiatry, 185*, 46–54.

Rostom, A., O'Connor, A., Tugwell, P., & Wells, G. (2002). A randomized trial of a computerized versus an audio-booklet decision aid for women considering post-menopausal hormone replacement therapy. *Patient Education and Counseling, 46*(1), 67–74.

Schmitz, J. M., Sayre, S. L., Stotts, A. L., Rothfleisch, J., & Mooney, M. E. (2005). Medication compliance during a smoking cessation clinical trial: A brief intervention using MEMS feedback. *Journal of Behavioral Medicine, 28*(2), 139–147.

Seligman, M. E. P., Steen, T. A., Park, N., & Peterson, C. (2005). Positive psychology progress: Empirical validation of interventions. *American Psychologist, 60*(5), 410–421.

Shannon, C. E. (1948). A mathematical theory of communication. *The Bell System Technical Journal, 27*, 379–423, 623–656.

Stevens, V. J., Severson, H., Lichtenstein, E., Little, S. J., & Leben, J. (1995). Making the most of a teachable moment: A smokeless-tobacco cessation intervention in the dental office. *American Journal of Public Health, 85*(2), 231–235.

Tate, D. F., Jackvony, E. H., & Wing, R. R. (2003). Effects of Internet behavioral counseling on weight loss in adults at risk for type 2 diabetes: A randomized trial. *Journal of the American Medical Association, 289*(14), 1833–1836.

Tate, D., & Zabinski, M. F. (2004). Computer and Internet applications for psychological treatment: update for clinicians. *Journal of Clinical Psychology, 60*(2), 209–220.

Tjora, A., Trung, T., & Faxvaag, A. (2005). Privacy vs usability: A qualitative exploration of patients' experiences with secure Internet communication with their general practitioner. *Journal of Medical Internet Research, 7*(2), e15.

Towle, A., Godolphin, W., Manklow, J., & Wiesinger, H. (2003). Patient perceptions that limit a community-based intervention to promote participation. *Patient Education and Counseling, 50*(3), 231–233.

Walters, S. T., Hester, R. K., Chiauzzi, E., & Miller, E. (2005). Demon rum: High-tech solutions to an age-old problem. *Alcoholism: Clinical and Experimental Research, 29*(2), 270–277.

Webb, M. S., Simmons, V. N., & Brandon, T. H. (2005). Tailored interventions for motivating smoking cessation: Using placebo tailoring to examine the influence of expectancies and personalization. *Health Psychology, 24*(2), 179–188.

Whitlock, E. P., Williams, S. B., Gold, R., Smith, P. R., & Shipman, S. A. (2005). Screening and interventions for childhood overweight: A summary of evidence for the us preventive services task force. *Pediatrics, 116*(1), e125–e144.

Wiener, N. (1948) *Cybernetics, or control and communication in the animal and the machine*. New York: Wiley.

Wofford, J. L., Smith, E. D., & Miller, D. P. (2005). The multimedia computer for office-based patient education: A systematic review. *Patient Education and Counseling*, 59(2), 148–157.

Zhao, X., Fei, D.-Y., Doarn, C. R., Harnett, B., & Merrell, R. (2004). A telemedicine system for wireless home healthcare based on Bluetooth and the Internet. *Telemedicine Journal and e-Health, 10*(Suppl 2), S110–S116.

Section V

Secondary Relational Approaches

Nonconventional interventions have gained a great deal of acceptance during the last generation. According to the Center for Disease Control and Prevention Advanced Data Report (2004), the ten most common complementary and alternative medicine therapies are: prayer for one's own health, prayers by others for one's own health, participation in a prayer group for one's own health, natural products (reviewed in Section II), deep-breathing exercises, meditation, and yoga (reviewed in Section III), chiropractic care (not reviewed at all), diet-based therapies (reviewed in Section II), and massage (reviewed in this Section).

With few exceptions, most of these interventions are rather inexpensive and easily available. By the same token, a treatise on health psychology (Camic & Knight, 1998) included only two chapters pertaining to health-oriented interventions, family, friends, and community (Rhodes, 1998) as well as spirituality and religion (Chapter 22) (Potts, 1998). In contrast, in this Section not only we have chapters overlapping with those two topics (Chapters 19 and 20) but we have also a chapter on forgiveness (Chapter 21), as well as others relating to close physical contact between mother and infant (Chapter 16), massage (Chapter 17) and non-erotic contact (Chapter 18).

Consequently, the purpose of this section it to review low-cost interventions related to relationships between self and others. For a detailed and up-to-date review of how relationships effect and are effected by physiological factors, the reader is referred to the exhaustive review by Diamond and Hicks (2004). By the same token, the closer the relationship, the greater the chances of higher levels of subjective well-being. Married couples, for instance, report highest levels of subjective well-being followed by individuals in cohabiting relationships, steady dating relationships, casual dating relationships, and individuals who dated infrequently or not at all. Individuals in happy relationships tend to report higher levels of subjective well-being than individuals in unhappy relationships, irrespective of relationship status (Kamp-Dush & Amato, 2005).

All these relatively new approaches speak to the incompleteness of traditional medical interventions, not because of inherent defects in themselves but because one profession cannot be held responsible to deal with all the many aspects of life as well as all the many ills that beset humanity. Many other professions will need to take responsibility for the very realms of physical and mental health that cannot possibly be covered by medical specialties, as discussed in Chapter 1.

Changes in the need for alternative, non-traditional approach parallel changes in priorities between men and women. While the latter have entered the workforce in increasing numbers, men have increasing taking communal, care-taking roles traditionally reserved to women. These changes signal a fourth stage in the evolution of marriage, family, and intimate relationships (Young & Willmott, 1973). Originally, women in the home attended to the three Ks (kooking, kirchen, und kinder), while men were out in the jungle hunting and procuring money and foods to fulfill basic human needs. With the industrial revolution of the nineteenth century, women went out of the house into factories, and therefore, a second stage in the man–woman relationship began and continued until the middle of last century.

With women receiving more education and becoming involved in earning a living without the help of men, the rate of divorces increased to signify a third stage in the evolution of couple relationships. Men were not able to fulfill the many communal requests for emotional availability and sharing in homework demanded by women, who were also earning a living and were able to manage both home and work responsibilities. While these changes have occurred in USA earlier than other countries, some countries, especially in North Europe, are beginning to match our statistics in the number of divorces, single mothers, same-sex relationships, and other aspects of changes in intimate relationships (L'Abate, 2004, 2005).

These changes in roles speak to a fourth stage in the evolution of the family where traditional, legally formed relationships need to reach a more equalitarian and less formal accommodation to take care of both communal and instrumental responsibilities. Hence, chapters in this Section cover the very aspects of intimate relationships that need to be enacted for individuals, couples, and families in intimate relationships, not only to survive materially but also to survive well emotionally and physically, with enjoyment. Other sections of this Handbook cover more instrumental tasks and interventions.

References

Camic, P., & Knight, S. (Eds.) (1998). *Clinical handbook of health psychology*. Seattle, WA: Hogrefe & Huber.

Diamond, L. M., & Hicks, A. M. (2004). Psychobiological perspectives on attachment: Implications for health over the lifespan. In W. S. Rholes, & J. A. Simpson (Eds.), *Adult attachment: Theory research, and clinical implications* (pp. 240–263). New York: Guilford.

Kamp-Dush, C. M., & Amato, P. R. (2005). Consequences of relationship status and quality of subjective well-being. *Journal of Social and Personal Relationships, 22*, 607–627.

L'Abate, L. (2004). La lenta scomparsa della famiglia: Chi prendera' il suo posto? (The slow disappearance of the family: Who will replace it?). *Saggi: Child Development & Disabilities, 30*, 23–34.

L'Abate, L. (2005). *Personality in intimate relationships: Socialization and psychopathology*. New York: Springer Science.

Potts, R. G. (1998). Spirituality, religion, and the experience of illness. In P. Camic, & S. Knight (Eds.), *Clinical handbook of health psychology* (pp. 495–522). Seattle, WA: Hogrefe & Huber.

Rhodes, J. E. (1998). Family, friends, and community: The role of social support in promoting health. In P. Camic, & S. Knight (Eds.), *Clinical handbook of health psychology* (pp. 481–493). Seattle, WA: Hogrefe & Huber.

Young, M., & Willmott, P. (1973). *The symmetrical family*. New York: Pantheon Books.

16

Maternal-Infant Contact and Child Development: Insights from the Kangaroo Intervention

Ruth Feldman

Low-Cost Interventions; Some Preliminary Thoughts

A "low-cost intervention" must, by definition, capitalize on the resources available in the natural ecology. Yet, transforming natural substances, behaviors, or patterns of relatedness into an organized intervention that can be subjected to scientific scrutiny requires more than the use of nature's offerings. As a first step, one must establish that the specific substance or activity advocated as intervention is not just "good for you", but that there are specific, theoretically-based, and empirically proven links between "cause" and "care". Second, the mechanisms by which the proposed intervention improves the level of functioning must be laid out for empirical testing. In this context, it is important to distinguish between natural resources that promote well-being in general from the use of these same resources for the treatment of a pathological state (i.e., use as prevention versus use as intervention). Third, specific outcomes of the intervention should be proposed and tested, not only a global promotion of well-being and development. Such specificity may further define chains of cause-care-cure in the case of low-cost interventions. Finally, at least in the domain of infant development, the role of the natural resource in shaping specific brain systems and its effects on structure-function relationship is an important aspect of the intervention. Thus, applying a "sensitive period" approach, which underscores the need for specific environmental inputs during unique time-windows in structure-function relationship, is likely to increase the scientific value, testability, and generalizability of the proposed intervention.

In this chapter, I will describe the use of maternal-infant skin-to-skin contact as a form of low-cost intervention for premature infants in the neonatal period. Mother–infant contact is not only a prevalent, immediately available, and natural phenomenon, but the very image of "motherhood." It is depicted in countless drawings, sculptures, poems, and novels throughout history and across cultural communities, and is rooted in the physical union between mother and child. Maternal-infant contact lies at the basis of our collective unconscious, and possibly for good evolutionary reasons. In proposing mother–infant contact as an intervention strategy, I will follow each of the four guidelines detailed above. First, on the basis of research in humans and animal models, I will demonstrate that maternal touch and contact in the postpartum period is not only a positive experience; it provides the foundation for maternal care that is essential for infant growth and survival. Second, the mechanisms that mediate the effects of early physical contact on the child's later development will be outlined, including the centrality of maternal proximity for the infant's biobehavioral regulatory systems that support the emergence of attention, exploration, and emotion regulation capacities. Similarly, the effects of maternal-infant contact on the development of mothering, which in turn supports infant growth, will be detailed. Third, the specific improvements following early contact intervention for premature infants will be presented on the basis of our longitudinal study that now spans 9 years. Finally, a "sensitive period" perspective will be utilized in addressing the effects of touch on the development of premature infants during a critical period of maternal deprivation. Because premature infants are separated from their mothers immediately after birth and placed in incubators and full maternal-infant contact is prevented, prematurity provides the only human model to examine the effects of maternal deprivation on the infant's emerging biobehavioral systems during a critical period for infant growth. As such, the beneficial provision of maternal proximity and contact in the context of typical infant development (touch as prevention) are differentiated from the curative use of contact as a low-cost intervention for premature infants (touch as intervention).

Maternal-Infant Touch and Contact; Its Role in Early Development

Touch-and-Contact in the Postpartum: The Mother's Perspective

In all mammals, including humans, the birth of an infant triggers a set of species–specific maternal behaviors aimed at assuring survival, promoting optimal growth, providing care, and soothing during times of distress (Carter & Keverne, 2002; Fleming, O'Day, & Kraemer, 1999; Leckman et al., 2004). The emergence of the maternal behavior repertoire depends upon the immediate availability of maternal-infant contact, which starts the process of mothering and the species–specific forms of touch and contact (Meaney, 2001). Immediate maternal contact with the newborn is also critical for the formation of the mother's "bond" to her infant (Klaus & Kenell, 1976) and initiatcs a cascadc of ncurological, hormonal, bchavioral, and cognitive changes in the mother that follow childbirth and are required for the onset of mothering. The specific maternal behavioral repertoire in humans includes the mother's holding or rocking of the infant, gazing at the infant's face and body, smiling, "motherese" (i.e., high-pitched, rhythmical) vocalizations, and affectionate touch (e.g., caressing, stroking, kissing), a behavior akin to the licking-and-grooming behavior of other mammals. The frequencies of maternal affectionate touch and specific maternal behaviors in the immediate postpartum period have profound effects on the infant's neurobiological, cognitive, and social-emotional development (Feldman & Eidelman, 2003; Feldman, Eidelman, & Rotenberg, 2004; Goldberg, Perrotta, Minde, & Corter, 1986). Moreover, because the human infant is innately prepared to orient to the mother's face and to detect contingencies in social behavior (Eckerman, Oehler, Hannan, & Molitor, 1995), mothers often adjust their maternal behavior to the infant's scant moments of attention. While holding the infant in their arms, mothers pay close attention to the infant's momentary alertness and, by providing coordinated behavior to the infant state, augment episodes of engagement and introduce infants to a very rudimentary form of reciprocal social relationships. This early experience of social contingency is critical for the development of mother–infant synchrony, which provides the foundation for the infant's self-regulation, socialization, empathy, and moral orientation across infancy and up to adolescence (Feldman & Greenbaum, 1997; Feldman, Greenbaum & Yirmiya, 1999; Feldman, 2005; Jaffee, Beebe, Feldstein, Crown, & Jasnow, 2002). Importantly, social contingencies between the mother and her newborn impact not only on the development of mothering but also on the father–child relationship and on the development of synchrony between father and child (Feldman & Eidelman, 2007).

Due to the centrality of maternal behavior for survival and evolutionary adaptation, maternal behavior is genetically programmed and is highly conserved across mammalian species. Lesion studies in rodents have implicated brainstem and limbic areas, including the bed nucleus of the stria terminalis, the medial preoptic area, and brainstem nuclei such as ventral tegmental area, and locus ceruleus in the expression of maternal behavior (Leckman & Herman, 2002), pointing to the participation of subcortical, nonconscious and homeostatic brain systems in the emergence of maternal behavior. However, although programmed, maternal behavior is highly susceptible to epigenetic influences, and hence to risk conditions. For instance, Meaney (2001) used naturally occurring variations between dams who provided high or low levels of licking-and-grooming to breed groups of high- and low- touch-and-contact moms. In cross-fostering studies, daughters of low licking-and-grooming dams were raised by high licking-and-grooming moms and vice versa and the results demonstrated that early experience, rather than genetics, determined the formation of maternal behavior. Female pups reared by high licking-and-grooming dams provided high levels of touch-and-contact to their own infants. In addition, high levels of maternal touch and contact had a profound effect on the infant brain development in terms of both structure (e.g., oxytocin receptor density) and function (e.g., HPA functioning) and pups who received more licking-and-grooming showed better stress management throughout life. These findings underscore two important points in the present context. First, touch-and-contact is the central organizing framework for the emergence of maternal behavior and the key element through which such behavior is transmitted to the next generation. Second, consistent with Bowlby's (1969) formulations on "internal working models", the internalized schema that supports the sense of safety and security throughout life is built upon repeated patterns of maternal care, touch, and contact in early infancy that shape the infant's neurobiological mechanisms of relatedness throughout life.

The initiation of maternal behavior is a unique process and possibly depends on different hormonal systems than the maintenance of such behavior (Pedersen, 1999). Thus, the first postbirth moments appear to be critical for the onset of motherhood and trigger the emergence of maternal behavior. Oxytocin, a neuropeptide released during uterine contractions and milk ejection, has been implicated in processes of bonding – at the pair, flilial, and parental bonding levels – and plays an important role in the initiation of maternal behavior (Carter & Keverne, 2002). Oxytocin is a key hormone in the expression of a range of maternal behavior across a variety of mammalian species and its role in social affiliation, stress management, social cognition, fear reduction, and interpersonal trust and empathy has been demonstrated (Heinrichs, Baumgartner, Kirschbaum, & Ehlert, 2003; Insel, 1997; Nelson & Panksepp, 1998). Importantly, mother–infant touch and contact stimulate oxytocin release. Newborn infants placed on their mother's chest initiated oxytocin release through hand movement and suckling (Matthiesen, Ransjo-Arvidson, Nissen, & Uvnas-Moberg, 2001), and mother–infant skin-to-skin contact immediately after birth elevated maternal oxytocin levels (Nissen, Lilja, Widstrom, & Uvnas-Moberg, 1995). Oxytocin increase was observed following breast massage in lactating women (Yokoyama, Ueda, Irahara, & Aono, 1994), and a comparable increase in oxytocin was found following breast pumping and breastfeeding (Zinaman, Hughes, Queenan, Labobok, & Albertson, 1992). This suggests that expressing breast milk may be one way to initiate the "oxytocinergic" bonding system when contact is unavailable. Touch and oxytocin, therefore, seem to function as a feedback loop: touch leads to oxytocin release which, in turn, further increases the mother's tendency to provide touch and contact, with its ensuing sense of trust, affiliation, and interpersonal bond. The role of oxytocin in reducing anxiety and depression (Carter, 1998) similarly facilitates the mother's calm state and availability to her infant.

In two recent studies we demonstrated the effects of oxytocin on maternal behavior and on the mother's postpartum depression. In the first (Feldman & Eidelman, 2003), we examined 86 mothers of premature infants in three matched groups; those providing minimal (< 25% of infant nutrition), moderate (25–75%), and high (> 75%) doses of breast milk. Pre-term infants in this study received the mother's milk by bottle, not through direct contact. Still, because breast pumping and nursing elicit equal amounts of oxytocin release, the amount of expressed milk can serve as a proxy for oxytocin levels. At term age (37 weeks gestational age), mothers and infants were videotaped in a 15-minute session of natural interactions, infant neurobehavioral development was assessed with the Neonatal Behavior Assessment Scale (Brazelton, 1973), and maternal depressive symptoms were self-reported. At 6 months, infants' mental and motor skills were tested with the Bayley Scale of Infant Development (Bayley, 1993). Mothers in the high maternal milk group showed more maternal behavior: they looked, smiled, vocalized, and provided affectionate touch to their infants more frequently during interactions. These mothers also reported less depressive symptoms, possibly due to the effects of oxytocin on maternal mood, and their infants showed better neurobehavioral and cognitive development at 6 months. Associations were found between higher levels of maternal depression and lower levels of maternal touch, indicating that maternal postpartum depression may be related to decreased maternal ability to maintain physical intimacy with their infants. This difficulty leads to disruptions in the mothering system, which in turn decreases the infant's involvement and reliance on the mother.

Associations between maternal depression and reduced touch and contact were found in several other studies we conducted in normative and at-risk populations. For instance, among clinically-referred infants with a range of social-emotional disorders of infancy (e.g., sleep disorders, feeding disorders, attachment disorders, and mood disorders) higher maternal depression was associated with less maternal affectionate touch, less infant touch, and reduced physical proximity between mother and child during naturalistic interactions, with mother's placing infants more frequently out of arms' reach during play so that no accidental contact would occur (Feldman, Keren, Gross-Rozval, & Tyano, 2004). Similarly, comparing the parent-infant and family interactions in Israeli and Palestinian families, it was found that in both cultures, higher maternal depression was associated with less affectionate touch and physical contact between mothers and fathers and their 5-month-old infants and less contact was also observed between spouses when mothers were depressed (Feldman, Masalha, & Alony, 2006).

In a second study, the first to examine plasma oxytocin across pregnancy and early postpartum in relation to maternal behavior in humans, we followed 63 healthy women at 3 time-points: in the first trimester of pregnancy, in the last trimester, and in the first postpartum month (Feldman, Levine, Zagoory-Sharon, & Weller, 2006). At each time-point oxytocin was essayed from plasma and mothers reported anxiety and depression. In the first postbirth month, mothers were videotaped in a natural interaction and were interviewed regarding their experience as mothers. Higher oxytocin in the first trimester predicted more maternal behavior, particularly higher frequencies of affectionate touch, pointing to the priming role of oxytocin for the development of bonding which possibly functions, among other modes, by means of increasing touch and contact. Women who were depressed in the first trimester of pregnancy showed lower levels oxytocin during pregnancy and engaged in less maternal behavior in the postpartum. Immediate touch and contact, therefore, appear to be central for the mother, both in terms of initiating the neuropeptide oxytocin system implicated in bonding and for the development of early relational behaviors and social contingencies that provide a necessary foundation for the infant's growth and development.

In addition to the physiological and behavioral manifestation of bonding – which is found in all mammals – attachment in the human mother is organized by a specific set of mental representations that depend on the availability of immediate mother–infant contact. Contact helps the mother transform the fantasies she had during pregnancy from the "imagined" infant to the real infant, and such images build around the child a mental system of thoughts, representations, worries, and wishes, which are critical for the infant's mental and social-emotional development (Stern, 1995). Hinde (1989) argues that, unlike other mammals, bond formation in humans is organized by cognitive and meta-cognitive processes that coordinate responses at the biological, perceptual, and behavioral levels. Important to note that in all mammals, maternal bonding involves the integration of two seemingly polarized processes: those related to the activation of *fear* systems, including heightened awareness, vigilance, and anxiety; and those related to *reward* systems, implicated in hedonic homeostasis, motivation, and the incentive value invested in the object of love. In humans, however, in addition to processes that activate the fear system (which are mediated by brainstem and limbic structures) bonding also includes preoccupations and worries about the physical health and emotional well-being of the infant. Similarly, the reward component considers the motivational and incentive value placed on the loved person and is mediated in part by midbrain, thalamic, and hypothalamic structures. In humans, it is expressed not only in selective contact, hormonal release, and affiliative touch, but also in attachment representations and thoughts concerning the self, the infant, and the future relationship (Leckman et al., 2004).

During the first postpartum weeks, the mother's mental state has been described by Winnicott (1956) as that of "primary parental preoccupation," a state that resembles an obsessive-compulsive condition. Mothers are completely preoccupied with thoughts and worries about the infant's well-being and safety and the future relationship. At the same time, dyad-specific, relationship-building behaviors and mental representations begin to emerge. They include singing or talking to the infant in a special way, nursing or bathing the child in a special position, looking for resemblances between the infant and other family members, or engaging in pleasant thoughts of the infant as the most perfect baby ever born. During the bonding period, mothers are unable to go for more than 15 minutes without the intrusion of thoughts or worries about the infant's well-being and safety (Leckman, et al., 1999). Using fMRI technology, Swain and colleagues (2004) found that the level of maternal anxious-intrusive thoughts in the postpartum were associated with activation in arousal and emotion brain centers – particularly in the midbrain and amygdala – when mothers were exposed to their own infant cry versus a standard baby cry.

The bonding-related maternal cognition and mental state depends on the availability of immediate touch and contact. When contact is precluded, for instance after premature birth, the nature and frequency of the bonding-related cognitions are diminished or altered. Because the mother's representations and preoccupations are related to both the physiological and behavioral levels, disruptions to the neurobiological foundation of bonding are likely to affect the mother's mental investment. We found that the degree of maternal pleasant thoughts of the infant and the emergence of relationship-building behaviors were related to maternal oxytocin levels in early pregnancy and the postpartum. Immediate maternal-infant contact, therefore, appears to function as a trigger for the initiation of maternal bonding at the biological, behavioral, and cognitive-mental levels. This "maternal bonding" constellation is coordinated with specific inborn neurobehavioral sensitivities of the infant to maternal cues, including the mother's voice, touch, body rhythms, and odor. Over time, autonomic, neurological, and endocrinological systems in each partner are sensitized to the temporal patterns of the other, leading to the formation of a unique mother–infant bond (Fleming et al., 1999) that provides the basis for the infant's physical growth, emotional security, and the capacity to form meaningful ties throughout life.

Prematurity: A Break in Maternal Bonding

Premature birth disrupts the formation of maternal bonding. Following premature birth, full maternal-infant contact is not available as infants are placed in incubators, nursing is typically not possible, and birth is often not vaginal. Such conditions disrupt the proper functioning of the neuropeptide oxytocin system. For mothers who delivered full-term infants by Cesarean section and did not nurse them, the oxytocinergic system is typically initiated through maternal-infant touch and contact, which starts the system's feedback loop. Unfortunately, in the case of prematurity, all avenues for the proper functioning of the systems are shut. As such, any intervention that may "initiate" the oxytocin bonding system at the critical postbirth period – whether through touch, contact, or nursing – is likely to have a major impact on the entire maternal bonding constellation.

On the behavioral level, mothers of premature infants tend to display less looking, vocalizing, and touch-and-contact behavior toward their infants and report lower levels of relationship-building behaviors and attachment representations in the postpartum even when discharged from the hospital (Davis & Thoman, 1988; Feldman et al., 1999; Minde, 2000). At the same time, the infant's neurological immaturity decreases its capacity for social responsiveness and contingency detection, and mothers of premature neonates are less able to coordinate their interactive behavior with the infant's momentary alertness (Eckerman et al., 1995; Feldman & Eidelman, 2007). This creates a paradoxical state: the premature infant depends on the mother's sensitive approach to a greater extent than the full-term infant in order to reach developmental milestones (Belsky, 1998). However, the decrease in the mother's postpartum behavior and the infant's unclear social signals often result in less sensitive parenting among mothers of premature infants (Lester, Hoffman, & Brazelton, 1985). Because the mother's sensitivity is formed in the first weeks of life and remains relatively stable across infancy and childhood, it is especially important to target mothers of premature infants in the immediate postpartum period. Thus, interventions that may promote maternal sensitivity and increase maternal behavior in the postpartum may place the mother–infant relationship at a better starting point. Maternal sensitivity is among the central predictors of children's cognitive, social, and emotional growth, and thus, higher maternal sensitivity is likely to lead to better outcomes for the fragile premature infant (Feldman et al., 2004).

On the representational level, following premature birth, the mother's bonding-related representations appear to "shut down" to a certain extent. Mothers of very low birth weight infants, whose infants went through a period of life-threatening illness, report lower levels of preoccupations and worries about the infant's well-being, health, and growth, less of the typical relationship-building behaviors, and lower levels of pleasurable attachment representations (Feldman et al., 1999). The condition such mothers report mirrors the infant state of "loss," described by Bowlby (1969). In this condition, infants whose mothers are physically or emotionally unavailable for a lengthy period, and the behavioral repertoire of the "protest" stage was not successful in bringing the mother back, the infant sinks into a depressed-like state characterized by social withdrawal, motor retardation, introversion, and sadness. Mothers of sick preterm infants may similarly enter a state of apathy, depression, and lower investment in the infant. From an evolutionary perspective mothers may be preserving their emotional resources for the next, more viable offspring. Important to mention that premature birth often increases the mother's depression, anxiety, guilt, and sense of helplessness (Keren, Feldman, Eidelman, Sirota, & Lester, 2003). When asked about their experience in the Neonatal Intensive Care Unit (NICU), mothers described feelings that the infant is not "theirs" but belongs to the staff, fears of becoming attached to a fragile child, and a sense of "estrangement" from the infant. When the premature infant is not a firstborn, mothers often describe a very different experience from their emotions toward the previous full-term infant. Contact with the child at that formative stage, in addition to its contribution to the biological and behavioral levels, is important in order to increase the mother's involvement, attachment representations, and sense of bonding and care for her child.

Maternal Proximity and Contact; The Infant's Perspective

Since the early works of Spitz (1946), the negative effects of early maternal separation on the infant's physical and emotional growth have been well-known. The extensive work of Hofer (for review; Hofer, 1995), spanning over 30 years of research in animal models, helped specify the effects of maternal proximity and physical contact on the development of biobehavioral regulation in the pup. In a series of studies, the researchers separated and experimentally manipulated specific components of the "maternal proximity" constellation; such as the mother's body heat, nursing, odor, or licking-and-grooming behaviors and showed their effects on specific physiological regulatory systems in the pup, such as sleep-wake cyclicity, thermoregulation, or autonomic regulation, with each maternal feature directly impacting a specific regulatory function. Other researchers extended this work and pointed to the role of maternal proximity for the regulation of arousal, attention, and exploration, and in the management of the stress response (Lehmann, Stohr, & Feldon, 2000).

Considerable evidence points to the effects of maternal proximity on the regulation of emotion and behavior and on the relations between maternal separation, arousal disregulation, and behavior disorganization. Anand and Scalzo (2000) describe two pathways by which prematurity disrupts behavior organization. Maternal separation leads to apoptosis (programmed cell-death) in multiple areas of the immature brain, while pain exposure causes excessive excitatory amino acid activation that result in excitotoxic damage to developing neurons. Behaviorally, both conditions are expressed in disturbed reactivity, difficulties in sustained attention, and inability to self-regulate. Rodents separated from their mothers showed changes in the prelimbic prefrontal areas, causing increased excitation and hyper-reactivity (Poeggel, et al., 1999), and early separation was found to alter HPA and corticotropin-releasing hormone (CRH) pathways, compromising stress-management capacities throughout life (Francis, Diorio, Plotsky, & Meaney, 2002). These studies highlight the construct of "maternal proximity" – the mother's physical presence in its entirety, including her smell, touch, voice, nursing, biological rhythms, body heat, and unique interactive style – as a central regulatory framework for the infant's growth and development in the first postbirth period.

As suggested by the "sensitive period" perspective, when early maternal proximity is unavailable – due to prematurity, maternal illness, or maternal depression – the missing maternal contact has a lifelong impact on the development of regulatory functions in the cognitive and social-emotional domains. Moreover, because higher mechanisms of cognitive control (such as executive functions and causal reasoning) depend on the proper regulation of lower cognitive abilities (such as the regulation of attention, perception, and memory) deficits in the first months of life related to maternal deprivation are likely to exert a lifelong impact on the infant's higher cognitive skills. Similarly, the regulation of complex emotions in later childhood and adolescence depends upon the child's acquired capacity to modulate basic emotions in the first months of life, which is shaped in the context of the infant's initial closeness to the mother.

The soothing effect of maternal touch and contact on the infant during moments of distress can be seen in studies employing the "still-face" procedure. In this procedure, which has been used to assess the young infant's self-regulatory capacities in the face of maternal unavailability, mothers play with the infant naturally and then refrain from interacting and maintain a still face for 2 minutes, before resuming natural play. During maternal still-face infants react with distress and a marked decrease in social behavior, including gazing, positive affect, and vocalization toward the mother. However, when mothers were able to maintain touch of the infant while performing the still-face, the infant's distress was substantially reduced, suggesting that touch may uphold the mother–infant communication when other channels are unavailable (Stack & Muir, 1992). Cross-cultural research shows that mothers in non-Western societies provide more touch and contact to their infants and these infants show lower levels of negative emotionality (Tronick, 1995). Maternal contact is thought to provide an "external regulation" (Field, 1994), a protected arena for the practice self-regulatory skills. From a psychoanalytic perspective, maternal touch and contact provide the "holding environment" (Winnicott, 1956), the safe haven where infants can develop the differentiation of self and other, form selective and enduring bonds to significant others, and gain a sense of trust in the world. The holding environment is also the place from which play, creativity, imagination, and the appreciation for culture, art, and spirituality grow and consolidate.

Prematurity: A Double Risk for the Fragile Immature Infant

Prematurity is a condition that involves both immaturity of physiological systems and disruption to the mother–infant relationship. Premature birth truncates the normal development of neurological systems responsible for the regulation and fine-tuning of basic physiological processes, such as sleep and wakefulness, sucking and feeding, thermo-regulation, stress management, attention, and the organization of social encounters, functions that lay the foundation for the emergence of emotion regulation (Feldman et al., 2004). Birth alters the developmental course of brain maturation and, since even the most optimal incubator conditions cannot mimic the intrauterine environment, delays the maturation process of the various physiological regulators. In addition, prematurity involves early and persistent maternal separation, as infants are placed in incubators immediately after birth and are deprived of the essential inputs of the mother's physical presence. Consequently, premature infants typically exhibit difficulties in regulatory functions, such as organizing attention, regulating negative affect, maintaining optimal thresholds of reactivity, moderating social interactions, and sustaining exploration of the environment. In later childhood and adolescence, children who were born prematurely, tend to show higher levels of conduct disorders, more attention and hyperactivity problems, low frustration tolerance and poor social skills (Malatesta, Grigoryev, Lamb, Albin, & Culver, 1986; McCormick, Workman-Daniels, & Brooks-Gunn, 1996; Ruff, 1986; Sigman, Cohen, Beckwith, & Parmelee, 1986; Thoman, Denenberg, Sievel, Zeidner, & Becker, 1981).

Parent–Infant Skin-to-Skin Contact (Kangaroo Care)

Similar to other forms of natural interventions, the Kangaroo Care (KC) method emerged out of necessity. Confronted with a shortage of incubators in Bogota, Columbia, the medical staff used parents as natural incubators. Premature infants in stable medical condition were placed naked between the mother's breasts, to facilitate nursing, while body temperature was regulated through the maternal body heat. Infants remained attached to the mother around the clock until they matured and were able to maintain their own body heat in the external environment, and fathers and other family members often participated in the KC intervention for parts of the day. A series of randomized clinical trials in Columbia showed that the "kangaroo mother intervention" was safe in caring for low birth-weight premature infants and did not increase mortality or morbidity rates as compared to infants cared for by standard incubator care (Charpak, Ruiz, de Calume, & Charpak, 1997; Sloan, Camacho, Rojas, & Stern, 1994).

In the last decade, the benefits of early maternal-infant contact for the premature infant became apparent, and the Kangaroo Care intervention changed from being a method used out of necessity in developing countries to a method of choice used in many hospitals in industrialized countries. Once the infant's medical condition stabilized, parents and infants were offered the option to spend a portion of their day in the kangaroo position. Infants were placed naked (wearing a diaper and sometimes a cap) in the kangaroo position while still being attached to the monitoring devices. The kangaroo position afforded parents the only opportunity for a full body contact with their premature infant, and the experience was thought to help facilitate the maternal infant bond and the working through of the trauma of premature birth (Affonso, Bosque, Wahlberg, & Brady, 1993).

As the KC method was introduced to Western NICUs, evidence of the benefits of skin-to-skin contact for the development of premature infants was beginning to accumulate. Research throughout the 1990s showed – mainly through anecdotal and studies in small samples – that the KC intervention has a positive impact on infant development and the maternal-infant bonding. Three main areas were discussed as showing improvement following KC: the regulation of the infant's physiology and behavior, increasing nursing rates and maternal lactation, and improving the mother's mood and sense of parenting. These early studies were important because they pointed to the dimensions that might improve following mother–infant bodily contact. However, these studies were not rigorous methodologically, often relied on case reports, and no observations of mother–infant interactions took place

(Charpak, Ruiz-Palaez, & de Calume, 1996). Importantly, infants were not followed after discharge and no longitudinal data on the long-term effects of KC on infant development or parenting behavior was available.

Recently, several follow-up studies of infants who received KC in the neonatal period in comparison with controls have been reported. Our longitudinal research, which is among the most comprehensive follow-ups of the KC intervention, examined 146 infants from birth to 6 months, a select group of KC and controls infants were seen until the age of 5 years, and we are currently observing all infants that are able and willing to come at age nine. We suggest that the KC intervention provides a unique paradigm to examine key theoretical issues in a human model, including the short- and long-term effects of maternal separation, the positive impact of touch and contact on self-regulatory systems, the role of early experiences in infant development, and the effects of minor variations in maternal bonding on later growth. Research in animal models supports the hypothesis that early contact during periods of maternal separation has positive and lasting effects on the development of attention and emotion-regulation, and on stress management throughout life (Francis, Diorio, Plotsky, & Meaney, 2002; Weizman, et al., 1999). On the basis of our longitudinal findings, we suggest that mother–infant contact has an impact on four domains of development; (1) improving the regulation of infant arousal, attention, and emotion, (2) accelerating neuro-maturation, (3) improving the mother's mood, and (4) promoting the parent–infant relationship and the coregulation of social interactions. These improvements in self- and coregulatory skills in the first year of life predict better cognitive and social-emotional development for the treated infants.

It is important to note that recently, the KC intervention has been applied to other high-risk conditions for the mother–infant bonding, including maternal depression, anxiety, and grief following stillbirth (Burkhammer, Anderson, & Chiu, 2004). It thus seems that the kangaroo intervention is gradually expanding and being applied to various conditions that may compromise the mother–infant bonding, either for maternal or child biological reasons. Similarly, applying kangaroo contact to term neonates in the immediate postbirth hours improves the infant's neurobehavioral maturation (Ferber & Makhoul, 2004), findings that emphasize the importance of early bodily contact for all infants.

The Longitudinal Kangaroo Care Project; Effects on Mother and Child

Our longitudinal Kangaroo Care Project followed 146 low birth-weight premature infants and their families born in the Jerusalem and Tel-Aviv areas in Israel. All infants were born with a birth weight below 1750 gram and gestational age of 33 weeks or less to two-parent families of middle-class background. Of these, 73 infants received KC for at least 1 hour per day for a period of at least 2 weeks and 73 served as controls, matched for gender, birth-weight, gestational age, the degree of medical risk, and family demographic (including maternal and paternal age and education and birth order). No differences between groups were found on Apgar 1 and 5 scores, the ratio of vaginal to Cesarean delivery, and the family's social support network.

The KC was targeted to a period when the infant was still incubated and full maternal-infant bodily contact was precluded for medical reasons. Infants and their parents were seen at four time-points; at pre-kangaroo (controls were observed at 32 weeks GA, matched to the mean age of the initiation of KC); at term age; and at 3 and 6 months corrected age. A subsample (N = 70) was also observed at 12 and 24 months of age and at 5 years. We are now in the process of following all children whom we are able to locate and are willing to come at 9 years, and data for this follow-up is being collected.

The pre-kangaroo and term observations took place in the hospital, the 3-month observation was conducted in the family home, and the 6-month assessment took place in a developmental laboratory, to allow for the assessment of infant behavior in different settings and contexts. Following, the 1, 2, 5, and 9 years assessments all took place in a developmental laboratory. Multiple outcome measures were collected, including physiological indices, standard tests, attention and perception measures, observations of infant reaction to stimuli, mother–infant, father–infant, and family interactions, and parental interviews and self-reports. Results of these multiple assessments indicated that KC had a positive, multi-dimensional impact on child development, which led to lasting gains in infants' cognitive and social-emotional development. In the following, I present the main findings under four headings; infant self-regulation, neuromaturation and biobehavioral processes, maternal mood and lactation, and the parent–child relationship. Each topic is introduced with a general overview, followed by review of previous KC studies on the topic and finally, data from out longitudinal project in each domain is presented.

Maternal-Infant Contact and the Development of Self-Regulatory Functions

Hofer's work on the contribution of maternal proximity to the formation of regulatory structures suggests that providing kangaroo contact is likely to improve physiological and behavior regulation. Indeed, since its introduction in Bogota, Columbia, the kangaroo method was found to have a stabilizing effect on the infant's physiological systems (Fischer, Sontheimer, Scheffer, Bauer, & Linderkamp, 1998; Ludington and Golant, 1993). Studies of before, during, and after skin-to-skin contact showed that during contact infants spent more time in quiet sleep, heart rate was lower and more stable, episodes of apnea and bradycardia decreased, body temperature was maintained, and oxygenation and gas exchange improved (Acolet, Sleath, & Whitelaw, 1989; Bauer, Sontheimer, Fischer, & Linderkamp, 1996; Bier et al., 1996; Bosque, Brady, Affonso, & Wahlberg, 1995; Fohe, Dropf, & Avenarius, 2000; Ludington-Hoe & Swinth, 1996; Tornhage, Stude, Lindberg, & Serenius, 1998). Skin-to-skin contact was also found to improve arousal regulation and stress reactivity. Michelsson and colleagues (1996) showed that infants in cots cried ten times as much as infants who were being held by their mothers and spectographic cry analysis showed the cry of held infants to be less distressful. A reduction in beta-endorphin was found following KC, suggesting that kangaroo contact attenuates the stress response (Mooncey, Giannakoulopoulos, Glober, Acolet, & Modi, 1997). These findings demonstrate the effects of early maternal contact on behavior organization, arousal regulation, and physiological stability.

The effects of skin-to-skin contact were found to persist even after contact ended. Following kangaroo contact premature infants slept longer and their sleep was more restful and organized (Gale, Frank, & Lund, 1993). Interestingly, kangaroo-contact improved not only sleep but also alert states, as shown by the findings that infants spent longer periods in alert states after KC (Gale & Vandenberg, 1998). Skin-to-skin contact reduced infant negative emotionality, and infants treated by KC were reported by their mothers to cry less as compared to controls at 6 months (Whitelaw, Heiserkamp, Sleath, Acolet, & Richards, 1988). Faster growth rates and earlier discharge from the hospital were also reported for infants treated with KC in India (Kambarami, Chidede, & Kowo, 1998), pointing to the positive impact of skin-to-skin contact on growth and maturation. A recent review summing up 25 years since the introduction of the Kangaroo Mother Intervention shows that, overall, studies pointed not only to the safety of the intervention but to its beneficial effects in regulating the infant's systems and in improving the mother–infant and family relationship in later infancy (Charpak et al., 2005).

Self-regulatory functions; Findings from the KC longitudinal study

Among the most basic regulatory functions is the regulation of sleep and wakefulness. The organization of the biological clock is thought to provide the foundation for the development of attention, arousal, and behavior regulation (Dahl, 1996). Due to the role of maternal proximity in organizing the biological clock in mammals, KC was expected to promote more organized sleep-wake cyclicity in the neonatal period, which, in turn, would lead to better arousal modulation, emotion regulation, and exploratory behavior across infancy.

To assess sleep-wake cyclicity, 4 hours of infant state were observed at pre-kangaroo and again at term age. As the sleep-wake cycle of newborns has been shown to last between 60 and 70 minutes, this time-frame enabled the detection of several sleep-wake cycles. States were defined according to Brazelton (1973) and included quiet sleep, active sleep, sleep-wake transition, unfocused alertness, alert wakefulness, and cry. A coder sat at the infant's bedside and marked infant state for each 10-second epoch. The distribution of states across the 4-hour period was examined and sleep-wake cyclicity was measured with spectral analysis, with higher amplitudes indicating better organization of the biological clock. No differences were found at the pre-kangaroo observation. At term age, infants who received KC showed longer periods of quiet sleep and alert wakefulness and shorter periods of active sleep and their sleep-wake cycle was more organized. The consolidation of the sleep-wake cycle is required for the later fine-tuning of the arousal system and its regulation into micro-patterns of activity and rest, observed in tasks such as attention shifting, arousal modulation, and attention maintenance (Feldman, Weller, Sirota & Eidelman, 2002). As suggested, more organized sleep-wake cyclicity is an index of maturity in terms of more optimal balance between the reactive and regulatory aspects of the state system, which is the system that provides the global framework for experience, growth, and learning in the neonatal period (Brazelton, 1990).

At 3 months corrected age, infants' arousal modulation and emotion regulation were assessed with a procedure where infants are presented with 17 stimuli and stimuli increase in the magnitude of intrusiveness, ranging from a simple unimodel stimulus (light, soft sound) to multi-modal, high-impact stimuli (a car flashing lights and making loud noises approaching the infant). Each stimulus was presented for 10 seconds with a 20-second break between stimuli. Infants who received skin-to-skin contact showed an improved performance on two aspects of emotion regulation. First, their "threshold" to negative emotionality was higher, meaning that they were able to tolerate more aversive stimuli. And second, the Kangaroo Care infants were better able to modulate their arousal to the onset and offset of stimulation. They showed medium reactivity – an optimal mode for information intake – during periods of "stimulus on" and low reactivity during periods of "stimulus off". The ability to shift between optimal reactivity during information intake and utilize the period of stimulus offset for rest and processing is an index of an efficient, task-specific and mature information processing system (Feldman & Mayes, 1999) and the findings suggest that kangaroo contact impacted the infants' emotion regulation and arousal modulation capacities. These results point to the role of maternal proximity in providing a barrier for outside stimulation and in increasing the threshold to negative reactivity, a central determinant of emotion regulation. The findings also underscore the role of early contact in promoting mature, task-specific information processing by organizing infant arousal to more optimal levels to quickly respond to changing inputs (Feldman et al., 2002).

At 6 months corrected age, the infant's exploratory behavior was assessed during mother–infant interaction. Mothers were provided with six new toys in a basket and asked to play with the infant using these toys. Microanalysis of the interactions focused on the direction of maternal and infant gaze, maternal and infant affect, infant exploratory behavior, and the mother's modes of demonstrating toys to the infant. Shared visual attention was defined as periods when both mother and infant were simultaneously looking at the same object. Infant sustained exploration was coded when the infant explored the toy with two hands, showed visible interest, and the exploration lasted at least 2 seconds. Mothers and infants in the KC group spent longer periods in shared visual attention and the latency to the first episode of shared attention was shorter. Mothers of controls spent more time in introducing new toys, whereas mothers of KC infants spent more time jointly manipulating and exploring the toy with their child. More sustained exploration was found in the KC group, both in terms of longer durations of sustained exploration and shorter latencies to the first exploratory bid. These findings demonstrate a link between self-regulatory processes, observed in the infant's ability to quickly settle into exploratory play, and maternal coregulation of infant exploration, observed in the KC mothers' improved ability to present stimulation in a synchronous and appropriate manner and to jointly engage in gaze and exploration with their infants (Feldman et al., 2002).

Findings at 1 and 2 years suggest that infants who received kangaroo contact as infants functioned better on the fine-tuned measures of self-regulation. For instance, at 1 year infants were tested in a sensory integration paradigm where they were familiarized to different shapes (e.g., square, circle, etc.) through the modality of touch but had to recognize these "learned" objects on the basis of vision in a visual novelty responsiveness paradigm. Infants in the KC group were able to better integrate the modalities of touch and vision and showed higher novelty preference in this intermodal task (i.e, looked longer at the novel figure when familiarization was by touch). These infants were also better able to manage separation distress during a separation-reunion paradigm with their mothers. At the end of the visit, mothers were asked to leave the room and the infant remained with a stranger for several minutes. The child's behavior, affect, distress, and ability to maintain exploration were microcoded. Similar to the findings for the emotional stimuli at 3 months, KC infants showed less distress and were better able to maintain exploration of the environment during periods of maternal absence.

Findings from 2 and 5 years similarly show that the main long-term effects of skin-to-skin contact are in the area of self-regulation, in both the attention and emotional domains. At 2 years, infants in the Kangaroo Care group showed better executive functions, which refer to the child's ability to inhibit a dominant response in order to allow for a sub-dominant response. At 5 years, we found that infants who received kangaroo contact did not differ from the controls on measures of global intelligence and language development. However, similar to the findings for 2 years, subtle differences in tasks requiring inhibitions, self-restraint, attention shifting, and emotion regulation were found and children in the KC group showed a better performance.

At present, we are testing the cohort at 9 years of age and attempting to reach the entire group of 146 children. We are particularly interested in the fine-grained measures of emotion regulation and cognitive control. The children's response to different emotions are observed, executive functions are tested, and sleep patterns are assessed over several nights to examine whether early contact has a long-lasting effect on the unfolding of regulatory behavior in time. We expect that the sleep patterns in the KC group, as measured by actigraphs, would be more organized, that their behavioral and physiological response to anger and distress would be more modulated, and that their ability to perform complex cognitive tasks requiring the participation of higher cortical mechanisms would be more integrated.

Mother–Infant Contact and Infant Neuromaturation

According to Goetlieb's (1991) theory, the development of the senses is organized in a sequential order with the primary senses – touch and proprioception – preceding the development of the secondary senses, vision and audition. Infants in the immediate post-birth period should receive substantially more information to the primary senses than to the secondary senses. Moreover, infants should receive visual and auditory stimuli while being held in their mothers' arms to buffer against excessive stimulation. Following premature birth, the sequential development of the senses is disturbed. Typical Western NICUs bombard infants with continuous light and nonstop noise, which their immature systems cannot process or ward off (Als, 1991). Animal research has shown that nursery conditions have an irreversible effect on neuromaturation. Simulating the continuous lights and sounds of a typical nursery and exposing newborn animals to these conditions resulted in permanent damage to the biological clock and in disturbances in information-processing and learning (Hao & Rivkees, 1999; Sleigh & Lickliter, 1998). Similarly, exposure to excessive pain has been shown to result in permanent damage to brain maturation, in terms of both structural and functional development (Grunau, 2002).

Intervention programs that provide separate components of the "maternal proximity" construct, such as massage, rhythmic stimulation, or minimal handling to filter overwhelming stimulation, improve neuromaturation in terms of physical growth, motor maturity, and physiological organization in premature infants (Feldman & Eidelman, 1998). It thus appears that any component of the mother's presence may serve to organize the infant's physiology and behavior during a period when full maternal contact is precluded. Consistent with the "sensitive period" perspective in neuro-development (Schore, 2001; Tucker, 1992), interventions applied during a specific time-window in brain-behavior relationship can have a lasting impact on the development of emotion regulation, arousal modulation, and stress management throughout life (Laviola & Terranova, 1998).

Skin-to-skin contact was found to promote neurodevelopment in premature infants. Ludington-Hoe & Swinth (1996) suggested that skin-to-skin contact contributes to stability and maturation in each of the five neuro-behavioral systems that are compromised by premature birth, including autonomic, motor, state, attention-interaction, and self-regulation. KC also functions as a buffer of the experience of pain and was found to be a useful method of pain reduction in full-term neonates. Kangaroo contact was used as an analgesic during painful medical procedures (Gray, Watt, & Blass, 2000) and assisted in the recovery process after heart surgery in full-term neonates (Gazzolo, Masetti, & Meli, 2000). Faster growth rates and maturation was observed following KC, and treated infants were discharged earlier from the hospital (Kambarami et al., 1998), which points to KC's positive impact on neuromaturation.

Neuromaturation; Findings from the KC longitudinal study

In our longitudinal study, the effect of KC on the maturation of the autonomic nervous system was operationalized by cardiac vagal tone (Porges, 1985), which was measured at pre-kangaroo and at term age and is now being assessed at 9 years. Cardiac vagal tone assesses the effects of respiration on heart-rate variability as mediated through the parasympathetic system and is a measure of the integrity and maturity of the autonomic nervous system in premature infants. Porges (1996) suggested that vagal tone indexes the mammalian brainstem organization and its adaptive capacity to mobilize or save energy in response to external or internal stresses. Vagal tone has been used as a physiological marker of the infant's emotion regulation capacities and has shown to predict infant development in full-term infants (Fox and Porges, 1985). In preterm infants, vagal tone has been associated with the degree of medical risk (DiPietro & Porges, 1991) and the resting vagal tone at term age was found to predict infant development up to 6 years of age (Doussard-Roosevelt, McClenny, & Porges, 2001). Neonatal vagal tone provides the neurological basis for the emergence of infant social behaviors and relatedness, and premature infants show lower vagal tone than full-term infants, due to the immaturity of neurological systems. This immaturity of the vagal system is associated with lower infant social alertness in the neonatal period and with lower levels of mother–infant synchrony at 3 months. We found that the resting vagal tone at term age was associated with the amount of maternal behavior in the postpartum, but only among preterm, not among full-term infants. Premature infants with low vagal tone received the lowest amount of maternal behavior, which places them at a higher risk for a range of developmental outcomes. As such, it is clear that interventions that can impact on the maturation of the vagal tone are likely to have an important impact on the infant's neurodevelopmental maturation.

Vagal tone index was extracted from 10 minutes of ECG recording according to a system developed by Porges at pre-kangaroo and again at 37 weeks GA. Whereas vagal maturation during this period was observed for all infants, those receiving KC showed a higher vagal tone at 37 weeks GA, indicating a quicker maturation of the autonomic nervous system (Feldman & Eidelman, 2003a). Thus, kangaroo contact appears to accelerate neuro-maturation rate during a period of rapid brain development as measured by objective physiological indices. Such findings point to the pervasive impact of maternal contact during periods of early separation on the maturation of neuro-functions in premature infants.

Longitudinal associations were found between resting vagal tone at term age and the development of emotion regulation in the first year, attention regulation in the second year, and self-regulation skills at age five, including the capacity for self-restraint, lower levels of externalizing and internalizing symptoms, and better executive functions. At 9 years, we are currently measuring the children's vagal tone at baseline and during challenging tasks, one in the cognitive and one in the emotional domain. In the cognitive domain, infants' vagal tone is assessed during the "Tower of London" test, which measures neurocognitive skills, and in the emotional domain, children assessed in a procedure where they listen and reflect on a tape of an interadult angry exchange. Consistent with previous research (El-Sheik, 2001), we expect the Kangaroo Care group, who showed better regulatory skills across infancy and early childhood, to have higher baseline vagal tone, higher vagal withdrawal during challenging stimuli, and a quicker recovery of the ANS system.

In addition, neurodevelopmental maturation in the KC and control groups was assessed with the NBAS (Brazelton, 1973) at term age. Following kangaroo contact infants received higher scores on the orientation and habituation clusters of the NBAS. Of the NBAS clusters, disturbances in orientation and habituation are those most associated with a variety of risk signals. Poorer orientation is correlated with higher stress reactivity and negative emotionality (Auerbach et al., 1999; Spangler & Scheubeck, 1993) and habituation is related to pathological conditions such as prenatal exposure to cocaine (Mayes, Granger, Frank, Schottenfeld, & Bornstein, 1993). These findings are consistent with those of a Japanese sample, which similarly showed that following KC infants' orientation scores were higher (Ohgi et al., 2002). Orientation indexes the infant's ability to mobilize sufficient internal resources to attend to visual and auditory environmental stimuli. These capacities mark a mature and organized internal system, which enable efficient information processing and later learning. These findings point to the role of the maternal contact in organizing infant orientation to the environment, possibly leading to more mature neurodevelopmental profiles. Vagal tone and sleep-wake cyclicity were both related to infant orientation, indicating that proper functioning of the autonomic nervous systems and the biological clock shape the infant's first approach to its environment. The capacity to orient to the environment appears therefore to be related to smooth and synchronous functioning of the various regulators (Feldman & Eidelman, 2003a).

Mother–Infant Contact and Maternal Well-Being, Mood, and Lactation

Apart from its contribution to the infant's physiological stability and stress reactivity, skin-to-skin contact is among the stimulants of maternal lactation following premature birth. Although breast milk is especially important for the vulnerable premature infant, all to often mothers of premature infants give up nursing when faced with the difficulties of expressing milk (Killersreiter, Grimmer, Buhrer, Dudenhausen, & Oblade, 2002). Breast milk consists of proteins, enzymes, micronutrients, lipids, and particularly long-chain polyunsaturated fatty acids, which are critical for the growth and development of premature infants (Heird, 2001). In addition, breast milk has long-term effects on cognitive development (Horwood, Darlow, & Mogridge, 2001), neurobehavioral maturation, and mother–infant interaction in premature infants (Feldman & Eidelman, 2003). Given these findings, intervention strategies that may increase nursing rates among mothers of preterm infants are valuable.

Skin-to-skin contact was found to increase nursing among mothers of premature infants. Evaluating the correlates of lactations in mothers of very low birthweight infants, Furman and colleagues (2002) found that KC was related to continuing maternal nursing beyond forty weeks gestational age, and skin-to-skin contact has shown to increase the volume of maternal milk (Hurst, Valentine, & Renfro, 1997). A study in New Delhi, India reported that low birthweight premature infants who received 4 hours of KC per day had faster weight gains, were discharged earlier from the hospital, and their mothers were more likely to be exclusively breastfed as compared to controls (Ramanathan, Paul, Deorari, Taneja, & George, 2001). Following the initial cohort of the infants who received KC in Bogota, Columbia, Charpak and colleagues (2001) found that more infants in the kangaroo intervention group were breastfed by 3 months corrected age as compared to incubator-cared infants. In addition, Meyer and Anderson (1999) began to use the kangaroo position with mothers of full-term infants who were experiencing difficulties in nursing, expanding the KC intervention beyond the care of premature infants.

By affording touch and contact and stimulating breast milk, skin-to-skin contact increases maternal oxytocin levels, thereby promoting maternal behavior. Because oxytocin functions to reduce stress and depression (Carter, 1998), skin-to-skin contact also provides a buffer against post-partum depression. Indeed, Dombrowski and colleagues (2001) applied the KC intervention successfully with a woman who suffered post-partum depression. Mothers who provided KC reported more positive feelings toward the infant, lower parental stress, and better sense of the parenting role (Affonso et al., 1993; Neu, 1999). Although no observations were made of mother–infant interactions, these reports suggest that KC may help reverse some of the negative effects of premature birth on the mother, her identity as a competent parent, and reduce the guilt and anxiety that typically accompany premature birth (Brooten, Gennaro, Brown, Butts, Gibbons, Bakewill-Sachs, & Kumar, 1988).

Finally, another important dimension of the KC intervention is its contribution to maternal well-being in developing countries. Reports from Zimbabwe (Kambarami, Chidede, & Kowo, 1999) or Papua New Guinea

(McMaster & Vince, 2000), among others, describe the positive effects of KC on maternal and infant well-being. These findings highlight the KC intervention as a natural, cost-free intervention, which does not require long training or sophisticated methodologies but carries a significant benefit to the infant and the mother–infant dyad.

Maternal Well-Being; Findings from the KC longitudinal study

In line with previous case reports, KC was expected to have a positive effect on maternal depression and on the mother's perception of her premature infant. Upon discharge, maternal depression was lower among KC mothers, and an interaction effect of group and medical risk indicated that KC improved maternal mood especially among those with low-risk premature infants. Mothers of low-risk preterm infants were able to achieve full contact with their infants only several days after birth and this experience possibly improved the negative effects of infant incubation (Feldman et al., 2002). At term age, KC mothers also perceived their infants as less different than the average full-term neonate. Although maternal anxiety at term age did not differentiate the groups, at 6 months KC mothers reported lower separation anxiety. Mothers of premature infants often suffer higher levels of anxiety and depression (Brooten et al., 1988) and perceive their infant as very different from the normal healthy child (Levy-Shiff, Sharir, & Mogilner, 1989). The findings thus suggest that following KC mothers are better prepared for the maternal role.

Findings from ages 1, 2, and 5 show that no differences in mothers' moods or well-being were detected between the KC and control mothers. However, maternal depression in the neonatal period had a negative impact on aspects of the children's cognitive, social, and emotional development until 5 years of age, findings consistent with much previous research (Goodman & Gottlieb, 1999). Thus, the improvement in maternal mood and depressive symptomatology following Kangaroo contact may help put the mother–infant relationship on a more favorable trajectory, which, in turn, has a positive effect on the child's ultimate development.

Maternal–Infant Contact and the Development of the Mother–Infant and Family Relationship

As suggested above, premature birth alters the context of the mother–infant relationship and the reasons are related to both the disruption in the maternal bonding and the immaturity of the infant's neurological systems. Difficulties in the mother–infant coregulation may also be related to the premature infant's limited self-regulation capacities. Premature infants have difficulties maintaining visual attention during play (Eckerman, Hsu, Molitor, Leung, & Goldstein, 1999), and their emotional expressions are often unclear (Malatesta et al., 1986), conditions which make it difficult for the mother to read and interpret the infant's communicative signals. Because premature infants are less regulated, prone to negative emotionality, and less able to modulate arousal, they are less rewarding social partners. Although there are no previous studies documenting the effects of KC on the mother–infant interaction patterns, its reported effects on maternal lactation, mood, and sense of parenting suggest a potential impact on maternal behavior.

Mother–Child and Family Relationships; Findings from the KC longitudinal study

Skin-to-skin contact may promote the mother's ability to provide a more sensitive framework for infant development. Close contact increases the mother's familiarity with the infant and her improved mood may increase maternal investment. The development of the mother–infant relationship relies on the mother's gradual learning of the infant's interactive signals, which mothers typically acquire during moments of physical intimacy. The infant's improved self-regulation and shared attention skills following KC may also contribute to the structuring of the interaction, leading to more reciprocal exchange.

Mother–infant interactions were videotaped and coded at term age in the hospital and at 3 and 6 months corrected age. Because social processes are dialectical, more optimal interactions in the neonatal period are likely to continue in a mutually-reinforcing way and lead to improved interactions at later stages. In the newborn period, mother–infant interactions were subjected to micro-coding of maternal and infant behavior, which focused on maternal gaze, affect, touch, vocalization, and adaptation to infant signal, and on the infant's state and interactive alertness. Mothers in the KC group showed more affectionate touch to their infant, were more adaptive to infant signals, and their infants were more alert during social interactions (Feldman et al., 2002), indicating that the mother–infant dyad was off to a better start following the KC intervention.

Mother–infant interaction in the KC group continued to be more positive at 3 and 6 months. At these ages mother–infant interaction was coded with the Coding Interactive Behavior Manual (CIB; Feldman, 1998). The CIB is a global coding system of adult–infant interaction that includes 42 scales summarized into six parent, infant, and dyadic composites. The system which has shown reliability and validity, was applied to a range of healthy and at risk populations. The system also has shown sensitivity to infant age, interacting partner, cultural variability, and biological and social-emotional risk conditions (Feldman & Klein, 2003; Feldman, Masalha, & Nadam, 2001; Feldman et al., 2004; Feldman, Keren et al., 2004).

Mothers of KC infants were more sensitive and less intrusive during mother–infant interactions and infants showed higher social involvement and lower negative emotionality. The level of dyadic reciprocity between KC mothers and their infants was higher as compared to controls (Feldman, Weller, Eidelman, & Sirota, 2003). It is important to note that improvements in the mother–infant interaction were observed on those dimensions reported to be compromised by premature birth, i.e., reduced maternal sensitivity, increased intrusiveness, lower reciprocity, and lower infant involvement. These findings may suggest that KC functions to reverse some of the negative effects of premature birth on the mother–infant relationship. The dialectical relationship between self- and coregulation was observed in the findings that higher maternal affectionate touch and adaptation in the neonatal period were related to better arousal modulation at 3 months and to better cognitive development at 6 months. Results in the opposite directions were also found; improved sleep-wake cyclicity at term age correlated with higher maternal sensitivity at 3 months and dyadic reciprocity at 6 months.

At 6 months mother–infant interaction continued to show lower levels of infant negative affect and higher levels of maternal sensitivity and dyadic reciprocity in the KC group (Feldman et al., 2002). As maternal sensitivity is considered a stable attribute throughout infancy, the early effects of KC on maternal sensitivity appear to be critical in shaping more optimal mother–infant relational patterns.

Follow-up at 1 and 2 years showed that infants who received KC were more involved, creative, and socially alert during interactions and the dyadic relationship was more reciprocal. Toddlers who received KC in the neonatal period also exhibited less behavior problems, in terms of both externalizing and internalizing behavior symptoms. These findings point to a persistent effect of early contact on better behavior organization and socialization across infancy. kangaroo contact, therefore, appears to have a lasting impact on the child's social-emotional development and on the mother–infant relationship across infancy. These improvements during the toddler stage, a period when the child's social and symbolic world is quickly expanding, place the treated infants at a better starting point for growth and development and better adaptation in the social world. Findings from 5 years show that the improved relationships between mother and child in dyads engaged in kangaroo contact were maintained only for procedures that had a stressful component, for instance, when children had to comply to maternal requests in a "toy pick-up" procedure or had to refrain from actions mothers prohibited and not touch sweets until they were allowed. The long-term effect of kangaroo contact on the mother–child relationship, therefore, was specific to the co-regulatory component in early relationships in tasks that require child socialization and regulation in the context of the maternal commands.

Assessment of the father–child and family interaction patterns was conducted at 3 months during a home visit. Father–child interactions in the kangaroo families were more optimal, in terms of higher sensitivity, lower intrusiveness, and higher father–child (not only father–son) reciprocity. Such findings are surprising, as fathers did not perform skin-to-skin contact. It is possible that the decrease in the infant's negative emotionality during social interaction – related to the effects of KC on the infant's self-regulation and stress management – increased the father's involvement in the interaction. Another possibility is that fathers learn the paternal role in part through observing and imitating the mother's behavior and thus, better mothering may have a spillover effect to more optimal fathering (Feldman et al., 2003). Similar to the findings for mothers, fathers whose wives provided KC were more sensitive and less intrusive during interactions and the level of dyadic reciprocity between father and child was higher as compared to controls. Although the mechanisms for this improvement are not fully understood, it is possible that a more positive atmosphere between the mother and the infant may have contributed to a better home atmosphere and facilitated more optimal fathering.

In addition to the relationships between each parent and the infant we also observed triadic interactions between mother, father, and child. Infants as young as 3 months of age are able to coordinate social signals with both mother and father and to respond to non-verbal communications between mother and father (Fivas-Depeursinge & Corboz-Warnery, 1999). Interactions in the family triad provide infants the first opportunity to participate in a group experience, and this experience colors their later social competence in group settings. The mother–father–infant interactions were microcoded for gaze and affect of each family member, proximity position between each two members, and touch patterns between each two family members (mother–infant, father–infant, mother–father). The family atmosphere as a whole was globally coded on the dimension of coherence – the level of harmony, reciprocity, and unity in the triad – and intrusiveness – the degree to which members interfere with each other's communications. Families in the kangaroo groups showed better functioning on both the microanalytic and global assessments. Infants who received kangaroo contact showed lower levels of gaze aversion and less negative affect in a triadic context. In addition, both mothers and fathers of KC infants touched their infants affectionately more often during triadic interactions. As touch is among the central regulatory components of the mother–infant coregulatory system (Tronick, 1995) and affectionate touch is unique to parents as compared to other caregivers (Miller & Holditch-Davis, 1992), more affectionate touch in the family context contributes to infant self-regulation and development. Triadic interactions of KC families were described as more harmonious and less intrusive, possibly as a result of both improvements in the infant's self-regulation and the mother's familiarity with the infant that expanded to the triadic context. Family processes, which are dynamic and multidimensional, are sensitive to changes in each family member and these individual changes lead to better organization, harmony, and coherence in the triad following intervention. Thus, Kangaroo Care seems to have an impact on a large array of developmental processes, which extend beyond the mother–infant dyad and much beyond the neonatal period. The early improvements seem to have a positive effect on fathering and family processes, as well as the child's later cognition, learning, and social adaptation.

Summary

Touch, perhaps similar to the air we breathe, is readily available in any intimate relationship and represents the most natural activity between human beings. Mother–infant touch and contact provides the foundation for the child's physical growth, self-regulation, and social fittedness. However, in order for touch to functions as an intervention, it must be applied in a theoretically-driven way that posits direct links between specific components of the touch-and-contact experience and specific risk conditions in which these components are missing. The findings presented here demonstrate that skin-to-skin contact in early infancy functions primarily to organize the infant's physiological, attentional, and emotional systems and to promote the maternal bonding processes that were truncated due to the premature birth. Similar to the findings for other mammals, the effects of skin-to-skin contact in the immediate post-birth period were observed in several dimensions up to the age of 5 years. Children who received contact in infancy were better able to regulate their negative emotions, performed better on complex neurocognitive tasks that required attention shifting and organization, and showed better behavioral control. Long-term effects of the KC intervention were also observed for the mother–child relationship, particularly in encounters that required maternal control of child behavior and the child's socialized conduct. Touch and contact in early infancy may thus be considered a prototypical example of a "low-cost intervention". It capitalizes on a natural, available, free of charge resource; its application is theoretically based and its implementation – when provided during the system's sensitive period – may go a long way and have a substantial impact on the growth and development of the fragile premature infant.

Acknowledgements: Research at Ruth Feldman's laboratory is supported by the Israeli Science Foundation (01/945), the Bi-national Science Foundation (2001-241), and the March of Dimes Foundation (#12-FY04-50).

References

Acolet, D., Sleath, K., & Whitelaw, A. (1989). Oxygenation, heart rate and temperature in very low birth infants during skin-to-skin contact with their mothers. *Acta Paediatrica Scandinavica, 78*, 189–193.

Affonso, D., Bosque, E., Wahlberg, V., & Brady, J. P. (1993). Reconciliation and healing for mothers through skin-to-skin contact provided in an American tertiary level intensive care nursery. *Neonatal Network, 12*, 25–32.

Als, H. (1991). Neurobehavioral organization of the newborn: Opportunity for assessment and intervention. *NIDA Research Monograph, 114*, 106–116.

Anand, K. J., & Scalzo, F. M. (2000). Can adverse neonatal experiences alter brain development and subsequent behavior? *Biology of the Neonate, 77*, 69–82.

Auerbach, J., Geller, B., Lezer, S., Shinewell, E., Belmaker, R. H., Levin, J., & Ebstein R. (1999). Dopamine D4 receptor (D4DR) and serotonin transporter promoter (5-HTTLPR) plymorphisms in the determination of temperament in 2-month-old infants. *Molecular Psychiatry, 4*, 369–373.

Bauer, J., Sontheimer, D., Fischer, C., & Linderkamp, O. (1996). Metabolic rate and energy balance in very low birth weight infants during kangaroo holding by their mothers and fathers. *Journal of Pediatrics, 129*, 608–611.

Bayley, N. (1993). *Bayley scales of infant development*. Administering and scoring manual. New York, NY: The Psychological Corporation.

Belsky, J. (1998). Theory testing, effect-size evaluation, and differential susceptibility to rearing influence: The case of mothering and attachment. *Child Development, 68*, 598–600.

Bier, J. A., Ferguson, A. E., Morales, Y., Liebling, J. A., Archer, D., Oh, W., & Vohr, B. R. I. (1996). Comparison of skin-to-skin contact with standard contact in low-birth-weight infants who are breast-fed. *Archives of Pediatrics and Adolescent Medicine, 150*, 1265–1269.

Bosque, E. M., Brady, J. P., Affonso, D. D., & Wahlberg, V. (1995) Physiologic measures of kangaroo versus incubator care in a tertiary-level nursery. *Journal of Obstetric, Gynecologic, and Neonatal Nursing, 24*, 219–226.

Bowlby, J. (1969). *Attachment and loss. Vol.1: Attachment*. New York: Basic.

Brazelton, T. B. (1973). *Neonatal behavioral assessment scale*. Philadelphia, PA: J. B. Lippincott Co.

Brazelton, T. B. (1990). Saving the bathwater. *Child Development, 61*, 1661–1671.

Brooten, D., Gennaro, S., Brown, L., Butts, P., Gibbons, A., Bakewill-Sachs, S., & Kumar, S. P. (1988). Anxiety, depression, and hostility in mothers of preterm infants. *Nursing Research, 37*, 213–216.

Burkhammer, M. D., Anderson, G. C., & Chiu, S. H. (2004). Grief, anxiety, stillbirth, and perinatal problems: Healing with Kangaroo Care. *Journal of Obstetric, Gynecological, and Neonatal Nursing, 33*, 774–782.

Carter, S. C. (1998). Neuroendocrine perspectives on social attachment and love. *Psychoneuroendocrinology, 23*, 779–818.

Carter, S. C., & Keverne, E. B. (2002). The neurobiology of social affiliation and pair bonding. *Hormones, Brain and Behavior, 1*, 299–339.

Charpak, N., Ruiz, J. G., de Calume, Z. F., & Charpak, Y. (1997). Kangaroo mother versus "traditional" care for newborn infants $\leq$ 2000 grams. A randomized, controlled trial. *Pediatrics, 100*, 682–688.

Charpak, N., Ruiz, J. G., Zupan, J., Cattaneo, A., Figueroa, Z., Tessier, R., Cristo, M., Anderson, G., Ludington, S., Mendoza, S., Mokhachane, M., & Worku, B. (2005). Kangaroo mother care: 25 years after. *Acta Paediatrica, 94*, 514–522.

Charpak, N., Ruiz-Palaez, J. G., & de Calume, Z. F. (1996). Current knowledge of kangaroo mother intervention. *Current Opinion in Pediatrics, 8*, 108–112.

Charpak, N., Ruiz-Palaez, J. G., Figueroa de, C. Z., & Charpak, Y. A. (2001). Randomized, controlled trial of kangaroo mother care: Reulsts of follow-up at 1 year of corrected age. *Pediatrics, 108*, 1072–1079.

Dahl, R. E. (1996).The regulation of sleep and arousal: Development and psychopathology. *Development and Psychopathology, 8*, 3–27.

Davis, D. H., & Thoman, E. B. (1988). The early social environment of premature and full term infants. *Early Human Development, 17*, 221–232.

DiPietro, J. A., & Porges, S. W. (1991). Vagal responsiveness to gavage feeding as an index of preterm status. *Pediatric Research, 29*, 231–236.

Dombrowski, M. A., Anderson, G. C., Santori, C., & Burkhammer, M. (2001). Kangaroo (skin-to-skin) care with a postpartum woman who felt depressed. *American Journal of Maternal and Child Nursing, 26*, 214–216.

Doussard-Roosevelt, J. A., McClenny, B. D., & Porges, S. W. (2001). Neonatal cardiac vagal tone and school-age developmental outcome in very low birth weight infants. *Developmental Psychobiology, 38*, 56–66.

Eckerman, C. O., Hsu, H. C., Molitor, A., Leung, E. H., & Goldstein, R. F. (1999). Infant arousal in an en-face exchange with a new partner: Effects of prematurity and perinatal biological risk. *Developmental Psychology, 35*, 282–293.

Eckerman, C. O., Oehler, J. M., Hannan, T. E., & Molitor, A. (1995). The development prior to term age of very prematurely born newborns' responsiveness in an en face exchanges. *Infant Behavior and Development, 18*, 283–297.

El-Sheik, M. (2001). Parental drinking problems and children's adjustment vagal regulation and emotional reactivity as pathways and moderators of risk. *Journal of Abnormal Psychology, 110*, 499–515.

Feldman, R. (1998). Coding Interactive Behavior (CIB) Manual. Unpublished Manual. Bar-Ilan University.

Feldman, R. (2004). Mother-infant skin-to-skin contact and the development of emotion regulation. In S. P. Shohov (Ed.), *Advances in psychology research*, Vol. 27 (pp. 113–131). Hauppauge, NY: Nova Science.

Feldman, R. (2005). Mother-infant synchrony and the development of moral orientation in childhood and adolescence: Direct and indirect mechanisms of developmental continuity. Manuscript submitted for publication.

Feldman, R., & Eidelman, A. I. (1998). Intervention methods for premature infants: How and do they affect development. *Clinics in Perinatology, 25*, 613–626.

Feldman, R., & Eidelman, A. I. (2003). Direct and indirect effects of maternal milk on the neurobehavioral and cognitive development of premature infants. *Developmental Psychobiology, 43*, 1–12.

Feldman, R., & Eidelman, A. I. (2003a). Mother-infant skin-to-skin contact (Kangaroo Care) accelerates autonomic and neurobehavioral maturation in premature infants. *Developmental Medicine and Child Neurology, 45*, 274–280.

Feldman, R., & Eidelman, A. I. (2007). Maternal postpartum behavior and the emergence of infant-mother and infant-father synchrony in preterm and full-term infants: The role of neonatal vagal tone. *Developmental Psychobiology, 49*.

Feldman, R., Eidelman, A. I., & Rotenberg, N. (2004). Parenting stress, infant emotion regulation, maternal sensitivity, and the cognitive development of triplets: A model for parent and child influences in a unique ecology. *Child Development, 75*, 1774–1791.

Feldman, R., Eidelman, A. I., Sirota, L., & Weller, A. (2002). Comparison of skin-to-skin (Kangaroo) and traditional care: Parenting outcomes and preterm infant development. *Pediatrics, 110*, 16–26.

Feldman, R., & Greenbaum, C. W. (1997). Affect regulation and synchrony in mother-infant play as precursors to the development of symbolic competence. *Infant Mental Health Journal, 18*, 4–23.

Feldman, R., Greenbaum, C. W., & Yirmiya, N. (1999). Mother-infant affect synchrony as an antecedent to the emergence of self-control. *Developmental Psychology, 35*, 223–231.

Feldman, R., Keren, M., Gross-Rozval, O., & Tyano, S. (2004). Mother and child's touch patterns in infant feeding disorders: Relation to maternal, child, and environmental factors. *Journal of the American Academy of Child and Adolescent Psychiatry, 43*, 1089–1097.

Feldman, R., & Klein, P. S. (2003). Toddlers' self-regulated compliance with mother, caregiver, and father: Implications for theories of socialization. *Developmental Psychology, 39*, 680–692.

Feldman, R., Masalha, S., & Alony, D. (2006). Micro-regulatory patterns of family interactions: Cultural pathways to toddlers' self-regulation. *Journal of Family Psychology, 20*, (December), 614–623.

Feldman, R., Masalha, S., & Nadam, R. (2001). Cultural perspective on work and family: Dual-earner Jewish and Arab families at the transition to parenthood. *Journal of Family Psychology, 15*, 492–509.

Feldman, R., & Mayes, L. C. (1999). The rhythmic organization of infant attention during habituation is related to infants' information processing. *Infant Behavior and Development, 22*, 37–49.

Feldman, R., Weller, A., Leckman, J. F., Kuint, J., & Eidelman, A. I. (1999). The nature of the mother's tie to her infant: Maternal bonding under conditions of proximity, separation, and potential loss. *Journal of Child Psychology and Psychiatry, 40*, 929–940.

Feldman, R., Weller, A., Eidelman, A. I., & Sirota, L. (2003). Testing a family intervention hypothesis: The Contribution of mother-infant skin-to-skin contact (Kangaroo Care) to family interaction and touch. *Journal of Family Psychology, 17*, 94–107.

Feldman, R., Weller, A., Sirota, L., & Eidelman, A. I. (2002). Skin-to-skin contact (Kangaroo Care) promotes self-regulation in premature infants: Sleep-wake cyclicity, arousal modulation, and sustained exploration. *Developmental Psychology, 38*, 194–207.

Feldman, R., Levine, A., Zagoory-Sharon, O., & Weller, A. (2006). Evidence for a neuropeptide foundation for human affiliation; Plasma oxytocin levels across pregnancy and the postpartum predict maternal-infant bonding. *Manuscript submitted for publication.*

Ferber, S. G., & Makhoul, R. I. (2004). The effect of skin-to skin contact (kangaroo care) shortly after birth on the neurobehavioral responses of the full-term newborn: A randomized controlled trial. *Pediatrics, 113*, 858–865.

Field, T. (1994). The effects of mother's physical and emotional unavailability on emotion regulation. *Monographs of the Society for Research in Child Development, 59* (serial no. 240), 208–228.

Fischer, C. B., Sontheimer, D., Scheffer, F., Bauer, J., & Linderkamp, O. (1998). Cardiorespiratory stability of premature boys and girls during kangaroo care. *Early Human Development, 52*, 145–153.

Fivas-Depeursinge, E., & Corboz-Warnery, A. (1999). *The primary triangle.* New York: Basic.

Fleming, A. S., O'Day, D. H., & Kraemer, G. W. (1999). Neurobiology of mother-infant interaction: Experience and central nervous system plasticity across development and generations. *Neuroscience and Biobehavioral Review, 23*, 673–685.

Fohe, K., Dropf, S., & Avenarius, S. (2000). Skin-to-skin contact improves gas exchange in premature infants. *Journal of Perinatology, 20*, 311–315.

Fox, N. A., & Porges, S. W. (1985). The relation between neonatal heart period patterns and developmental outcome. *Child Development, 56*, 28–37.

Francis, D. D., Diorio, J., Plotsky, P. M., & Meaney, M. J. (2002). Environmental enrichment reverses the effects of maternal separation on stress reactivity. *Journal of Neuroscience, 22*, 7840–7843.

Furman, L., Minich, N., & Hack, M. (2002). Correlates of lactation in mothers of very low birth weight infants. *Pediatrics, 109*(4), e57.

Gale, G., Frank, L., & Lund, C. (1993). Skin-to-skin (kangaroo) holding of the incubated premature infant. *Neonatal Network, 12*, 49–57.

Gale, G., & Vandenberg, K. A. (1998). Kangaroo care. *Neonatal Network, 17*, 69–71.

Gazzolo, D., Masetti, P., & Meli, M. (2000). Kangaroo care improves post-extubation cardiorespiratory parameters in infants after open heart surgery. *Acta Paediatrica Scandinavica, 89*, 728–729.

Goldberg, S., Perrotta, M., Minde, K., & Corter, C. (1986). Maternal behavior and attachment in low-birth-weight twins and singletons. *Child Development, 57*, 34–46.

Goodman, S. H., & Gottlieb, I. H. (1999). Risk for psychopathology in the children of depressed mothers: A developmental model for understanding mechanisms of transmission. *Psychological Review, 106*, 458–490.

Gottlieb, G. (1991). Experiential canalization of behavioral development: Theory. *Developmental Psychology, 27*, 4–13.

Gray, L., Watt, L., & Blass, E. (2000). Skin-to-skin contact is analgesic in healthy newborn. *Pediatrics, 105*, e14–e24.

Grunau, R. (2002). Early pain in preterm infants. A model of long-term effects. *Clinics in Perinatology, 29*, 373–394.

Hao, H., & Rivkees, S. A. (1999). The biological clock of very premature primate infants is responsive to light. *Proceedings of the National Academy of Sciences USA, 96*, 2426–2429.

Heinrichs, M., Baumgartner, T., Kirschbaum, C., & Ehlert, U. (2003). Social support and oxytocin interact to suppress cortisol and subjective responses to psychosocial stress. *Biological Psychiatry, 54*, 1398–1398.

Heird, W. C. (2001). The role of polyunsaturated fatty acids in term and preterm infants and breastfeeding mothers. *Pediatic Clinics of North America, 48*, 173–188.

Hinde R. A. (1989). Ethological and relationship approaches. *Ann Child Dev, 6*, 251–285.

Hofer, M. A. (1995). Hidden regulators: Implications for a new understanding of attachment, separation, and loss. In S. Golberg, R. Muir, & J. Kerr (Eds.), *Attachment theory: Social, developmental, and clinical perspectives* (pp. 203–230). Hillsdale, NJ: Analytic Press.

Horwood, L. J., Darlow, B. A., & Mogridge, N. (2001). Breast milk feeding and cognitive ability at 7–8 years. *Archives of Diseases in Childhood Fetal and Neonatal Edition, 84*, F23–F27.

Hurst, N., Valentine, C., & Renfro, L. (1997). Skin-to-skin holding in the neonatal intensive care unit influences maternal milk volume. *Journal of Perinatology, 17*, 213–217.

Insel, T. R. (1997). A neurobiological basis of social attachment. *American Journal of Psychiatry, 154*, 726–735.

Jaffee, J., Beebe, B., Feldstein, S., Crown, C. L., & Jasnow, M. D. (2002). Rhythms of dialogue in infancy: Coordinated timing in development. *Monographs of the Society for Research in Child Development, 66*, 1–132.

Kambarami, R. A., Chidede, O., & Kowo, D. T. (1998). Kangaroo care versus incubator care in the management of well preterm infants-a pilot study. *Annals of Tropical Paediatrics International Child Health, 18*, 81–86.

Kambarami, R. A., Chidede, O., & Kowo, D. T. (1999). Kangaroo care for well low birth weight infants at Harare Central hospital maternity unit- Zimbabwe. *Central African Journal of Medicine, 45*, 56–59.

Keren, M., Feldman, R., Eidelman, A. I., Sirota, L., & Lester, B. (2003). Clinical interview for high-risk parents of premature infants (CLIP): Relations to mother-infant interaction. *Infant Mental Health Journal, 24*, 93–110.

Killersreiter, B., Grimmer, I., Buhrer, C., Dudenhausen, J. W., & Oblade M. (2002). Early cessation of breast milk feeding in very low birth weight infants. *Early Human Development, 60*, 193–205.

Klaus, M. H., & Kenell, J. H. (1976). *Maternal-infant bonding*. St. Louis, MO: Mosby.

Laviola, G., & Terranova, M. L. (1998). The developmental psychobiology of behavioral plasticity in mice: The role of social experiences in the family unit. *Neuroscience Biobehavioral Review, 23*, 197–213.

Leckman, J. F., Feldman, R., Swain, J. E., Eichler, V., Thompson, N., & Mayes, L. C. (2004). Primary parental preoccupation: Circuits, genes, and the crucial role of the environment. *Journal of Neural Transmission, 11*, 753–771.

Leckman, J. F., & Herman, A. E. (2002). Maternal behavior and developmental psychopathology. *Biological Psychiatry, 51*, 27–43.

Leckman, J. F., Mayes, L. C., Feldman, R., Evans, D., King, R. A., & Cohen, D. (1999). Early parental preoccupations and behaviors and their possible relationship to the symptoms of obsessive-compulsive disorder. *Acta Psychiatrica Scandinavica (supplementum), 100*(396), 1–26.

Lehmann, J., Stohr, T., & Feldon, J. (2000). Long-term effects of prenatal stress experiences and postnatal maternal separation on emotionality and attentional processes. *Behavior and Brain Research, 107*, 133–144.

Lester, B. M., Hoffman, J., & Brazelton, T. B. (1985). The rhythmic structure of mother-infant interaction in term and preterm infants. *Child Development, 56*, 15–27.

Levy-Shiff, R., Sharir, H., & Mogilner, M. B. (1989). Mother- and father-preterminfant relationship in the hospital preterm nursery. *Child Development, 60*, 93–102.

Ludington, S. M. & Golant, S. K. (1993). *Kangaroo care: The best you can do for your preterm infant*. New York: Bantum Press.

Ludington-Hoe, S. M., & Swinth, J. Y. (1996). Developmental aspects of kangaroo care. *Journal of Obstetric, Gynecologic, and Neonatal Nursing, 25*, 691–703.

Malatesta, C. Z., Grigoryev, P., Lamb, C., Albin, M., & Culver, C. (1986). Emotion socialization and expressive development in preterm and full-term infants. *Child Development, 57*, 316–330.

Matthiesen, A. S., Ransjo-Arvidson, A. B., Nissen, E., & Uvnas-Moberg, K. (2001). Postpartum maternal oxytocin release by newborns: effects of infant hand massage and sucking. *Birth, 28*, 13–19.

Mayes, L. C., Granger, R. H., Frank, M. A., Schottenfeld, R., & Bornstein M. H. (1993). Neurobehavioral profiles of neonates exposed to cocaine prenatally. *Pediatrics, 91*, 778–783.

McCormick, M. C., Workman-Daniels, K., & Brooks-Gunn, J. (1996). The behavioral and emotional well-being of school-age children with different birth weight. *Pediatrics, 97*, 18–25.

McMaster, P., & Vince, J. D. (2000). Outcome of neonatal care in Port Moresby, Papua New Guinea; A 19-year review. *Journal of Tropical Pediatrics, 46*, 57–61.

Meaney, M. J. (2001). Maternal care, gene expression, and the transmission of individual differences in stress reactivity across generations. *Annual Review of Neuroscience, 24*, 1161–1192.

Meyer, K., & Anderson, G. C. (1999). Using kangaroo care in a clinical setting with fullterm infants having breastfeeding difficulties. *American Journal of Maternal and Child Nursing, 24*, 190–192.

Michelsson, K., Christenson, K., Rothganger, H., & Winberg, J. (1996). Crying in separated and non-separated newborns: Sounds spectrographic analysis. *Acta Paediatrica Scandinavica, 85*, 471–475.

Miller, D.B., & Holditch-Davis, D. (1992). Interactions of parents and nurses with high-risk preterm infants. *Research in Nursing and Health, 15*, 187–197.

Minde, K. (2000). Prematurity and serious medical conditions in infancy: Implications for development, behavior, and intervention. In C. H. Zeanah (Ed.), *Handbook of infant mental health* (pp. 176–194). New York: Guilford.

Mooncey, S., Giannakoulopoulos, X., Glober, V., Acolet, D., & Modi, N. (1997). The effect of mother-infant skin-to-skin contact on plasma cortisol and beta endorphin concentration in preterm infants. *Infant Behavior and Development, 20*, 553–557.

Nelson, E. E., & Panksepp, J. (1998). Brain substrates of infant-mother attachment: Contributions of opioids, oxytocin, and norepinephrine. *Neuroscience and Biobehavioral Reviews, 22*, 437–452.

Neu, M. (1999). Parents' perception of skin-to-skin care with their preterm infants requiring assisted ventilation. *Journal of Obstetric, Gynecologic, and Neonatal Nursing, 28*, 157–164.

Nissen, E., Lilja, G., Widstrom, A. J., & Uvnas-Moberg, K. (1995). Elevation of oxytocin levels early post partum in woman. *Acta Obstetricia et Gynecologica Scandinavica, 74*, 530–533.

Ohgi, S., Fukud, M., Moriuchi, H., Kusumoto, T., Akiyama, T., Nugent, J. K., Brazelton, T. B., Arisawa, K., Takahashi, T., & Saitoh, H. (2002). Comparison of kangaroo care and standard care; behavioral organization, development, and temperament in healthy, low-birth-weight infants through 1 year. *Journal Perinatology, 22*, 374–379.

Orzalesi, M. (1987). Vitamins and the premature infant. *Biology of the Neonate, 52* (suppl. 1), 97–112.

Pedersen, C. A. (1999). Oxytocin control of maternal behavior: Regulation of sex steroids and offspring stimuli. In C. S. Carter, I. I. Lederhendler, & B. Kirkpatrick (Eds.), *The Integrative Neurobiology of Affiliation* (pp. 301–320). Cambridge: MIT Press.

Poeggel, G., Lange, E., Hase, C., Metzger, M., Gulyaeva, N., & Braun, K. (1999). Maternal separation and early social deprivation in Octodon degua: Quantitative changes of nicotinamide adenine dinucleotide phosphate-diaphorase- reactive neurons in the prefrontal cortex and nucleus accumbens. *Neuroscience, 94*, 497–504.

Porges, S. W. (1985). Method and apparatus for evaluating rhythmic oscillations in a periodic physiological response system. (Patent No. 4,510,944, April 16, 1985).

Porges, S. W. (1996). Physiological regulation in high-risk infants: A model for assessment and potential intervention. *Development and Psychopathology, 8*, 43–145.

Ramanathan, K., Paul, V. K., Deorari, A. K., Taneja, U., & George, G. (2001). Kangaroo mother care in very low birth weight infants. *Indian Journal of Pediatrics, 68*, 1019–1023.

Ruff, H. A. (1986). Attention and organization of behavior in high-risk infants. *Journal of Developmental and Behavioral Pediatrics, 7*, 298–301.

Schore, A. N. (2001). Effects of a secure attachment relationship on right brain development, affect regulation, and infant mental health. *Infant Mental Health Journal, 22*, 7–66.

Sigman, M., Cohen, S. E., Beckwith, L., & Parmelee, A. H. (1986). Infant attention in relation to intellectual abilities in childhood. *Developmental Psychology, 22*, 788–792.

Sleigh, M. J., & Lickliter, R. (1998). Timing of presentation of prenatal auditory stimulation alters auditory and visual responsiveness in bobwhite quail chicks (colinus virginianus). *Journal of Comparative Psychology, 112*, 153–160.

Sloan, N., Camacho, L. W. L., Rojas, E. P., & Stern, C. (1994). Kangaroo mother method: Randomised controlled trial of an alternative method of care for stabilized low-birth weight infants. *Lancet, 344*, 782–785.
Spangler, G., & Scheubeck, R. (1993). Behavioral organization in newborns and its relation to adrenocortical and cardiac activity. *Child Development, 64*, 622–633.
Spitz, R. (1946). Anaclitic depression. *Psychoan Study Child, 2*, 313–342.
Stack, D. M., & Muir, D. W. (1992). Adult tactile stimulation during face-to-face interactions modulates five-month-olds' affect and attention. *Child Development, 63*, 1509–1525.
Stern, D. N. (1995). *The motherhood constellation.* New York: Basic Books.
Swain, J. E., Leckman, J. F., Mayes, L. C., Feldman, R., Constable, R. T., & Schultz, R. T. (2004). Neural substrates of human parent-infant attachment in the postpartum. *Biological Psychiatry, 55*, 153S.
Thoman, E. B., Denenberg, V. H., Sievel, J., Zeidner, L. P., & Becker, P. (1981). State organization in neonate: Developmental inconsistency indicates risk for developmental dysfunction. *Neuropediatrics, 12*, 45–54.
Tornhage, C. J., Stude, E., Lindberg, T., & Serenius, F. (1998). First week kangaroo care in sick very preterm infants. *Acta Paediatrica, 88*, 1402–1404.
Tronick, E. Z. (1995). Touch in mother-infant interaction. In T. M. Field (Ed.) *Touch in early development* (pp. 53–65). Mahwah, NJ: Erlbaum.
Tucker, D. M. (1992). Developing emotions and cortical networks. In M. R. Gunnar & C. A. Nelson (Eds.) *Developmental behavioral neuroscience: The minnesota symposia on child psychology*, Vol. 24. Hillsdale, NJ: Erlbaum.
Weizman, R., Lehmann, J., Leschiner, S., Allmann, I., Stoehr, T., Heidbreder, C., Domeney, A., Feldon, J., & Gavish, M. (1999). Long-lasting effects of early handling on the peripheral benzodiazepine receptor. *Pharmacology, Biochemistry, and Behavior, 64*, 725–729.
Whitelaw, A., Heiserkamp, G., Sleath, K., Acolet, D., & Richards, M. (1988). Skin-to-skin contact for very low birth weight infants and their mothers. *Archives of Disease in Childhood, 63*, 1377–1381.
Winnicott D. W. (1956). *Collected papers: Through pediatrics to psychoanalysis.* New York: Basic Books.
Yokoyama, Y., Ueda, T., Irahara, M., & Aono, T. (1994). Releases of oxytocin and prolactin during breast massage and suckling in puerperal women. *European Journal of Obstetrics Gynecology and Reproductive Biology, 53*, 17–20.
Zinaman, M. J., Hughes, V., Queenan, J. T., Labobok, M. H., & Albertson, B. (1992). Acute prolactin and oxytocin responses and milk yields to infant suckling and artificial methods of expression in lactating women. *Pediatrics, 89*, 437–440.

17

Touch Interventions Positively Affect Development

Nancy Aaron Jones and Krystal D. Mize

Greater and more loving types of touch are expected to enhance the relationship between dyads. While touch behaviors have been shown to have a positive impact on infants' physiological and psychological development (Field et al., 1996), only recently have empirical studies investigated the mechanisms and systems involved in touch behaviors that impact infant and child development. This chapter will explore the recent evidence implicating touch behaviors and touch interventions in optimal developmental outcomes (Field, 1998). The first section will outline the variety of terms employed when referring to touch behaviors and will provide a brief overview of the history of touch in medicine, psychological theory and research. The second section is a presentation of the evidence that touch behaviors provide advantages for mother-infant interactions and for an infant's brain development.

The third section is an examination of the role of touch behaviors and touch interventions in infants "at risk." Specifically, the advantages (and potential disadvantages) of touch for premature infants, for infants of depressed mothers, and other high-risk groups of children will be noted. The next section is a brief report of a recent study in which we demonstrated that touch behaviors increased in mother-infant dyads who breastfeed, even dyads in which mothers were depressed. The implications of these findings for the development of the frontal lobes of the brain will also be discussed. Finally, the last section will discuss future avenues for research and will attempt to consolidate the research evidence linking touch behaviors to optimal developmental outcomes, ultimately supporting the advantage of touch during infancy as a low-cost intervention.

Defining Touch and the History of Touch

Definition of Types of Touch and Touch Interventions

A number of definitions have been used to refer to a variety of micro- and macro-analytic behaviors that a person may experience as touch. Among the different definitions is that touch can be referred to as a physical or sensory quality, processed in the brain by the somatosensory cortex and mediated by the skin (Kaas, 2000; Merzenich, 1984). The functions of the skin are to reconcile sensations and help maintain the body's homeostatic functioning. Some refer to this more micro-component of touch as physical contact or tactile sensations (Hertenstein & Campos, 2001; Perez, 2001).

Touch can also be conceptualized as an emotional process or feeling state, aptly accompanied by the specific neural activity associated with emotional experiences (Fox, 1991; Tomkins, 1982). A fundamental advantage of touch is that it promotes a sense of security and closeness and alleviates distress, i.e., a sense of feeling positively influenced by another person.

In addition, when touch is combined with other modalities (e.g., vision, hearing) and is consistently presented across development, it can be viewed as a part of a larger communication process between mothers and their infants (Herrera, Reissland, & Shepherd, 2004; Moreno, Posada, & Goldyn, 2006). These more macro-analytic communication processes are part of affiliative system that potentially influence the development of complex processes such as emotion regulation (Herenstein & Campos, 2001; Moreno et al., 2006), self-competence (Muir & Lee, 2003), and learning (Weiss, 1990).

Finally, touch can be utilized as a form of intervention or therapy. For instance, massage (Field, 1998) and skin-to-skin contact (Ferber & Makhoul, 2004) have been employed as interventions to promote and sustain an individual's well-being during early development and across the lifespan (Field, 1998; Feldman, this volume).

Historical Use of Touch in Medicine

Although the empirical investigation of mother-infant touch behaviors have only arisen in the last 50 years, touch as a therapy or an intervention has been around since before 2000 BC (Fritz, 1999; Salvo, 1999). In fact, touch therapies were a primary form of medical treatment prior to the annexation by the pharmaceutical industry during the 1940s. Initially touch behaviors had been employed as methods of therapy in a variety of Mediterranean and Asian ancient cultures. Documented reports indicate that notable figures in history like Hippocrates and others wrote about the medicinal and therapeutic benefits of massage and other complementary techniques such as bathing, anointing, acupuncture, and exercise for promoting health and reducing pain (Elton, Stanley, & Burrows, 1983).

Later in medical history, touch therapies were relegated into the domain of folk medicine as massage was considered to be an imperfect treatment for the medical community (Salvo, 1999). Currently, medical research on the benefits of touch and massage are compartmentalized under the rubric of complementary and alternative medicines (Moyer, Rounds, & Hannum, 2004).

History of Touch in Psychological Theories

With increasing support for the connection between the mind and body, noting the negative effects of stress on health (Chesney et al., 2005), the benefits of touch have been reemerging in scientific endeavors, primarily in the realm of psychological theory and research. Both animal and human studies have provided support for the idea that touch is a necessary component for psychological well-being and is particularly important during development (see Feldman, this volume for a review). In general, studies have supported the primacy and importance of touch behaviors during infancy. Infants receiving appropriate levels of tactile contact from parents developed a sense of safety, and security during socialization whereas those infants who had been deprived of touch because of parental absence experienced enduring periods of despair and grief (Bowlby, 1969).

Ainsworth and her colleagues (Ainsworth, Blehar, Waters, & Wall, 1978; Bell & Ainsworth, 1972) later suggested that the quality of touch was even more important than the quantity of touching and holding. In essence, the quality of touch conveys information to infants enabling them to be able to discern the caretakers who genuinely "care" for them versus those that do not. Most notably these ideas have been used in contemporary psychology within the ethological-evolutionary theory of mother-infant attachment (Ainsworth et al., 1978) and bonding (Kennel & Klaus, 1984). Moreover, these ideas are the basis for interventions like infant massage training (Field, 1998) and kangaroo care (Ferber & Makhoul, 2004).

Touch Behaviors Provide Benefits for Infants

As Feldman has discussed previously (Chapter 16 of this volume), touch is a sophisticated sense that involves communication, both stemming from and thereby affecting sensory and physiological functioning. Empirical evidence suggests that infants can retain memory traces of early sensory experiences, mentally processing information about themselves and their early interactive experiences with caregivers as a function of their experiences with and about touch (Schore, 1996; Siegel, 1999). Touch is physical and has a physiological impact that exceeds the immediate sensation. In addition, touch is uniquely experienced by both members of the dyad. Touch helps infants with affective and cognitive development, helps mothers with parental competence and decreases depression, and helps the dyad with bonding and adaptive socialization experiences. Overall, exposure to touch during development has the potential to influence a variety of outcomes including mother-infant attunement, dyadic co-regulation and infant brain development and plasticity.

Mother-Infant Interaction

Touch is universally experienced, (Eibl-Eibesfeldt, 1996), is inherently reciprocal in dyadic interaction, is multidimensional (Montagu, 1986; Sachs, 1988) and is likely more primary (Schopler, 1965) than any other developmental processes. We first learn to communicate with our environment via touch and then through other sensory modalities. For example, the mother's soothing voice and her expression of concern in combination with her caressing touch settles the distressed infant. In later development, a mother's compassionate words and expression of concern becomes a substitute for positive touch and the words and/or face alone may ultimately calm the infant's distress. In point of fact, Jahromi, Putnam, and Stifter, (2004) recently reported that touching behaviors decreased from 2 to 6 months while using vocalization and distracting behaviors as soothing methods increased in frequency as the infant matured.

Touch not only conveys meaning but has a variety of positive and negative messages that can be used to either sooth or to elicit distress. Developmental studies (Tronick, 1995; Weinberg, 1992) investigating the frequency of specific touching behaviors between mothers and their infants showed that the most frequent tactile behaviors were positive, including stroking, touching, and tapping compared to rhythmic movements, holding, and tickling. Infrequent positive tactile behaviors included repositioning, kissing and sucking. However, the least frequent tactile behaviors were more negative types of touch like poking, jabbing, pulling, and pinching.

In other developmental work, a collection of studies (LePage & Stack, 1993; Stack & Muir, 1992) also examined the effects of touch during the classic maternal still-face paradigms, situations that typically produces distress in infants (as the mother is asked to be unresponsive to her infant). In these studies, touch appears to act as a protective mechanism. Findings showed that tactile stimulation attenuates or eliminates the negative responses produced by still-face paradigms because it is a positive mode of communication between infants and adults. Furthermore, touch is as effective as facial and vocal expressions for mother-infant communication (Stack & Muir, 1992). For example, LePage and Stack (1993) found that mothers can elicit smiling from their infants using only touch as the impetuous for the resultant behavior. Moreover, touch alone was as effective as the combination of face, touch, and voice for eliciting smiling in infants. In essence, touch *expressions* performed like (and in some cases were superior to) facial or vocal expressions and thus are used to carry on mutually reciprocal exchanges between parents and their infants (Stack & Muir, 1992).

Researchers (Pelaez-Nogueras et al., 1996b) have also demonstrated that tactile stimulation augments other positive behaviors during the mother-infant interactive experience. In several studies (Pelaez-Nogueras, 1996a; Pelaez-Nogueras et al., 1996b), infants between 1- and 4-months-old who received touch as a stimulus spent more time in eye-contact, displayed more smiles and vocalizations while also exhibiting less crying and fretting than infants who didn't receive the touch stimulation.

In addition, to increasing positive behaviors between mothers and their infants, Blass and Ciaramitaro (1994) demonstrated that touch may help inhibit neural pathways for pain during infant inoculations, suggesting that touch protects infants from negative physical experiences as well. Their finding showed that touch decreased pain by lessening the intensity of crying at 2 months and later during development combinations of holding and rocking along with vocalizations were needed to sooth infants during painful inoculation. Field (1998) has argued that infants need a particular level of touch intervention, specifically massage, to protect them from negative outcomes, with massaged infants exhibiting less crying during painful procedures. Evidence also supports the benefits of massage, in that massage leads to more optimal sleep patterns, and soothability, more optimal arousal and attentiveness, and more positive interactive relationships (Field, 1998; Field et al., 2004b).

Ultimately, exposure to touch and touch intervention during infancy profoundly influences a variety of outcomes. Ottenbacher and colleagues (1987), in their meta-analytic review of 19 massage studies of infants/children, demonstrated that tactile stimulation was beneficial for motor, cognitive, social, physiological, and development, in general. Wyschograd (1981) and Weber (1990) even posit that quality touch is a primary factor in the socialization of higher-order emotional processes like sympathy and empathy.

Infant Brain Development

Touch perception is the earliest sense to form during embryological development and is a fundamental part of the emerging organism and mother-infant communication system. For example, in animal studies, Schanberg and his colleagues (Schanberg & Field, 1987; Schanberg & Kuhn, 1985) have shown that brain development in rat pups was determined by the specific patterns of stroking while the lack of touch produced a decrease in the growth hormone, ornithine decarboxylase. Moreover, in primate studies Suomi (1995) showed a positive relationship between early touch experiences and adaptive immunological functioning.

In neonates, touch responses can be observed as a sensory-perceptual capacity in the brain. Development of the infant progresses rapidly, evolving into an integrated system of emotional feelings and finally to an affection-transmitting, communication system between dyads. During that same period of time, behavioral neuroscientists (Bell, 1998; Goldman-Rakic, 1987) have contended that key functions of the infant's brain are also forming and changing. While the neonate's brain is protracted in course during the first several years of life, it is logical to theorize that touch and tactile experiences are both influenced by and have an influence on the brain circuitry of the infant. Maternal touch has also been implicated as an essential regulator of infant physiology and bio-behavioral development (Field et al., 2004c). Therefore, changes in cortical organization and activation are likely to occur simultaneously with emerging mother-infant tactile interaction, and these changes implicate touch as an important variable in contemporary research on brain plasticity.

Brain plasticity is not uni-dimensional and includes change to the functional organization of the somatosensory cortex (Burton & Sinclair, 1996; Cholewiak & Collins, 1991; Stevens & Green, 1996), change in the neural biochemical compositions (Kuhn & Schanberg, 1998), change in gene *expression* (Schanberg, 1995; Schanberg, Ingledue, Lee, Hannun, & Bartolome, 2003; Wang, Bartolome, & Schanberg, 1996), and change in the hemispheric patterns of regional EEG activity as a consequence of touch experiences (Jones & Field, 1999; Jones et al., 1998a). For example, we (Jones et al., 1998a) have shown that infant tactile stimulation at 1-month positively impacts the brain electrical activity patterns implicated in approach motivation and also promotes more positive infant behaviors. In essence, developmental experiences may coalesce to influence higher-order regions of the brain devoted to motivational systems for communication and affect. These ideas are consistent with Field and her colleagues' (Field, 1998; Field et al., 2004c) view that maturation of cortico-limbic and frontal systems are experience-dependent and highly responsive and malleable during early interactive experiences. Thus, touch behaviors are expected to stimulate more optimal patterns of brain organization and biobehavioral regulation. However, the mechanisms by which touch-quality interacts to alter the developing cognitive and emotional processes in the brain is still elusive.

Touch Behaviors in Infants Deemed "At Risk" During Development

Unlike typically developing infants, infants in high-risk groups present a special challenge to those studying touch behaviors. While tactile interaction between mothers and their infants should benefit healthy infants and infants of well mothers, the scientific literature is replete with additional concerns when examining other, more diverse groups. Two "at-risk" groups that have been studied in greater depth are premature infants and infants of depressed mothers. In the former group, the concern seems to surround the added physical contact, inasmuch as premature infants' nervous systems are under-developed so they may be hypersensitive to environmental stimulation and there is the added concern that the greater environmental exposure leads to the potential for exposing the fragile infant to environmental toxins. In the latter group, psychologically ill mothers are perceived as lacking the appropriate perspective or the "judgment" to provide appropriate levels of stimulation for their infants. A number of other high-risk groups have been studied and these results will also be noted.

Premature Infants

Prematurity is associated with both short and long-term problems including low birth weight, cognitive deficits, self-regulation problems, disturbed sleep patterns, social and cognitive deficits, and decreased scores on developmental measures (see Feldman this volume; Field et al., 2004c). In recent years, many hospitals have had a minimal touch policy with premature infants. However, a growing body of research has demonstrated that tactile stimulation can be beneficial for these infants. Researchers have found a variety of touch therapy effects including increased weight gain, increased active wake time, better performance on infant development scales, earlier discharge from intensive care units, and facilitation of mother-infant interactions (Cigales, Field, Lundy, Cuadra, & Hart, 1997; Dieter, Field, Hernandez-Reif, Emory, & Redzepi, 2003; Ferber et al., 2005). Two types of touch have been investigated in these studies, massage and skin-to-skin contact (KC) in which the mother holds the undressed infant between her breasts. This section will review the research addressing the benefits of massage for preterm infants (see Feldman, this volume for a review of KC).

Generally, preterm infants require extended hospitalization at great expense to the family. After medical stabilization, the most important factor for discharge of preterm infants from the hospital is adequate weight gain (Field et al., 2004c). Studies have found accelerated weight gain ranging from 28% to 53% (Dieter et al., 2003; Field et al., 1986; Scafidi, Field, & Schanberg, 1993) in infants receiving massage relative to control groups of infants. Furthermore, Field, Scafidi, and Schanberg, (1987) found that at age one, premature infants who had received massage maintained a long-term weight advantage over premature infants not receiving massage. Hernandez-Reif and Field (2000) have suggested that there is a sensitive period, when the infant weighs between 900 and 1500 grams, for beginning massage intervention, to achieve optimal weight gain. This weight-gain advantage reduces the length of hospitalization, which is beneficial for the infant and the parents, both financially and emotionally.

In addition to increased weight gain, tactile stimulation of preterm infants has been found to promote self-regulation or stability in preterm infants. Studies (Dieter et al., 2003) have found that infants who receive massage are more physiologically stable and better able to regulate their sleep cycles. The benefit of physiological stability is twofold. First, the infant benefits from the stabilization of its biological functions. Second, the stability in the sleep cycle specifically increases the infant's alertness which allows caregivers the opportunity to provide additional stimulation, thus promoting optimal development in the infant (Tessier et al., 2003). Collectively, research supports that massage (and KC as is noted by Feldman, this volume) promotes neurobehavioral development in the infant which in turn improves the child's overall outcome (Weiss, Wilson, & Morrison, 2004).

Infants of Depressed Mothers

Maternal emotional state has been shown time and time again to influence the quality of mother-infant interaction across the first year of life (Cicchetti & Toth, 1998; Dawson, Ashman, & Carver, 2000). Touch has been identified as a sensory characteristic that can potentially compensate for other interactive disturbances in depressed groups (Field, 1998). Yet an awareness of the benefits of touch must be tempered by the recognition of the potential for negative outcomes, as touch can be perceived as over-stimulating, excessive, intrusive, and abusive (Cohn, Matias, Tronick, Connell, & Lyons-Ruth, 1986; Malphurs, Raag, Field, Pickens, Pelaez-Nogueras, 1996). Among the issues investigated previously are whether depressed mothers use the appropriate quantity and quality of touch as well as whether depressed mothers who are trained to massage their infants showed advantages in interactive patterns across development (Field, 1998; Field et al., 2004c).

Touch is particularly important to infants of depressed mothers because touch has been shown to be related to the infant's ability to regulate neurobehavioral systems, a process that has been dysregulated in infants of depressed mothers (Jones et al., 1998a; Jones et al., 1998b). Diminished *quantities* of maternal touch towards their infants have been documented in mothers with postpartum depression (Field, 1998; Onozawa, Glover, Adams, Modi, & Kumar, 2001; Stepakoff, 1999) and even those with postpartum blues (Ferber & Makhoul, 2004). For example, Stepakoff (1999) found that depressed mothers demonstrated less tactile contact with their infants whereas non-depressed mothers had three times more touching as depressed mothers.

In other studies, depressed mothers have also been reported to touch too much, resulting in over-stimulation of their infants (Herrera et al., 2004). Perhaps, the excessive touch behavior of depressed mothers is due to their unconscious ambivalence toward their infants. Alternatively, lack of maternal understanding of developmental changes may be the pivotal factor here, as depressed mothers touched their infants less at 6-months and more at 10-months (Herrera et al., 2004), in contrast to other developmental studies where non-depressed mothers show reductions in touch behaviors across age (Jahromi, Putnam, & Stifter, 2004).

Touch-quality is also altered in depressed mothers (Ferber, 2004; Stepakoff, 1999). For example, in one recent study, Ferber (2004) demonstrated that experienced mothers who were only mildly-depressed showed more firm touching compared to first-time, mildly-depressed mothers, suggesting that experienced mothers are cognizant of the need for touch but depressed mothers are less organized and supportive in their touch style than non-depressed groups. That infants of depressed mothers are exposed to less affectionate touch is significant in that it also helps expose the mothers' nonverbal socialization patterns, ones that are influential in the development of communication patterns between dyads (Herrera et al., 2004).

In addition to lower quality touch behaviors, Herrera and colleagues (2004) also demonstrated that depressed mothers showed less affectionate and informative speech toward their infants, implicating a dysfunction of the entire communication system. Speech and touch are important in interactive communication between mothers and their infants, and depressed mothers may not use an optimal style of communicating information to their infants resulting in interactive difficulties. The different types of interactive behaviors, exhibited by depressive mothers, may be a reflection of the withdrawal of the mother from her infant even during the newborn period and would be expected to produce negative outcomes in the infant's physiological and behavioral adjustment.

Further, depressed mothers relative to non-depressed mothers exhibit more object-mediated touch (i.e. using a soft object) rather than touching with their hands (Stepakoff, 1999). Speculations as to why mothers may use objects in touch interactions range from the mother's need for the object for their own comfort to a lack of confidence in their mothering abilities. So perhaps, the material things or objects are used as a substitute for the affection that depressed parents feel they are inadequately providing for their children. Depressed mothers may also have unclear understanding of the potentially positive effects of appropriate touch (or they may be uncomfortable providing the intimacy of contact) and/or they may inhibit their own touch because they observe the infant is more often self-soothing. Finally, biological factors involved in depression (i.e., low levels of serotonin, left hemisphere hypoactivation patterns) may lower approach motivation implicit in the desire to provide adequate and appropriate tactile simulation in depressed mothers (Field et al., 2004a; Field, Diego, Hernandez-Reif, Gil, & Vera, 2005), a process that may also impact an infant's temperament and subsequent socio-emotional development.

Each of these explanations may be likely as primary factor or mediators of interactive behaviors of depressed mothers and their infants. Ultimately, however, these studies suggest that depressed mothers demonstrate a need for training in appropriate touch and communication patterns tailored to the developmental levels of their infants.

Traditional therapies for depressed mothers have only minimal effects on the interactive experience of the depressed mother-infant pair, as a one-person-centered therapy does not directly modulate the relationship difficulties. However, massage studies have demonstrated positive outcomes for depressed mothers and her infant, with depressed mothers reporting less depression and anxiety when they have been trained in infant massage and their infants exhibit significantly improve dyadic vocalization, soothability and affect, as well as decreases in restlessness and delayed sleep (Field, 1998; Onozawa et al., 2001). Field's Touch Therapy Model (1998) suggests that changes in brain activity and biochemistry or vagal tone (mediated by the parasympathetic system) could feedback to change mood and enhance the mother-infant dyad.

Though massage clearly reduces maternal depression symptoms, promotes optimal changes infant brain patterns and improves mother-infant interaction quality, it is unclear what specific factors in the massage session ameliorates the effects of depression for the dyads.

Other High-Risk Groups

Benefits of touch interventions have also been found in other high-risk infant groups. Autistic children are known to have problems with social interactions due to communication issues and atypical behavioral patterns. Touch intervention in this group have been associated with increased communication skills and decreased touch aversion (Cullen, Barlow, & Cushway, 2005) as well as a decrease in off-task and stereotypical autistic behaviors (Field et al., 1996).

Massage served to reduce stress behaviors, increase weight gain and increase scores on the Brazelton motor and orientation scales for cocaine-exposed preterm infants (Wheeden et al., 1993). Massage was also found to reduce spasticity in infants suffering from Cerebral Palsy (Hernandez-Reif et al., 2005). Orphaned infants suffer many of the same attachment issues as preterm infants (Kim, Shin, White-Traut, 2003) and massage has been found to moderate those issues in this group of high-risk infants as well. Overall, the research seems to support using touch as a low-cost medical intervention for preterm infants, infants of depressed mothers, and other high-risk infants and their families.

Brief Report of a Study on Nurturing Touch in Depressed Mothers who Breastfeed

In a short-term longitudinal study examining the relationship between the development of brain electrical activity, temperamental style, infant feeding, and maternal depression, we (Jones, Gagnon, & Mize, 2006) observed a variety of mother-infant interactive behaviors, including touching within two contexts. The purpose of this study was to investigate nurturing behaviors, including touch behaviors in a sample of infants of depressed and non-depressed mothers who elected to breastfeed versus those mothers that formula fed their infants. As human touch is believed to be an essential element of healthy infant development and is designed to promote optimal mother-infant interactive patterns so too has breastfeeding been shown to positively affect the physiological (Jones, McFall, & Diego, 2004) and social-interactive experiences of infants (Kuzela, Stifter, &Worobey, 1990). However, depressed mothers have been reported to provide fewer instances of nurturing touch (Field, 1998) and depressed mothers also are less likely to maintain stable breastfeeding patterns (Allen, Lewinsohn, & Selley, 1998; Jones et al., 2004).

Utilizing data from a pilot sample, 54 infants and their mothers (18 depressed and 36 non-depressed) were examined during a play interaction and during feeding session when the infants were 1 and 3 months of age. In order to be classified as depressed, mothers reported more depressive symptoms on a self-report depression scale (Center for Epidemiological Studies, Depressions Scale, CES-D, (Radloff, 1977) score of ≥ 16) and also met criteria for dysthymia or major depressive disorder within an interview

(Diagnostic Interview Schedule, DIS, Robins et al., 1981). Mothers assigned to the non-depressed group had few depressive symptoms (score of ≤ 12 on the CES-D) and a negative family history of depression. All infants in the study were physically healthy (> 9 on 5-minute APGAR and within normal range on the Infinib (Ellison, Horn, & Brown 1985) developmental scales).

Mothers were interviewed as to the duration and quality of breastfeeding with higher scores indicating a longer duration of breastfeeding (or expected breastfeeding) and fewer supplements added to their infant feeding regimen. Videotapes of the dyadic interactions were assessed by two research assistants who were uninformed as to the mother's depression status. All interactions were scored on a 1 to 5 scale, with higher scores indicating more optimal interaction patterns. Specifically, both infants and their mothers were assessed on their affect, vocalization, attention/gaze, touch quality, and mutually responsive behaviors. 25% of the videotapes were coded by both assistants to establish measurement reliability (Cohen's Kappa's ranged from .86–92).

The results of the correlational analyses showed relationships between more optimal touching behaviors and breastfeeding duration and quality, with more nurturing touch related to a longer duration of breastfeeding, $r(52) = .42$, $p < .05$, and a higher quality (i.e., exclusive) breastfeeding, $r(52) = .53$, $p < .05$. In addition, a 2 (depression status) by 2 (feeding status) repeated-measures ANOVA using the summed and standardized percentage of optimal/nurturing touch behaviors across the two ages and the two contexts as the dependent variables was conducted. Results showed significant differences across age and but not across contexts. As expected, the dyads' optimal/nurturing touch behaviors increased by approximately 20% from 1 to 3 months of age. Significant Depression Group by Feeding Group interactions were obtained during the feeding, $F(3, 50) = 10.76$, $p < .05$, and play-based interactive contexts, $F(3, 50) = 9.65$, $p < .05$ (Figure 17.1). Specifically, the depressed group that was formula fed exhibited the least nurturing touch patterns. Interestingly, the depressed mothers who also breastfed demonstrated similar percentages of nurturing touch as the two non-depressed groups, suggesting that breastfeeding during infancy enhances nurturing touch behaviors even in families with a depressed mother.

As past studies (Malphurs et al., 1996) have reported that depressed mothers demonstrate more negative/intrusive touch behaviors toward their infants, it is informative that breastfeeding, depressed mothers exhibited more nurturing touch compared to depressed mothers who formula fed. It appears that breastfeeding and maternal emotional status may jointly contribute to the quality of nurturing touch provided by mothers to their infants. In addition, in our previous work (Jones et al., 2004) we have demonstrated that infants of depressed mothers who are breastfed also showed more optimal EEG patterns, patterns that suggest greater approach motivation and interactive attunement with their environments. That breastfeeding, nurturing touch, and EEG patterns indicative of approach-type motivational styles occur in combination is not surprising, even for depressed mother-infant dyads, as all these processes are adaptive and provide the opportunity for experiencing positive interactive experiences.

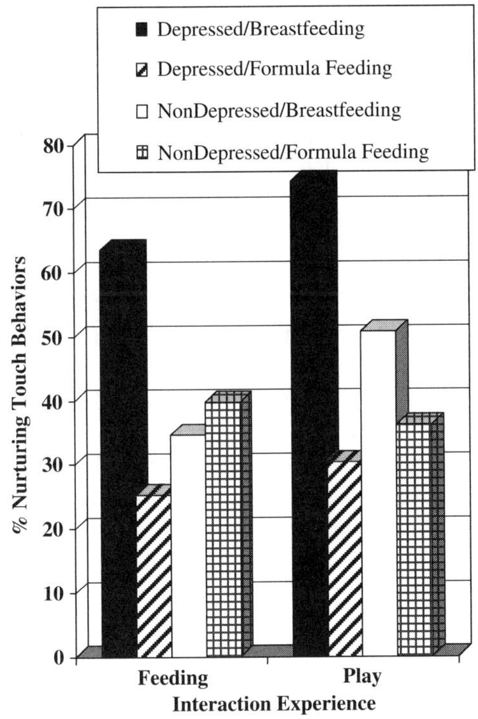

Figure 17.1. Touch Behaviors during Interactions and Feeding

Discussion

Theories of the mechanism for the effectiveness of touch and massage have prompted study in many areas of psychology. Currently we know that touch is not a unitary construct, as touch affects numerous systems during development. Most notably for normative and at-risk groups, touch and touch interventions have positively influence physiology, biochemistry, interpersonal behaviors, attention, emotion regulation, and mother-infant attunement. In addition, our own work has shown that touch can be a protective factor, providing infants of depressed mothers who are touched within the context of breastfeeding, additional interactive benefits and advantages in bio-behavioral regulation (Jones et al., 2004, 2006).

Although these findings are compelling, a number of the meaningful questions have not been addressed. For instance, investigations have not determined: (1) how the mechanism for adaptive-types of touch assists the interactive relationship between mothers and their infants; (2) what the factors involved in touch are that provide benefits and/or the possibility of risks to these dyads; and (3) what scientific evidence is available or needed in future studies to further argue for the use of touch as a low-cost relational vaccine.

In addition, questions arise that are specifically relevant to high risk families. For example, what are the limits of touch for providing beneficial outcomes and could infants in high-risk groups be the ones most benefited by touch and touch interventions? It would be informative to understand whether scientists could effectively track the dose/response levels of touch, as is necessary for understanding any intervention. In addition, is touch experienced in the same way for individuals "at risk?" Although Modi and Glover (1995) have attempted to "view" the experience of touch using fMRIs, science has not progressed far enough to truly understand the qualitative experiences derived from touch during development. Moreover, it may be that the physiological dysregulation (Jones et al., 1998b) reported in infants exposed to risk during intervention also influence their experiences associated with touch. During what circumstances (or at what level) does maternal touch produce negative outcomes in high-risk groups and can this or should this be altered? Depressed mothers may be using objects to touch because that is beneficial for them and their infants, as is the self-touch demonstrated by their infants. Should we intervene and will the intervention help this dyad or other high-risk groups in their future functioning? This we do not know or understand, as of yet.

From another perspective, can sensory and physiological studies inform us as to the excessive nature of touch and how do we use this information to provide optimal developmental outcomes for these high-risk groups? Finally, additional high-risk groups should be the subjects of further study. For example, we know relatively little about touch and touch interventions in maltreated children, in young children who are later diagnosed with ADHD or with comorbid psychological and physiological disorders.

The available evidence suggests that parent-child dyads may benefit from preventative or remedial interventions employed to enhance their ability to engage in appropriate direct and affectionate forms of tactile contact. It remains to be seen whether or not touch interventions can significantly improve sensitivity, skillfulness of nonverbal communication, and empathy development. This latter factor is important to study, as we know that empathy may be a protective factor for human relationships (Jones, Field, & Davalos, 2000).

Conclusion

The massage method used in the studies reviewed above is not complicated and anyone, including parents, can be trained to administer it. Touch interventions are not only easy and inexpensive to implement, but they have been shown to decrease hospitalization time and expense when used remedially (Field et al., 2004c). Furthermore, it seems reasonable to infer that touch could be a potent avenue for intervention in that tactile communication is pervasive in several realms of social interaction (e.g breastfeeding and soothing behaviors) and touch interventions are easier to learn to moderate than are facial, verbal and other emotional behaviors on their own.

Acknowledgements

This paper was supported by an NIMH research Grant (#MH61888) to Nancy Aaron Jones, Correspondence and requests for reprints should be sent to Nancy Aaron Jones, Florida Atlantic University, 5353 Parkside Drive, Jupiter Florida 33458. Telephone: 561-799-8632, E-mail: njones@fau.edu

References

Ainsworth, M. D. S., Blehar, M. C., Waters, E., & Wall, S. (1978). *Patterns of attachment: A psychological study of the strange situation*. Hillsdale, NY: Lawrence Erlbaum.

Allen, N. B., Lewinsohn, P. M., & Selley, J. R. (1998). Prenatal and perinatal influences on risk for psychopathology in childhood and adolescence. *Development and Psychopathology, 10*, 513–529.

Bell, M. A. (1998). Frontal lobe function during infancy: Implications for the development of cognition and attention. In J. E. Richards (Ed.), *Cognitive neuroscience of attention: A developmental perspective* (pp. 287–316). Mahwah NJ: Lawrence Erlbaum Associates.

Bell, S. M., & Ainsworth, M. D. S. (1972). Infant crying and maternal responsiveness. *Child Development, 43*, 1171–1190.

Blass, E. M., & Ciaramitaro, V. (1994). Tones and states. *Monographs of the Society for Research in Child Development, 59*(1), 97–101.

Bowlby, J. (1969). *Attachment and Loss* (Vol.1) New York, NY: Basic Books.

Burton, H., & Sinclair, R. (1996). Somatosensory cortex and tactile perceptions. In L. Kruger (Ed.), *Pain and touch* (pp. 105–177). San Diego, CA: Academic Press.

Chesney, M. A., Darbes, L. A., Hoerster, K., Taylor, J. M., Chambers, D. B., & Anderson, D. E. (2005). Positive emotions: Exploring the other hemisphere in behavioral medicine. *International Journal of Behavioral Medicine, 12*(2), 50–58.

Cholewiak, R. W., & Collins, A. A. (1991). Sensory and physiological bases of touch. In M. A. Heller, & W. Schiff (Eds.), *The psychology of touch* (pp. 23–60). Hillsdale, NJ: Lawrence Erlbaum.

Cicchetti, D., & Toth, S. L. (1998). The development of depression in children and adolescents. *American Psychologist, 53*, 221–241.

Cigales, M., Field, T., Lundy, B., Cuadra, A., & Hart, S. (1997). Massage enhances recovery from habituation in normal infants. *Infant Behavior & Development, 20*(1), 29–34.

Cohn, J., Matias, R., Tronick, E., Connell, D., & Lyons-Ruth, K. (1986). Face-to-face interactions of depressed mothers and their infants. In E. Tronick, & T. Field (Eds.), *Maternal depression and infant disturbance*. San Francisco: Jossey-Bass.

Cullen, L. A., Barlow, J. H., & Cushway, D. (2005). Positive touch, the implication for parents and their children with autism: An exploratory study. *Complementary Therapies in Clinical Practice, 11*(3), 182–189.

Dawson, G., Ashman, S. B., & Carver, L. J. (2000). The role of early experience in shaping behavioral and brain development and its implications for social policy. *Development and Psychopathology, 12*, 695–712.

Dieter, J. N. I., Field, T., Hernandez-Reif, M., Emory, E. K., & Redzepi, M. (2003). Stable preterm infants fain more weight and sleep less after five days of massage therapy. *Journal of Pediatric Psychology, 28*, 403–411.

Eibl-Eibesfeldt, E. (1996). *Love and hate*. (G. Strachan Translation). Hawthorne, NY: Aldine de Gruyter.

Ellison, P. H., Horn J. L., & Brown C. A. (1985). Construction of an infant neurological international battery (Infanib) for the assessment of neurological integrity in infancy. *Physical Therapy, 65*, 16–31.

Elton, D., Stanley, G., & Burrows, G. (1983). *The psychological control of pain*. New York, NY: Grune & Stratton.

Ferber, S. G. (2004). The nature of touch in mothers experiencing maternity blues: The contribution of parity. *Early Human Development, 79*(1), 65–75.

Ferber, S. G., Feldman, R., Kohelet, D., Kuint, J., Dollberg, S., Arbel, E., & Weller, A. (2005). Massage therapy facilitates mother-infant interaction in premature infants. *Infant Behavior & Development, 28*, 74–81.

Ferber, S. G., & Makhoul, R. I. (2004). The effect of skin-to-skin contact (Kangaroo Care) shortly after birth on the neurobehavioral responses of the full-term newborn: A randomized controlled trial. *Pediatrics, 113*, 858–865.

Field, T. (1998). Massage therapy effects. *American Psychologist, 53*(12), 1270–1281.

Field, T., Diego, M., Dieter, J., Hernandez-Reif, M., Schanberg, S., Kuhn, C., Yando, R., & Bendell, D. (2004a). Prenatal depression effects on the fetus and the newborn. *Infant Behavior and Development, 27*, 216–229.

Field, T., Diego, M. A., Hernandez-Reif, M., Gil, K., & Vera, Y. (2005). Prenatal maternal cortisol, fetal activity and growth. *International Journal of Neuroscience, 115*, 423–429.

Field, T., Grizzle, N., Scafidi, F., Abrams, S., Richardson, S., Kuhn, C., & Schanberg, S. (1996). Massage therapy for infants of depressed mothers. *Infant Behavior & Development, 19*, 107–112.

Field, T., Hernandez-Reif, M., Diego, M., Feijo, L., Vera, Y., & Gil, K. (2004b). Massage therapy by parents improves early growth and development. *Infant Behavior & Development, 27*, 435–442.

Field, T., Hernandez-Reif, M., & Freedman, J. (2004c). Stimulation programs for preterm infants. *Social Policy Report, 18*(1), 3–19.

Field, T., Lasko, D., Mundy, P., Henteleff, T., Talpins, S., & Dowling, M. (1996). Autistic children's attentiveness and responsivity improved after touch therapy. *Journal of Autism and Developmental Disorders, 27*, 329–334.

Field, T., Scafidi, F., & Schanberg, S. (1987). Massage of preterm newborns to improve growth and development. *Pediatric Nursing, 13*, 385–387.

Field, T. M., Schanberg, S. M., Scafidi, F., Bauer, C. R., Vega-Lahr, N., Garcia, R., Nystrom, J., & Kuhn, C. M. (1986). Tactile/kinesthetic stimulation effects on preterm neonates. *Pediatrics, 77*, 654–658.

Fox, N. A. (1991). If it's not left, it's right: Electroencephalogram asymmetry and the development of emotion. *American Psychologist, 46*, 863–872.

Fritz, S. (1999). *Mosby's Fundamentals of Therapeutic Massage*. St. Louis, MO: Mosby.

Goldman-Rakic, P. S. (1987). Development of cortical circuitry and cognitive function. *Child Development, 53*(3), 601–622.

Hernandez-Reif, M., & Field, T. (2000). Preterm infants benefit from early interventions. In J. Osofsky & H. Fitzgerald (Eds.) *WAIMH Handbook of infant mental health* (pp. 296–325). New York, NY: John Wiley & Sons.

Hernandez-Reif, M., Field, T., Largie, S., Diego, M., Manigat, N., Seoanes, J., & Bornstein, J. (2005). Cerebral palsy symptoms in children decreased following massage therapy. *Early Child Development and Care, 175*(5), 445–456.

Herrera, E., Reissland, N., & Shepherd, J. (2004). Maternal touch and maternal child-directed speech: Effects of depressed mood in the postnatal period. *Journal of Affective Disorders, 81*(1), 29–23

Hertenstein, M. J., & Campos, J. J. (2001). Emotion regulation via maternal touch. *Infancy, 2*(4), 549–566.

Jahromi, L. B., Putnam, S. P., & Stifter, C. A. (2004). Maternal regulation of infant reactivity from 2 to 6 months. *Developmental Psychology, 40*(4), 477–487.

Jones, N. A., & Field, T. (1999). Massage and music therapies attenuate frontal EEG asymmetry in depressed adolescents. *Adolescence, 34*, 529–534.

Jones, N. A., Field, T., & Davalos, M. (1998a). Massage therapy attenuates right frontal EEG asymmetry in one-month-old infants of depressed mothers. *Infant Behavior & Development, 21*(3), 527–530.

Jones, N. A., Field, T., & Davalos, M. (2000). Right frontal EEG asymmetry and lack of empathy in preschool children of depressed mothers. *Child Psychiatry and Human Development, 30*, 189–204.

Jones, N. A., Field, T., Fox, N. A., Davalos, M., Lundy, B., & Hart, S. (1998b). Newborns of mothers with depressive symptoms are physiologically less developed. *Infant Behavior and Development, 21*, 537–541.

Jones, N. A., Gagnon, C. M. & Mize, K. D. (2006). Nurturing touch is beneficial for depressed mothers and their infants. Paper presented at the International Conference of Infant Studies, Kyoto, Japan.

Jones, N. A., McFall, B. A., & Diego, M. A. (2004). Patterns of brain electrical activity in infants of depressed mothers who breastfeed and bottle feed: The mediating role of infant temperament. *Biological Psychology, 67*, 103–124.

Kaas, J. J. (2000). Touch: Biological organization. In A. E. Kazdin (Ed.), *Encyclopedia of psychology*, Vol. 8. (pp. 94–98), Washington DC, American Psychological Association. New York, NY: Oxford University Press.

Kennell, J. H., & Klaus, M. H. (1984). Mother-infant bonding: Weighing the evidence. *Developmental Review, 4*(3), 275–282.

Kim, T. I., Shin, Y. H., White-Traut, R. C. (2003). Multisensory intervention improves physical growth and illness rates in Korean orphaned newborn infants. *Research in Nursing and Health, 26*, 424–433.

Kuhn, C., & Schanberg, S. (1998). Responses to maternal separation: Mechanisms and mediators. *International Journal of Developmental Neuroscience, 16*(3/4), 261–270.

Kuzela, A. L., Stifter, C. A., & Worobey, J. (1990). Breastfeeding and mother-infant interactions. *Journal of Reproductive and Infant Psychology, 8*, 185–194.

LePage, D. E., & Stack, D. M. (1993). *Manipulation of maternal touch during mother-infant still-face interactions: Differential effects on infant affect and attention*. Paper presented at the Society for Research in Child Development, New Orleans, LA.

Malphurs, J. E., Raag, T., Field, T., Pickens, J., & Pelaez-Nogueras, M. (1996). Touch by intrusive and withdrawn mothers with depressive symptoms. *Early Development and Parenting, 5*(2), 111–115.

Merzenich, M. M. (1984). Functional "maps" of skin sensations. In C. C. Brown (Ed.), *The many facets of touch* (Vol. 10). Skillman, NJ: Johnson and Johnson Pediatric Round Table.

Modi, N., & Glover, J. (1995). Massage therapy for preterm infants. Paper presented at the Touch Research Symposium, Providence, Rhode Island.

Montagu, A. (1986). *Touching: The human significance of the skin* (3rded.). New York, NY: Harper & Row.

Moreno, A. J., Posada, G. E., & Goldyn, D. T. (2006). Presence and quality of touch influence coregulation in mother-infant dyads. *Infancy, 9*(1), 1–20.

Moyer, C. A., Rounds, J., & Hannum, J. W. (2004). A meta-analysis of massage therapy research. *Psychological Bulletin, 130*(1), 3–18.

Muir, D., & Lee, K. (2003). The still-face effect: Methodological issues and new applications. *Infancy, 4*(4), 483–491.

Onozawa, K., Glover, V., Adams, D., Modi, N., & Kumar, R.C. (2001). Infant massage improves mother-infant interaction for mothers with postnatal depression. *Journal of Affective Disorders, 63*, 201–207.

Ottenbacher, K. J., Muller, L., Brandt, D., Heintzelman, A., Hojem, R., & Sharpe, P. (1987). The effectiveness of tactile stimulation as a form of early intervention: A quantitative evaluation. *Developmental and Behavioral Pediatrics, 8*, 68–76.

Pelaez-Nogueras, M., Field, T., Hossain, Z., & Pickens, J. (1996a). Depressed mothers' touching increases infants' positive affect and attention in still-face interactions. *Child Development, 67*, 1780–1792.

Pelaez-Nogueras, M., Gewirtz, J., Field, T., Cigales, M., Malphurs, J., Clasky, S., & Sanchez, A. (1996b). Infants' preference for touch stimulation in face-to-face interactions. *Journal of Applied Developmental Psychology, 17*, 199–213.

Perez, H. (2001). Types and amplitudes of touch as reinforcing stimuli in operant conditioning of infant behavior. *Dissertation Abstracts International: Section B: The Sciences and Engineering, 61*(10-B), 5546.

Radloff, L. S. (1977). The CES-D Scale: A self-report symptoms scale to detect depression in a community sample. *American Journal of Psychiatry, 137*, 1081–1083.

Robins, L., Helzer, J., Croughan, J., & Ratcliff, K. (1981). National Institute of Mental Health Diagnostic Interview Schedule. *Archives of General Psychiatry, 38*, 381–390.

Sachs, F. (1988). The intimate sense: Understanding the mechanics of touch. *The Sciences, 1*, 28–34.

Salvo, S. G. (1999). *Massage therapy: Principles and practice*. Philadelphia, PA: Saunders.

Scafidi, F., Field, T., & Schanberg, S. (1993). Factors that predict which preterm infants benefit most from massage therapy. *Journal of Developmental and Behavioral Pediatrics, 14*, 176–180.

Schanberg, S. (Ed.). (1995). *The genetic basis for touch effects*. Hillsdale, NJ, England: Lawrence Erlbaum Associates, Inc. xii, 121 pp. Retrieved January 6, 2006, from PsycINFO database.

Schanberg, S., & Field, T. (1987). Sensory deprivation stress and supplemental stimulation in the rat pup and preterm human neonate. *Child Development, 58*, 1431–1447.

Schanberg, S., & Kuhn, C. (1985). The biochemical effects of tactile deprivation in neonatal rats. *Perspectives in Behavioral Medicine, 2*, 133–148.

Schanberg, S. M., Ingledue, V. F., Lee, J. Y., Hannun, Y. A., & Bartolome, J. V. (2003). PKCα mediates maternal touch regulation of growth-related gene expression in infant rats. *Neuropsychopharmacology, 28*(6), 1026–1030.

Schopler, E. (1965). Early infantile autism and receptor processes. *Archives of General Psychiatry, 13*, 327–335.

Schore, A. N. (1996). The experience-dependent maturation of a regulatory system in the orbital prefrontal cortex and the origin of developmental psychopathology. *Developmental and Psychopathology, 8*, 59–87.

Siegel, D. J. (1999). *The developing mind: Toward a neurobiology of interpersonal experience*. New York, NY: Guilford.

Stack, D. M., & Muir, D. W. (1992). Adult tactile stimulation during face-to-face interactions modulates five-month-olds affect and attention. *Child Development, 63*, 1509–1525.

Stepakoff, S. A. (1999). Mother-infant tactile communication at four-months: Effects of infant gender, maternal ethnicity and maternal depression. *Dissertation Abstracts International: Section B: The Sciences and Engineering, 9951115*. New York: St. John's University.

Stevens, J. C., & Green, B. G. (1996). History of research on touch. In L. Kruger (Ed.), *Pain and Touch* (pp. 1–23). San Diego, CA: Academic Press.

Suomi, S. (1995). Touch and the immune system in rhesus monkeys. In T. Field (Ed.), *Touch in Early Development* (pp. 53–65). Mahwah, NJ: Lawrence Erlbaum.

Tessier, R., Cristo, M. B., Velez, S., Giron, M., Nadeau, L., de Calume, Z. F., & Ruiz-Palaez, J. G. (2003). Kangaroo mother care: A method for protecting high-risk low-birth-weight and premature infants against developmental delay. *Infant Behavior & Development, 26*, 384–397.

Tomkins, S. S. (1982). *Affect, imagery, consciousness* (Vol. 3). New York, NY: Springer.

Tronick, E. (1995). Touch in mother-infant interaction. In T. Field (Ed.), Touch in Early Development (pp. 53–65). Mahwah, NJ: Lawrence Erlbaum.

Wang, S., Bartolome, J. V., & Schanberg, S. M. (1996). Neonatal deprivation of maternal touch may suppress ornithine decarboxylase via downregulation of the proto-oncogenes c-myc and max. *Journal of Neuroscience, 16*(2), 836–842.

Weber, R. (1990). A philosophical perspective on touch. In K. Barnard & T.B. Brazelton (Eds.), Touch: The foundation of Experience (pp. 11–43). Madison, CT: International Universities Press.

Weinberg, K. (1992). Sex differences in 6-month-old infants' affect and behavior: Impact on maternal caregiving. *Dissertation Abstracts International: Section B: The Sciences and Engineering*, University of Massachusetts at Amherst.

Weiss, S. J. (1990). Parental touching: Correlates of a child's body concept and body sentiment. In K. E. Barnard & T. B. Brazelton (Eds.), *Touch: The foundation of experience* (pp. 425–459). Madison: International Universities Press.

Weiss, S. J., Wilson, P., & Morrison, D. (2004). Maternal tactile stimulation and the neurodevelopment of low birth weight infants, *Infancy, 5*(1), 85–107.

Wheeden, A., Scafidi, F.A., Field, T., Ironson, G., Bandstra, E., Schanberg, S., & Valdeon, C. (1993). Massage effects on cocaine-exposed preterm neonates. *Journal of Developmental and Behavioral Pediatrics, 14*, 318–322.

Wyschograd, E. (1981). Empathy and sympathy as tactile encounter. *Journal of Philosophy, 6*, 25–43.

18

Non-Erotic Physical Affection: It's Good for You

Andrew K. Gulledge, Michael Hill, Zephon Lister, and Carolyn Sallion

> Affection is responsible for nine-tenths of whatever solid and durable happiness there is in our lives.
>
> –C.S. Lewis

Do it. That's right; do it. Physical affection is good for you, and it is good for your close relationships. This chapter outlines the extant studies that support this notion (given certain parameters and limitations), and it provides a cohesive theoretical and practical framework for understanding physical affection in the context of individual and relational betterment. Also, while something like a kiss may range from harmlessly "peckish" to ravenously sexual, the main focus of this chapter is on *non-erotic* physical affection. Consult other chapters in this volume that deal with issues peripherally related to physical affection (such as touch, close physical contact in children, love, sex, and intimacy). Thus the main point of this chapter on physical affection is that you should *do it*, and we'll tell you why.

Theory

This section covers various theoretical issues regarding physical affection. It addresses the various subjective meanings that can be attached to physical affection, across a broad range of dimensions. It offers a brief discussion of the *pursuer-distancer* pattern of relational interaction, in regard to physical affection. The section also introduces a model of relational interaction known as *social attunement*, which explains how behavioral assumptions are built and maintained in a relational context. It then goes on to explain how to use this model to enhance the degree to which physical affection can benefit individual relationships.

Physical Affection and Meaning

It should be plainly evident that physical affection can hold no one meaning across the dimensions of time, circumstance, quantity, quality, motivation, macroculture, microculture, relationship and individual. Certainly the interpretive meaning of physical affection is as subject to individual and societal interpretation as most any behavior in the context of a romantic relationship.

That is, a hundred different people engaged in the same type of physical affection might reasonably have a hundred different experiences regarding the same.

Macroculture has been determined in the research literature to affect some elements of physical affection. Studies have targeted the following populations:

- Dominican and Puerto Rican mother/child dyads (Calzada & Eyberg, 2002)
- French and American adolescents (Field, 1999, 2002)
- Asian and Latino couples (Regan, Jerry, Narvaez, & Johnson, 1999)
- Public interactions in England, France, the Netherlands, Italy, Greece, Scotland, and Ireland (Remland, Jones, & Brinkman, 1995)

In short, these studies find that cultural influences *do* affect physical affection across a range of nationalities, relationship status, and research methodologies.

Circumstance might very well color the meanings associated with romantic physical affection. When I (Gulledge) kiss my wife at the gym (in front of the many flirtatious personal trainers), it has a completely different meaning than when we kiss on a romantic evening at the beach. Thus the circumstance of "hands off, fellas" is much different than that of "it's just us, and I love you."

Quantity and quality are also dimensions of physical affection that are likely to affect the meanings associated with it. A one-second kiss is not necessarily one tenth of a ten-second kiss. Furthermore, a one hour massage is not necessarily six times as good as a ten minute massage. A five-second passionate kiss is not necessarily equal in meaning to a five-second forced kiss. A "dead fish" handholding experience will likely not mean the same thing as a more engaged one. Given the theoretically influential nature of physical affection *quality*, future studies using self-report methodologies should consider measuring this dimension of physical affection.

Motivation is also an important factor in attributing meaning to romantic physical affection. If I am giving you a ten-minute massage because you won a bet, the massage will probably not be as likely to be attributed to affection and love. Couples that thus use physical affection as "legal tender" in their relationships (e.g. massaging each other with an egg timer on hand) are probably not as likely to attribute the same meaning to the physical affection as if they had done it for a more loving motivation. *A gift born of necessity holds a different meaning than one born of love.*

The meanings associated with physical affection are thus to be determined, as should be self-evident, by the partners themselves, given a wide range of influencing factors, *some* of which have been considered above. Suffice it to say that the subjective meanings behind physical affection play an overarching role in determining how "good" physical affection is for you.

The Pursuer/Distancer Relationship: Playing Cat and Mouse with Physical Affection

The common theme of the so-called *pursuer/distancer* relationship is quite applicable to physical affection. If there is a significant imbalance in the partners' respective desires for physical affection (quantity and/or quality), then a pattern of pursuing and distancing is likely to follow. (The image of a small child trying to cuddle an unwilling cat comes to mind. Without belaboring the point, suffice it to say that too much of this kind of interaction (especially the one-sided kind, without an equitable trade-off of roles) is most likely detrimental to the individuals, and to the couple. A little chasing once in a while might be fun, but too much can be harmful.

Social Attunement: A Model for the Development of Interpersonal Propriety

Gulledge, and Louw (2004) proposed a model of social attunement, which describes how couples come to understand the propriety of behavior within the context of their relationship. It forms the set of unspoken assumptions and guidelines by which couples govern their relational interaction. It is about the unwritten rules that guide how we behave around each other. In other words, it is how couples come to "just know" certain things about the way they should interact.

When a couple first meets, they have *implicit rules* that guide how they are to act around each other. These rules come from their prior socialization. A man doesn't go up to a woman at the library and ask in a suave voice, "May I have this dance?" Why not? This is because he "just knows" that this kind of behavior is inappropriate to that context. Now, what if a couple had watched a movie depicting a romantic scene in which a man did, in fact, approach a woman at the library in this manner. Then, let's say the man, in real life, unexpectedly bumps into his wife at the library. Now he says, "May I have this dance?" They both share a good laugh.

Having watched the romantic movie changed the implicit attunement of this couple, as to the propriety of greeting in a library in this manner. Surely, the couple didn't have to sit down after watching the movie and agree, "Okay, if we are to ever meet unexpectedly in a library, let's greet this way; only it won't be weird, it'll be funny since we saw it in the movie." Rather, this attunement "just happens" in the background. The implicit rules guiding this couple's behavior has changed, without their having discussed it (or even consciously recognizing it!).

Consider another situation:

> A recently married couple reunites one evening in a loving kiss. The husband is suddenly surprised by his wife's bad breath. He makes some slight comment regarding this, and the wife withdraws with hurt feelings, not wanting to kiss for the moment. The husband feels somewhat guilty about the whole thing; and both parties turn to other activities.
>
> The next night, they greet and kiss again. The wife has bad breath again. The husband doesn't say anything this time since he doesn't want to repeat the last night's sequence of hurt feelings for both him and her. He kisses for a little while, then discreetly moves on to some other activity. The wife doesn't notice anything out of the ordinary. He still kissed her, after all.
>
> After a short while, when the couple greets, the husband gives his wife a huge bear hug and a couple of light pecks on the lips, but nothing very passionate. He then moves on to his other activities. The wife doesn't notice anything particularly wrong.
>
> After a while, the couple seldom kisses each other passionately, but they could not tell you why.

This sequence demonstrates how a couple, without overtly discussing it, has "socially attuned" with each other to avoid kissing passionately during their evening greetings. This kind of negotiation is a nonverbal pattern of social interaction, subtle enough to be veritably invisible to the attuning parties. Someone might ask this couple later why they don't kiss passionately as often. And they might very well respond, "I don't know. We *just don't*." In fact, it would be rare indeed to have a couple that could target and cite a specific pattern of interactive behavior that led to an underlying assumption as to the propriety of their relational interaction. In other words, we tend to not notice the underlying social attunement in our relationships. It just sort of happens.

Intentional Attunement: Talk About It!

The quantity and quality of romantic physical affection should be determined as a matter of deliberate, purposeful social attunement. This attunement can, and should, involve both verbal and nonverbal communication. Phrases like, "Honey, I don't really like that," or, "Oh baby, that was great!" can help the couple to thus attune. A purr, or perhaps even just a crooked grin, can also serve well to communicate the message nonverbally, facilitating this kind of attunement. With time, and patience, partners can come to "just know" what kinds of physical affection (and how much) the other likes. This would be more likely to lead to a happier couple than if they were misattuned to each other's physical affection wants (or even attuned to not be physically affectionate at all!).

It thus follows that if a couple never talks about (much less participates in) physical affection, this attunement will remain underdeveloped (or, more correctly, developed to underdevelopment). Put another way, the couple will proactively attune to *not* give each other physical affection. "Why don't we ever kiss? I don't know. *We just don't*."

Incidentally, if a poorly attuned couple did try to spark up this physical affection out of nowhere, they would be less likely to know what and how much their partner likes (due to their poor level of attunement). One could imagine how awkward this might look. And, in a behavioristic vein, if they thus have an unsatisfactory experience, they are unlikely to continue since it would be more punishing than reinforcing. (Behavioristic theory posits that we tend towards an increase in behavior that is perceived to be reinforcing, and a decrease in behavior that is perceived to be punishing; see Mazur, 2001; Gulledge, 2004).

In short, talk about what kinds of physical affection you like. Talk about what kind of cuddling, kissing, or backrubs you like. Talk about frequency, intensity, and technique. You need not be a professional massage therapist to give a good massage. If your partner is giving you a massage, give a deep, "Mmmm," when it feels good. Say, "Oww," if it hurts (e.g. if they are massaging you too hard, or in the wrong place). In other words, give clear feedback as to what you like, and what you don't like.

Make specific requests if you feel so inclined. "Darling, could you do it like you did the other time? You know, right in the middle of my lower back there? That'd be—ooh! Aaaaaaahhh! That's the ticket." My wife and I (Gulledge) call it "The *Money* Spot," as in the phrase, "Right on the Money." Now I need only say, "Sweetheart, could you do me on the *Money* spot?" And, even more frequently, I need not say anything at all because we have come to the level of attunement where she *just knows* how I like the massages.

She knows how hard and where I like them. (The same goes, I hope, for how I massage her.) And, incidentally, our massages are better now than they have ever been, due to this kind of active attunement on our parts.

We will inevitably attune to each other, regardless of any deliberate effort. Why not at least be conscious of this attunement, and direct it in a way to our liking (and, incidentally, favorable to our relational stability and happiness)? *After all, not talking about it is to attune to not talking about it.* And, if a couple is unable to talk about it (due to the implicit rule they inadvertently laid down by not talking about it), then there is less of a chance that they will get what they want out of the relationship. And, if couples are thus unsatisfied in their relationship, they are subject to all the vicissitudes inherent in relational dissatisfaction, and possible dissolution (should said dissatisfaction endure or even worsen).

Research

This section outlines various research issues dealing with physical affection. The first part describes the pressing issue of theoretical and operational definitions of physical affection, including its many subtypes. The next part cites a number of studies about physical affection, including a discussion on the emerging research literature on oxytocin.

Defining the Beast

One definition of physical affection (and, consequently, the one we use herein) is "any touch intended to arouse feelings of love in the giver and/or the recipient" (Gulledge, Gulledge, & Stahmann, 2003, p. 234; Gulledge, Stahmann, & Wilson, 2004; Hill, 2004). Thus, *romantic* physical affection might rightly be described as "any touch intended to arouse feelings of *romantic* love in the giver and/or the recipient." Or, more generally, romantic physical affection could be described as any physical affection (as defined previously) that occurs within the context of a romantic relationship.

It bears mention, however, that these definitions are more *theoretical* (or subjective) in nature than *empirical* (or objective). That is, one could not conduct a sound *observational* study of physical affection based upon these descriptions. Clearly, any "[intention] to arouse feelings of love" is not an observable quality. Notwithstanding, this definition may be of scientific use when applied to self-report survey research.

The simple definition of physical affection, for example, can easily be provided on the survey instrument (so that participants, reading the survey can understand what is meant when the survey questions refer to *physical affection*). This approach would do more to achieve a uniformity in responses with self-report data. Incidentally, it is possible that one could define physical affection, or perhaps a certain *type* of physical affection, with the strictest of empirical descriptions. But this approach would be more likely to confuse the typical survey respondent than to be of any significant scientific value.

We use the term *physical affection*, yet others have used terms such as touch, affection, affectionate behavior, and romantic behavior. Others refer to specific types of physical affection only, such as kissing, hugging, or patting on the back. Still others lump a handful of these typologies into a single unit of measurement, such as "hugging and kissing." In both the common vernacular and in scientific terminology, people use varying words and phraseologies to refer to (what we simply call) *physical affection*.

The same is true of different *typologies* of physical affection. Spanier's (1976) Dyadic Adjustment Scale includes a Likert-type item on kissing. Landau (1989) refers to kissing, hugging, and patting. Field (1999) uses observational coding to distinguish between such behaviors as hugging, kissing, leaning, and stroking. Regan and colleagues (1999) talk about hand holding and one-armed embracing. Hill (2004) measures some 29 distinct types of physical affection, including such items as dancing, grooming, napping, and various forms of sexual physical affection. Gulledge et al. (2003) distinguish between backrubs/massages, caressing/stroking, cuddling/holding, holding hands, hugging, kissing on the face, and kissing on the lips.

One problem with this variance is that relating empirical findings on one uniquely defined topic may not necessarily be directly comparable to empirical findings on another. For example, a simple replication using a different operational or theoretical definition may not produce equivalent findings. The researcher, however, would be hard pressed to determine if this disparity is due to unreliable conclusions, or to inconsistent definitions and measurement. Furthermore, this problem is compounded severely when studies regarding a given topic are sparse, as in the case of physical affection. The logical solution of uniformity in definition and measurement might solve the problem of varying terminologies in physical affection research, but it would also present another problem – a lack of scientific creativity. That is, researchers who are bound to the operational and theoretical templates of the past can only make limited progress in scientific advancement. Stale replications (or bland rehashing) might thus be a waste of time, energy, and shelf space. Dynamic replications, on the other hand, can provide invaluable verification, generalization of findings (or the lack thereof), and intellectual prodding. (By *dynamic*, we mean using elements in one's study that are both comparable and novel, not just novel.)

It's Good for You

Physical affection has been associated with the following:

- Relationship satisfaction (Bell, Daly, & Gonzalez, 1987; Gulledge et al., 2003; Hill, 2004)
- Intimacy (Cooper & Bowles, 1973; Guerrero and Andersen, 1999; Hill, 2004; Jourard & Friedman, 1970; Mackey, Diemer, & O'Brien, 2000)
- Feeling understood (Flaherty, 1999)
- Relationship unity (Gurevitch, 1990)
- Respectful behavior (Gaines, 1996)
- Increased self-disclosure/openness (Cooper & Bowles, 1973; Flaherty, 1999)
- Increased self-esteem (Barber & Thomas, 1986)
- Increased religious self-evaluation (Barber & Thomas, 1986)
- Increased empathy (Adams, Jones, Schvaneveldt, & Jenson, 1982; Field, 2002)
- Social sensitivity development (Adams et al., 1982)

- Cardiovascular arousal modulation (Diamond, 2000; Fishman, Turkheimer, & DeGood, 1995)
- Stress relief (Fishman et al., 1995)
- Pain relief (Fishman et al., 1995)
- Decreased blood pressure (Fishman et al., 1995)
- Increased oxytocin levels (Carter, 1998; Field, 2002)
- Decreased cortisol levels (Field, 2002)
- Decreased dopamine levels (Field, 2002)
- Decreased anxiety (Field, 2002; Olson & Sneed, 1995)
- Decreased aggression (Field, 1999, 2002; Shuntich, Loh, & Katz, 1998)
- Improved mood (Field, 2002)
- Positive emotional responsiveness (Olausson, Lamarre, Backlund, Morin, Wallin, Starck, et al., 2002)
- Developing attachment bonds (Diamond, 2000; Landau, 1989)
- Reduced sexual dysfunction (in the context of behavioral sex therapy; Brender, Libman, Burstein, & Takefman, 1983; McCarthy, 2001; Sollod, 1975)
- Decreased couple/parental conflict (Gulledge et al., 2003; Shuntich et al., 1998)
- Enhanced conflict resolution (Gulledge et al., 2003)

Studies have examined physical affection in reference to the following groups:

- Couples (Bell et al., 1987; Flaherty, 1999; Gaines, 1996; Gulledge et al., 2003; Gulledge et al., 2004; Hall & Veccia, 1990; Hill, 2004; L'Abate 2001; Regan et al., 1999; Shuntich et al., 1998; Van Horn, Arnone, Nesbitt, Desllets, Sears, Giffin, et al., 1997)
- Children (Adams et al., 1982; Barber & Thomas, 1986; Calzada & Eyberg, 2002; Deatrick, Brennan, & Cameron, 1998; Felson & Zielinski, 1989; Field, Diego, & Sanders, 2001; Hartup, 1960; L'Abate, 2001; Landau, 1989; McHale, 1997; Shuntich et al., 1998)
- Adults (Cooper & Bowles, 1973; Diamond, 2000; Field, 1999, 2002; Fishman et al., 1995; Remland, Jones, & Brinkman, 1995)

In reference to the above association between physical affection and couple conflict, note that parental conflict has detrimental effects upon children (for a review, see Cummings & Davies, 2002), including the development of the following:

- Insecure and/or disorganized attachment bonds (Owen & Cox, 1997)
- Negative perceptions of conflict (El-Sheikh, 1997)
- Lower levels of well-being (Jekielek, 1998; Vandewater & Lansford, 1998)
- "Severe behavior problems" (Radovanovic, 1993)
- Diminished competence (Radovanovic, 1993)
- Later anxiety and depression/withdrawal (Jekielek, 1998)
- Sensitization to future conflicts (Davies, Myers, Cummings, & Heindel, 1999; El-Sheikh, 1997)

In other words, *do it*. It's good for you.

Physical Affection and Oxytocin

An area of particular interest is oxytocin. Oxytocin is a hormone that has been implicated in mammalian bonding (Bales & Carter, 2003; Bielsky & Young, 2004; Carter, 1998, 1999; Cho, De Vries, Williams, & Carter, 1999; Insel, 2000; Insel, Preston, & Winslow, 1995; Liu, Curtis, & Wang, 2001; Porges, 1998; Young, 2002). Although the precise mechanisms by which pair bond formation occurs are not specifically delineated, it is safe to say that oxytocin does help couples to form lasting relationship bonds. (It should be noted that the presence of oxytocin alone is probably not sufficient for pair bond formation to occur.)

Oxytocin has receptor sites in the limbic system of the brain, which is responsible for controlling human emotions (Carter, 1998). The release of oxytocin has been linked to feelings of positive emotions as well as lowering blood pressure (Light, Grewen, & Amico, 2005), decreasing stress (Field, 2002; Heinrichs, Baumgartner, Kirschbaum, & Ehlert, 2003), lowering stress hormones (Field, 2002; Heinrichs et al., 2003), and possibly even speeding the healing of wounds (Stock, Fastborn, Bjorkstrand, Ungerstedt, & Uvnas-Mober, 1990). While far from being conclusive, there is emerging evidence that oxytocin imbalances in the brain may be linked to eating disorders (Demitrach et al., 1990; Frank, Kaye, Altemus, & Greeno, 2000), depression (Arletti & Bertolini, 1987; Uvnas-Mober, 2003), anxiety (Bale, Davis, Auger, Dorsa, & McCarthy, 2001), or even autism and schizophrenia (Insel, 2000).

Oxytocin can be released through a variety of different ways. Sexual contact tends to induce the largest release of oxytocin (Williams, Catania, & Carter, 1992; Winslow, Hastings, Carter, Harbaugh, & Insel, 1993). Yet nonsexual physical affection such as backrubs and hugs also induce the release of oxytocin (Shermer, 2004). Women who have received more hugs from their partners in the past have been shown to have higher levels of oxytocin and significantly lower blood pressure than women who have not been hugged much by their partners in the past (Light et al., 2005).

In terms of how oxytocin may help relationships to form and to be maintained, oxytocin may play an important role, especially in the serious dating and committed stages. Couples who are casually dating may not participate in as much physical affection due to the lack of trust and commitment. However once the relationship becomes more established, physical affection increases, increasing oxytocin levels which in turn aids in feelings of commitment. Once commitment has been achieved, be it through serious dating, cohabitation, engagement, or marriage, etc., continued physical affection would be important to the survival of the relationship, as it would constantly reinforce the pair bond.

Practice

This section describes how to make use of the theory and research outlined above. The main idea is, "Do it!" but some more detailed guidelines are given as well. In short, this section describes how to apply the behavioral vaccine of non-erotic physical affection to your own relationship, and to those with whom you work.

Some Practical Considerations

Make sure you don't have bad breath. Love and affection aside, it is difficult to kiss someone with bad breath for any considerable length of time, or with any considerable amount of passion. Use mouthwash, chewing gum, or breath mints as appropriate (and regular tooth-brushing!).

Bathe. It might be difficult to comfortably cuddle up next to someone with poor general hygiene. If your partner likes cologne or perfume, use it. If, on the other hand, your partner could care less about personal hygiene, then I suppose you don't need to worry about it as much.

If you have clammy hands (sometimes we can't help it), try not to hold hands. Consider giving a massage or some other type of physical affection first (on *top* of the clothing, please). Then, when the blood is flowing better in your extremities, go ahead and hold hands.

Give good massages. Don't expect massaging to help your relationship if you give poor ones. The first rule of thumb is to give them a massage you think you would like to have if you were on the receiving end. This is a good foundation, but not the ending point. Then, as you gain more experience in massaging your partner, you will be able to attune with them to understand better what they like and don't like. Thus you will get better, not only at giving massages in general, but at giving *your partner* massages, which is what really matters.

Physical Affection as a Behavioral Vaccine

As mentioned previously, physical affection is good for you. However, since the majority of studies presented herein are correlative in nature (and not causational), one cannot strictly determine the direction of causality. That is, studies on this topic have not traditionally used appropriate experimental designs to establish a time-order relationship between physical affection and outcome (e.g. relationship satisfaction, couple conflict).

Thus, it is not firmly established in the research literature if an increase in romantic physical affection will precede individual and relational betterment. We would think, however, from the wealth of information showing positive (correlative) associations with physical affection, that it couldn't hurt. (Of course, as mentioned before, this statement assumes a nonviolent, noncoercive, and otherwise safe relationship.)

Couples therapists and marriage educators could thus "prescribe" physical affection to their couples as a behavioral vaccine. True, doing it "just because our therapist said so" is not the same as "doing it just for the hell of it," but it's a start. Couples might decide they enjoy massaging each other – that it actually feels good! They might learn (through personal, albeit coached, experience) that a tight hug can go far in diffusing a potentially volatile situation.

If the couples can thus have a positive experience in giving each other physical affection, then there is an increased likelihood that they will continue their physically affectionate behavior. If this is the case, then true *second-order change* might be said to have taken place – not just "more of the same," but actual therapeutic movement (see Bateson, 2000).

Therapists and marriage educators can also help couples to actively attune to each other's feelings and desires (as suggested by the above discussion on *social attunement*). A therapy session or workshop might serve as a good platform for having couples discuss what they like or dislike about their physical affection (assuming they don't talk about it in private). Again, if they have a positive and enlightening experience in attuning to one another, they will be more likely to talk about it in the future. And, if they make the shift to talking about it more, then we have, once again, obtained a solid *second-order change* in the relationship (see Bateson, 2000).

Unlike many other interventions and task prescriptions, physical affection is relatively easy to implement. Couples don't need a sophisticated understanding of the science and theory related to the topic. (After all, they will be the masters of their own wants anyway.) They don't need any equipment or materials. And they don't even need special classes or workshops! All they need to do is *do it*!

Many couples already do it. For those who do, they can do it better. For those couples that don't do it, they can simply talk about what they like and dislike about it. They can try it out, then talk about it.

Conclusion

We have discussed some of the positive aspects of physical affection as related to the individual and to the relationship. We have also discussed a number of theoretical, research-related, and practical issues regarding physical affection. Limitations have been discussed. Future research considerations have been proposed. Yet the overarching conclusion remains the same. Physical affection is good for you. And, unlike many other types of interventions, it is also relatively easy to implement. So do it.

References

Adams, G. R., Jones, R. M., Schvaneveldt, J. D., & Jenson, G. O. (1982). Antecedents of affective role-taking behaviour: Adolescent perceptions of parental socialization styles. *Journal of Adolescence, 5*(3), 259–265.

Arletti, R., & Bertolini, A. (1987). Oxytocin acts as an antidepressant in two animal models of depression. *Life Science, 41*, 1725–1730.

Bale, T., Davis, A., Auger, A., Dorsa, D., & McCarthy, M. (2001). CNS region-specific oxytocin receptor expression: Importance in regulation of anxiety and sex behavior. *Journal of Neuroscience, 21*, 2546–2552.

Bales, K., & Carter, C. S. (2003). Developmental exposure to oxytocin facilitates partner preferences in male prairie voles (microtus ochrogaster). *Behavioral Neuroscience, 117*, 854–859.

Barber, B. K., & Thomas, D. L. (1986). Dimensions of fathers' and mothers' supportive behavior: The case for physical affection. *Journal of Marriage and the Family, 48*, 783–794.

Bateson, G. (2000). *Steps to an ecology of mind: Collected essays in anthropology, psychiatry, evolution, and epistemology*. Chicago: University of Chicago Press.

Bell, R. A., Daly, J. A., & Gonzalez, M. C. (1987). Affinity-maintenance in marriage and its relationship to women's marital satisfaction. *Journal of Marriage and the Family, 49*, 445–454.

Bielsky, I., & Young, L. (2004). Oxytocin, vasopressin, and social recognition in mammals. *Peptides, 25*, 1565–1574.

Brender, W., Libman, E., Burstein, R., & Takefman, J. (1983). Behavioral sex therapy: A preliminary study of its effectiveness in a clinical setting. *Journal of Sex Research, 19*, 351–365.

Calzada, E. J., & Eyberg, S. M. (2002). Self-reported parenting practices in Dominican and Puerto Rican mothers of young children. *Journal of Clinical Child and Adolescent Psychology, 31*(3), 354–363.

Carter, C. S. (1998). Neuroendocrine perspectives on social attachment and love. *Psychoneuroendocrinology, 23*, 779–818.

Carter, C. S. (1999). Stress and soothing: An endocrine perspective. In M. Lewis & D. Ramsay (Eds.), *Soothing and Stress* (pp. 3–18). Mahwah, NJ: Lawrence Erlbaum Associates.

Cho, M., De Vries, A., Williams, J., & Carter, C. S. (1999). The effects of oxytocin and vasopressin on partner preferences in male and female prairie voles (microtus ochrogaster). *Behavioral Neuroscience, 113*, 1071–1079.

Cooper, C., & Bowles, D. (1973). Physical encounter and self-disclosure. *Psychological Reports*, 33, 451–454.

Cummings, E. M., & Davies, P. T. (2002). Effects of marital conflict on children: Recent advances and emerging themes in process-oriented research. *Journal of Child Psychology and Psychiatry, 43*(1), 31–63.

Davies, P. T., Myers, R. L., Cummings, E. M., & Heindel, S. (1999). Adult conflict history and children's subsequent responses to conflict: An experimental test. *Journal of Family Psychology, 13*(4), 610–628.

Deatrick, J. A., Brennan, D., & Cameron, M. E. (1998). Mothers with multiple sclerosis and their children: Effects of fatigue and exacerbations on maternal support. *Nursing Research, 47*(4), 205–210.

Demitrach, M. A., Lesem, M. D., Listwak, S. J., Brandt, H. A., Jimerson, D. C., & Gold, P. W. (1990). CSF oxytocin in anorexia nervosa and bulimia nervosa: Clinical and pathophysiological considerations. *American Journal of Psychiatry, 147*, 882–886.

Diamond, L. M. (March, 2000). Are friends as good as lovers? Attachment, physical affection, and effects on cardiovascular arousal in young women's closest relationships, *Dissertation Abstracts International*, Section B: The Sciences and Engineering, *60*(8-B), 4272.

El-Sheikh, M. (1997). Children's responses to adult-adult and mother-child arguments: The role of parental marital conflict and distress. *Journal of Family Psychology, 11*(2), 165–175.

Felson, R. B., & Zielinski, M. A. (1989). Children's self-esteem and parental support. *Journal of Marriage and the Family, 51*, 727–735.

Field, T. (1999). American adolescents touch each other less and are more aggressive toward their peers as compared with French adolescents. *Adolescence*, 34, 753–758.

Field, T. (2002). Violence and touch deprivation in adolescents. *Adolescence, 37*(148), 735–749.

Field, T., Diego, M., & Sanders, C. (2001). Adolescent depression and risk factors. *Adolescence, 36*(143), 491–498.

Fishman, E., Turkheimer, E., & DeGood, D. (1995). Touch relieves stress and pain. *Journal of Behavioral Medicine, 18*, 69–79.

Flaherty, L. M. (1999). Communication expectations, feeling understood, and relationship development (Doctoral dissertation, 1999). *Dissertation Abstracts International*, Section A: Humanities and Social Sciences, *60*(1-A), 0020.

Frank, G. K., Kaye, W., Altemus, M., & Greeno, C. G. (2000). CSF oxytocin and vasopressin levels after recovery from bulimia nervosa and anorexia nervosa, bulimic subtype. *Biological Psychiatry, 48*, 315–318.

Gaines, S. O. (1996). Impact of interpersonal traits and gender-role compliance on interpersonal resource exchange among dating and engaged/married couples. *Journal of Social and Personal Relationships, 13*(2), 241–261.

Guerrero, L. K., & Andersen, P. (1994). Patterns of matching and initiation: Touch behavior and touch avoidance across romantic relationship stages. *Journal of Nonverbal Behavior, 18*, 137–153.

Guerrero, L. K., & Andersen, P. (1999). Public touch behavior in romantic relationships between men and women. In L. Guerrero, J. DeVito, & M. Hecht (Eds.), *The nonverbal communication reader* (pp. 202–210). Prospect Heights, IL: Waveland Press.

Gulledge, A. K. (2004). *The art of persuasion: A practical guide to improving your convincing power.* Lincoln, NE: iUniverse.

Gulledge, A. K., Gulledge, M. H., & Stahmann, R. F. (2003). Romantic physical affection types and relationship satisfaction. *The American Journal of Family Therapy, 31*(4), 233–242.

Gulledge, A. K., & Louw, K. (2004). *The process of social attunement.* Unpublished manuscript, Loma Linda University.

Gulledge, A. K., Stahmann, R. F., & Wilson, C. M. (2004). Seven types of nonsexual romantic physical affection among Brigham Young University students. *Psychological Reports, 95*, 609–614.

Gurevitch, Z. (1990). On the element of non-distance in human relations. *The Sociological Quarterly*, 31, 187–201.

Hall, J., & Veccia, E. (1990). More "touching" observations: New insights on men, women, and interpersonal touch. *Journal of Personality and Social Psychology*, 59, 1155–1162.

Hartup, W. W. (1960). Nurturance in pre-school children and its relation to dependency. *Child Development, 31*, 681–689.

Heinrichs, M., Baumgartner, T., Kirschbaum, C., & Ehlert, U. (2003). Social support and oxytocin interact to suppress cortisol and subjective responses to psychosocial stress. *Biological Psychiatry, 54*, 1389–1398.

Hill, M. T. (2004). *Romantic physical affection and relationship satisfaction across romantic relationship stages.* Unpublished master's thesis, University of North Dakota, Grand Forks, North Dakota.

Insel, T. R. (2000). Toward a neurobiology of attachment. *Review of General Psychology, 4*, 176–185.

Insel, T. R., Preston, S., & Winslow, J. T. (1995). Mating in the monogamous male: Behavioral consequences. *Physiology & Behavior, 57*, 615–627.

Jekielek, S. M. (1998). Parental conflict, marital disruption and children's emotional well-being. *Social Forces, 76*(3), 905–935.

Jourard, S., & Friedman, R. (1970). Experimenter-subject distance and self-disclosure. *Journal of Personality and Social Psychology*, 15, 278–282.

L'Abate, L. (2001). Hugging, holding, huddling and cuddling (3HC): A task prescription in couple and family therapy. *Journal of Clinical Activities, Assignments & Handouts in Psychotherapy Practice, 1*(1), 5–18.

Landau, R. (1989). Affect and attachment: Kissing, hugging, and patting as attachment behaviors. *Infant Mental Health Journal*, 10, 59–69.

Light, K., Grewen, K., & Amico, J. (2005). More frequent partner hugs and higher oxytocin levels are linked to lower blood pressure and heart rate in premenopausal women. *Biological Psychology, 69*, 5–21.

Liu, Y., Curtis, J. T., & Wang, Z. (2001). Vasopressin in the lateral septum regulates pair bond formation in male prairie voles (microtus ochrogaster). *Behavioral Neuroscience, 115*, 910–919.

Mackey, R. A., Diemer, M. A., & O'Brien, B. A. (2000). Psychological intimacy in the lasting relationships of heterosexual and same-gender couples. *Sex Roles, 43*(3/4), 201–227.

Mazur, J. E. (2001). *Learning and behavior* (5th ed.). Upper Saddle River, NJ: Prentice Hall.

McCarthy, B. (2001). Integrating sex therapy strategies and techniques into marital therapy. *Journal of Family Psychotherapy, 12*, 45–53.
McHale, J. P. (1997). Overt and covert coparenting processes in the family. *Family Process, 36*(2), 183–201.
Olausson, H., Lamarre, Y., Backlund, H., Morin, C., Wallin, B., Starck, G., Ekholm, S., Strigo, I., Worsley, K., Vallbo, A., & Bushnell, M. (2002). Unmyelinated tactile afferents signal touch and project to insular cortex. *Nature Neuroscience*, 5, 900–904.
Olson, M., & Sneed, N. (1995). Anxiety and therapeutic touch. *Issues in Mental Health Nursing*, 16, 97–108.
Owen, M. T., & Cox, M. J. (1997). Marital conflict and the development of infant-parent attachment relationships. *Journal of Family Psychology, 11*(2), 152–164.
Porges, S. W. (1998). Love: An emergent property of the mammalian autonomic nervous system. *Psychoneuroendocrinology, 23*, 837–861.
Radovanovic, H. (1993). Parental conflict and children's coping styles in litigating separated families: Relationships with children's adjustment. *Journal of Abnormal Child Psychology, 21*(6), 697–713.
Regan, P. C., Jerry, D., Narvaez, M., & Johnson, D. (1999). Public displays of affection among Asian and Latino heterosexual couples. *Psychological Reports, 84*, 1201–1202.
Remland, M. S., Jones, T. S., & Brinkman, H. (1995). Interpersonal distance, body orientation, and touch: Effects of culture, gender, and age. *Journal of Social Psychology, 135*(3), 281–297.
Shermer, M. (2004). A bounty of science. *Scientific American, 290*, 33.
Shuntich, R. J., Loh, D., & Katz, D. (1998). Some relationships among affection, aggression, and alcohol abuse in the family setting. *Perceptual and Motor Skills, 86*, 1051–1060.
Sollod, R. (1975). Behavioral and psychodynamic dimensions of the new sex therapy. *Journal of Sex & Marital Therapy, 1*, 335–340.
Spanier, G. (1976). Measuring dyadic adjustment: New scales for assessing the quality of marriage and similar dyads. *Journal of Marriage and the Family, 38*, 15–28.
Stock, S., Fastbom, J., Bjorkstrand, E., Ungerstedt, U., & Uvnas-Mober, K. (1990). Effects of oxytocin on in vivo release of insulin and glucagons studied by micro-dialysis in the rat pancreas and autoradiographic evidence for [3H] oxytocin binding sites within the islets of Langerhans. *Regulatory Peptides, 30*, 1–13.
Uvnas-Moberg, K. (2003). *The oxytocin factor: Tapping the hormone of calm, love, and healing*. Cambridge, MA: Merloyd Laurence/DuCapo Press.
Vandewater, E. A., & Lansford, J. E. (1998). Influences on family structure and parental conflict on children's well-being. *Family Relations, 47*, 323–330.
Van Horn, R., Arnone, A., Nesbitt, K., Desllets, L., Sears, T., Giffin, M., & Brudi, R. (1997). Physical distance and interpersonal characteristics in college students' romantic relationships. *Personal Relationships, 4*, 25–34.
Williams, J. R., Catania, K. C., & Carter, C. S. (1992). Development of partner preferences in female prairie voles (Microtus ochragaster): The role of social and sexual experience. *Hormones and Behavior, 26*, 339–349.
Winslow, J. T., Hastings, N., Carter, C. S., Harbaugh, C. R., & Insel, T. R. (1993). A role for central vasopressin in pair bonding in monogamous prairie voles. *Nature, 365*, 545–548.
Young, L. J. (2002). The neurobiology of social recognition, approach, and avoidance. *Biological Psychiatry, 51(1)*, 18–26.

19

Sex, Sexuality, and Sensuality

Chad L. Cross* and Gerald R. Weeks

There are few words that pique our interest more than *sex*, and few words of passion that are filled with more innate sensation and emotion than *sensuality*. Yet, amazingly, relatively little is known about the inherent benefits of sexuality and sensuality on our physical, emotional and mental well-being. Some scientists have, however, begun exploring the relationship of sex on longevity and sex as a form of exercise – the benefits of which are akin to any brief, but rigorous, physical activity. Further, more is being learned from the field of endocrinology and the effects of sex on hormonal functioning and from the field of neuropsychology and the influence of sex and sensuality on the brain.

It is our intention in this chapter is to review what little scientific information is known about sex, sexuality and sensuality and how these are related to physical and mental health. Interestingly, anecdotal evidence, case studies of participants, and stories make up the bulk of what is known about sex and its relationship to human health. However there is an inherent sense that sex, sexuality and sensuality play a key role in our lives and that therefore physical and mental health are enhanced by relationships that allow expression of the most intimate emotions and acts.

We begin the chapter with some basic definitions and background information, and then proceed through a topical discussion of the current state of knowledge of sex, sexuality and sensuality as it relates to human health. We also discuss areas of research that we believe may add to this small literature. It should be noted that our discussions of touch and of exercise are meant as a brief review of these topics in relation to sex and sensuality, as these topics are covered in depth in other chapters.

Definitions and Background

Many definitions of sex and sexuality have been operationalized in the literature; the variation stems from the type of science involved in investigating it. Sex, in a pure biological sense, is defined as a trait specific to an individual's

*Corresponding Author: Chad L. Cross, Ph.D., NCC, School of Public Health, University of Nevada Las Vegas, 4505 Maryland Parkway, M/S 3064, Las Vegas, NV 89154-3064, chad.cross@unlv.edu

genotypic expression that is used to categorize individuals (e.g., "male" or "female"; Crews, 2003). When used in a colloquial or conversational sense, however, most individuals immediately imagine sex as defined by an act such as coitus or other physical expression. Sexuality, on the other hand, is a more complex suite of characteristics inherent in an individual. These characteristics may be related to morphology, behavioral characteristics, or other physiological mechanisms that occur over an individual's lifespan (Crews, 1999, 2003). Human sexuality involves age, gender, cultural influences, family background and history, religious proclivities, and any myriad of other personal experiences. These factors shape individual attitudes concerning sexuality and sexual expression (Sandowski, 1989). The involvement of the senses (touch, smell, taste, etc.) in the expression of sexuality is defined as "sensuality."

Research on human sex and sexuality has a strikingly recent history. Much biological research and speculation on the roles of sex and sexual reproduction was mostly limited to investigations of plants and animals, with humans simply characterized as expressing sexuality with the same ideals and motivations as their phylogenetic cousins (e.g., Darwin's *Origin of Species*). It was not until midway through the twentieth century that Alfred Kinsey, a zoology professor, discovered that very little was available on human sexual behavior and began collecting data. This led to the formation of the Institute for Sex Research at Indiana University (eventually to become the Kinsey Institute). Kinsey's 1948 tome, *Sexual Behavior in the Human Male*, became a leading publication in the field of human sexuality. Today the Kinsey Institute is still the premier research organization on human sexuality, but interest in sex and sexuality has spread to many other disciplines, including psychology, medicine, neuroscience, and endocrinology.

Sex, Sexuality, and Health

Emotion and Behavior

Few emotions are felt as deeply as love and few behaviors are as deeply satisfying as sex (Kluger, 2004). The feelings and emotions that humans place on sex and sexual expression are much more than simply the physicality of the act. Indeed, sex functions multifariously "as a way to reduce boredom or anxiety, to provide reassurance of our self worth,. . ., provides comfort from loss or pain, and forges emotional bonds between individuals" (Brown & Ceniceros, 2001, p. 171).

The extent of emotional involvement in sexuality and the role that it plays in the lives of individuals and partners is a function of life experience and expectation. Those with strong moral and/or a strong sense of religiosity, for example, may perceive the act of sex and of sexual expression to be procreative, hence restricting sex to marriage and for the sole purpose of reproduction. Others, however, may view sex as a physical expressive act meant largely for pleasure and bonding (Brown & Ceniceros, 2001). Perhaps it is this disparity of views and the difficulty inherent in studying sexuality from these perspectives that led early researchers to focus on the biological response of humans before, during, and after sex (Masters & Johnson, 1970) as opposed to focusing on the psychological motivations of the act.

Sexuality and Sensuality

Intimacy, Commitment and Passion

Over 15 years have passed since Sternberg published his work on the triangular theory of love (1988), and the ideas of intimacy, commitment and passion became a staple of marital therapy. The importance of intimacy in relationships cannot be overstated, as becomes apparent when working with participants who seek counseling – the majority of whom report unfulfilling sex lives as problematic to their marriage. There is ample anecdotal evidence and some research (addressed below; Bachand & Caron, 2001) suggesting that happily married couples tend to have increased longevity and enhanced happiness and emotional well-being. What is less known is how strongly intimacy and sexuality are related. One would venture to suggest that a strong correlation must, by definition, exist. Further research in this area would greatly enhance our understanding of human health and intimate bonding.

Sternberg's model has been extraordinarily valuable in clinical practice. Weeks and Treat (2001), for example, have integrated the model into comprehensive couples treatment. When couples are asked to define intimacy, commitment and passion, it is not uncommon for sexuality and sensuality to be categorized as important in any, and all, three parts of the triangle. In one case example a couple that had been married for six years was struggling with making a decision about separation and divorce and hence, both reported mild depressive thinking and a sense of loss. After several sessions it became apparent that the husband defined intimacy as sex and that sex meant commitment. His wife favored sensual touching – cuddling, hugging, and kissing – which she defined as being the passion in the marriage; sex to her was important for defining intimacy, but was not necessary for maintaining a sense of commitment in the marriage. Integrating Sternberg's model using the ideas from Weeks and Treat (2001) became invaluable in helping the couple define, together, what sex and sexuality meant to them and how to add and maintain sensuality in their marriage. The end result was a couple with improved mental and emotional health functioning. As will become apparent in this chapter, intimacy, commitment, and passion throughout the lifespan is important for mental and emotional balance.

Pleasure and Happiness

Pleasure and happiness, and the behaviors associated with them, can be defined, listed, and discussed (Argyle, 1987). However, it is quite something else to define the state of "being" happy (Cleare & Wessely, 1997). Though the idea of happiness and pleasure may not seem to spark the interest of many researchers, potentially there are serious health considerations that may result if these issues are not addressed. This is precisely the philosophy of a valuable clinical model, the Practical Application of Intimate Relationship Skills (PAIRS) program, which recognizes the need for pleasure in the couple relationship, because happiness in relationships promotes both mental and physical well-being (DeMaria & Hannah, 2003).

An important component of the PAIRS program is a focus on Sexuality and Sensuality. Problems with happiness in relationships often surface in an obvious fashion when couples withdraw from one another physically and emotionally. Reconnecting sexually and sensuality, then, is of utmost importance to reestablishing emotional balance (Adams & Azevedo, 2003).

Physical intimacy is not necessarily the primary desire of regaining a positive relationship, however. Many couples are misinformed about physical intimacy, expectations, and the nature of sensuality in their relationships. This can lead to any number of relationship-related psychological issues owing to decreased intimacy, emotional separation, and depressive thinking (Weeks & Treat, 2001), which have been related to many health problems (e.g., Laumann, Paik, & Rosen, 1999).

The body of literature that supports the idea of a strong correlation between depression and marital distress continues to grow. In a recent review, it became apparent that the literature strongly supports the idea that depression and marital discord or distress are highly correlated (Gilliam & Cottone, 2005). Additional research has shown that marital therapy for depression has proven to be just as effective as individual therapy for depression that stems from marital problems.

Touch

No discussion on sexuality and sensuality would be complete without a consideration of touch. The most well-known work on healing touch dates back over 30 years ago (Krieger, 1975, 1979). It found its way into the nursing profession as a means of energy-based healing – though this type of touch may be more in the metaphysical, not physical, sense. The importance of touch, of course, is not new. In fact, ancient writings from many cultures (Egyptian, Greek, Asian) mention the healing powers of touch (Krieger, 1975; Stahlman, 2000). More recent, popular works also stress the significance of the skin and of touch in human development and functioning (Montagu, 1986).

Humans are sexual beings throughout their lifespan – and, as Sandowski (1989) points out, "everyone has sexual needs, including the need to be close, to touch and be touched" (p. 24). Not only is direct, physical touch an important aspect of sexuality, it is also the essence of overt sensual pleasure. The pleasure associated with touch can be seen in something as innocent as friend sharing a comforting embrace, a couple holding hands or walking arm-in-arm, or can be as intimate as cuddling and sexual foreplay. The point is that touch plays a key role in how we communicate with one another sensually and, at times, sexually. For some, touch and sensual pleasure may be the only option available – for instance when one is disabled or suffering from a debilitating disease. There is a growing literature that emphasizes the importance of sensuality and sexuality in special populations (Sandowski, 1989); this literature provides a sound argument that expressive sexuality is important for overall physical and mental well-being of those with disabilities. She also discusses the idea of expressing sexuality in ways that do not require the touch sensate. Many participants with spinal cord injuries, for example, may have limited senses of touch; however, the psychological nature of sexuality, even physicality, is not necessarily hampered or lessened by this disability. Indeed, "a paralyzed person is very much a sexual being, who still has a need for the closeness of a physical relationship, even in the absence of tactile sensation" (p. 88). This strengthens the notion that sexuality and sensuality play a particularly important role in the maintenance of psychological health, regardless of one's personal circumstances.

In therapy, women often complain that the man is too interested in sex and greatly distressed that he is not more interested in affection and sensuality.

From a clinical perspective, women are usually much more concerned and distressed about the lack of touch than sex. They relate touch to being loved. Men, on the other hand, tend to focus on sex and receive touch via sex. Many women we have treated are so upset over the lack of touch that they report feeling unloved, depressed, deprived, and some even consider it so essential that the prospect of divorce is raised.

Sex and Exercise

The physicality of sex immediately brings to mind the idea of sex as a specialized form of exercise; indeed, Butt (1990) refers to sex as one of the most basic forms of exercise and likens it to a sport with intense exertion. The benefits of exercise for improving physical and mental health are well known. In fact, one of the first interventions when treating depressed participants is simply to get them motivated to begin a basic exercise routine. One would imagine, then, that much research has been done linking the positive benefits of sex and its influence on human health. Unfortunately those who study exercise have not accepted the sexual response as physical exercise – a problem that Butt (1988) calls the "ostrich effect." One available study, however, does provide some controlled laboratory results relating coitus to measures of physical exercise and conditioning (e.g., heart rate and oxygen uptake; Bohlen, Held, Sanderson, & Patterson, 1984).

There is quite a literature relating exercise to mood (Butt, 1990), and presumably if exercise were studied more extensively as an exercise phenomenon, it would become clear that the physical activity during sex elevates mood and hence is associated with enhanced psychological well-being. Some interesting research is available to support such a claim, and comes from the biological sciences and neurophysiological literature. Some argue that those that are physically fit tend to be more extroverted than those who are not, and are more likely to have higher rates of sexual activity (Butt & Beiser, 1987). This argument is based on the contention that those who are extroverts tend to have intercourse more frequently than others and have overt sexual behaviors outside of coitus (Eysenck, Nias, & Cox, 1982). There may be some validity to this argument given that a recent poll of over 1000 Americans suggests that over 40% of men and over one-third of women state that exercise is very important to them because it allows them to have better sex lives (Miranda & Park, 2005).

Sex and Aging

There is a well-documented relationship between sex and age – namely that sexual functioning declines with age regardless of gender (Brown & Ceniceros, 2001; Renshaw, 1996). A large body of literature documents declining fertility and fecundity in both men and women as age increases (Kidd et al., 2001; Menken et al., 1986; Ng et al., 2004; Schwartz & Mayaux, 1982). This is not necessarily to be taken negatively, however. Many older adults will remain sexually active well into elderly years, with over 80% of married couples, three-quarters of single men, and half of single women being sexually active in their seventies (Brown & Ceniceros, 2001). Obviously the majority of elderly adults maintain a healthy sex life well into advanced age, the effects of which have been found to be inversely related to mortality

(Palrnore, 1982). The likelihood of sexual dysfunction, particularly in aging men, may be an important consideration (discussed below).

Human longevity has also been challenged by evolutionary theorists as coming with a high cost; namely infertility or impaired reproductive success (Westendorp & Kirkwood, 1998). As above, this would seem to suggest that sexual expression and aging are inversely correlated and that the energy demands of reproduction are deleterious to overall health. Though there may be some support for this argument, Gavrilova, Gavrilov, Semyonova and Evdokushkina (2004) have countered the work of Westendorp and Kirkwood (1998) and have found no such relationship.

To further the support of arguments for the independence of human longevity and reproductive output, the idea of living in a marital relationship where sexuality and sensuality are expressed has been shown to enhance longevity, particularly for men married to younger women (Foster, Klinger-Vartabedian, & Wispe, 1984). This supports the claim that being in intimate relationships may lead to increased vitality and provide for better physical and emotional health. Apparently, at least for humans, evolution has favored those with a penchant for maintaining intimate relationships, regardless of any possible reduction in longevity owing to reproductive success.

As a case example, an older woman presented to therapy because her sex drive was much higher than that of her husband. For years they had both lacked sexual interest. She had developed MS, and for a period of a couple of years had withdrawn from life and stopped being active. She reported that her level of desire had suddenly increased just after starting physical therapy. Of course, the physical therapy alone may not be the only contributing factor since she had to be ready to psychologically accept the therapy and she was considering the fact that she was now the healthiest that she would probably be and did not want to miss out on having some sex life before her MS became worse.

Clinical experience has show us that the elderly, even those in homes, continue to have a desire for sex and physical contact in spite of the fact that it has nothing to do with reproduction or bonding for purposes of marriage. Their activity runs counter to the notion that the elderly have or should not have any interest in sex. Obviously, something is driving this need for a sexual connection.

Sex and Mortality

There are several longitudinal studies that have suggested a link between sexual activity and death, in particular noting the inverse relationship between sexual activity and mortality (Drory, 2002; Palnrore, 1982; Smith, Frankel, & Yarnell, 1997). Further the data indicate that frequency of intercourse for men, and quality of intercourse for women, are the indicative variables of longevity – although findings can be confounded by smoking status and general health status at the time of interview (Smith et al., 1997). Also supportive of this claim is that cessation of sexual activities prior to the age of 70 has been linked with an increased risk of mortality (Persson, 1981; Smith et al., 1997). Knoll (1997) provides an interesting neurobiological look at sexual performance and longevity, suggesting that catecholamines are important in this process.

Sexual activity, however, has been linked with adverse health effects as well, such as an increased risk of myocardial infarction and cardiac arrhythmia

(Drory, 2002). It should be noted, however, that this increased risk is small, and that those individuals that lead a healthy lifestyle have the least health risk. Further, mean peak heart rates during intercourse are not significantly different from normal, daily activities and hence the risk of cardiac problems should be minimal (Drory, Fisman, Shapira, & Pines, 1996; Drory, Shapira, Fisman, & Pines, 1995).

Sex and Health

An important consideration in terms of mental and physical health is the prevalence, cause, and etiology of sexual dysfunction. Most research in this area has been done on erectile dysfunction (ED) and the aging male (Feldman, Goldstein, Hatzichristou, Krane, & McKinlay, 1994; Laumann et al., 1999). Weeks and Gambescia (2000) discuss psychological impacts and treatment considerations of ED, providing a thorough coverage of the topic. Of particular importance to the issue of sex and physical health, ED can be caused by emotional problems, high stress levels, and/or cardiovascular problems (Drory, 2002; Laumann et al., 1999). If this is the case, the increased risk of health problems associated with sex may be dramatic (Drory, 2002), just as overt physical exercise can be dangerous for those predisposed to cardiovascular disease. In this sense sex and health are linked in an important way – namely sexual health and mental/physical health require, and lead to, increased happiness, longevity, and well-being (Cleare & Wessely, 1997).

The inextricable nature of this general health fact make it extraordinarily important that health practitioners take a proactive stance in discussing sexual health with their participants (Nusbaum & Hamilton, 2002). Unfortunately, experience has shown us that the vast majority of clinicians we supervise are poorly trained in sexuality and sex therapy and do not make the issue a part of therapy. In some cases, the participant or couple clearly wants to talk about sex, and the therapist may provide no information, misinformation, avoid the topic, or skim over it as if the issue has been covered.

Neurochemistry and Neurobiology

Neurosciences are an exciting field of investigation and, with the development of brain-scanning technology, scientists are learning much about how certain thoughts, behaviors, and actions are processed, catalogued, and recalled. In particular, research investigating the chemistry of love and lust and what makes sexually compatible partners find one another has been investigated since the early 1980s (e.g., Liebowitz, 1983). The brain, of course, is very complex, and pin-pointing areas of brain activity in the process of love and love-making is not a straightforward task. Two interesting popular review articles (Fisher, 2004; Lemonick, 2004) explore these topics, but certainly there is much more to be learned. Further investigations into brain neurochemistry would be interesting in that such research may shed light on why "being in love" or why physical acts of sex are reported to enhance mood, improve mental well-being, and result in an overall improvement in physical health.

As clinicians, we often note that when the couple's sexual relationship begins to return, the couple seems more relaxed, emotionally connected, and happier. It is such a noticeable effect that during a course of sex therapy the couple will present nonverbally in such a way that it is clear they are feeling better. When the clinician points out that they are looking better or happier, they will then confirm that they had a good week sexually. This phenomenon has been noted in many of the couples we have treated where sex was the issue at hand.

Conclusion

A full consideration of sex, sexuality and sensuality brings one immediately to the conclusion that there is something interesting, important and controversial to be found in terms of conceptually linking physical and mental health to human sexuality. We have provided some evidence of a correlative relationship, but certainly there is nothing definitive that currently exists in the literature. Speculation and observation are at the heart of all good scientific inquiry, and these are exactly what we are left with after reviewing the literature on this topic.

In conversations with many researchers on the topic of sex and human health, there appears to be a strong sense that those with a fulfilling sex life and those that have an understanding of the roles that sexuality and sensuality play in their lives simply are happier and more fulfilled – and hence, ultimately healthier individuals. Frustratingly, however, there seems to be no smoking gun and the literature is sparse at best. With the current advances in the possibilities for scientific investigation, the future of research in this area seems ripe. The ultimate goal, of course, is to find a way to tie all of the apparently disparate pieces of information together and to find a definitive link between sexuality – and all of its expressions – and emotional, physical, and mental health.

References

Adams, D., & Azevedo, D. (2003). Sensuality and Sexuality. In DeMaria R., & Mo T. Hannah (Eds.), *Building intimate relationships: Bridging treatment, education, and enrichment through the PAIRS program* (pp. 149–162). New York, NY: Brunner-Routledge.

Argyle, M. (1987). *The psychology of love*. London, England: Methuen.

Bachand, L., & Caron, S. (2001). Ties that bind: A qualitative study of happy long-term marriages. *Contemporary Family Therapy, 23*, 105–121.

Bohlen, J., Held, J., Sanderson, M., & Patterson, R. (1984). Heart rate, rate-pressure produce, and oxygen uptake during four sexual activities. *Archives Internal Medicine, 144*, 1745–1748.

Brown, G., & Ceniceros, S. (2001). Human sexuality in health and disease. In Wedding D. (Ed.), *Behavior & medicine* (pp. 171–183). Seattle, WA: Hogrefe & Huber.

Butt, D. (1988). Physical activity, well-being and sexual behavior in adulthood: The ostrich effect. *Canadian Journal of Sport Science, 13*, 48–49.

Butt, D. (1990). The sexual response as exercise: A brief review and theoretical proposal. *Sports Medicine, 9*, 330–343.

Butt, D., & Beiser, M. (1987). Successful aging: A theme for international psychology. *Psychology and Aging, 2*, 87–94.

Cleare, A., & Wessely, S. (1997). Just what the doctor ordered – more alcohol and sex (editorial). *British Medical Journal, 315*, 1637–1638.

Crews, D. (1999). Sexuality: The environmental organization of phenotypic plasticity. In K. Wallen and J. Schneider (Eds.), *Reproduction in Context*. Cambridge, MA: M.I.T. Press.
Crews, D. (2003). Sex determination: Where environment and genetic meet. *Evolution & Development, 5*, 50–55.
DeMaria, R., & Hannah, Mo T. (2003). *Building intimate relationships: Bridging treatment, education, and enrichment through the PAIRS program*. New York, NY: Brunner-Routledge.
Drory, Y. (2002). Sexual activity and cardiovascular risk. *European Heart Journal Supplements, 4*, H13–H18.
Drory, Y., Fisman, E., Shapira, Y., & Pines, A. (1996). Ventricular arrhythmias during sexual activity in patients with coronary artery disease. *Chest, 109*, 922–924.
Drory, Y., Shapira, Y., Fisman, E., & Pines, A. (1995). Myocardial ischemia during sexual activity in patients with coronary artery disease. *American Journal of Cardiology, 75*, 835–837.
Eysenck, H., Nias, D., & Cox, D. (1982). Sport and personality. *Advances in Behavioral Research and Therapy, 4*, 1–56.
Feldman, H., Goldstein, I., Hatzichristou, D., Krane, R., & McKinlay, J. (1994). Impotence and it medical and psychosocial correlates: Results of the Massachusetts Male Aging Study. *Journal of Urology, 151*, 54–61.
Fisher, H. (2004). Your brain in love. *Time Archive*, January 19, 2004. Downloaded May 26, 2005 from http://www.time.com/time/archive.
Foster, D., Klinger-Vartabedian, L., & Wispe, L. (1984). Male longevity and age differences between spouses. *Journal of Gerontology, 39*, 117–120.
Gavrilova, N., Gavrilov, L., Semyonova, V., & Evdokushkina, G. (2004). Does exceptional human longevity come with a high cost of infertility?: Testing the evolutionary theories of aging. *Annals of the New York Academy of Sciences, 1019*, 513–517.
Gilliam, C., & Cottone, R. (2005). Couple or individual therapy for the treatment of depression? An update of the empirical literature. *American Journal of Family Therapy, 33*, 265–272.
Kidd, S. A. (2001). Effects of male age on semen quality and fertility: A review of the literature. *Fertility and Sterility, 75*, 237–248.
Kluger, J. (2004). The power of love. *Time Archive*, January 19, 2004. Downloaded May 26, 2005 from http://www.time.com/time/archive.
Knoll, J. (1997). Sexual performance and longevity. *Experimental Gerontology, 32*, 539–552.
Krieger, D. (1975). Therapeutic touch: The imprimatur of nursing. *American Journal of Nursing, 75*, 784–787.
Krieger, D. (1979). *The therapeutic touch: How to use your hands to help or to heal*. Englewood Cliffs, NJ: Prentice-Hall.
Laumann, E., Paik, A., & Rosen, R. (1999). Sexual dysfunction in the United States: Prevalence and predictors. *Journal of the American Medical Association, 281*, 537–544.
Lemonick, M. (2004). The chemistry of desire. *Time Archive*, 19 January 2004. Downloaded 26 May 2005 from http://www.time.com/time/archive.
Liebowitz, M. (1983). *The chemistry of love*. Boston, MA: Little, Brown & Co.
Masters, W., & Johnson, V. (1970). *Human sexual inadequacy*. New York, NY: Little & Brown.
Menken, J., Trussell, J., & Larsen, U. (1986). Age and infertility. *Science, 233*, 1389–1394.
Mirnda, C. A., & Park, A. (2005). Getting fit: The shape of the nation. *Time*, June 6, 48–50.
Montagu, A. (1986). *Touching: The human significance of the skin*. New York, NY: Harper Paperbacks.

Ng, K., Donat, R., Chan, L., Lalak, A., Di Pierro, I., & Handelsman, D. (2004). Sperm output of older men. *Human Reproduction, 19*, 1811–1815.

Nusbaum, M., & Hamilton, C. (2002). The proactive sexual health history. *American Family Physician, 66*, 1705–1712.

Palrnore, E. (1982). Predictors of the longevity difference: A 25-year follow-up. *Gerontologist, 6*, 513–518.

Persson, G. (1981). Five-year mortality in a 70-year-old urban population in relation to psychiatric diagnosis, personality, sexuality and early parental death. *Acta Psychiatric Scandanavia, 64*, 244–253.

Renshaw, D. (1996). Sexuality and aging. In J. Sadavoy, L. Lazarus, L. Jarvik, & G. Grossberg (Eds.), *Comprehensive Review of Geriatric Psychiatry-II* (pp. 713–730). Washington, DC: American Psychiatric Press.

Sandowski, C. (1989). *Sexual concerns when illness or disability strikes.* Springfield, IL: Charles C. Thomas.

Schwartz, D., & Mayaux, M. J. (1982). Female fecundity as a function of age: Results of artificial insemination in 2193 nulliparous women with a zoospermic husbands. Federation CECOS. *New England Journal of Medicine, 306*, 404–406.

Smith, G., Frankel, S., & Yarnell, J. (1997). Sex and death: Are they related? Finding from the Caerphilly cohort study. *British Medical Journal*, 1641–1644.

Stahlman, J. (2000). A brief history of therapeutic touch. In B. Scheiber, & C. Selby (Eds.), *Therapeutic touch* (pp. 21–51). Amherst, NY: Prometheus Books.

Sternberg, R. (1988). *The triangle of love: Intimacy, passion, commitment.* Philadelphia, PA: Basic Books.

Weeks, G., & Gambescia, N. (2000). *Erectile dysfunction: Integrating couple therapy, sex therapy, and medical treatment.* New York, NY: W. W. Norton & Company.

Weeks, G., & Treat, S. (2001). *Couples in treatment* (2nd ed.). New York, NY: Brunner-Routledge.

Westendorp, R., & Kirkwood, T. (1998). Human longevity at the cost of reproductive success. *Nature, 396*, 743–746.

20

Intimacy and Fear of Intimacy

Anita L. Vangelisti and Gary Beck

Intimacy is a phenomenon that is both sought-after and feared. People often spend a great deal of time and effort pursuing intimacy – they frequent singles bars, join church groups, respond to personal ads, peruse online dating services, and get their friends to introduce them to potential partners. Although these, and other, related activities can be precursors to close, intimate relationships, they also can be associated with fear and anxiety. Those seeking intimate partners may worry about whether they will succeed, whether they are using the right techniques, and whether, if they do find a partner, they ultimately will be happy. For many, difficult childhood experiences and failed adult relationships reinforce their fear that intimacy is illusive or that it is inevitably fraught with pain and disappointment. Yet research suggests that, at least in the U.S., intimacy has become more important to people over time (Veroff, Douvan, & Kulka, 1981). Indeed, close, supportive relationships are associated with both greater physical and mental well-being (Cohen & Syme, 1985).

In spite of the efforts individuals expend seeking out intimacy and the importance of intimacy to people's physical and psychological health, researchers still struggle with how to define the concept. Most agree that intimacy involves feelings of closeness, affection, and mutual understanding (see Perlman & Fehr, 1987) but many disagree about the specific ways that intimacy should be conceptualized. Some view it as a capacity that is possessed to varying degrees by different individuals; others regard it as a form of social interaction. Some see it as a motivation that influences people's behavior; others consider it to be a quality of interpersonal relationships. The purpose of the current chapter is to synthesize existing literature on intimacy and, in doing so, to highlight the utility of viewing intimacy as a dyadic process – a process that is enacted in the context of interpersonal relationships and influenced by individual, interactional, and relational variables. The chapter begins with a description of the various ways that intimacy has been conceptualized in the research literature. In the first two sections, common components of these conceptualizations are noted and models that have been put forth treating intimacy as an interpersonal process are discussed. The literature reviewed in these first sections serves as the basis for the next portion of the chapter which points to the need for researchers, theorists, and practitioners to rethink current, relatively individualistic conceptions of intimacy and to ask questions that reflect the interactive, processual nature of the phenomenon. Then, a selective review of research is provided which demonstrates the importance of intimacy to individuals' well-being. Finally, a brief discussion of some of the techniques that couples might employ to increase relational intimacy is offered.

How has Intimacy been Conceptualized?

Research suggests that people who have close, intimate relationships experience greater physical and psychological well-being than do those who lack them (Reis, 1984). Although this general pattern of findings has been replicated using different methods and samples, it is important to acknowledge that the ways scholars have conceptualized intimacy can vary widely from study to study. Indeed, Laurenceau and Kleinman (2006) argue that intimacy has been examined on three different levels of analysis. More specifically, these researchers note that intimacy has been conceptualized: (a) at the individual level, as a quality of persons; (b) at the interactional level, as a quality of interactions between persons; and (c) at the relational level, as a quality of ongoing associations between persons.

Individual Level

At the level of the individual, intimacy typically is viewed in terms of variations in the capacity of people to develop and maintain close relationships. Researchers have examined a number of individual differences that reflect this capacity. Perhaps one of the most commonly studied of these is attachment. Attachment theory suggests that early interactions between infants and their caregivers serve as a context for the development of beliefs and expectations about the responsiveness of others in relation to the self (Bowlby, 1969, 1973). Although these beliefs and expectations – also termed *inner working models* – can and do change over time, they are relatively stable and have influenced people's close relationships in adulthood (Pietromonaco, Laurenceau, & Feldman Barrett, 2002). Indeed, people with secure attachment orientations have a greater tendency to engage in behaviors associated with intimacy than do people with avoidant attachment orientations. For instance, those who are secure engage in more self-disclosure (Kobak & Hazan, 1991; Mikulincer & Nachshon, 1991) and are more likely to offer and accept social support (Collins & Feeney, 2000; Simpson, Rholes, & Nelligan, 1992) than are those who are avoidant. Secure people also tend to report higher needs for closeness and lower needs for distance (Feeney, 1999), and are more likely to report higher levels of intimacy and positive emotion in their daily interactions (Tidwell, Reis, & Shaver, 1996) than are their avoidant counterparts.

Another individual difference that affects people's capacity to develop and maintain close relationships is the fear of intimacy (Descutner & Thelen, 1991). Firestone and Catlett (1999) suggest that the fear of intimacy is rooted in negative attitudes toward the self and others that develop early in life. Like the inner working models advanced by attachment theorists, these negative attitudes comprise a part of people's identity, are somewhat resistant to change, and influence people's intimate relationships. For instance, individuals who fear intimacy have a restricted capacity to form and maintain close ties with others (Firestone & Firestone, 2004). There also may be a curvilinear association between individuals' fear of intimacy and their desire for closeness. More specifically, Mashek and Sherman (2004) found that people who want less closeness and those who want more closeness in their relationships with others are more fearful of intimacy than are those who are relatively satisfied with the degree of closeness they have in their relationships. In explaining their findings, the researchers note the possibility that some who fear intimacy may desire less closeness because they associate intimacy with anxiety, whereas others who fear intimacy may desire more closeness, but may lack the social skills and confidence to seek out and develop intimate relationships.

Closely related to the fear of intimacy is another concept that was initially examined by Pilkington and Richardson (1988): risk in intimacy. Risk in intimacy involves people's sensitivity to the hazards or dangers associated with close, intimate relationships. In developing a measure of this concept, Pilkington and Richardson found that individuals' tendency to perceive risk in intimacy was associated with having fewer close friends and less trust in others. Those who scored high on the risk in intimacy scale also were relatively unlikely to be involved in romantic relationships, had less assertiveness in dating, and were more likely to endorse attitudes toward love that could be construed as hesitant. Pilkington and Woods (1999) later used response times and ratings of hypothetical relationship events to evaluate the accessibility of risk in intimacy schemas. Their studies showed that, in many cases, risk in intimacy schemas were more accessible to those who scored high on the risk in intimacy scale than those who scored low. For instance, people with high risk in intimacy scores tended to rate relationship events as more dangerous and tended to believe that risky relationship events were more likely to occur than did those with low scores. The findings associated with response times were mixed, however, those who scored high on risk in intimacy did report that negative outcomes were more likely in ambiguous relationship situations than did those who scored low.

Although all of the aforementioned variables have been conceived as relatively stable individual differences, researchers also have argued that variables associated with the propensity to form and maintain intimate relationships may be less stable. A case in point is the argument put forth by Mashek and her colleagues concerning the desire for less closeness. Mashek and Sherman (2004) suggest that

> unlike individual difference variables (e.g., attachment orientation), the desire for less closeness seems to be a reaction to a specific relationship (vs. an attribute characterizing a person's perception of all of her or his relationships) and seems to be bounded by time (that is, I might desire less closeness with my partner today, but desire more closeness with her two weeks from now). (p. 349)

In describing this variable, Mashek and Sherman note that the desire for less closeness involves feeling that another person's influence over the self is too strong or inappropriate. The desire for less closeness, thus, is likely to occur when individuals sense a threat to their personal control or their personal identity. In both of these situations, people feel a need to reduce the degree to which they are influenced by their relational partner and anticipate that they can do this by being less close to him or her. Because the desire for less closeness has only recently been formally conceived and measured, research examining its causes and consequences is limited. As more studies are conducted, this variable may offer a useful way to explain some of the fluctuations in intimacy that occur in relationships over time.

Interactional Level

Although variables examined at the level of the individual can serve as important predictors of the behaviors that people engage in as they establish and maintain intimate relationships, they do not offer much information about the behaviors themselves. Examining intimacy at the level of the interaction can provide such information. At the interactional level, intimacy is conceptualized in terms of behaviors that have a tendency to encourage or create intimate relationships. Three of the behaviors most widely acknowledged for their contributions to intimacy are: self-disclosure, responsiveness, and perceived partner responsiveness.

Self-disclosure has long been regarded by researchers as a means for individuals to develop intimate relationships (Jourard, 1964). Indeed, one of the first theories of relationship development – social penetration theory – placed self-disclosure at center stage (Altman & Taylor, 1973). According to Altman and Taylor, relationships become more intimate as partners increase the breadth and depth of their disclosures to one another. More specifically, as the breadth (the number of topics disclosed) and depth (the degree to which the topics are personally relevant) of disclosures increase, the relationship between interacting partners is likely to become more intimate.

Although self-disclosure has been defined in a number of different ways (Derlega, Metts, Petronio, & Margulis, 1993; Perlman & Fehr, 1987; Rosenfeld, 2000), most researchers agree that it involves interactions in which one person willingly divulges personally relevant information to another (Greene, Derlega, & Mathews, 2006). Thus conceived, self-disclosure emphasizes the depth of information given over the breadth of topics discussed. The disclosure of personally relevant information can be either verbal or nonverbal, but its potential to create feelings of intimacy is defined more in terms of quality (personal relevance) than quantity (number of topics). In line with this perspective, researchers and theorists generally regard the disclosure of feelings as more integral to the development of intimacy than the disclosure of facts. For example, in marriage, the tendency of spouses to communicate feelings is more closely associated with relational satisfaction than is their tendency to communicate facts (Fitzpatrick, 1986).

Of course, one person disclosing personally relevant information to another does not comprise an intimate relationship. Reciprocal disclosures are thought to be particularly important to the development of intimacy early in relationships. If one person's disclosures are not reciprocated by the other (or if they are not perceived as such), the chance of an intimate relationship developing is relatively low. There is some evidence that as relationships become more established, the importance of reciprocal disclosures seems to decline (Morton, 1978). One explanation for this pattern of findings is that partners in established relationships perceive a more extended time period within which they can reciprocate each other's disclosure (Knapp, 1984); another is that many partners in established relationships develop a communal orientation toward their relationships (Clark & Mills, 1979) and, as a consequence, feel less of a need to immediately reciprocate disclosures.

Although the association between self-disclosure and intimacy is relatively clear, at least two qualifications are in order. First, it is important to note that even though self-disclosure often is closely associated with the development of intimacy, the two concepts are distinct (Waring & Chelune, 1983). Both theoretical (Reis & Shaver, 1988) and empirical (Laurenceau, Feldman Barrett, & Peitromonaco, 1998) work support the claim that self-disclosure is an integral component of intimacy, but that intimacy involves more than disclosure. Second, a number of researchers have implicitly cautioned against assuming that the association between self-disclosure and intimacy is a positive, linear one. Gilbert (1976) and Cozby (1973) both argue that the association between disclosure and satisfaction may be curvilinear, such that extremely high levels of self-disclosure may reduce satisfaction. The same may be true for the relationship between self-disclosure and intimacy. Too much disclosure or disclosures that are repeated over and over again may be negatively associated with intimacy. These researchers and others further suggest that the degree to which disclosure is viewed as appropriate is important. They note that disclosure that is inappropriate or ill-timed may discourage, rather than encourage, intimacy. Similarly, disclosure that is elicited under pressure (e.g., when someone feels compelled to disclose, but does not want to do so) may be associated with less intimacy.

Another key component of intimate interactions is *responsiveness*. Responsive behaviors demonstrate that a disclosure made by one individual is met by the other with attentiveness, understanding, and validation (Prager & Roberts, 2004; Reis & Patrick, 1996). Miller and Berg (1984) suggest, more specifically, that responsiveness involves the tendency of one person to address the other's previous behaviors, communication, needs, or wishes. These researchers also distinguish between conversational responsiveness and relational responsiveness. They note that the former involves behaviors that indicate interest in, and understanding of, another's communication; whereas the latter involves behaviors that show concern for another's outcomes or needs. Although these two types of responsiveness are distinct, both "are means through which one person indicates understanding of another and concern with him or her" (Berg, 1987, p. 103).

In the absence of responsiveness, the link between self-disclosure and intimacy becomes quite tentative. In fact, self-disclosure that is not met with responsiveness may be associated with decreased intimacy. When one person reveals personal information to another, he or she is placed in a position of vulnerability (Derlega et al., 1993). If that vulnerability is not met by the other with concern and validation, the lack of concern and lack of validation may be viewed as an indication that the other is an unfit candidate for intimate interaction. Indeed, the demand for responsiveness may be so strong that, in certain situations, people may feign responsiveness in order to present themselves as fit conversational or relational partners. The influence of such feigned responsiveness on intimacy is quite complex. Partners may be able to create a temporary illusion of intimacy by feigning responsiveness, but maintaining that illusion over time is likely another matter.

Responsiveness, as such, not only validates prior disclosures, it encourages future ones. For example, responsiveness is positively associated with communication and interpersonal attraction (Davis, 1982). It also facilitates reciprocity in disclosure, liking, and closeness (Berg & Archer, 1982).

The association between responsiveness and disclosure has been highlighted by studies examining variables associated with the elicitation of disclosure. For instance, Miller, Berg, and Archer (1983) developed a measure, called the Opener Scale, to assess the degree to which people are able to elicit disclosure from others. They found that people who were "high openers" were more well-liked than others and suggested this may be the case because high openers tend to be relatively responsive. Purvis, Dabbs, and Hopper (1984) confirmed that there are differences in the responsive behavior of high and "low openers." They examined the nonverbal behavior of high and low openers during conversation and found that high openers smiled more, gazed at each other more, used more back channels, and nodded their heads more than did low openers.

Of course, if responsiveness is to be effective in creating intimacy, it must be perceived. Reis and Shaver (1988) suggest that while responsive behaviors can be objectively described, the subjective interpretation of behaviors as responsive can matter more than their objective descriptions. Reis, Clark, and Holmes (2004) elaborate on the centrality of perceived responsiveness to intimacy. These researchers define *perceived partner responsiveness to the self* "as a process by which individuals come to believe that relationship partners both attend to and react supportively to central, core defining features of the self" (p. 203). They argue that perceived partner responsiveness, like responsiveness, contributes significantly to the formation and maintenance of intimate relationships.

Relational Level

Although most researchers and theorists agree that intimate interactions are key to the formation and maintenance of intimate relationships, many also suggest that there are important distinctions to be made in conceptualizing intimacy at the level of the interaction and intimacy at the level of the relationship. Prager (1995) is one of a number of scholars who has discussed the differences between interactional and relational intimacy. She suggests that intimate interactions are essential to intimate relationships, but argues that the two are distinct in that intimate relationships are not confined to specific interactions and/or behaviors. Intimate relationships, thus conceived, are influenced by intimate interactions, but they also are affected by other variables.

There are several different perspectives on which variables are essential to intimate relationships. For instance, Prager and Roberts (2004) suggest that intimate relationships come into being through one person's accumulation of shared knowledge or understanding of the other. They note, more specifically, that intimate relationships are "characterized by mutual, accumulated, shared personal knowledge" (p. 46). This conception of relational intimacy fits nicely with the work of Planalp and Benson (1992; Planalp, 1993) which indicated that mutual knowledge is a primary factor distinguishing the conversations of acquaintances and friends. Assuming that, on average, friends' relationships are more intimate than those of acquaintances, the findings of Planalp and Benson suggest that mutual knowledge may be a particularly important determinant of intimacy.

Other definitions of relational intimacy focus more on shared experiences than shared knowledge. For instance, Schaefer and Olson (1981) note that an intimate relationship "is generally one in which an individual shares intimate experiences in several areas, and there is the expectation that the experiences and relationship will persist over time" (p. 50). Based on this definition, they identified five different types of intimacy: emotional, social, sexual, intellectual, and recreational.

Waring and his colleagues emphasize particular qualities or characteristics of relationships in their definition of relational intimacy (Waring, 1984; Waring, McElrath, Lefcoe, & Weisz, 1981; Waring & Reddon, 1983). They suggest that intimacy can be defined in terms of eight different components. These include: affection, cohesion, conflict resolution, compatibility, expressiveness, sexuality, autonomy, and identity. A number of other measures assessing intimacy similarly tap broad dimensions of relationships such as romantic love, supportiveness, ease of communication (Tesch, 1985), and trust (Guerney, 1977).

Clearly, the variables central to intimate relationships are still under discussion. The difficulties associated with establishing a coherent definition of relational intimacy – one that accounts for the differences that individuals, couples, and members of particular social groups bring to their relationships – are considerable. Addressing the ways in which these differences unfold over time complicates matters further. Challenges such as these have encouraged a number of scholars to formulate process models of intimacy.

Bringing it all Together: Process Models

Although research focused on each of the aforementioned levels of analysis provides useful information about intimacy and intimate relationships, it also offers a picture of intimacy that is somewhat fragmented. Intimacy is conceived as a capacity possessed to varying degrees by individuals, as behaviors that encourage or discourage a particular relational state, or as a quality of interpersonal relationships. Research integrating these various levels of analysis and examining the possible associations between them is scarce. In part as a response to the fragmented nature of this literature, several scholars have advocated conceiving of intimacy as an interpersonal process (e.g., Chelune, Robinson, & Kommor, 1984; Duck & Sants, 1983; Hatfield, 1984; Prager, 1995; Schaefer & Olson, 1981) – dynamic, interactive, and influenced by the characteristics that individuals bring to it, the way partners communicate, and the unique quality of partners' relationships.

Some of the early efforts to conceptualize intimacy as a process did so in terms of equilibrium models. These models suggest that there are optimal levels of intimacy and that individuals strive to maintain a balance between achieving enough intimacy and avoiding too much of it. For instance, Argyle and Dean (1965) claim that intimacy involves both the nonverbal behaviors that people engage in as well as the topics they discuss. These scholars argue that if there is a change in one of these two components of intimacy, the other will change in the opposite direction. As such, individuals maintain equilibrium in the degree of intimacy that they experience. Patterson (1976, also see 1984) elaborated on Argyle and Dean's model by noting that people label their affective reactions to increases in intimacy. Thus when one partner increases eye contact or reveals something of a personal nature, the other labels his or her affective response to this change in equilibrium. If the affective response is labeled by the other as negative, he or she will reduce intimacy by engaging in compensatory behavior. If the response is viewed as positive, he or she will establish a new (higher) level of intimacy by reciprocating the intimate behavior.

Another well-known effort to conceptualize intimacy as a process is a model put forth by Reis and Shaver (1988; also see Reis & Patrick, 1996). Reis and Shaver define intimacy as "an interpersonal process that involves communication of personal feelings and information to another person who responds warmly and sympathetically" (p. 375). The integrative model of intimacy proposed by these researchers has several components: self-disclosure, partner responsiveness, reaction to partner responsiveness, and both partners' motives, needs, goals, and fears. According to Reis and Shaver, the process of intimacy begins when one individual reveals personal information to another. This disclosure may be either verbal or nonverbal and it may be intentional or unintentional. Next, the recipient of the disclosure interprets the information that he or she has received and responds in some way. The recipient's interpretation and response are influenced by his or her own motives, needs, goals, and fears. Reis and Shaver argue that intimacy only occurs when the response put forth by the recipient is perceived by the individual who originally engaged in disclosure as attentive and caring. The final step in the process, thus, involves the discloser's interpretation of, and response to, the recipient's reaction – both of which are influenced by the discloser's motives, needs, goals, and fears.

Prager and Roberts (2004) propose a model of intimate interactions that has a number of similarities to the one put forth by Reis and Shaver (1988). Prager and Roberts suggest that intimate interactions are characterized by self-revealing behavior, positive involvement with the other, and shared understandings. They note that self-revealing behavior involves the disclosure of personal, private information and that it can be either verbal or nonverbal. They also argue that intimate interactions require individuals to be positively involved with each other. According to these researchers, positive involvement is defined both by attending to the interaction and by having a positive regard for the other that is conveyed through verbal and/or nonverbal communication. The final component of this model is shared understanding. Prager and Roberts suggest that shared understanding occurs when both partners know or understand each other's inner experiences. They argue that shared understanding extends beyond the boundaries of single interactions and makes subsequent interactions more intimate than they would be otherwise. According to these researchers, it is the frequency of intimate interactions and the accuracy of accumulated shared understanding that distinguishes intimate from nonintimate relationships.

A theoretical model proposed by Cusinato and L'Abate (1994) offers yet another way to understand fluctuations in intimacy. This model includes both sharing and responsiveness – components that are viewed as central to intimacy – but it also suggests that there are prerequisites to intimacy and specifies the issues that should be the focus of individuals' sharing and responsive behaviors. More particularly, Cusinato and L'Abate argue that there are three prerequisites for intimacy. They claim that partners must be committed to the importance of the relationship; that they must see themselves as having equally important, but complementary functions; and that they must demonstrate reciprocity and mutuality in dealing with each other. These three requirements serve as the basis for six processes that, according to Cusinato and L'Abate, create a "positive, upward spiral of growth in the relationship" (p. 36). The first process involves the communication of personal values. Partners who convey their personal beliefs and opinions to each other are relatively likely to develop an intimate relationship. The second process focuses on respect for each other's personal feelings. According to Cusinato and L'Abate, individuals who have a positive regard for the personal feelings of their partner are more likely than others to develop intimacy. Acceptance of each other's personal limitations is the third process. By acknowledging and accepting what their partner cannot do, people create an atmosphere of respect that allows intimacy to grow. The fourth process involves the affirmation of both partner's potentialities. In addition to accepting each other's limitations, Cusinato and L'Abate suggest that intimate partners support each other's hopes, dreams, and goals. Sharing of hurts is the fifth process. When they share their hurt feelings, people make themselves vulnerable. If a partner responds to this vulnerability with concern, the potential for intimacy increases. The sixth and final process is the forgiveness of errors. Cusinato and L'Abate note that people who are able to forgive their partner for his or her mistakes create the foundation for a more intimate relationship.

Although process models such as those put forth by Argyle and Dean (1965), Patterson (1976), Reis and Shaver (1988), Prager and Roberts (2004), and Cusinato and L'Abate (1994) have been well-received, research testing and elaborating on these models has been limited (for exceptions see, e.g., Cusinato & L'Abate, 2005a, 2005b; Laurenceau et al., 1998). Much of the empirical work on intimacy still treats it as a relatively static relational state that is achieved by individuals engaging in or avoiding particular behaviors. Such an approach can inform researchers and theorists about how to identify individuals who may have problems with intimacy or how to predict behaviors that are likely to discourage intimacy. However, it offers a limited understanding of the ways in which intimacy is initiated, maintained, and dissolved. If researchers and theorists are going to conceive of intimacy as a dynamic process, they need to begin asking questions that treat it as such.

Treating Intimacy as a Process

Process models provide a means to integrate empirical work that has examined intimacy from the vantage point of different levels of analysis. They allow for the consideration of individual and relational characteristics. At the same time, they create a framework for studying intimacy as a dynamic phenomenon that is jointly constructed through social interaction. Although these models offer a conceptual base for what could be a burgeoning new area of study, scholars have yet to fully exploit the strengths of the models.

There are a number of questions that researchers and theorists might address as they begin to study the dyadic nature of intimacy. One very basic question involves the degree to which intimacy is jointly experienced. If, as suggested by some process models, people experience intimacy when they perceive that a relational partner is responsive to their personal disclosures, it is entirely possible that, in a given interaction, one partner may feel a sense of intimacy while the other does not (e.g., one partner may perceive the other was responsive when the other did not intend to be responsive). Laurenceau and Kleinman (2006) take issue with this scenario in their critique of the literature on intimacy. They suggest that even though process models typically include the behavior of two people (sharing and responsiveness), most are "decidedly one-sided". These authors argue that intimacy involves more than one partner self-disclosing and then feeling validated by the other's responsiveness. Indeed, they suggest that people may experience intimacy while providing understanding and validation as well as when receiving it. Although the tendency of people to experience intimacy jointly or individually is a very basic issue, it has profound theoretical and methodological implications. For instance if, as suggested by Laurenceau and Klineman, intimacy is a joint experience, then some process models need to be modified to account for the possibility that people may feel intimacy when they provide understanding and validation to a relational partner as well as when they receive it. By contrast, if intimacy is a relatively individualistic experience, the models characterized by Laurenceau and Klineman as "one-sided" may be sufficient. However, even if this is the case, researchers will need to be very cautious about assuming that one partner's reports of intimacy can be generalized to the other. Furthermore, examining intimacy at the level of the relationship will require researchers to collect data from both partners. Discrepancies in the degree to which relational partners experience intimacy will need to be examined because partners who both experience similar levels of intimacy may evaluate their relationship differently than those who experience dissimilar levels of intimacy.

Another issue that researchers and theorists might usefully address as they begin to study intimacy as a process involves the tendency of intimacy to fluctuate over time. What predicts fluctuations in intimacy within relationships? How is intimacy maintained over time? How do positive and negative changes in intimacy influence the quality of relationships? Laurenceau and his colleagues have used daily-diary methods to find that behaviors typically associated with intimacy vary a great deal over time (Laurenceau et al., 1998). When this group of researchers examined the impact of disclosure and responsiveness on intimacy, they found that both self-disclosure and partner-disclosure predicted spouses' ratings of intimacy and that the influence of self- and partner-disclosure on intimacy was affected by perceived partner responsiveness (Laurenceau, Feldman-Barrett, & Rovine, 2005). Although this work provides an important glimpse of the variables that may influence fluctuations in intimacy, it is limited in at least two ways. Both of the limitations pose interesting questions for future research. First, participants reported on individual behaviors, as opposed to sequences of behavior. Of course this, in and of itself does not represent a flaw in the study, but it does raise questions about the behavioral sequences that may be associated with intimacy. Prager and Roberts (2004) suggest that there are three types of intimacy regulation sequences: (a) an intimacy engage sequence, in which there is an intimacy approach by one partner and intimacy reciprocation by the other; (b) an intimacy withdrawal sequence, in which one partner withdraws from intimacy and the other either complies with the withdrawal or resists it; and (c) a decline intimacy sequence, in which there is an intimacy approach, a decline in response to the approach, and then a response to the decline. The way these sequences are enacted may affect relational intimacy: "the more often initiations are offered and reciprocated, the more relational intimacy; the more quickly partners withdraw from intimate interactions, the less relational intimacy" (Prager & Roberts, 2004, pp. 54–55). Although the claims made concerning the influence of these behavioral sequences on intimacy are compelling, they have yet to be empirically tested. Exploring the influence of these, and other behavioral sequences, on intimacy offers a potentially important agenda for future research.

The second limitation of the Laurenceau et al. (2005) study that raises interesting questions is that the data were collected over a six-week time period. Once again, this does not represent a problem with the study or its findings; instead, it sets the stage for researchers to question the predictors of intimacy over longer, more sustained time periods. For instance, researchers know relatively little about how self-disclosure changes over the life course of relationships. Much of the literature presumes that intimacy is associated with high levels of self-disclosure. Although studies do suggest that reciprocal disclosure facilitates the development of intimacy, there is little evidence indicating that high levels of reciprocal disclosure are maintained throughout the course of intimate relationships. As previously noted, at least one study indicates that reciprocal disclosures decline as relationships become more established (Morton, 1978). Another found that self-disclosures are much less frequent in everyday conversations than the literature (particularly laboratory studies) suggests they are (Duck, Rutt, Hoy Hurst, & Strejc, 1991). Some scholars argue that high levels of reciprocal disclosure are necessary in the early stages of relationships as partners initially get to know and trust each other, but that disclosure is much less important in the later stages of relationships because partners already have (or believe they have) a great deal of information about each other (Knapp, 1984). It also is possible that the amount of disclosure couples engage in surges during particular periods – e.g., when partners experience a crisis or a transition of some sort – because the circumstances create a context for sharing new experiences or updating old ones.

In addition to examining fluctuations in intimacy over time, researchers and theorists who are interested in studying the dyadic, processual nature of intimacy should begin to look at the outcomes associated with various patterns of intimate interactions. Theoretically, intimate interactions differ in terms of variables such as their frequency, duration, and intensity. Similarly, partners involved in intimate relationships likely differ with regard to the frequency, duration, and intensity of intimate interactions they engage in. A layperson might predict positive, linear associations among these variables. Yet, a close reading of the literature suggests that the associations are likely more textured and nuanced than that. Self-disclosure and shared knowledge do not always encourage feelings of closeness and intimacy (Parks, 1982). Indeed, partners in intimate relationships often withhold information from each other and avoid discussing particular issues (Petronio, 1991; Vangelisti, 1994). For instance, although the number of topics that couples explicitly declare off-limits is negatively related to satisfaction, this negative association only is significant among people who are relatively uncommitted or moderately committed to their relationship (Roloff & Ifert, 1998). Similarly, the association between topic avoidance and relational dissatisfaction is moderated by individuals' motivations for avoidance: The negative influence of avoidance on satisfaction is less pronounced for those who avoid topics to protect their relationship (Caughlin & Afifi, 2004). Findings such as these suggest that there may very well be times, places, and circumstances where avoiding intimate interactions actually facilitates intimacy. Exploring the outcomes associated with different patterns of intimate interactions would enable researchers and theorists to begin to identify situations when intimate interactions promote intimacy and when they do not.

Why Study Intimacy?

Given the questions that can be raised about current research on intimacy and the challenges associated with addressing these questions, laypeople might wonder about the value of studying intimacy. Why have researchers and theorists devoted time to investigating this seemingly elusive concept? Why do practitioners encourage people to establish and maintain intimate relationships? The response to queries such as these can be found in studies that have examined the psychological and physical benefits of intimacy and the costs associated with its absence.

Researchers have argued that the need to form and maintain interpersonal relationships is a fundamental human motivation (Baumeister & Leary, 1995; Ryan & Deci, 2000). People seek out and initiate social relationships without a great deal of prompting and they tend to resist the dissolution of social bonds. A relatively large body of literature suggests that intimate relationships are associated with individuals' psychological development and well-being. The capacity for intimacy has been identified by many theorists as one of the primary indicators of psychological adjustment (Erikson, 1963; Maslow, 1968; Sullivan, 1953). Intimate relationships between infants and their caregivers provide infants with a secure base from which to explore their social world (Bowlby, 1969, 1973). Secure intimate attachment in infancy, in turn, is associated with the development of confidence and self-esteem (Ainsworth, Blehar, Waters, & Wall, 1978). Similarly, intimate relationships during adolescence and early adulthood are the basis for emotional integration (Erikson, 1963; Sullivan, 1953).

In adulthood, the availability of close social relationships serves as a buffer against stress (Cohen, Sherrod, & Clark, 1986). Indeed, older adults who have an intimate friend tend to maintain a greater sense of well-being than those who do not (Lowenthal & Haven, 1968). Relational intimacy is positively associated with individual need fulfillment (Prager & Buhrmester, 1998) and well-being (Baumeister, 1991). Even the motivation to seek intimacy is positively linked to the psychosocial adjustment of adults (McAdams & Vaillant, 1982).

Conversely, difficulties with intimacy and with establishing close, intimate relationships are associated with a wide variety of mental health problems, including general maladjustment and personality disorders (Firestone & Catlett, 1999; Fisher & Stricker, 1982; Horowitz, 1979; Jones & Carver, 1991). For instance, children who experience rejection display a relatively high incidence of psychopathology (Bhatti, Derezotes, Kim, & Specht, 1989). Adults who are divorced or separated have a higher rate of admission to mental hospitals than do those who are married (Bloom, White, & Asher, 1979). Those who are single, divorced, or widowed also are more likely to commit suicide than are their married counterparts (Rothberg & Jones, 1987; also see Durkheim, 1897/1963). Women who lack an intimate relationship with a spouse or partner have a greater tendency to be depressed than do others (Brown & Harris, 1978; Costello, 1982). People who lack close, satisfying relationships also are relatively likely to be chronically lonely (Cutrona, 1982). In fact, loneliness is positively associated with a fear of intimacy (Descutner & Thelen, 1991). Inasmuch as a fear of intimacy contributes to loneliness, individuals who are lonely are at a particular disadvantage when it comes to remedying their problem because they fear the very thing they desire.

In addition to being associated with psychological well-being, intimacy is linked to people's physical well-being. Studies suggest that the presence or absence of intimate relationships affects the individuals' health. For example, Lynch (1977) used data from a number of investigations to argue that mortality rates for all causes of death are lower for people who are married than they are for those who are single, divorced, or widowed. In line with his argument, Lynch found that married individuals were less likely to have fatal heart attacks than were others. Kiecolt-Glaser and her colleagues (1987) similarly found that women who experienced divorce, separation, or dissatisfying marriages had poor immune function compared to their married counterparts.

One of the most common approaches that researchers have taken to studying the associations between intimacy and physical health has been to examine the support that individuals receive from members of their social network. Although social support is conceived and measured in a variety of ways, a number of theorists view intimacy as a central characteristic of support (e.g., Brown & Harris, 1978; Reis & Shaver, 1988). Researchers have found that support from others often is associated with positive health outcomes (Cohen & Syme, 1985). Indeed, social support has been demonstrated to have a positive influence on a long list of physical health-related variables including: mortality (House, Landis, & Umberson, 1988); recovery from surgery (Kulik & Mahler, 1989); pregnancy and childbirth (Collins, Dunkel-Schetter, Loebel, & Scrimshaw, 1993); recovery from stroke; hip fracture; and myocardial infarction (Wilcox, Kasl, & Berkman, 1994); and caregiver health (Goode, Haley, Roth, & Ford, 1998).

Intimacy as Practice

The benefits of intimacy to individuals' physical and psychological well-being have encouraged practitioners to make a number of recommendations for how intimacy might be increased in relationships. Suggestions for the application of theoretically grounded interpersonal research emerge from a body of work that, as noted by Bradbury (2002), exerts its influence on therapeutic practices "indirectly by producing measures of important concepts or by refining the theoretical system as it is translated into treatments for couples in distress" (p. 581). Given this, a reasonable translation of the findings presented earlier in this chapter will be positioned as tentative advice in the following paragraphs.

A modest starting place for developing or fostering increased intimacy in a partnership is to perform an assessment of the relationship. Differences in partners' perceptions of how long the relationship has lasted, how many days out of the week partners see each other (or how many hours of the day), and how often the couple has time to talk about intimate issues or concerns might not be realized by partners as they move through their day to day routines. Yet, there is a substantial literature which shows that discrepancies between desired and undesired (or expected and unexpected) outcomes is closely associated with relational satisfaction (Beck, 1988; Duck, 1990; Epstein & Eidelson, 1981; Fletcher, Simpson, & Thomas, 2000; Lederer & Jackson, 1968; Vangelisti & Daly, 1997). Further, because relationships are dynamic, partners' goals may change over time. Conducting a status-check on the individual goals of each partner can help to minimize discrepancies between desired and undesired relational practices and, thus, can be a vital part of increasing relational intimacy.

With similar intent, L'Abate and his colleagues (e.g., Baggett & L'Abate, 2005; L'Abate, 1999) suggest that partners generate written assessments of their relationship and of repetitive behaviors that each feels are negative (for a discussion of how couples can use homework assignments and workbooks to achieve similar goals, see Kazantzis & L'Abate, 2005; L'Abate & Goldstein, Chapter 14). Instead of raising the same topics and repeating the same negative behaviors time and time again, couples can record and assess their feelings about their relationship and thus make progress toward resolving concerns that each partner sees as problematic. By setting aside time to engage each other through writing, relationship partners can increase their awareness of cognitive and behavioral patterns that might inhibit intimacy, re-examine their common interests, and prioritize what each values in the relationship (see L'Abate, Chapter 1).

Like written and oral assessments, the ways partners communicate provide an opportunity to increase relational intimacy. Although findings about how much self-disclosure couples should engage in are influenced by relationship stage and other situational variables, the value that partners place on responsiveness is a bit clearer. As an indicator of attentiveness, understanding, and validation, responsiveness reflects concern for the needs expressed by one relationship partner to the other. Developing a pattern of interaction in which the expression of each partner's relationship interests and needs is met by responsiveness on the part of the other is likely to encourage intimacy in relationships (Prager & Roberts, 2004; Reis & Shaver, 1988).

Conclusion

The present chapter synthesizes extant literature on intimacy and points to the utility of viewing intimacy as an interactive process. In the first portions of the chapter, various conceptualizations of intimacy are discussed and several models that present intimacy as a process are covered. Then, a case is made for researchers and theorists to further exploit the strengths of process models and several questions are put forth that would, if examined, increase understanding of the interactive, processual nature of intimacy. Next, research illustrating the centrality of intimacy to individuals' well-being is reviewed. Finally, a brief discussion is offered concerning some of the ways that partners might increase intimacy in their relationships.

Intimacy can profoundly influence individuals and their relationships. It affects physical and mental well-being and shapes the way people communicate and relate to each other. Although it is frequently sought by individuals and relational partners, intimacy is not yet clearly understood by researchers and theorists. The current chapter suggests that conceptualizing intimacy as a process addresses many of the gaps in the literature. In advocating a conceptualization of intimacy that is interactive and processual, we do not suggest that researchers and theorists set aside the findings of earlier studies. Rather, it is our hope that they employ process models to integrate prior work and to study the ways in which individual, interactive, and relational variables operate together in the initiation, maintenance, and dissolution of intimacy.

References

Ainsworth, M. D. S., Blehar, M. C., Waters, E., & Wall, S. (1978). *Patterns of attachment: Assessed in the strange situation and at home*. Hillsdale, NJ: Lawrence Erlbaum.

Altman, I., & Taylor, D. A. (1973). *Social penetration: The development of interpersonal relationships*. New York: Holt, Rinehart, & Winston.

Argyle, M., & Dean, J. (1965). Eye contact, distance, and affiliation. *Sociometry, 28*, 289–304.

Baggett, M. S., & L'Abate, L. (2005). *Still fighting! Does talk work? Try writing! Help for troubled couples cheaper than talk therapy*. Manuscript submitted for publication.

Baumeister, R. F. (1991). *Meanings of life*. New York: Guilford Press.

Baumeister, R. F., & Leary, M. R. (1995). The need to belong: Desire for interpersonal attachments as a fundamental human motivation. *Psychological Bulletin, 117*, 497–529.

Beck, A. T. (1988). *Love is never enough: How couples can overcome misunderstandings, resolve conflicts, and solve relationship problems through cognitive therapy*. New York: Harper & Row.

Berg, J. H. (1987). Responsiveness and self-disclosure. In V. J. Derlega, & J. H. Berg (Eds.), *Self-disclosure: Theory, research, and therapy* (pp. 101–130). New York: Plenum Press.

Berg, J. H., & Archer, R. L. (1982). Responses to self-disclosure and interaction goals. *Journal of Experimental Social Psychology, 18*, 501–512.

Bhatti, B., Derezotes, D., Kim, S., & Specht, H. (1989). The association between child maltreatment and self-esteem. In A. M. Mecca, N. J. Smelser, & J. Vasconcellos (Eds.), *The social importance of self-esteem* (pp. 24–71). Berkeley: University of California Press.

Bloom, B. L., White, S. W., & Asher, S. J. (1979). Marital disruption as a stressful life event. In G. Levinger & O. C. Moles (Eds.), *Divorce and separation: Context, causes, and consequences* (pp. 184–200). New York: Basic Books.

Bowlby, J. (1969). *Attachment and loss, Vol. 1: Attachment*. New York: Basic Books.

Bowlby, J. (1973). *Attachment and loss, Vol. 2: Separation anxiety and anger*. New York: Basic Books.

Bradbury, T. N. (2002). Invited program overview: Research on relationships as a prelude to action. *Journal of Social and Personal Relationships, 19*, 571–599.

Brown, G. W., & Harris, T. (1978). *Social origins of depression: A study of psychiatric disorder in women*. New York: Free Press.

Caughlin, J. P., & Afifi, T. D. (2004). When it topic avoidance unsatisfying? Examining moderators of the association between avoidance and dissatisfaction. *Human Communication Research, 30*, 479–513.

Chelune, G. J., Robinson, J. T., & Kommor, M. J. (1984). A cognitive interactional model of intimate relationships. In V. J. Derlega (Ed.), *Communication, intimacy, and close relationships*. (pp. 11–40). New York: Academic Press.

Clark, M. S., & Mills, J. (1979). Interpersonal attraction in exchange and communal relationships. *Journal of Personality and Social Psychology, 37*, 12–24.

Cohen, S., & Syme, S. L. (1985). *Social support and health.* Orlando, FL: Academic Press.

Cohen, S., Sherrod, D. R., & Clark, M. S. (1986). Social skills and the stress-protective role of social support. *Journal of Personality and Social Psychology, 50,* 963–973.

Collins, N. L., Dunkel-Schetter, C., Loebel, M., & Scrimshaw, S. C. M. (1993). Social support in pregnancy: Correlates of birth outcomes and postpartum depression. *Journal of Personality and Social Psychology, 65,* 1243–1258.

Collins, N. L., & Feeney, B. C. (2000). A safe haven: An attachment theory perspective on support seeking and caregiving in intimate relationships. *Journal of Personality and Social Psychology, 78,* 1053–1073.

Costello, C. G. (1982). Social factors associated with depression: A retrospective community study. *Psychological Medicine, 12,* 329–339.

Cozby, P. C. (1973). Self-disclosure: A literature review. *Psychological Bulletin, 79,* 73–91.

Cusinato, M., & L'Abate, L. (1994). A spiral model of intimacy. In S. M. Johnson & L. S. Greenberg (Eds.), *The heart of the matter: Perspectives on emotion in marital therapy* (pp. 108–123). New York: Brunner/Mazel.

Cusinato, M., & L'Abate, L. (2005a). The dyadic relationships test: Creation and validation of a model-derived, visual-verbal instrument to evaluate couples Part I of II. *The American Journal of Family Therapy, 33,* 195–206.

Cusinato, M., & L'Abate, L. (2005b). The dyadic relationships test: Creation and validation of a model-derived, visual-verbal instrument to evaluate couple relationships. Part II. *The American Journal of Family Therapy, 33,* 1–16.

Cutrona, C. E. (1982). Transition to college: Loneliness and the process of social adjustment. In L. A. Peplau & D. Perlman (Eds.), *Loneliness: A sourcebook of current theory, research, and therapy* (pp. 291–309). New York: Wiley-Interscience.

Davis, D. (1982). Determinants of responsiveness in dyadic interaction. In W. Ickes & E. S. Knowles (Eds.), *Personality, roles, and social behavior* (pp. 85–139). New York: Springer-Verlag.

Derlega, V. J., Metts, S., Petronio, S., & Margulis, S. T. (1993). *Self-disclosure.* Newbury Park, CA: Sage.

Descutner, C. J., & Thelen, M. H. (1991). Development and validation of a fear-of-intimacy scale. *Psychological Assessment, 3,* 218–225.

Duck, S. W. (1990). Relationships as unfinished business: Out of the frying pan and into the 1990's. *Journal of Social and Personal Relationships, 7,* 5–28.

Duck, S., Rutt, D. J., Hoy Hurst, M., & Strejc, H. (1991). Some evident truths about conversations in everyday relationships: All communications are not created equal. *Human Communication Research, 18,* 228–267.

Duck, S. W., & Sants, H. K. A. (1983). On the origins of the specious: Are personal relationships really interpersonal states? *Journal of Clinical and Social Psychology, 1,* 27–41.

Durkheim, E. (1897/1963). *Suicide.* New York: Free Press. (Original work published in 1897).

Epstein, N., & Eidelson, R. J. (1981). Unrealistic beliefs of clinical couples: Their relationship to expectations, goals, and satisfaction. *The American Journal of Family therapy, 9,* 13–22.

Erikson, E. H. (1963). *Childhood and society* (2nd ed.). New York: W. W. Norton.

Feeney, J. A. (1999). Issues of closeness and distance in dating relationships: Effects of sex and attachment style. *Journal of Social and Personal Relationships, 16,* 571–590.

Fisher, M., & Stricker, G. (1982). *Intimacy.* New York: Plenum Press.

Firestone, R. W., & Catlett, J. (1999). *Fear of intimacy.* Washington, DC: American Psychological Association.

Firestone, R. W., & Firestone, L. (2004). Methods for overcoming the fear of intimacy. In D. J. Mashek & A. Aron (Eds.), *Handbook of closeness and intimacy* (pp. 375–395). Mahwah, NJ: Lawrence Erlbaum.
Fitzpatrick, M.A. (1986). Self disclosure in marriage. In V. Derlega and J. Berg (Eds.), *Self disclosure*, New York: Plenum Press.
Fletcher, G. J. O., Simpson, J. A., & Thomas, G. (2000). Ideals, perceptions, and evaluations in early relationship development. *Journal of Personality and Social Psychology, 79*, 933–940.
Gilbert, S. J. (1976). Empirical and theoretical extensions of self-disclosure. In G. R. Miller (Ed.), *Explorations in interpersonal communication* (pp. 197–215). Beverly Hills, CA: Sage.
Goode, K. T., Haley, W. E., Roth, D. L., & Ford, G. R. (1998). Predicting longitudinal changes in caregiver physical and mental health: A stress process model. *Health Psychology, 17*, 190–198.
Greene, K., Derlega, V. J., & Mathews, A. (2006). Self-disclosure in personal relationships. In A. L. Vangelisti & D. Perlman (Eds.), *Cambridge handbook of personal relationships* (pp. 409–427). New York: Cambridge University Press.
Guerney, B. G. (1977). *Relationship enhancement*. San Francisco: Jossey-Bass.
Hatfield, E. (1984). The dangers of intimacy. In V. J. Derlega (Ed.), *Communication, intimacy, and close relationships* (pp. 207–220). New York: Academic Press.
Horowitz, L. M. (1979). On the cognitive structure of interpersonal problems treated in psychotherapy. *Journal of Consulting and Clinical Psychology, 47*, 5–15.
House, J. S., Landis, K. R., & Umberson, D. (1988). Social relationships and health. *Science, 241*, 540–545.
Jones, W. H., & Carver, M. D. (1991). Adjustment and coping implications of loneliness. In C. R. Snyder & D. R. Forsyth (Eds.), *Handbook of social and clinical psychology: The health perspective* (pp. 395–415). New York: Pergamon Press.
Jourard, J. M. (1964). *The transparent self* (1st ed.). New York: D. Van Nostrand.
Kazantzis, N., & L'Abate, L. (2005). Theoretical foundations. In N. Kazantzis, F. P. Deane, K. R. Ronan, & L. L'Abate (Eds.), *Using homework assignments in cognitive behavior therapy* (pp. 9–34). New York: Routledge.
Kiecolt-Glaser, J. K., Fisher, L. D., Ogrocki, P., Stout, J. C., Speicher, C. E., & Glaser, R. (1987). Marital quality, marital disruption, and immune function. *Psychosomatic Medicine, 49*, 13–34.
Knapp, M. L. (1984). *Interpersonal communication and human relationships*. Boston: Allyn & Bacon.
Kobak, R., & Hazan, C., (1991). Attachment in marriage: Effects of security and accuracy of working models. *Journal of Personality and Social Psychology, 60*, 861–869.
Kulik, J. A., & Mahler, H. I. M. (1989). Social support and recovery from surgery. *Health Psychology, 8*, 221–238.
L'Abate, L. (1997). *The self in the family: A classification of personality, criminality, and psychopathology*. New York: Wiley.
L'Abate, L. (1999). Taking the bull by the horns: Beyond talk in psychological interventions. *The Family Journal: Therapy and Counseling for Couples and Families, 7*, 206–220.
Laurenceau, J-P., Feldman Barrett, L. A., & Pietromonaco, P. R. (1998). Intimacy as an interpersonal process: The importance of self-disclosure and perceived partner responsiveness in interpersonal exchanges. *Journal of Personality and Social Psychology, 74*, 1238–1251.
Laurenceau, J-P., Feldman Barrett, L. A., & Rovine, (2005). The interpersonal process model of intimacy in marriage: A daily-diary and multilevel modeling approach. *Journal of Family Psychology, 19*, 314–323.

Laurenceau, J-P., & Kleinman, B. M. (2006). Intimacy in personal relationships. In A. L. Vangelisti & D. Perlman (Eds.), *Cambridge handbook of personal relationships* (pp. 637–653). New York: Cambridge University Press.

Lederer, W., & Jackson, D. O. (1968). *The mirages of marriage*. New York: Norton.

Lowenthal, M. F., & Haven, C. (1968). Interaction and adaptation: Intimacy as a critical variable. *American Sociological Review, 33*, 20–30.

Lynch, J. J. (1977). *The broken heart: The medical consequences of loneliness*. New York: Basic Books.

Mashek, D. J., & Sherman, M. D. (2004). Desiring less closeness with intimate others. In D. J. Mashek & A. Aron (Eds.), *Handbook of closeness and intimacy* (pp. 343–356). Mahwah, NJ: Lawrence Erlbaum.

Maslow, A. H. (1968). *Toward a psychology of being* (2nd ed.). New York: D. Van Nostrand.

McAdams, D. P., & Valliant, G. E. (1982). Intimacy motivation and psychosocial adjustment: A longitudinal study. *Journal of Personality Assessment, 46*, 586–593.

Mikulincer, M., & Nachshon, O. (1991). Attachment styles and patterns of self-disclosure. *Journal of Personality and Social Psychology, 61*, 321–331.

Miller, L. C., & Berg, J. H. (1984). Selectivity and urgency in interpersonal exchange. In V. J. Derlega (Ed.), *Communication, intimacy, and close relationships* (pp. 161–205). Orlando, FL: Academic Press.

Miller, L. C., Berg, J. H., & Archer, R. L. (1983). Openers: Individuals who elicit intimate self-disclosure. *Journal of Personality and Social Psychology, 44*, 1234–1244.

Morton, T. L. (1978). Intimacy and reciprocity of exchange: A comparison of spouses and strangers. *Journal of Personality and Social Psychology, 38*, 72–81.

Parks, M. R. (1982). Ideology in interpersonal communication: Off the couch and into the world. In M. Burgoon (Ed.), *Communication yearbook 6* (pp. 79–107). Beverly Hills, CA: Sage.

Patterson, M. L. (1976). An arousal model of interpersonal intimacy. *Psychological Review, 83*, 235–245.

Patterson, M. L. (1984). Intimacy, social control, and nonverbal involvement: A functional approach. In V. J. Derlega (Ed.), *Communication, intimacy, and close relationships* (pp. 105–132). New York: Academic Press.

Perlman, D., & Fehr, B. (1987). The development of intimate relationships. In D. Perlman & S. W. Duck (Eds.), *Intimate relationships: Development, dynamics, and deterioration* (pp. 13–42). Beverly Hills, CA: Sage.

Petronio, S. (1991). Communication boundary management: A theoretical model of managing disclosure of private information between marital couples. *Communication Theory, 1*, 311–335.

Pietromonaco, P. R., Laurenceau, J- P., & Feldman Barrett, L. (2002). Change in relationship knowledge representations. In A. L. Vangelisti, H. T. Reis, & Fitzpatrick, M. A. (Eds.), *Stability and change in relationships* (pp. 5–34). New York: Cambridge University Press.

Pilkington, C. J., & Richardson, D. R. (1988). Perceptions of risk in intimacy. *Journal of Social and Personal Relationships, 5*, 503–508.

Pilkington, C. J., & Woods, S. P. (1999). Risk in intimacy as a chronically accessible schema. *Journal of Social and Personal Relationships, 16*, 259–263.

Planalp, S. (1993). Friends and acquaintances conversations II: Coded differences. *Journal of Social and Personal Relationships, 10*, 339–354.

Planalp, S., & Benson, A. (1992). Friends and acquaintances conversations I: Perceived differences. *Journal of Social and Personal Relationships, 9*, 483–506.

Prager, K. J. (1995). *The psychology of intimacy*. New York: Guilford Press.

Prager, K. J., & Buhrmester, D. (1998). Intimacy and need fulfillment in couple relationships. *Journal of Social and Personal Relationships, 15*, 435–469.

Prager, K. J., & Roberts, L. J. (2004). Deep intimate connection: Self and intimacy in couple relationships. In D. J. Mashek & A. Aron (Eds.), *Handbook of Closeness and Intimacy* (pp. 43–60). Mahwah, NJ: Lawrence Erlbaum.

Purvis, J. A., Dabbs, J. M., Jr., & Hopper, C. H. (1984). The "opener": Skilled user of facial expression and speech pattern. *Personality and Social Psychology Bulletin, 10*, 61–66.

Reis, H. T. (1984). Social interaction and well-being. In S. Duck (Ed.), *Personal Relationships 5: Repairing personal relationships* (pp. 21–45). London: Academic Press.

Reis, H. T., Clark, M. S., & Holmes, J. G. (2004). Perceived partner responsivenss as an organizing construct in the study of intimacy and closeness. In D. J. Mashek & A. Aron (Eds.), *Handbook of closeness and intimacy* (pp. 201–225). Mahwah, NJ: Lawrence Erlbaum.

Reis, H. T., & Patrick, B. C. (1996). Attachment and intimacy: Component processes. In H. T. Higgins, & A. W. Kruglanski (Eds.), *Social psychology: Handbook of basic principles* (pp. 523–563). New York: Guilford Press.

Reis, H. T., & Shaver, P. (1988). Intimacy as an interpersonal process. In S. W. Duck (Ed.), *Handbook of personal relationships* (pp. 367–389). Chicester, England: Wiley.

Roloff, M. E., & Ifert, D. (1998). Antcedents and consequences of explicit agreements to declare a topic taboo in dating relationships. *Personal Relationships, 5*, 191–205.

Rosenfeld, L. B. (2000). Overview of the ways privacy, secrecy, and disclosure are balanced in todays society. In S. Petronio (Ed.), *Balancing the secrets of private disclosures* (pp. 3–17). Mahwah, NJ: Lawrence Erlbaum.

Rothberg, J. M., & Jones, F. D. (1987). Suicide in the U.S. army: Epidemiological and periodic aspects. *Suicide and Life-Threatening Behavior, 17*, 119–132.

Ryan, R. M., & Deci, E. L. (2000). Self-determination theory and the facilitation of intrinsic motivation, social development, and well-being. *American Psychologist, 55*, 68–78.

Schaefer, M. T., & Olson, D. H. (1981). Assessing intimacy: The PAIR inventory. *Journal of Marital and Family Therapy, 7*, 47–60.

Simpson, J. A., Rholes, W. S., & Nelligan, J. S. (1992). Support seeking and support giving within couples in an anxiety-provoking situation: The role of attachment styles. *Journal of Personality and social Psychology, 62*, 434–446.

Sullivan, H. S. (1953). *The interpersonal theory of psychiatry*. New York: Norton.

Tesch, S. A. (1985). The psychosocial intimacy questionnaire: Validational studies and an investigation of sex roles. *Journal of Social and Personal Relationships, 2*, 471–488.

Tidwell, M. C. O., Reis, H. T., & Shaver, P. R. (1996). Attachment, attractiveness, and social interaction: A diary study. *Journal of Personality and Social Psychology, 71*, 729–745.

Vangclisti, A. L. (1994). Family secrets: Forms, functions, and correlates. *Journal of Social and Personal Relationships, 11*, 113–135.

Vangelisti, A. L., & Daly, J. A. (1997). Gender differences in standards for romantic relationships. *Personal Relationships, 4*, 203–219.

Veroff, J., Douvan, E., & Kulka, R. A. (1981). *The inner American*. New York: Basic Books.

Waring, E. M. (1984). The measurement of marital intimacy. *Journal of Marital and Family Therapy, 10*, 185–192.

Waring, E. M., & Chelune, G. J. (1983). Marital intimacy and self-disclosure. *Journal of Clinical Psychology, 39*, 183–190.

Waring, E. M., McElrath, D., Lefcoe, D., & Weisz, D. (1981). Dimensions of intimacy in marriage. *Psychiatry, 44*, 169–175.

Waring, E. M., & Reddon, J. R. (1983). The measurement of intimacy in marriage: The waring intimacy questionnaire. *Journal of Clinical Psychology, 39*, 53–57.
Wilcox, V. L., Kasl, S. V., & Berkman, L. F. (1994). Social support and physical disability in older people after hospitalization: A prospective study. *Health Psychology, 13*, 170–179.

21

Low-Cost Interventions for Promoting Forgiveness

Lindsey M. Root and Michael E. McCullough

It is a truism of social and clinical psychology that norm-violating interpersonal behavior can cause behavioral, psychological, health-related problems for victims. Serious life events caused by other people—violent crime, for example—can of course have long-standing effects, but even less overtly harmful events such as hurt feelings (Leary, Springer, Negel, Ansell, & Evans, 1998), social exclusion (Leary, Cottrell, & Phillips, 2001; Twenge, Catanese, & Baumeister, 2003), and rejection (Nolan, Flynn, & Garber, 2003) can elicit sadness, depression, anger, anxiety, and other negative outcomes. For example, discovering that one's spouse has been sexually unfaithful is associated with a sixfold increase in the likelihood of being diagnosed with a major depressive disorder (Cano & O'Leary, 2000) and being humiliated is associated with a 70% increase in the likelihood of major depressive disorder (Kendler, Hettema, Butera, Gardner, & Prescott, 2003).

Perhaps because of the pervasive norm of reciprocity (Gouldner, 1960), which dictates that people respond in kind when others harm them, transgressions frequently stimulate two negative motivations: the motivation to avoid and the motivation to seek revenge against the transgressor (McCullough et al., 1998; McCullough, Worthington, & Rachal, 1997). These transgression-related interpersonal motivations, or TRIM*s*, may be accompanied by reduced benevolent motivation toward the transgressor (McCullough et al., 1997). Although these motivational reactions to transgressions may be present in the human behavioral repertoire because they are (or were) functional (Bushman, Baumeister, & Phillips, 2001; Lerner, Gonzalez, Small, & Fischoff, 2003; McCullough, Bellah, Kilpatrick, & Johnson, 2001), they can have insidious societal and relational effects: Feeling avoidant and vengeful toward one's transgressor impedes the restoration of that relationship (McCullough et al., 1998). In addition, feeling vengeful after suffering a perceived interpersonal harm underlies a considerable amount of destruction and human aggression (Baumeister, 1996), including workplace aggression (Douglas & Martinko, 2001), school violence/adolescent aggression (Delveaux & Daniels, 2000; Pfefferbaum & Wood, 1994), driver aggression (Wiesenthal, Hennessy, & Gibson, 2000), and even arson (Masayuki, 1995; Prins, 1995; Swaffer & Hollin, 1995).

In addition to these relational and societal effects, avoidant and vengeful interpersonal motivations after a transgression may (a) increase risk for psychopathology and other mental health problems; (b) increase anger and stress-related physiological responses; and (c) impair cognitive performance. First, maintaining a negative motivational stance toward a transgressor may increase one's risk for mental disorders. People who tend to feel vengeful or unforgiving after transgressions are prone to depressive symptoms (Brown, 2003) and are more likely to be diagnosed with Major Depression, Generalized Anxiety Disorder, Phobias, and Panic Disorder (Kendler, Liu et al., 2003).

Second, resentment about the transgressions one has suffered is an important aspect of hostility. Hostility and resentment are correlates of cardiovascular reactivity, which in turn is a risk factor for a wide range of cardiovascular difficulties (Miller, Smith, Turner, Guijarro, & Hallet, 1996; Smith, Gallo, & Ruiz, 2003). Not surprisingly, thoughts of revenge are among the strongest elicitors of angry affect (DiGiuseppe & Froh, 2002), and entertaining one's grudges and thoughts of revenge lead to cardiovascular and sympathetic nervous system arousal (Witvliet, Ludwig, & Vander Laan, 2001).

Third, the anger associated with suffering a negative interpersonal event impairs cognitive performance. People who experience anger after being demeaned by another person are more likely to disengage from performance tasks (Herrald & Tomaka, 2002), so it is likely that when angry thoughts regarding a transgression are activated, people will experience cognitive interference that inhibits goal pursuits. Conversely, dissipating one's anger and anger-related motivations such as revenge may free up cognitive resources that are needed to perform optimally in performance situations.

Because negative motivational responses to interpersonal harms appear to impact the risk for psychopathology, anger, stress-related physiological responses, and cognitive performance, interventions that help to alleviate people's negative motivational responses to interpersonal harms could have considerable clinical value. In the last decade, a variety of researchers have explored interventions for promoting *forgiveness* as a way of addressing this goal. In this chapter we will describe the theory, research, and practice that relates to the potential of forgiveness to improve mental and physical health outcomes. First, we will define forgiveness and briefly review some of the theoretical models that have guided clinical research and practice in recent years. Second, we will explore existing research on the forgiveness-health connection, including both basic and intervention studies. Finally, we will examine issues related to implementing low-cost forgiveness interventions.

Theory

A Conceptualization of Forgiveness

To understand what forgiveness is, it is useful to distinguish it from a variety of related concepts. Freedman (1998) proposed that forgiveness is distinct from reconciliation, which requires two people (or groups) to reenter a relationship. Most researchers seem to agree with this distinction (Fincham & Beach, 2002b; McCullough, Pargament, & Thoresen, 2000).

The majority also concur with Enright and Coyle (1998), who distinguish forgiveness from pardoning (which is a legal term), condoning (which implies justifying the offence), excusing (which implies that the transgressor had a good reason for the transgression), forgetting (which implies a decaying or missing memory), and denying (which implies an inability or unwillingness to face the present circumstances; McCullough et al., 2000).

Despite the consensus about what forgiveness is not, researchers have defined forgiveness in slightly different ways. For example, Enright, Gassin, and Wu (1992) defined forgiveness as "the overcoming of negative affect and judgment toward the offender, not by denying ourselves the right to such affect and judgment, but by endeavoring to view the offender with compassion, benevolence, and love..." (p. 101). Exline and Baumeister (2000) defined forgiveness as the "cancellation of a debt" by "the person who has been hurt or wronged" (p. 133). Finally, McCullough et al. (1997) defined forgiveness as "the set of motivational changes whereby one becomes (a) decreasingly motivated to retaliate against an offending relationship partner; (b) decreasingly motivated to maintain estrangement from the offender; and (c) increasingly motivated by conciliation and goodwill for the offender, despite the offender's hurtful actions" (pp. 321–322).

Despite the differences among such definitions, they are all based on the proposition that forgiveness involves prosocial change regarding a transgressor on the part of the transgression recipient. Most theorists concur that when people forgive, their responses (i.e., thoughts, feelings, behavioral inclinations, or actual behaviors) toward a transgressor become more positive and/or less negative. This point of consensus led McCullough et al. (2000) to propose that *intraindividual prosocial change toward a transgressor* is a foundational and uncontroversial feature of forgiveness.

McCullough and Witvliet (2002) proposed that forgiveness can be conceptualized as a construct that operates at three distinct social-psychological levels. First, forgiveness can be viewed as a response: a prosocial change in a person's thoughts, feelings, or behaviors toward a specific transgressor (McCullough et al., 2000). Second, forgiveness can be viewed as a personality disposition, or the proclivity to forgive others across a wide variety of situations (e.g., Berry, Worthington, Parrott, O'Connor, & Wade, 2001; McCullough et al., 2001; Mullet, Houdbine, Laumonier, & Girard, 1998). Finally, forgiveness can be viewed as an attribute of social units in the same way that intimacy and trust are characteristics of some dyads or groups (e.g., Fincham, 2000; Hargrave & Sells, 1997).

Theoretical Models that have Guided Intervention Research

More than a decade ago, McCullough and Worthington (1994) reviewed over twenty theoretical models that had been proposed for making sense of forgiveness and its clinical applications. In the years since the publication of that review, a much smaller number of models guided empirical research on interventions for facilitating forgiveness. Space does not permit a comprehensive review of these models, so we describe a few of the more prominent ones here. More detailed treatments of these approaches, and others, appear in Worthington (2005).

Enright et al.'s Process Model of Forgiveness

Enright and colleagues (Enright & the Human Development Study Group, 1991; Freedman, Enright, and Knutson, 2005) have developed a model that they call the "Process Model" of forgiveness. The Process Model consists of 20 steps. Enright and colleagues describe these 20 steps as "a flexible set of processes with feedback and feed-forward loops" (Enright, Freedman, & Rique, 1998, p. 12), allowing for variation in how individuals forgiven specific transgressions. They divide the 20 steps into four phases: (a) the uncovering phase, (b) the decision phase, (c) the work phase, and (d) the outcome phase.

The "uncovering phase," comprising steps 1–8, is the phase in which the victim acknowledges and/or re-experiences the pain that he or she encountered and recognizes the injustice that occurred. Units 9–11 constitute a "decision-making phase," as an individual spends time considering and exploring forgiveness, which ultimately results in a commitment to forgive. The "work phase" includes steps 12–16, and is the phase in which the individual attempts to understand the context of the transgression and the transgressor, designed to lead to the development of empathy, compassion, and acceptance. Finally, during the "outcome phase," comprising steps 17–20, the individual experiences and acknowledges the healing that results from forgiveness.

Worthington et al.'s REACH Model

Worthington (2001) developed the Pyramid Model to REACH Forgiveness. The REACH acronym represents the five steps that Worthington has put forth as the key elements of the forgiveness process. First, an individual must *recall* the hurt and recognize the pain that the situation has caused him or her. Second, he or she *empathizes* with the transgressor, attempting to understand the perspective of the transgressor, perhaps by writing a letter from the offender's point of view or brainstorming his or her motives for the hurtful actions. Third, the hurt individual chooses to *altruistically* grant forgiveness, recalling times in which he or she have might have needed forgiveness and was freely granted forgiveness by someone whom he or she hurt. Fourth, the individual *commits* publicly to forgiveness, designed to cement the decision to forgive. Additionally, it provides a tangible reminder of the forgiveness he or she has granted the transgressor. Finally, the last step of this intervention is *holding* onto forgiveness, as individuals will naturally remember the hurts they have experienced. Some of the components of this model have been validated in intervention research (e.g., McCullough et al., 1997).

Other Approaches

Other conceptualizations have emphasized different elements as necessary or helpful on the path to forgiveness. Luskin and his colleagues (Luskin & Thoresen, 1998; Luskin et al., 2001) have incorporated relaxation, meditation, guided imagery, and techniques from cognitive behavioral and rational emotive therapies. They have used their model with people who have experienced the death of a loved one due to murder with mixed results (Luskin & Bland, 2000, 2001). Rye and colleagues (Rye & Pargament, 2002; Rye et al., 2005) have focused their approach on failed relationships. Rye and colleagues have also begun to investigate religiously integrated treatments. Their approach, which also incorporates more relaxation than does the average forgiveness intervention, has been effective (Wade, Worthington, & Meyer, 2005).

Finally, researchers and clinicians have focused on forgiveness within couples and families (e.g., Gordon, Baucom, & Snyder, 2005; Hargrave, 1994; L'Abate & Baggett, 1997). For example, Gordon and colleagues (Gordon et al., 2005; Gordon & Baucom, 1998; Snyder, Gordon, & Baucom, 2004) have developed a model of forgiveness specifically for working with couples in which one partner has betrayed the other partner's trust in a serious way (e.g., sexual infidelity). In Gordon's model, forgiveness consists of three basic components: (a) acquiring a realistic view of the relationship; (b) freeing oneself from the control of negative emotions and hurt toward one's partner; and (c) decreasing one's desire to punish one's partner. Gordon and colleagues believe that their model leaves room for the development of more positive emotions toward the partner, but emphasize that forgiveness can occur without reconciliation.

Basic and Applied Research on Forgiveness, Mental Health, and Physical Health

The links between forgiveness and health have been assessed using basic research (i.e., correlational research, experimental research) and intervention studies. In basic research, researchers have examined the associations between the disposition to forgive and individual differences in forgiveness for specific transgressions and a variety of measures of physical and mental health. They have also tried to manipulate forgiveness experimentally to examine its association with measures of health and well-being. Additionally, several groups of researchers have enrolled individuals in counseling intervention programs designed to facilitate forgiveness (for recent reviews and meta-analyses, see Baskin and Enright, 2004; Wade et al., 2005). Later in this chapter, we will consider the empirical research on the efficacy of these interventions for promoting forgiveness, mental health, and physical health.

Associations of Forgiveness with Mental and Physical Health

Basic Research

Studies examining the relationship between forgiveness and mental health have consistently suggested a positive association. Although this literature is limited almost exclusively to depression, anxiety, broadly defined mental health, and broadly defined well-being, the associations are consistent (Toussaint & Webb, 2005). For example, research has repeatedly revealed that the propensity to forgive others is negatively associated with depression (e.g., Brown, 2003; Maltby, Macaskill, & Day, 2001; Mauger et al., 1992). Specifically, Brown (2003) found that among 70 undergraduates, those who reported a greater propensity to forgive others had lower scores on the Centers for Epidemiological Studies-Depression scale than did those who did not report a strong propensity to forgive. Additionally, unforgiving participants were more likely to be depressed if they valued forgiveness highly or if their scores were both low on the tendency to forgive and low in vengeance-seeking; Brown hypothesized that those who are unlikely to forgive and unlikely to seek revenge may feel powerless against their offenders, as hopelessness and low self-efficacy are strongly tied to depression (e.g., Peterson, Maier, & Seligman, 1993; Alloy, Abramson, & Francis, 1999).

Similarly, Maltby et al. (2001) examined links between mental health and individual differences in the propensity to forgive others and the propensity to forgive oneself. Using Mauger et al.'s (1992) Failure to Forgive Self (FFS) and Failure to Forgive Others (FFO) scales, Maltby and colleagues correlated 324 participants' forgiveness ratings with their scores on a general mental health questionnaire. For both male and female undergraduates, high scores on the FFS scale (indicative of unwillingness to forgive the self) were positively correlated with symptoms of depression and anxiety. High FFO scores (indicative of a weak tendency to forgive others) were associated with higher levels of depression for both men and women.

Additional studies across more diverse populations have paralleled these findings. Seybold, Hill, Neumann, and Chi (2001) found that higher levels of forgiveness were correlated with lower anxiety and lower depression in community residents. In a study of twin pairs, Kendler, Liu et al. (2003) found that high forgiveness was associated with a decreased risk of externalizing disorders (i.e., substance use or dependence and nicotine dependence) and that low vengefulness was associated with a lower risk of internalizing disorders (i.e., generalized anxiety disorder, phobia, major depression, and bulimia nervosa). Finally, Witvliet, Phipps, Feldman, and Beckham (2004) asked veterans with PTSD to complete the Failure to Forgive Self (FFS) and Failure to Forgive Others (FFO) scales (Mauger et al., 1992). Dispositional difficulty forgiving oneself was associated with PTSD severity and symptoms of depression and anxiety. Dispositional difficulty forgiving others was associated with PTSD severity and depression.

Researchers have also shown that more general measures of mental health and well-being are associated with forgiveness. In a study of forgiveness within romantic relationships, Berry and Worthington (2001) assessed general mental health. Thirty-nine participants were classified as happy or unhappy with their romantic relationships. Participants imagined scenes typical of their relationship for five minutes and then completed several questionnaires, including a health survey and two trait forgiveness questionnaires: the Transgression Narrative Test of Forgiveness (TNTF) and the Trait Unforgiveness-Forgiveness (TUF) scale. High scores on the TUF measure, indicating high dispositional forgiveness, were correlated with better mental health (as measured by the SF-36 Health Survey; Hays, Sherbourne, & Mazel, 1995).

Using a two-level approach for analyzing longitudinal data, Bono, McCullough and Root (under review) explored the relationship between within-persons changes in people's transgression-related interpersonal motivations (TRIMs: Avoidance, Revenge, and Benevolence) toward specific transgressors who harmed them and within-persons changes in four measures of general well-being (satisfaction with life, positive affect, negative affect, and psychosomatic symptoms). Participants began this longitudinal study within seven days of experiencing a transgression and completed questionnaires on the aforementioned variables five times (approximately every 14 days). On measurement occasions when individuals were more forgiving than would be expected (i.e., occasions when they were more forgiving than was typical for them) they reported greater satisfaction with life, greater positive affect, less negative affect, and fewer physical symptoms than was typical for them.

The connection between forgiveness and physical health has not received as much attention as has the relationship between forgiveness and mental health. Thoresen, Harris, and Luskin (2000) challenged researchers to examine whether forgiveness promotes better physical health, which they deemed "an unanswered question" (p. 254)—a situation that has not, by their reckoning, improved very much in the five years that have ensued (Harris & Thoresen, 2005). Still, the small body of research examining both trait and specific trangression forgiveness and their relationships with health variables provides some provocative preliminary evidence.

In the study of forgiveness in romantic relationships discussed above, Berry and Worthington (2001) also assessed measures of physical health and physiological functioning. Samples of salivary cortisol (a hormone highly responsive to perceived physical and psychosocial threats; Dickerson & Kemeny, 2004) from saliva were taken at baseline and in the fifth minute of the five-minute imagery task. Participants also completed a self-reported measure of physical health. Cortisol reactivity was inversely related to both personality variables (high trait forgiveness, low trait anger) and relationship variables (high liking of the partner, high happiness in the relationship). Berry and Worthington speculated that the personality variables indirectly influenced cortisol reactivity through relationship quality: People who tended to be forgiving had higher-quality relationships and, as a result, when they imagined typical scenes from these relationships they experienced smaller increases in salivary cortisol. Higher trait forgiveness scores were associated with better physical health (as measured by the SF-36 Health Survey; Hays et al., 1995), indicating that forgiveness as a dispositional trait might be related to better general physical health.

Using data from a national probability survey, Toussaint, Williams, Musick, and Everson (2001) examined the links between dispositional forgiveness and self-reported health in young (ages 18–44), middle (ages 45–64), and old (65 and older) participants. They measured four dimensions of forgiveness: forgiveness of self, forgiveness of others, forgiveness by God, and proactive forgiveness (how actively a participant seeks granting or receiving forgiveness). For the young and middle-aged participants, only forgiveness of self was positively related to physical health. In contrast, forgiveness of self was not related to physical health in old participants, but forgiveness of others was associated with better physical health reports. These findings point to a relationship between trait forgiveness and health, although the correlation between forgiveness of others and health was obtained only in adults aged 65 and older.

Seybold et al. (2001), as mentioned above, also investigated the link between forgiveness and physical health by assessing a variety of physiological measures in community-dwelling adults. Blood pressure, heart rate, and the majority of the immune cell data they collected (e.g., total levels of lymphocytes, neutrophils, monocytes, T-cells) were not associated with forgiveness. Participants with lower forgiveness of others, however, had higher hematocrit levels, lower total white blood cell counts, lower lipoprotein toxicity preventing activity (TxPA) levels and higher T-helper/T-cytotoxic cell ratios.

These results present a somewhat mixed picture of the relationship of forgiveness with measures of physiological functioning. The inverse relationship between forgiveness and indices of blood viscosity (hematocrit, white blood cell count) suggests that people who score highly on measures of forgiveness may possess some cardiovascular risk factors; however, the hematocrit levels were within normal limits (Witvliet, 2001), so the clinical significance of these results may be limited. Conversely, Seybold et al. report that TxPA levels correlate directly with cardiovascular health and are known to decrease with psychological stress, suggesting that a lack of forgiveness is both psychologically stressful and may reduce cardiovascular health, whereas those individuals with high forgiveness scores may have better immune functioning (as indicated by T-helper/T-cytotoxic cell ratios). This is the first and only study examining the links between forgiveness and these variables. Moreover, all of the physiological measures were assessed on only one occasion: Repeated assessments would have allowed for more control of measurement error. Moreover, it may be useful to examine these relationships in contexts where reactivity rather than tonic physiological functioning can be assessed. Clearly, more research is needed to establish the relevance of these findings and how they fit into the forgiveness-health relationship.

Two published studies have examined the relationship between forgiveness and physiological reactivity (Lawler et al., 2003; Witvliet et al., 2001). Taken together, these studies suggest that people who do not forgive tend to experience cardiovascular responses to stress that are indicative of poor cardiovascular health.

In the first study, Witvliet et al. (2001) used a repeated measures design to examine the immediate emotional and physiological effects of forgiveness. When undergraduates imagined unforgiving responses (rehearsing the hurt, harboring a grudge) toward a real-life transgressor, heart rate reactivity, mean arterial pressure, corrugator EMG, and skin conductance levels were significantly greater than when they imagined forgiving responses (developing feelings of empathy, granting forgiveness). Both heart rate and mean arterial pressure indicate emotional arousal whereas corrugator tension is indicative of negative emotion and skin conductance levels indicate sympathetic nervous system arousal. Change score differences persisted into recovery periods for corrugator, heart rate, and skin conductance levels, suggesting that even when participants attempted to relax, arousal and negative affect persisted. These data provide a preliminary glimpse into the short-term effects of unforgiveness and forgiveness on physiological functioning.

Lawler et al. (2003) found that both state and trait forgiveness were associated with less cardiovascular reactivity. In their study, Lawler et al. (2003) interviewed participants about two real-life conflicts (one involving a parent and the other involving a friend or partner). Higher trait forgiveness was associated with lower systolic blood pressure (SBP), diastolic blood pressure (DBP), and mean arterial pressure (MAP) during the baseline, the interview, and recovery periods. Higher state forgiveness was also associated with lower SBP, DBP, and MAP, as well as heart rate and rate pressure product (RPP; SBP*heart rate; an indicator of myocardial oxygen demand and stress). In response to the interview about a parental conflict, participants with low trait forgiveness and low state forgiveness experienced the most cardiovascular reactivity and poorest recovery patterns. The only significant effect in response to the friend/partner conflict was smaller increases in RPP for highly forgiving women. For the recovery period, participants in high state forgiveness had lower DBP and MAP. These findings suggest that people who do not forgive specific transgressions, particularly if they are generally unforgiving, experience greater and more sustained cardiovascular reactivity when discussing those transgressions from their pasts.

In summary, the studies described above suggest associations between forgiveness and a wide variety of measures of mental and physical health. Although data examining the relationship between physical health outcomes and forgiveness are limited, the existing studies are quite provocative and call for more extensive research. We now turn to the existing intervention research for a more complete picture of the effects of forgiveness within a therapeutic context.

Intervention Research on Forgiveness

The published articles on forgiveness interventions provide persuasive evidence that these interventions are effective in producing important therapeutic outcomes. Researchers have focused predominantly on studying the effects of group interventions, with the exception of two studies that have examined the use of forgiveness interventions in individual counseling (e.g., Coyle & Enright, 1997; Freedman & Enright, 1996;). Two recent meta-analyses of these studies (Baskin & Enright, 2004; Wade et al., 2005) offer valuable insights into why these interventions are effective.

Baskin and Enright (2004) analyzed nine counseling interventions from six published studies that measured forgiveness quantitatively. They categorized the nine interventions into three groups: (a) decision-based interventions, (b) group process interventions, and (c) individual process interventions. *Decision-based* group interventions (Al-Mabuk, Enright, & Cardis, 1995; McCullough & Worthington, 1995, McCullough et al., 1997) consisted of a single session or partial intervention that focused only on the initial decision to forgive and commitment to that decision. *Group process* interventions (Hebl & Enright, 1993; Al-Mabuk et al., 1995; McCullough et al., 1997) consisted of groups that met for six to eight sessions and included multiple theoretically based steps designed to facilitate forgiveness. *Individual process* interventions (Coyle & Enright, 1997; Freedman & Enright, 1996) also included multiple theoretically based steps, but participants worked individually with a counselor for 12 or more sessions.

Each of these interventions used a control group of some kind (i.e., psychological placebo, support group, wait-list, or alternate intervention). Effect sizes were computed for each of the forgiveness interventions and a weighted mean was computed for each category. The decision based group total effect size was not statistically different from zero ($d = -0.04$), and suggested that those who received the intervention did not achieve more forgiveness than those who did not participate in the intervention. The mean effect size for the group process interventions was large ($d = 0.82$) and indicated that the average person in a group process intervention did as well or better than 75% of the control group. The mean effect size for the individual process interventions was very large ($d = 1.66$) and indicated that the average person in an individual process intervention did as well or better than 95% of the control group.

Baskin and Enright (2004) also examined whether these interventions were helpful on other mental health variables (e.g., anxiety, depression, self-esteem). Effect sizes were computed across variables for each intervention and weighted means were computed for each category. Again, the effect size for the decision based groups was not significantly different from zero ($d = 0.16$), which indicated that individuals in the intervention did not improve over those in the control group. The mean effect sizes for the group process interventions and individual process interventions ($ds = 0.59$ and 1.42, respectively) were again large and very large. Those in group process interventions did as well or better than 65% of the people in their respective control groups and those in the individual process interventions did as well or better than 92% of the people in their respective control groups.

The results of Wade and colleagues (Wade et al., 2005) more comprehensive meta-analysis are consistent with those of Baskin and Enright (2004), although Wade et al. go quite a bit further in explaining how forgiveness interventions facilitate forgiveness. Wade et al. included a total of 39 forgiveness interventions (i.e. theoretically grounded forgiveness interventions and forgiveness-oriented comparison interventions), 10 alternate treatment conditions (e.g., support groups, leadership interventions), and 16 no-treatment conditions (e.g., wait-list control groups) from 27 studies that included a quantitative measure of forgiveness. An effect size (ES) was computed for each condition by estimating the amount of pre-post gain in forgiveness that participants in that condition experienced on average. These pre-post effect sizes, expressed as standard change units, were used in all subsequent analyses. Theoretically grounded forgiveness interventions and forgiveness-oriented comparison interventions had the largest effect sizes ($ESs = 0.57$ and 0.43) and were not statistically different from each other. Alternative treatments ($ES = 0.26$) were significantly less effective than theoretically grounded treatments but not less effective than forgiveness-oriented comparison interventions. Any intervention (theoretically grounded, forgiveness-oriented comparison, or alternative) was more effective than a no-treatment control group ($ES = 0.10$). Additionally, full interventions ($ES = 0.77$), whether they were focused on forgiveness or not, were more effective than partial (e.g., early versions of a forgiveness treatment, a comparison group in a component analysis study; $ES = 0.28$) or no treatment ($ES = 0.10$). Regression analyses indicated that even when controlling for the amount of time spent in treatment, forgiveness interventions of any kind were more helpful than general treatments and full interventions were more helpful than partial interventions.

Several components were also significantly related to effect size (Wade et al., 2005). Specifically, empathizing with the offender, committing to forgiveness, and strategies like relaxation and anger management, were significantly related to outcome in an analysis that included only groups that explicitly attempted to facilitate forgiveness. These components may be particularly essential when promoting forgiveness.

The meta-analysis by Wade and colleagues (2005) clearly demonstrates that forgiveness interventions are able to promote forgiveness relative to no treatment at all and relative to alternative treatments that are not really expected to produce strong psychological effects. But this really doesn't say very much about the efficacy of *forgiveness* interventions *per se*. From the perspective of demonstrating efficacy, the critical question is whether forgiveness interventions are more effective than *bona fide* alternative treatments that do not explicitly facilitate forgiveness. Many of the comparison treatments were attention-only controls and not genuine treatments. Indeed, as Wade and colleagues note, the individual studies that used alternate treatments as control groups did not yield a statistically significant advantage for forgiveness interventions (e.g., Ripley & Worthington, 2002; Wade, 2002, stress reduction). This should be seen as a serious challenge to forgiveness research that should be taken up in the next generation of research. Baskin and Enright (2004) also comment on the present state of intervention research, calling for more rigorous standards so that forgiveness interventions are able to meet criteria for empirically supported treatments (Chambless & Hollon, 1998; Chambless & Ollendick, 2000; Crits-Christoph, 1996). Although the criteria for this designation have been met in separate studies, no specific two studies from two independent research settings have demonstrated all of the criteria (e.g., comparison with psychological placebo, comparison with established interventions, use of treatment manuals). We agree that the time has come to compare forgiveness interventions to established treatments for specific mental health difficulties (e.g., depression, anxiety), and continue to identify which components or processes present in forgiveness interventions are helpful.

Psychological Processes that Influence Forgiveness

As noted above, numerous authors have emphasized process models of forgiveness (e.g., Enright & the Human Development Study Group, 1991; Freedman et al., 2005; McCullough & Worthington, 1995; McCullough et al., 1997; Worthington, 2001). Whereas Enright and colleagues conceptualize 20 steps to forgiveness, Worthington puts forth only 5. Which of these processes are important and which are supported by empirical evidence? Various studies and meta-analyses have begun to shed some light on the specific processes that may be most helpful, or necessary, for facilitating forgiveness.

Deciding to Forgive and Making a Commitment to Forgiveness

Wade and colleagues (2005) found that the amount of time that participants spent on exploring the decision about whether to forgive and actually making a commitment to forgiveness were significantly related to effect size in their meta-analysis. Baskin and Enright (2004), however, found that decision-based models, which used these cognitive components without including more psychologically active components, were not effective at promoting forgiveness. Therefore, these processes do not appear sufficient for forgiveness, but they may be useful as part of a larger model.

Empathy

The experience of empathy for one's transgressor (and dispositional empathy more generally) is one of the best-studied and most reliable psychological predictors of forgiveness. McCullough and colleagues (McCullough et al., 1997, 1998, 2003) and Fincham and colleagues (Fincham, Paleari & Regalia, 2002; Paleari, Regtalia & Fincham, 2005) have consistently found positive associations between empathy and forgiveness. In a recent study on relationship quality, Paleari et al. (2005) collected data from married individuals at two time points at a six-month interval. Their analyses revealed that emotional empathy was predictive of concurrent forgiveness, which in turn predicted concurrent marital quality. Macaskill et al. (2002) also conducted a study with British undergraduates and found an association between forgiveness of others and dispositional empathy scores. It is worth noting as well that Wade and colleagues (2005) found that the amount of time that was devoted to helping transgression recipients develop empathy for their transgressors during forgiveness interventions was significantly related to effect size in their meta-analysis.

Rumination

Research suggests that rumination about a transgression is negatively related to forgiveness at the trait and specific transgression levels (e.g., Barber, Maltby & Macaskill, 2005; Berry, Worthington, O'Connor, Parrot & Wade, 2005; McCullough et al., 1998, McCullough et al., 2001). Berry and colleagues (2005) found that dispositional forgiveness was negatively correlated with vengeful rumination, and that rumination mediated the relationship between dispositional forgiveness and revenge motivation as well as trait and specific state anger. McCullough and colleagues (2001) found that when people focused on specific transgressions, rumination was related to revenge and avoidance motivations; in fact, those individuals who experienced decreases in rumination over time also experienced greater forgiveness. In a longitudinal study, McCullough, Bono, and Root (under review) asked participants to track their rumination and forgiveness daily for three weeks. In this sample, short-term increases in rumination were associated with short-term reductions in forgiveness, suggesting that rumination may interfere with forgiveness. In Paleari et al.'s (2005) study, rumination (along with empathy), was predictive of concurrent forgiveness, which was subsequently related to marital satisfaction. Additionally, Kachadourian, Fincham, and Davila (2005) found that rumination moderated the relationship between ambivalence and forgiveness, with greater ambivalence associated with less forgiveness only when a relationship partner was ruminating about the offense.

Benefit-Finding

McCullough, Root, and Cohen (in press) recent study indicated that encouraging individuals to focus on the benefits they have experienced as a result of a transgression may encourage forgiveness. Undergraduate participants (N = 300) were randomly assigned to writing conditions in which they wrote about one of the following: (a) the traumatic features of the most recent interpersonal transgression they had experienced, (b) the (realized or potential) benefits associated with their most recent interpersonal transgression, or (c) a non-emotional topic. Participants in the benefit-finding condition reported more forgiveness (i.e., less revenge and avoidance motivations, and more benevolence motivation) toward the transgressor. Given that this very simple, 20-minute task produced a group difference, this strategy may hold promise for more extensive use as an intervention component.

Generous Attributions Regarding the Transgressor

Another factor associated with the extent to which people forgive is the type of attributions they make about the transgression and the transgressor. For example, Bradfield & Aquino (1999) found that people who had forgiven their transgressors found them more likeable than those who had not forgiven. Similarly, Shapiro (1991) reported that people who had forgiven found their transgressors' explanations of the hurtful event more adequate and honest, and they reported that those transgressions were less severe than people who had not forgiven. Additionally, the tendency to forgive one's spouse was associated with lower responsibility attributions of his or her negative behavior. Although these findings are correlational and may reflect accurate perceptions of the transgressor and the transgression on the part of the victim, encouraging positive attributions might help to facilitate forgiveness.

Practice

Even though the superiority of forgiveness interventions to extant empirically based mental health treatments remains unclear, research shows that they are effective at fostering forgiveness and mental health. One clear and very encouraging lesson to draw from the existing research on forgiveness interventions (largely conducted in group format) is that they can be effectively administered in a low-cost manner. In this section, we consider two issues related to low-cost interventions for promoting forgiveness. First, what are the critical components to include in a group intervention for promoting forgiveness? Second, are there even more cost-effective approaches that can be used for fostering forgiveness, such as self-administered interventions?

What Components Should Be Included in a Group Intervention for Promoting Forgiveness?

In an earlier review, Worthington, Sandage, and Berry (2000) suggested several important components of psychoeducational group interventions that dovetail with more recent findings (Baskin and Enright, 2004; Wade et al., 2005). First, they highlighted the importance of helping participants arrive at a common understanding of what forgiveness is, emphasizing that a joint conceptualization is as important in group settings as it is in individual psychotherapy. Second, they noted that the goals of the therapy should be explicit. Third, they emphasized that the intervention should be theory-based. These recommendations resonate well with the findings we have already discussed. Those interventions that Wade et al. (2005) found to be most helpful (i.e., forgiveness-oriented interventions) are likely to contain these components.

Other elements should probably be present as well. First, helping participants develop empathy for their transgressors is consistently related to forgiveness, and was one of only three components to significantly predict effect size in the Wade et al. (2005) meta-analysis. Second, encouraging participants to make a decision to forgive or commit to forgiveness is a cognitive component of forgiving that was also related to effect size in the Wade et al. analysis. Although Baskin and Enright's (2004) results indicate that commitment alone is inadequate for facilitating forgiveness, it appears to be a necessary step. Finally, Wade et al. found that relaxation and anger management strategies were significantly related to effect size as well, indicating that these processes may facilitate forgiveness.

Three additional processes may also be useful. First, interventions that help participants to stop ruminating about the transgressions they have suffered would likely be useful. Kachadourian et al. (2005) also suggest that positive rumination, or intentionally considering a transgressors more positive qualities, could be particularly helpful in this regard. Second, encouraging positive and generous attributions of the transgression and the transgressor may also be helpful. Generous attributions have been linked with greater forgiveness for specific transgressions and a greater tendency to forgive in general (McCullough, 2001). Finally, helping participants to identify potential benefits to the self as a result of the transgressions they have suffered is another process that shows considerable promise (McCullough et al., in press). These three components should be explored more thoroughly in both research and practice.

Considerations for Future Intervention Strategies and Research

Fincham and Beach (2002a) have proposed a model for a public health intervention focused on forgiveness in close relationships. They suggest a writing program, similar to those used with individuals who have experienced trauma (for a review, see Esterling, L'Abate, Murray, & Pennebaker, 1999; for an early example of a written assignment on forgiveness, see L'Abate, 1986). This approach (a) would allow individuals to work through a transgression at their own rate, and (b) could be broadly disseminated through the print media and also through the Internet. Fincham and Beach describe four intervention components. In the first component, users would be able to determine whether the intervention was appropriate for them by initially clarifying their expectations and goals for the intervention and then comparing those expectations to the program's goals and definition of forgiveness.

The second component would lay the foundation for forgiveness by instructing participants to write about the transgression and subsequent hurt they experienced. Participants would then be encouraged to discuss the reasons behind the transgressor's actions and also write about the transgressor's positive qualities from the perspective of a friend or acquaintance. Presumably, both of these tasks will generate empathy, encourage positive attributions, and weaken the association between the transgressor and transgression.

Third, participants would begin to address forgiveness explicitly. In this component, users would write about events in the past in which they hurt another person and were grateful for the victim's forgiveness, or would have been grateful for it. In this stage, participants would also commit to forgiving the transgressor, either in writing or by confiding in a friend or confidant. A benefit-finding component, potentially in the form of a writing intervention, could be helpful here as well (McCullough et al., in press).

The final component would focus on maintenance of treatment gains. Participants would write about how they might react in the future if negative feelings and hurt resurface. Ideally, planning for such occurrences may help minimize their impact and encourage participants that they have not failed at forgiving if they encounter a setback. Additionally, participants would be encouraged to write about their forgiveness experience during the self-administered treatment. This task would help participants develop narratives about the experience and potentially help them find meaning both in the transgression and in their forgiveness of the transgressor.

While a self-administered intervention like the described above seems promising, to our knowledge, no published data have emerged examining such a program. Research on such a program would be extremely valuable. Although there are numerous self-help books, motivational speakers, and forgiveness workshops available for those who are looking, no program is as accessible, or as easily disseminated as this one could be.

Conclusion

Interpersonal transgressions routinely result in negative outcomes, including a heightened risk for psychopathology and stress-related physiological arousal. Promoting forgiveness may be one way to alleviate these negative outcomes. Researchers have repeatedly shown group interventions to be effective at promoting forgiveness, both within individual studies and meta-analyses. Alternatively, a writing intervention, like the one suggested by Fincham and Beach (2002a) may prove very useful and perhaps even more cost-effective than group interventions. Although many questions remain unanswered about forgiveness, its relation to health and well-being, the processes involved in producing forgiveness, and the best means for encouraging forgiveness in clinical settings, it seems clear that increasing forgiveness is a worthwhile goal within reach. We look forward to the next generation of clinical research on forgiveness, and we are particularly optimistic that new treatments will emerge that are both efficacious and cost-effective.

References

Al-Mabuk, R. H., Enright, R. D., & Cardis, P. A. (1995). Forgiveness education with parentally love-deprived late adolescents. *Journal of Moral Education, 24*, 427–444.

Alloy, L., Abramson, L., & Francis, E. L. (1999). Do negative cognitive styles confer vulnerability to depression? *Psychological Science, 4*, 128–132.

Barber, L., Maltby, J., & Macaskill, A. (2005). Angry memories and thoughts of revenge: The relationship between forgiveness and anger rumination. *Personality and Individual Differences, 39*, 253–262.

Baskin, T. W., & Enright, R. D. (2004). Intervention studies on forgiveness: A meta-analysis. *Journal of Counseling and Development, 82*, 79–90.

Baumeister, R. F. (1996). *Evil: Inside human violence and cruelty*. New York: Freeman.

Berry, J. W., & Worthington, E. L., Jr. (2001). Forgivingness, relationship quality, stress while imagining relationship events, and physical and mental health. *Journal of Counseling Psychology, 48*, 447–455.

Berry, J. W., Worthington, E. L., Jr, O'Connor, L. E., Parrott, L., III, & Wade, N. G. (2005). Forgivingness, venegeful rumination, and affective traits. *Journal of Personality, 73*, 183–225.

Berry, J. W., Worthington, E. L., Jr, Parrott, L., III, O'Connor, L. E., & Wade, N. G. (2001). Dispositional forgivingness: Development and construct validity of the transgression narrative test of forgivingness (TNTF). *Personality and Social Psychology Bulletin, 27*(10), 1277–1290.

Bono, G., McCullough, M. E., & Root, L. M. (under review). Forgiveness, feeling corrected to benefit others, and wellbeing: Two longitudinal studies.

Bradfield, M. & Aguino, K. (1999). The effects of blame attributions and offender likeableness on forgiveness and revenge in the workplace. *Journal of Management, 25*, 607–631.

Brown, R. P. (2003). Measuring individual differences in the tendency to forgive: Construct validity and links with depression. *Personality and Social Psychology Bulletin, 29*, 759–771.

Bushman, B. J., Baumeister, R. F., & Phillips, C. M. (2001). Do people aggress to improve their mood? Catharsis beliefs, affect regulation opportunity, and aggressive responding. *Journal of Personality and Social Psychology, 81*, 17–32.

Cano, A., & O'Leary, K. D. (2000). Infidelity and separations precipitate major depressive episodes and symptoms of nonspecific depression and anxiety. *Journal of Consulting and Clinical Psychology, 68*, 774–781.

Chambless, D. L., & Hollon, S. D. (1998). Defining empirically supported therapies. *Journal of Consulting and Clinical Psychology, 66*, 7–18.

Chambless, D. L., & Ollendick, T. H. (2001). Empirically supported psychological interventions: Controversies and evidence. *Annual Review of Psychology, 52*, 685– 716.

Coyle, C. T., & Enright, R. D. (1997). Forgiveness intervention with postabortion men. *Journal of Consulting and Clinical Psychology, 65*, 1042–1046.

Crits-Christoph, P. (1996). The dissemination of efficacious psychological treatments. *Clinical Psychology: Science and Practice, 3*, 260–263.

Delveaux, K. D., & Daniels, T. (2000). Children's social cognitions: Physically and relationally aggressive strategies and children's goals in peer conflict situations. *Merrill-Palmer Quarterly, 46*, 672–692.

Dickerson, S. S., & Kemeny, M. E. (2004). Acute stressors and cortisol responses: A theoretical integration and synthesis of laboratory research. *Psychological Bulletin, 130*, 355–391.

DiGiuseppe, R., & Froh, J. J. (2002). What cognitions predict state anger? *Journal of Rational-Emotive & Cognitive Behavior Therapy, 20*, 133–150.

Douglas, S. C., & Martinko, M. J. (2001). Exploring the role of individual differences in the prediction of workplace aggression. *Journal of Applied Psychology, 86*, 547–559.

Enright, R. D., & Coyle, C. T. (1998). Researching the process model of forgiveness within psychological interventions. In: E. L. Worthington Jr. (Ed.), *Dimensions of forgiveness: Psychological research and theological perspectives* (pp. 139–161). Philadelphia, PA: Templeton Foundation Press.

Enright, R. D., Freedman, S., & Rique, J. (1998). The psychology of interpersonal forgiveness. In: R. D. Enright, & J. North (Eds.), *Exploring forgiveness* (pp. 46–62). Madison, WI, US: University of Wisconsin Press.

Enright, R.D., Gassin, E.A., & Wu, C. (1992). Forgiveness: A developmental view. *Journal of Moral Education, 21*, 99–114.

Enright, R.D., & The Human Development Study Group (1991). The moral development of forgiveness. In: W. Kurtines & J. Gerwirtz (Eds.), *Handbook of moral behavior and development* (Vol. 1; pp. 123–152). Hillsdale, NJ: Lawrence Erlbaum.

Esterling, B. A., L'Abate, L., Murray, E. J., & Pennebaker, J. W. (1999). Empirical foundations for writing in prevention and psychotherapy: Mental and physical health outcomes. *Clinical Psychology Review, 19*, 79–96.

Exline, J. J., & Baumeister, R. F. (2000). Expressing forgiveness and repentance: Benefits and barriers. In: M. E. McCullough, K. I. Pargament & C. E. Thoresen (Eds.), *Forgiveness: Theory, research, and practice* (pp. 133–155). New York: Guilford.

Fincham, F. D. (2000). The kiss of the porcupines: From attributing responsibility to forgiving. *Personal Relationships, 7*, 1–23.

Fincham, F.D., & Beach, S. R. H. (2002a). Forgiveness: Toward a public health approach to intervention. In: J. H. Harvey & A. Wenzel (Eds.), *A clinician's guide to maintaining and enhancing close relationships*. New Jersey: Erlbaum.

Fincham, F. D., & Beach, S. R. H. (2002b). Forgiveness in marriage: Implications for psychological aggression and constructive communication. *Personal Relationships, 9*, 239–251.

Fincham, F. D., Paleari, F. G., & Regalia, C. (2002). Forgiveness in marriage: The role of relationship quality, attributions, and empathy. *Personal Relationships, 9*, 27–37.

Finkel, E. J., Rusbult, C. E., Kumashiro, M., & Hannon, P. A. (2002). Dealing with a betrayal in close relationships: Does commitment promote forgiveness? *Journal of Personality and Social Psychology, 82*, 956–974.

Freedman, S. (1998). Forgiveness and reconciliation: The importance of understanding how they differ. *Counseling and Values, 42*, 200–216.

Freedman, S. R., & Enright, R. D. (1996). Forgiveness as an intervention goal with incest survivors. *Journal of Consulting and Clinical Psychology, 64*, 983–992.

Freedman, S. R., Enright, R. D., & Knutson, J. (2005). A progress report on the process model of forgiveness. In E. L. Worthington, Jr. (Ed.), *Handbook of Forgiveness* (pp. 423–439). New York: Routledge.

Gordon, K. C., and Baucom, D. H. (1998). Understanding betrayals in marriage: A synthesized model of forgiveness. *Family Process, 37*, 425–450.

Gordon, K. C., Baucom, D. H., & Snyder, D. K. (2005). Forgiveness in couples: Divorce, infidelity, and couples therapy. In: E. L. Worthington, Jr. (Ed.), *Handbook of Forgiveness* (pp. 423–439). New York: Routledge.

Gouldner, A. W. (1960). The norm of reciprocity: A preliminary statement. *American Sociological Review, 25*, 161–178.

Hargrave, T. D. (1994). *Families and forgiveness: Healing wounds in the intergenerational family*. Philadelphia: Brunner/Mazel.

Hargrave, T. D., & Sells, J. N. (1997). The development of a forgiveness scale. *Journal of Marital and Family Therapy, 23*(1), 41–63.

Harris, A. H. S., & Thoresen, C. E. (2005). Forgiveness, unforgiveness, health, and disease. In E. L. Worthington, Jr. (Ed.), *Handbook of Forgiveness,* (pp. 321–334). New York: Brunner–Routledge.

Hays, R. D., Sherbourne, C. D., & Mazel, R. M. (1995). *User's manual for the Medical Outcomes Study (MOS) core measures of health-related quality of life* (Publication No. MR-162-RC). Santa Monica, CA: Rand.

Hebl, J. H., & Enright, R. D. (1993). Forgiveness as a psychotherapeutic goal with elderly females. *Psychotherapy, 30*, 658–667.

Herrald, M. M., & Tomaka, J. (2002). Patterns of emotion-specific appraisal, coping, and cardiovascular reactivity during an ongoing emotional episode. *Journal of Personality and Social Psychology, 83*, 434–450.

Kachadourian, L. K., Fincham, F., & Davila, J. (2005). Attitudinal ambivalence, rumination, and forgiveness of partner transgressions in marriage. *Personality and Social Psychology Bulletin, 31*, 334–442.

Kendler, K. S., Hettema, J. M., Butera, F., Gardner, C. O., & Prescott, C. A. (2003). Life event dimensions of loss, humiliation, entrapment, and danger in the prediction of onsets of major depression and generalized anxiety. *Archives of General Psychiatry, 60*, 789–796.

Kendler, K. S., Liu, X., Gardner, C. O., McCullough, M. E., Larson, D. B., & Prescott, C. A. (2003). Dimensions of religiosity and their relationship to lifetime psychiatric and substance use disorders. *American Journal of Psychiatry, 160*(3), 496–503.

L'Abate, L. (1986). *Systematic Family Therapy*. New York: Brunner/Mazel.

L'Abate, L, & Baggett, M. S. (1997). *The self in the family: A classification of personality, criminality, and psychopathology*. New York: Wiley.

Lawler, K. A., Younger, J. W., Piferi, R. L., Billington, E., Jobe, R., & Edmondson, K. et al. (2003). A change of heart: Cardiovascular correlates of forgiveness in response to interpersonal conflict. *Journal of Behavioral Medicine, 26*, 373–393.

Leary, M. R., Cottrell, C. A., & Phillips, M. (2001). Deconfounding the effects of dominance and social acceptance on self-esteem. *Journal of Personality & Social Psychology, 81*, 898–909.

Leary, M. R., Springer, C., Negel, L., Ansell, E., & Evans, K. (1998). The causes, phenomenology, and consequences of hurt feelings. *Journal of Personality & Social Psychology, 74*, 1225–1237.

Lerner, J. S., Gonzalez, R. M., Small, D. A., & Fischoff, B. (2003). Effects of fear and anger on perceived risks of terrorism: A national field experiment. *Psychological Science, 14*, 144–150.

Luskin, F., & Bland, B. (2000). *Stanford-Northern Ireland HOPE-1 project*. Unpublished manuscript, Stanford University, Palo Alto, CA.

Luskin, F., & Bland, B. (2001). *Stanford-Northern Ireland HOPE-2 project*. Unpublished manuscript, Stanford University, Palo Alto, CA.

Luskin, F., & Thoresen, C. (1998). *Effectiveness of forgiveness training on psychosocial factors in college-aged adults*. Unpublished manuscript, Stanford University, Palo Alto, CA.

Luskin, F., Thoresen, C., Harris, A. Benisovich, S., Standard, S., Bruning, J., et al. (2001). *Effects of group forgiveness interventions on perceived stress, state and trait anger, symptoms of distress, self-reported health, and forgiveness*. Unpublished manuscript, Stanford University, Palo Alto, CA.

Macaskill, A., Maltby, J., & Day, L. (2002). Forgiveness of self and others and emotional empathy. *Journal of Social Psychology, 142*, 663–665.

Maltby, J., Macaskill, A., & Day, L. (2001). Failure to forgive self and others: A replication and extension of the relationship between forgiveness, personality, social desirability and general health. *Personality and Individual Differences, 30*, 881–885.

Mauger, P. A., Perry, J. E., Freeman, T., Grove, D. C., McBride, A. G., & McKinney, K. E. (1992). The measurement of forgiveness: Preliminary research. *Journal of Psychology and Christianity, 11*, 170–180.

Masayuki, K. (1995). A basic study of rural arson in the last 18 years. *Japanese Journal of Criminal Psychology, 33*, 17–26.

McCullough, M.E. (2001). Forgiveness: Who does it and how do they do it? *Current Directions in Psychological Science, 10*, 194–197.

McCullough, M. E., Bellah, C. G., Kilpatrick, S. D., & Johnson, J. L. (2001). Vengefulness: Relationships with forgiveness, rumination, well-being, and the big five. *Personality and Social Psychology Bulletin, 27*, 601—610.

McCullough, M. E., Bono, G., & Root, L. M. (in press). Rumination, affect, and forgiveness: Three longitudinal studies. *Journal of Personality and Social Psychology*.

McCullough, M. E., Fincham, F. D., & Tsang, J. (2003). Forgiveness, forbearance, and time: The temporal unfolding of transgression-related interpersonal motivations. *Journal of Personality and Social Psychology, 84*, 540–557.

McCullough, M. E., Pargament, K. I., & Thoresen, C. E. (2000). The psychology of forgiveness: History, conceptual issues, and overview. In: M. E., McCullough, K. I., Pargament and C. E., Thoresen (Eds), *Forgiveness: Theory, Research, and Practice* (pp. 1–14). New York: Guilford.

McCullough, M. E., Rachal, K. C., Sandage, S. J., Worthington, E. L., Jr., Brown, S. W., & Hight, T. L. (1998). Interpersonal forgiving in close relationships II: Theoretical elaboration and measurement. *Journal of Personality and Social Psychology, 75*, 1586–1603.

McCullough, M. E., Root, L. M., & Cohen, A. D., (in press). Writing about the personal benefits of an interpersonal transgression facilitates forgiveness. *Journal of Consulting and Clinical Psychology*.

McCullough, M. E., and Witvliet, C. V., (2002). The psychology of forgiveness. In Snyder C. R. and Lopez S. J. (eds), *Handbook of Positive Psychology* (pp. 446–458) London: Oxford University Press.

McCullough, M. E. and Worthington, E. L., Jr. (1994). Encouraging clients to forgive people who have hurt them: Review, critique, and research prospectus. *Journal of Psychology and Theology, 22,* 3–20.

McCullough, M. E. and Worthington, E. L., Jr. (1995). Promoting forgiveness: A comparison of two brief psychoeducational group interventions with a waiting-list control. *Counseling and Values, 40*, 55–68.

McCullough, M. E., Worthington, E. L., Jr., and Rachal, K. C. (1997). Interpersonal forgiving in close relationships. *Journal of Personality and Social Psychology, 73*, 321–336.
Miller, T. Q., Smith, T. W., Turner, C. W., Guijarro, M. L., & Hallet, A. J. (1996). A meta-analytic review of research on hostility and physical health. *Psychological Bulletin, 119*, 322–348.
Mullet, E., Houdbine, A., Laumonier, S., & Girard, M. (1998). "Forgivingness": Factor structure in a sample of young, middle-aged, and elderly adults. *European Psychologist, 3*(4), 289–297.
Nolan, S. A., Flynn, C., & Garber, J. (2003). Prospective relations between rejection and depression in young adolescents. *Journal of Personality and Social Psychology, 85*, 745–755.
Paleari, F. G., Regalia, C., & Fincham, F. (2005) Marital quality, forgiveness, empathy, and rumination: A longitudinal analysis. *Personality and Social Psychology Bulletin, 31*, 368–378.
Peterson, C., Maier, S. F., & Seligman, M. E. (1993). *Learned Helplessness: A Theory for the Age of Personal Control*. New York: Oxford University Press.
Pfefferbaum, B., & Wood, P. B. (1994). Self-report study of impulsive and delinquent behavior in college students. *Journal of Adolescent Health*, (15), 295–302.
Prins, H. (1995). Adult fire-raising: Law and psychology. *Psychology, Crime & Law, 1*, 271–281.
Ripley, J. S., & Worthington, E. L., Jr., (2002). Comparison of hope-focused communication and empathy-based forgiveness group interventions to promote marital enrichment. *Journal of Counseling and Development, 80*, 452–463.
Rye, M. S., & Pargament, K. I. (2002). Forgiveness and romantic relationships in college: Can it heal the wounded heart? *Journal of Clinical Psychology, 54*, 419–441.
Rye, M. S., Pargament, K. I., Pan, W., Yingling, D. W., Shogren, K. A., & Ito, M. (2005). Can group interventions facilitate forgiveness of an ex-spouse? A randomizied clinical trial. *Journal of Consulting and Clinical Psychology, 73*, 880–892.
Seybold, K. S., Hill, P. C., Neumann, J. K., & Chi, D. S. (2001). Physiological and psychological correlates of forgiveness. *Journal of Psychology and Christianity, 20*(3), 250–259.
Shapiro, D. L., (1991). The effects of explanations on nagative reactions to detect. *Administration Science Quarterly, 36*, 614–630.
Smith, T. W., Gallo, L. C., & Ruiz, J. M. (2003). Toward a social psychophysiology of cardiovascular reactivity: Interpersonal concepts and methods in the study of stress and coronary disease. In J. Suls, & K. Wallston (Eds.), *Social Psychological Foundations of Health and Illness*. UK: Blackwell.
Swaffer, T., and Hollin, C. R. (1995). Adolescent firesetting: Why do they say they do it? *Journal of Adolescence, 18*, 619–623.
Synder, D. K., Gordon, K. C., & Baucom, D. H. (2004). Treating affair couples: Extending the written disclosure paradigm to relationship trauma. *Clinical Psychology: Science and Practice, 11*, 155–160.
Thoresen, C. E., Harris, A. H. S., & Luskin, F. (2000). Forgiveness and health: An unanswered question. In M. E. McCullough, K. I. Pargament & C. E. Thoresen (Eds.), *Forgiveness: Theory, research, and practice* (pp. 254–280). New York: Guilford.
Toussaint, L. L., & Webb, J. R. (2005). Theoretical and empirical connections between forgiveness, mental health, and well-being. In E. L. Worthington, Jr. (Ed.), *Handbook of Forgiveness* (pp. 349–362). New York: Routledge.
Toussaint, L. L., Williams, D. R., Musick, M. A., & Everson, S. A. (2001). Forgiveness and health: Age differences in a U.S. probability sample. *Journal of Adult Development, 8*(4), 249–257.

Twenge, J. M., Catanese, K. R., & Baumeister, R. F. (2003). Social exclusion and the deconstructed state: Time perception, meaninglessness, lethargy, lack of emotion, and self-awareness. *Journal of Personality and Social Psychology, 85*, 409–423.

Wade, N. G., (2002). Understanding reach: A component analysis of a group intervention to promote forgiveness. *Dissertation Abstracts International: Section B: The Sciences and Engineering, 63*, 2611.

Wade, N.G., Worthington, E. L., Jr., & Meyer, J. E. (2005). But do they work? A meta-analysis of group interventions to promote forgiveness. In E. L. Worthington, Jr. (Ed.), *Handbook of Forgiveness* (pp. 423–439). New York: Routledge.

Wiesenthal, D. L., Hennessy, D., & Gibson, P. M. (2000). The Driving Vengeance Questionnaire (DVQ): The development of a scale to measure deviant drivers' attitudes. *Violence & Victims, 15*, 115–136.

Witvliet, C. v. O. (2001). Forgiveness and health: Review and reflections on a matter of faith, feelings, and physiology. *Journal of Psychology and Theology, 29*(3), 212–224.

Witvliet, C. v. O., Ludwig, T. & Vander Laan, K. (2001). Granting forgiveness or harboring grudges: Implications for emotion, physiology, and health. *Psychological Science, 12*, 117–123.

Witvliet, C. v. O., Phipps, K. A., Feldman, M. E., & Beckham, J. C. (2004). Posttraumatic mental and physical health correlates of forgiveness and religious coping in military veterans. *Journal of Traumatic Stress, 17*, 269–273.

Worthington, E. L., Jr. (2001). *Five Steps to Forgiveness: The Art and Science of Forgiving*. New York: Crown Publishers.

Worthington, E. L., Jr. (Ed.). (2005). *Handbook of Forgiveness*. New York: Routledge.

Worthington, E. L., Sandage, S. J., & Berry, J. W. (2000). Group interventions to promote forgiveness: What researchers and clinicians ought to know. In M. E. McCullough, K. I. Pargament & C. E. Thoresen (Eds.), *Forgiveness: Theory, Research, and Practice*. (pp. 228–253). New York: Gilford Press.

22

Spirituality in Achieving Physical and Psychological Health and Well-Being: Theory, Research and Low Cost Interventions*

Len Sperry, Louis Hoffman, Richard H. Cox, and Betty Ervin Cox

Increasingly, the public has come to view spirituality and spiritual practices as ways of improving physical and psychological health and well-being. While not all clinicians and researchers share this view, an entire subspecialty of spiritually oriented counseling and psychotherapy has emerged, as well as lines of research that support it (Richards & Bergin, 1997; Sperry, 2002; Sperry & Shafranske, 2005). Common to many of these approaches is the therapist's use of traditional spiritual disciplines or practices as interventions within the context of formal counseling and psychotherapy. In fact, components or modules consisting of such spiritual practices are central to a few of these therapeutic approaches (D'Souza & Rodrigo, 2004; Cloninger, 2006). A basic premise of this book is that many therapeutic and similar interventions can be successfully applied or adapted to promote health and well-being outside the formal context of psychotherapy. It is our contention that, in given circumstances, a number of spiritual practices can be effectively employed outside the realm of psychotherapy to foster health and well-being as well as spiritual transformation.

This chapter begins with a brief discussion about the complexity of defining and operationalizing spirituality in a clinical context before reviewing some basic theory and research involving the link between spirituality and physical and psychological health. It suggests that achieving a measure of physical and psychological health and well-being is an intermediate step in the process of spiritual transformation. It then describes specific spiritual interventions that can be utilized both inside and outside the psychotherapuetic context to effect well-being and transformation. Finally, it suggests the kind of circumstances wherein such interventions are most likely to be efficacious and cost-effective.

* The authors would like to thank Patricia Schniedwind for her assistance in preparing this project.

Defining Spirituality

At the heart of much discussion about spirituality today is what has come to be called the "language of spirituality" debate. Basically, the debate centers on whether it is possible for clinicians and researchers to agree on the definition of spirituality, and two polar positions have emerged. On one side are those adopting a cultural relativity perspective wherein diversity and social construction of reality make a single definition or understanding of spirituality unlikely. Accordingly, clinicians are urged to seek to understand each individual's unique understanding of spirituality and respond accordingly (McSherry & Cash, 2004).

The opposite perspective is based on scientific naturalism which proposes to "reduce" and redefine psychology as a biological science and define spirituality in neurobiological terms. Several recent trade books, such as *The God Gene: How Faith Is Hardwired Into Our Genes* (Hamer, 2004) and *Looking for Spinoza: Joy, Sorrow, and the Feeling Brain* (Domasio, 2003), advocate such a biologically based definition of spirituality. Between these extremes are a plethora of definitions and views of spirituality.

For some spirituality is basically a feeling state (Domasio, 2003), while others contend it is an instinct (Hamer, 2004). Some consider it a basic trait, such as of character (Cloninger & Svrakic, 1994), a striving (Emmons, 1999), or spiritual transcendence (Cloninger, 2004; Piedmont, 1999; Reed, 1991). Others consider it a peak or mystical experience (Maslow, 1968), a search (Pargament, 1999), an insatiable spiritual longing (Rolheiser, 1999), spiritual practices (Walsh, 1999), a form of intelligence (Emmons, 2000), quantum change (Miller & C'de Baca, 2001), or spiritual transformation (StawAki, 2003).

Rather than choosing one of the many current definitions of spirituality, we contend that a systemic definition of the concept may have more theoretical and practical value. From this perspective, any definition of it can be characterized in terms of three systems theory variables: is spirituality portrayed as an input or antecedent variable, a mediating or process variable, or an output or dependent variable? Most current definitions usually reflect only one or two of these variables. For example spiritual longing (Rolheiser, 1999) is an antecedent variable while spiritual practices (Walsh, 1999) is a moderating variable, and spiritual transformation (Stawski, 2003) is an output or dependent variable. We propose that a systemic and composite definition is one that views spirituality as having input, moderating, and output variables or dimensions. Such a definition is more theoretically valuable and clinically useful then one that includes only one variable or dimension (Sperry, 2006).

Theory

Not surprisingly, definitional problems also plague much of the research which examines the relationship between spirituality and psychological health. One approach to resolving these issues places various religious variables into three categories: Organized Religious Activities (ORA), Non-organized Religious Activities (NRA), and Other Religious Variables (Ervin-Cox, Hoffman, & Grimes, 2005; Koenig, McCullough, & Larson, 2001). ORA include various communal aspects of religion, such as corporate worship and group scripture study. NRA are activities which individuals engage in on their own, including prayer and meditation. Lastly, among other religious variables are other ways of quantifying religiosity – spiritual well-being and religious orientation.

When examining the influence of spirituality on health, defined broadly, it becomes necessary to classify types of health. Two broad categories of physical health and psychological or mental health signify the most basic distinction. The choice of the word "health," which implies the attainment of health, is significant as it does not reduce health to the lack of pathology. Rather, a focus is maintained on the positive aspects of health with an implicit assumption that health avoids being overly diminished by pathology.

This broad categorization of spiritual and health variables quickly encounters several significant limitations. The inconsistency in empirical studies suggests a complex relationship between spirituality and health. More discrete definitions add to the understanding of the important nuances of the relationship. Therefore, a broad schema of the interrelationship between these variables is useful for the more nuanced studies and provides a framework for understanding the relevancy of spirituality for various forms of health.

Ervin-Cox et al. (2005) identified five implicit models revealed in previous research. Three levels of variables can be identified in this model: The implicit perception of being religious/spiritual, constructs of religious/spiritual activity or character, and constructs of health. An example of the first model is illustrated in Figure 22.1. This first model suggests the self-definition of being spiritual impacts various modes of being religious which in turn impacts psychological health. Physical health is only impacted through the spiritual influence on psychological health in a linear fashion.

The next three models continue with similar linear approaches to understanding the relationship between the six constructs. An important assumption of all of these models is that the primary influences of spirituality on health occurs through the intervening variables of religious activity (organized and nonorganized) and other spiritual characteristics (spiritual health, for

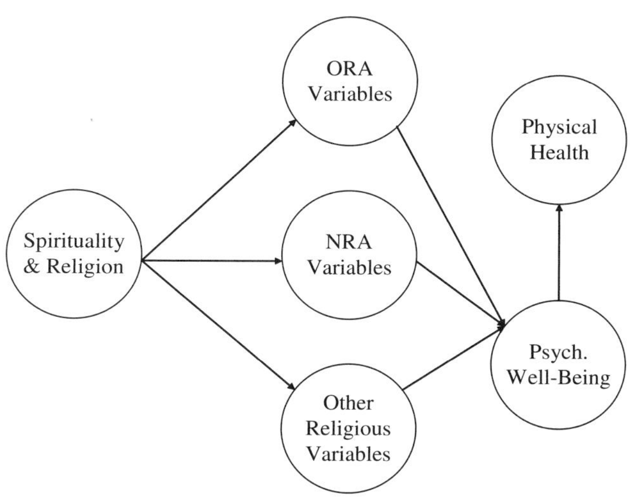

Figure 22.1. Linear Relationship of Spirituality to Health and Well-Being.

example). There is little room for a direct relationship between being spiritual and health.

The final model of the relationship of spirituality and health reflects a deeper level of complexity and is illustrated in Figure 22.2. It is a systemic or quantum model in which the multidirectional, interrelated assumptions are implicit. It addresses the limitations of a purely linear model and suggests that health impacts spirituality just as spirituality influences health. Finally, it reflects the systemic relationship of factors accounting for both direct and mediated relationships between and among spirituality and health.

A Multidimensional Definition of Spirituality

In short, there is both theoretical and clinical value in framing spirituality in an even broader systemic context. This broadened, systemic context involves a multidimensional view or model we propose which involves three dimensions, including the concept of spiritual transformation. So what is spiritual transformation? Spiritual transformation is defined as dramatic changes in world and self view, purposes, religious beliefs, attitudes and behavior. These changes are often linked to discrete experiences that can occur gradually or over relatively short periods of time (Stawski, 2003, p. 425). Spiritual transformation involves much more than increasing one's level of physical health and/or psychological well-being. Parenthetically, this definition of spiritual transformation has been operationalized in more than two dozen research studies funded by the Templeton Foundation and sponsored by the Spiritual Transformation Scientific Research Program (Katz, 2004). Similarly, spiritual transformation has been described as an output or dependent variable, and spiritual longing (Rolheiser, 1999) represents an antecedent or independent variable (Sperry, 2006). Linking spiritual longings and spiritual transformation are various spiritual transcending practices (Walsh, 1999) which are mediating variables or dimensions. These practices include prayer, meditation, mindfulness, fasting, and service. Figure 22.3, based on Sperry (2006),

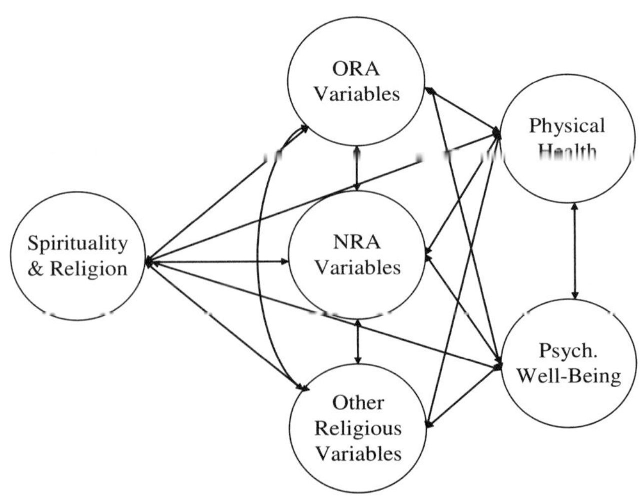

Figure 22.2. Model 2: Systemic Relationship of Spirituality to Health and Well-Being.

Spiritual Longing→ Self-Transcending Practices → Spiritual Transformation

Figure 22.3. A Multidimensional Model of Spirituality.

portrays this multidimensional model which articulates the relationship of these three variables. In short we define spirituality as a process that is activated by spiritual longings and fostered by self-transcending spiritual practices. It results in spiritual transformation, which is an ongoing process.

What relationship, if any, is there between this multidimensional model and the models of the relationship of spirituality and health portrayed in Figures 22.1 and 22.2? Essentially, the output dimension of these two models is physical health and psychological well-being which could be considered an intermediate step between spiritual practices and spiritual transformation. While neither model specifies the input dimension of spiritual longing, it is implicit. Similarly, neither model specifies transformation as the output variable, but neither is it incompatible. In addition to being more inclusive than the other two models, this multidimensional model provides a perspective for understanding the role of the various psychospiritual and spiritual practices or interventions in achieving health, well-being and transformation.

Research: General Studies

Religion/Spirituality and Mental Health

Early traces of interest in the relationship between spirituality and psychological health emerged in Freud's (1961) writings and continue to be controversial through contemporary times. Despite Freud's contentious view of religion, other influential early theorists such as James (1902), Jung (1958), and Maslow (1962) showed interest in the benefits of religion and spirituality. In the current literature, mixed empirical results continue to confuse many mental health practitioners. Despite the disparity, some themes do emerge.

Bergin's (1983) initial meta-analytic study of religiosity and mental health along with several subsequence studies supported the initial finding of a primarily small positive relationship between these constructs (Bergin, 1991; Hackney & Sanders, 2003; Sawatzky, Ratner, & Chiu, 2005). Bergin (1983) found 47% of the studies revealed positive outcomes between religion and mental health with an overall positive mean correlation of 0.09. Of the remaining studies, 30% found no correlation while 23% found a negative relationship.

A more recent meta-analysis conducted by Hackney and Sanders (2003) also reported significant overall positive findings between religiosity and mental health $r = 0.10$, $p < 0.0001$. Similar to Bergin, the results remained positive despite a high number of studies finding a negative relationship. This appears consistent with other reviews that reflect a trend which more favorably supports a positive, although small, relationship (Koenig & Larson, 2001; Sawatzky et al., 2005). Koenig and Larson (2001) found 80% of the 850 articles they reviewed revealed some positive associations while Sawatzky et al. (2005) found a moderate effect size in a meta-analysis of 59 studies.

The studies identified in this section represent a large sampling of the current literature. In attempting to understand the results, several important factors are important to consider. First, the trend toward more consistent positive findings likely result partially due to improved definitions and methodology. For example, studies on extrinsic versus intrinsic literature reveal a higher frequency of negative associations between religiosity and mental health among people scoring high on extrinsic religiosity scales (Koenig et al., 2001). The ability to control for negative forms of religiosity assists researchers in finding the positive correlates of being religious.

Research: Specific Studies

Religious Coping

Few areas of research on spirituality have received as much attention as religious coping. One of the challenges to understanding this literature is the large number of different measures, conceptualizations, and definitions of religious coping. In general, religious coping refers to the various attitudes, actions, and characteristics related to how an individual uses religion to deal with stressful or traumatic situations.

Ano and Vasconcellos (2005) conducted the most comprehensive meta-analysis of this literature thus far by grouping coping strategies into two broad categories of positive and negative religious coping. Outcomes of the coping were placed into the categories of positive and negative adjustment. The results indicated significant effects sizes with positive religious coping predicting positive adjustment while negative coping was related to negative adjustment.

One of the most extensive studies on religious coping compared three groups (college students, elderly adults, and individuals coping with the Oklahoma City bombings) and their use of religious coping (Pargament, Smith, Koenig, & Perez, 1999). Their results were consistent with the previously mentioned meta-analysis in terms of adjustment outcomes related to positive and negative religious coping. Additionally, the research identified a tendency toward individuals using positive approaches to religious coping.

Prayer

Many obstacles create challenges for empirical attempts to study prayer. Maybe the biggest challenges relate to the many different types of prayer which exist. Any serious research on prayer must take into account the different types of prayer in order to really understand the unique contributions of different aspects of prayer. Very few controlled studies have engaged in this challenge.

Probably the most significant research on prayer was Byrd's (1988) investigation of the effects of intercessory prayer. Individuals in this study were randomly assigned to one of two groups, one of which received prayer while the other group served as a control. This was a double blind study with neither the researchers nor the participants knowing who was receiving prayer. The subjects, who were coronary heart participants, did not know the individuals who were praying for them. Results indicated the participant being prayed for had better health outcomes on 21 of 26 health factors. Tloczynski and Fritzsch (2002) supported these findings in a second double blind study. However, despite the statistically significant results, this second study was limited small number of participants.

While these results are both important and impressive, several of the reviews of the literature on prayer found mixed results (Chamberlain & Hall, 2000; Ervin-Cox et al., 2005; Koenig et al., 2001). The mixed results may indicate the need for improved research and research methodologies in prayer research. Additionally, may of the studies reviewed have not taken into consideration the different types of prayer. Prayer still holds good promise of being a low-cost intervention and preventative measure.

Meditation

Meditation represents one popular spiritual approach which has been integrated with many therapies. An advantage of meditation is the easy access to receiving many forms of training which can be adapted to fit with the individual's personal religious values. Chapter 9 provides further background information on meditation and its relationship to relaxation methods.

Research suggests that meditation may be useful in treating anxiety disorders (Carlson, Bacaseta, & Simanton, 1998), heart disease (Leserman Stuart, Mamish, & Benson, as cited in Koenig et al., 2001), and increasing immune functioning (Sadsuang, Chentanez, & Veluvan, 1991, as cited in Koenig et al., 2001). The use of relaxation is often in conjunction with prayer, mindfulness, or other spiritual practices.

Mindfulness

The practice of mindfulness is often closely associated with meditation. Marlatt and Kristeller (1999) state, to be fully mindful in the present moment is to be aware of the full range of experiences that exist in the here and now. "Mindful awareness is based on an attitude of acceptance" (p. 68). In a sense, mindfulness is a heightened awareness and acceptance to what is happening to and around the individual. The practice, which parallels many themes of humanistic and existential psychotherapy, emerged primarily from Eastern religion and philosophy. However, in recent times many psychological and religious theories integrated mindfulness into their practice.

Teasdale, Segal, and Williams (1995) found that integrating mindfulness into relapse prevention along with cognitive therapy provides useful benefits for participants. One of the benefits of mindfulness practice is the focus on acceptance which, in addition to the change process in therapy, can assist participants in not overreacting to problematic situations. For example, mindfulness practice encourages individuals to be aware of their troubling thoughts, but not necessarily to seek to change them. Instead of changing the thought or event that result in discomfort, individuals are encouraged to change their attitudes toward their thoughts and emotional reaction. Retaining awareness of the discomfort while placing it in the context of acceptance allows the experience to become more tolerable.

Mindfulness-based Stress Reduction (MBSR) is nonreligious group approach which is intended to alleviate suffering. In a meta-analysis by Grossman, Niemann, Schmidt, and Walach (2003), this mindfulness-based approach was found to significantly reduce suffering with individuals struggling with a variety of physical and psychological health issues.

Communal Worship and Church Attendance

Participation in spiritual communities is one of the oldest measures of religiosity. As the model presented by Ervin-Cox et al. (2005) suggests, it may be difficult to distinguish between the direct impact of religious attendance upon mental health and the influence mediated by the social support offered through religious participation. Church or worship attendance is not a very sophisticated measure by itself and many of the studies utilizing this as a measure lack adequate controls. The power of this measure increases dramatically when combined with measures of intrinsic versus extrinsic religiosity or other constructs which may help explain the motivation for church attendance. Nonetheless, several studies have examined the impact of church attendance on mental health.

One significant study explored the relationship between church attendance and life satisfaction for 1,642 Finnish men and women (Hinikka et al., 2001). A strength of this study was that it controlled for the impact of social support, a common purported confounding variable. Regression analysis revealed that both social support and religious attendance contributed significant unique variance to life satisfaction. Another study explored the relationship between domestic violence and religious attendance (Ellison & Anderson, 2001). The results revealed that regular church attendance was a significant protective factor for both men and women. For men, church attendance was only successful in significantly decreasing domestic violence if attendance was weekly. However, for women even attending once a month provided achieved significance. As with many of the studies using church attendance as a variable, a weakness of this study was the lack of controls for social support and other potential mediating factors.

Spiritual Direction and Guidance

The potential for mutual enhancement between the fields of spiritual direction and psychotherapy has received increasing attention as evidenced by recent journals dedicated to exploring this relationship (Moon & Benner, 2002, 2003). Despite the promise of spiritual direction as an effective, low-cost enhancement of mental health, limited empirical research has been conducted on its effectiveness at the current time.

Forgiveness

Forgiveness has been the topic of a good deal of theory development in recent times. While many of the approaches to forgiveness are religious, some are not (Rye et al., 2000). Forgiveness is covered in more detail in Chapter 21.

Very Brief Spiritual Counseling/Therapy

The current climate of managed care necessitates that many therapists conduct therapy within a brief or focused format. While there are limitations to the brief approach to treatment, several therapeutic approaches demonstrate successful treatment for some participants. Included are several spiritually integrative approaches to treatment. For example, Tan (1987; Tan & Johnson 2005) integrate spiritual counseling with cognitive-behavioral therapy. The adaptation of cognitive-behavioral therapy to working with spiritual participants has received some empirical support (Propst, 1980; Propst, Ostrom, Watkins, Dean, & Mashburn, 1992). Similarly, Johnson, DeVries, Ridley, Pettorini, and Peterson (1994) found religiously oriented rational-emotive therapy to be similarly efficacious in a secular rational-emotive approach.

Much of the early work addressing spiritual approaches to brief therapy followed this format of applying secular brief therapy techniques to a spiritual setting. Early research attempted to demonstrate that spiritual approaches to brief counseling were no less effective than their secular counterparts (Hawkins, Tan, & Turk, 1999; McCullough, 1999; Propst et al., 1992; Tisdale et al., 1997). Over time, an increase of therapy applications emerged which are more uniquely Christian. For example, Pargament (1997) attempted to apply his extensive research on religious coping to therapeutic setting. While there is little outcome research which has been conducted on therapeutic application of religious coping, the theory emerged from a significant body of research. Similarly, Tan and Johnson (2005) integrate spiritual practices into well- established cognitive-behavioral therapy practices.

Practice

Prayer

Although we do not know the exact chronological origin of prayer as a human activity, it was certainly borne out of need. The word prayer is derived from a Latin root, *precari*, which means "dependent upon the will or favor of another person." In our time, the idea of praying to a p*erson* has for some given way to praying to an *entity* or *power*. Nevertheless, virtually everyone prays in the hope – and even at times without the belief-that someone or something will hear them! Prayer becomes a form of modifying and at times escaping the human condition. It becomes a metaphysical transcendence that permits the executive prefrontal cortex of the brain to engage the nebulous but firmly believed higher powers of human function that transports the otherwise chemical, electrical, and anatomical structure into the "spiritual" part of humanness.

The concept of the "therapeutic" is to treat that which is considered defective with the hope of changing that which is dysfunctional into healthy functioning. Perhaps nothing is more intentional in this regard than the petitioning plaintiff; a humbled human who in total inadequacy calls upon a "higher power" to literally take over when our resources have been depleted and at times even willingly squandered. Among other things, prayer provides the individual with a tool for achieving transcendence. For example, practicing intercessory prayer may be the deepest form of spiritual bonding. Prayer as such ceases to be a technique or tool, rather it becomes the demonstration of the human's yearning for connection to each other and the Eternal.

Prayer is a spiritual phenomenon that is central to most seekers' spiritual journey. Most individuals pray at least occasionally and many use prayer frequently for coping with life's difficulties. Prayer can serve as a journey marker for participants demarcating important struggles and events in their lives and as such is a marker of one's spiritual and psychosocial functioning.

Various types of prayer have been noted. Paloma and Pendleton (1989) describe four types: ritualistic prayer, i.e., reading from a prayer book; petitionary prayer, i.e, asking God to grant a request; colloquial prayer, i.e., prayer of thanksgiving; and meditative prayer, i.e., TM and centering prayer.

Meditation – Centering Prayer

Meditation has been described in many ways. It has been described as a means of relaxing the body/mind, as a way of training and strengthening awareness, as a method for centering and focusing the self, as well as a means of reducing high blood pressure and other cardiovascular conditions, relieving stress, bolstering self-esteem, and reducing the symptoms of anxiety and depression (Carrington, 1998). But, it is first and foremost, a spiritual practice. Because a previous chapter (Chapter 8) contains other background information on meditation and emphasizes TM meditation, this section will focus on another common form of meditation that is more closely associated with spirituality: centering prayer.

Centering prayer is a passive form of meditation in which a sacred word or an image is silently introduced when one becomes aware of thoughts. It is a method for centering or focusing on one's intention of consenting to God's presence. Since, it is not a concentrative form of meditation, it is not an exercise in *attention* which cultivates the faculty of the mind. Rather, it is an exercise of *intention* which cultivates the faculty of the will. In short, it is a spiritual practice for developing habits conducive to responding to the inspirations of the Spirit.

Centering prayer has been described as an initial form of contemplative prayer. Contemplative prayer is a process of interior transformation, a relationship initiated by God and leading to divine union. One's way of perceiving reality changes during this process. A restructuring of consciousness takes place that empowers one to perceive, relate to, and respond with increasing sensitivity to the divine presence and action in, through, and beyond everything that exists.

Centering prayer is not an end in itself but a beginning. It is not done to produce spiritual consolation but rather to increase the experience and expression of charity, joy, peace, self-knowledge, compassion, inner freedom, and humility. To achieve this end, centering prayer must be done regularly, preferably for a minimum of twenty minutes twice a day. To maximize the process, additional spiritual practices are recommended throughout the day. These might include: repetition of a prayer sentence, unconditional acceptance of others, and releasing upsetting emotions as soon as they arise (Keating, 1999).

Mindfulness

Mindfulness, as noted earlier was described as a basic of formal meditation practice, i.e., insight or mindfulness meditation. However, mindfulness can be, and is often, practiced outside of formal meditation. Mindfulness focuses on being fully mindful in the present moment, i.e., being fully aware and attentive to the full range of experiences that exist here and now, moment to moment. Four steps are typically involved in the practice of daily mindfulness.

First, assist the client in picking a given daily activity, such as eating, walking, watching, or listening, and a given time frame. Second, practice being totally present in the activity for that time frame. Third, observe and reflect on one's thoughts and feelings about this experience. Fourth, take these thoughts and feelings into the next activity. For example, an individual may want to be totally present and mindful during a 20-minute walk in the park. She is advised to gently look around and find something of beauty such as a child playing, a tree swaying in the wind, or a squirrel eating an acorn. If she chooses a tree, she may notice the swaying of branches, different colors and movements of individual leaves. At the same time, she becomes aware of thoughts and feelings such as pleasure and appreciation associated with that beauty. Finally, these pleasant thoughts and feelings are extended to other activities. Cf. Chapter 8 for additional information on mindfulness.

Communal Worship

Involvement in public worship or communal liturgical services provides the spiritual seeker with another venue, besides personal prayer and meditation, for communicating and worshiping with their deity. The psychological and spiritual dynamics of communal prayer and worship differ from personal prayer. Communal prayer and worship can provide considerable social, emotional, and spiritual support to members of a worshiping group or community (Pargament, 1997). Conversely, the psychosocial climate of some spiritual communities can be conflictual, hurtful or toxic. As noted in the research section, membership in a spiritual community can provide significant social support which probably accounts for increased longevity and protective effects with regard to disease, depression, and the like. It is not uncommon for spoken and sung prayer and praise, meditation, spiritual teachings, and even forgiveness and confession to occur in communal worship settings. Parenthetically, it may well be that communal prayer was the first form of group therapy.

Fasting

Fasting means abstaining from food or eating sparingly. There are various reasons for fasting: as a means of weight loss, detoxification the body for medical purposes, or as a spiritual practice. Done as a spiritual practice, fasting is abstention from food for the purpose of purification of one's motivation. All the great spiritual traditions recognize its merits. More than any other spiritual practice, fasting can surface and uncover not only the obvious but also the more subtle cravings and desires that control one's life. Food and other substances permit individuals to camouflage aspects of their inner life, which fasting quickly surfaces. Foster notes:

> If pride controls us, it will be revealed almost immediately. Anger, bitterness, jealousy, strife, fear-if they are within us, they will surface during fasting. At first we will rationalize that our anger is due to our hunger; then we will realize that we are angry because the spirit of anger is within us (Foster, 1988, p. 55).

There are other benefits as well. Fasting can foster balance in life. In addition to revealing cravings, it uncovers how nonessentials have taken precedence in our lives. This is important self-knowledge that might we might not otherwise become aware of. Fasting also helps increase our awareness of the plight of others. In commenting on the social dimension of fasting, Walsh says: "I try to use each feeling of hunger to remind me of the many hungry people around the world. That way each hunger pang not only reduces the craving but also elicits concerns and compassion for the hungry" (Walsh, 1999, p. 50).

Some guidelines for safely incorporating fasting as a spiritual practice are offered. The first is that, as with all the spiritual practice, a steady progression and moderation should be observed. That means beginning with a partial fast of no more than twenty-four hours. Fasting from lunch of one day to lunch of the next is the initial recommendation. This means that two meals are skipped, i.e., dinner and breakfast. Only water and fruit juices are taken during this period of fasting. This initial fast is recommended once a week for several weeks. The client should monitor both the physical and spiritual experience during each fast. Keeping a journal or log can be valuable. Particular attention should be directed at the inner attitude of the heart. As individuals go about their regular duties during this time of fasting, they are advised to inwardly pray and to be aware of thoughts and spiritual promptings and cultivate a "gentle receptiveness to divine breathings" (Foster, 1988, p. 57). This initial form of fasting is broken with a light meal of fresh fruits and vegetables. After two or three weeks of this form, the client may be ready for a fast in which only water is consumed. After completing several fasts with a degree of spiritual success, move on to a 36-hour fast: three meals. Fasts lasting longer than this probably should be medically supervised.

Spiritual Reading

Each of the major spiritual traditions in the east and the west view their sacred writings as a source of spiritual and moral wisdom. The purpose for reading sacred writings can differ by traditions and personal need. Some will study their tradition's sacred writings for intellectual reasons, to increase their doctrinal understanding of their tradition's theology or philosophy, while others will read them to find comfort or insight about particular concerns. Sacred writings can also be used for other purposes. These include: (a) challenging and modifying dysfunctional beliefs; (b) reframing and understanding life and problems from a spiritual perspective; (c) clarifying and enriching understanding of religious doctrines; and (d) seeking enlightenment, comfort, and guidance (Richards & Bergin, 1997).

However, a major reason spiritual seekers read and reflect on sacred writings is to put themselves into the presence of the divine. *Lectio divina* is a time-tested method of praying with Christian sacred writings, particularly scriptural texts, in hopes of experiencing the presence of the divine. It has been practiced in many forms by monks and other spiritual seekers for over a thousand years. Lectio divina has been described as the "art of letting God speak to us through his inspired and inspiring Word" (Pennington, 1998, p. xi) and then responding, since it is a two-way communication. The method for practicing lectio divina is a relatively straightforward and simple three-step process. The first is to take the sacred text and call upon the Holy Spirit. The second is to listen to the Lord speaking through the text for about ten minutes. Then reflect on it and respond. Third, choose a word or phrase from the text and reflect on it for the rest of the day.

Confession and Forgiveness

First, it should be noted that although there is some overlap, confession differs from forgiveness. Confession and/or forgiveness are noted to play a role in many spiritual traditions and religious denominations. In some traditions, confession is viewed as a necessary step in seeking forgiveness (Richards & Bergin, 1997). For most traditions and denominations, individuals confess their sins and transgressions directly to their deity, while in some, such as Roman Catholicism and Mormonism, individuals confess indirectly to God through another, such as a priest.

To confess, psychologically places the burden upon the plaintiff, thus therapeutically placing one in the position of being impotent and therefore dependent upon an external power for forgiveness. Therapists recognize the value of "ownership" in the process of psychological healing, and thus find value in the concept and practice of confession. While some religious groups have diminished the concept of confession, its practice and admitted value predates all religions. Psychologically, the admission of guilt places the human ego under the control of the super-ego in the psychoanalytic model, and places the human in need of a "higher power" in all models. The Freudian concept of "father confessor" is doubtless more theological than many, including Freud, might concede, and the early church concept of confession likewise is more therapeutic than its original practitioners understood.

In summary, it should be noted that the therapeutic value of prayer is efficacious in all areas of healing including, the physical, mental, relationships, and even environmental. There is no other addition to the clinician's armamentarium with the same power.

Service

Service is another spiritual practice. Whether called 'altruistic service' (Richards & Bergin, 1997), 'true service' (Foster, 1988) or 'awakened service' (Walsh, 1999), service involves doing something for others. Foster's distinction between 'self-righteous service' and 'true service' is worth noting. Self-righteous service is concerned with making impressive gains and achieving results, it usually requires the reward of recognition by others, picks and chooses whom to serve, and may be affected by moods and whims. True service, on the other hand, makes no distinction between big and small service, is contented with hiddeness, i.e., no recognition, and fosters such virtues as humility and gratitude (Foster, 1988).

Service can take numerous forms, such as providing food to the hungry or clothes and money to the poor, providing emotional support to those who are discouraged or grieving, visiting the sick, or volunteering in one's religious or spiritual community. The results of a national survey of volunteers across the United States found that individuals who helped others consistently reported better health than non-volunteers and that many believed that their health improved after beginning their volunteer service. Furthermore, the vast majority reported that service provided them with a sense of euphoria, greater calm, and relaxation (Luks, 1993).

How can service be utilized as a spiritual practice? Advise participants to select an hour, a morning, or a day for the spiritual practice of service. Five steps are suggested (Walsh, 1999): Begin by dedicating the time and what you will be doing during it. Second, look for ways to serve wherever you are, whoever you are with, and whatever you are doing. Third, try to accomplish the activity in a spirit of service. Fourth, be mindful of the intention to serve in such a way that you learn from each activity while releasing any attachments or bias you may have about those being served. Finally, reflect on how this experience affects your spiritual journey (Foster & Yanni, 1992).

Spiritual Direction, Very Brief Spiritual Counseling/Therapy, and Self Therapy

While spiritual direction, also called spiritual guidance, is usually associated with the Roman Catholic tradition, it is now increasingly common in other traditions, including Episcopal, Methodist, Orthodox, Pentecostal, and Judaism (Moon & Benner, 2004). In spiritual direction, the director assists the directee to listen and discern the presence and movement of God within the directee's life. Prayer often takes place within meetings with the director and prayer and other spiritual practices may be prescribed. In recent years, psychological concepts and psychotherapeutic techniques have increasingly influenced spiritual direction, and making a distinction between the two is sometimes difficult (Sperry, 2003).

As noted previously, the majority of the spiritual therapeutic applications incorporated spirituality into previously established therapeutic approaches. For example, Moriarty (2006) developed a brief therapy approach to working with the God image and depression. In reviewing the literature which suggests people with a negative God image (i.e., emotional experience of God) are more likely to have depressive symptoms, Moriarty proposes a treatment approach which targets helping people change the way they experience God. Previously, Tisdale et al. (1997) conducted research demonstrating the effectiveness of religiously based, object relationship therapy in treating distortions in the God image and issues of personal adjustment. Building from this research, Moriarty (2006) integrates brief psychodynamic and cognitive behavioral therapy to develop a brief approach that changes the God image. The therapist helps the client recognize their distorted beliefs about God, and then works through a process of helping them combat these beliefs through cognitive therapy and the utilization of the therapy relationship.

Another brief approach to spiritual therapy involves the integrating of intercessory prayer and other spiritual interventions with therapy (Tan & Dong, 2001). Many of these interventions may also be used in other context besides therapy as a separate treatment approach. While Tan (1991) also cautions regarding the potential ethical dangers of using spiritual interventions as an adjunct to therapy, he believes integrating them into brief therapy can enhance the effectiveness of the treatment (Tan, 1994; Tan & Johnson, 2005). Thus, by integrating spiritual practices into therapy and/or collaborating with religious professionals in the treatment process, it is possible to increase treatment effectiveness and decrease the length of treatment for many individuals.

Finally, there are individuals who want to engage in self-therapy, or who do not attend communal worship services, or have no affiliation with a religious denomination or spiritual group. What access and availability to spiritual resources is available to them? One such resource was developed by Luciano L'Abate, Ph.D. (L'Abate, 1996). It is a set of Spirituality Workbooks for a wide audience ranging from the religiously committed to the agnostic and atheist who seek greater meaning in their lives. These workbooks are based on three overlapping circles – church, religion, and spirituality – with whatever or whoever is attributed in the center, i.e., a deity, power, etc. The workbooks can be incorporated as an adjunct to therapy or used as self-therapy. They are titled the *CRS Sentences Workbook* and the *CRS Words Workbook* and can be found at *www.mentalhealthhelp.com.*

Utilizing Spiritual Practices as Low Cost Interventions

We have reviewed meditation, prayer, mindfulness communal worship, fasting, spiritual reading, communal worship, confession, and service as spiritual practices/interventions. We have noted their use in spiritual direction and very brief spiritual counseling/therapy. With the exception of spiritual direction which sometimes involves a donation, and brief spiritual counseling/therapy which almost always involves a fee, the spiritual practices/interventions discussed in this chapter can be essentially free of any fee or remuneration. These interventions can be practiced privately or communally. They can be learned from listening, reading, and modeling, at a seminar, a retreat or from a spiritual mentor – which might have begun in early life because of a parent, minister or teacher or later because of a spiritual community, minister or spiritual guru. They can all be self-administered or prescribed and monitored by a spiritual guide, spiritual director or therapist. An individual may become interested in spiritual practices as the result of a conversion or experience of intense spiritual longing. Whether the individual continues with such practices is dependent on a number of factors which include readiness to change, perceived positive change, social support of a spiritual community or the advice and validation of a spiritual guide, etc.

Concluding Note

A multidimensional model and definition of spirituality was described to serve as an organizing principle to aid in comprehending theory and research regarding physical health and psychological well-being as well as spiritual transcendence. In that model spiritual practice is a key dimension. The remainder of the chapter described the use of spiritual practices as adjuncts in spiritually attuned psychotherapy and counseling, or low-cost/no-cost interventions outside the context of therapy.

References

Ano, G. G., & Vasconcellos, E. B. (2005). Religious coping and psychological adjustment to stress: A meta-analysis. *Journal of Clinical Psychology, 61*, 461–480.

Bergin, A. E. (1983). Religiosity and mental health: A critical reevaluation and meta-analysis. *Professional Psychology: Research and Practice, 14*, 170–184.

Bergin, A. E. (1991). Values and religious issues in psychotherapy and mental health. *American Psychologist, 46*, 394–403.

Byrd, R. C. (1988). Positive therapeutic effects of intercessory prayer in a coronary care unit population. *Southern Medical Journal, 81*, 826–829.

Carlson, C. R., Bacaseta, P. E., & Simanton, D. A. (1988). A controlled evaluation of devotional meditation and progressive relaxation. *Journal of Psychology and Theology, 16*, 362–368.

Carrington, P. (1998). *The book of meditation*. Boston: Element Books.

Chamberlain, T. J., & Hall, C. A. (2000). *Realized religion*. Philadelphia, PA: Templeton Foundation Press.

Cloninger, C. R., & Svrakic, D. (1994). Integrative psychobiological approach to psychiatric assessment and treatment. *Psychiatry, 60*, 120–41.

Cloninger, C. R. (2004). *Feeling good: The science of well-being*. New York: Oxford University Press.

Cloninger, C. R. (2006). *The science of well-being: The essentials of psychophathology*. New York: Oxford University Press.

Domasio, A. (2003). *Looking for Spinoza: Joy, sorrow, and the feeling brain*. Orlando, FL: Harcourt.

D'Souza R., & Rodrigo, A. (2004). Spiritually-augmented cognitive behavioral therapy. *Australasian Psychiatry, 12*, 148–152.

Ellison, C. G., & Anderson, K. L. (2001). Religious involvement and domestic violence among U.S. couples. *Journal for the Scientific Study of Religion, 40*, 269–286.

Emmons, R. (1999). *The psychology of ultimate concerns: Motivation and spirituality in personality*. New York: Guilford.

Emmons, R. (2000). Is spirituality an intelligence? Motivation, cognition and the psychology of ultimate concerns. *International Journal of Psychology of Religion, 10*, 1, 3–26.

Ervin-Cox, B., Hoffman, L., & Grimes, C. S. M. (2005). Selected literature on spirituality and health/mental health. In R. H. Cox, B. Ervin-Cox, & L. Hoffman (Eds.), *Spirituality and psychological health* (pp. 262–283). Colorado Springs, CO: Colorado School of Professional Psychology Press.

Foster, R., & Yanni, K. (1992). *Celebrating the disciplines: A journal workbook*. San Francisco: HarperSan Francisco.

Foster, R. (1988). Celebration of discipline: *The path to spiritual growth. Revised and expanded edition*. San Francisco: HarperSan Francisco.

Freud, S. (1961). *The future of an illusion* (J. Strachey trans.). New York: Norton & Company. (Original work published in 1927)

Grossman, P., Niemann, L., Schmidt, S., & Walach, H. (2003). Mindfulness-based stress reduction and health benefits: A meta-analysis. *Journal of Psychosomatic Research, 57*, 35–43.

Hackney, C. H., & Sanders, G. S. (2003). Religiosity and mental health: A meta-analysis of recent studies. *Journal for the Scientific Study of Religion, 42*, 43–55.

Hamer, D. (2004). *The God gene: How faith is hardwired into our genes*. New York: Doubleday.

Hawkins, R. S., Tan, S.-Y., & Turk, A. A. (1999). Secular versus Christian cognitive-behavioral therapy programs: Impact on depression and spiritual well-being. *Journal of Psychology and Theology, 27*, 309–331.

Hinikka, J., Koskela, T., Kontula, O., Koskela, K., Koivumaa-Honkanen, H.-T., & Viinamaki, H. (2001). Religious attendance and life satisfaction in the Finnish general population. *Journal of Psychology and Theology, 29*, 158–164.

James, W. (1902). *The varieties of religious experience*. New York: The New American Library.

Johnson, W. B., DeVries, R., Ridley, C. R., Pettorini, D., & Peterson, D. R. (1994). The comparative efficacy of Christian and secular rational-emotive therapy with Christian clients. *Journal of Psychology and Theology, 22*, 130–140.

Jung, C. G. (1958). *Psychology and religion*. New Haven, CT: Yale University Press.

Katz, S. (2004). *The Spiritual Transformation Scientific research program*. Philadelphia, PA: Metanexus Institute on Religion and Science.

Keating, T. (1999). Practicing centering prayer. In Reininger, G. (Ed.). *The diversity of centering prayer* (pp. 16–26). New York: Continuum.
Koenig, H. G., & Larson, D. B. (2001). Religion and mental health: Evidence for an association. *International Review of Psychiatry, 13*, 67–78.
Koenig, H. G., McCullough, M. E., & Larson, D. B. (2001). *Handbook of religion and health.* New York: Oxford University Press.
L'Abate, L. (1996). *Workbooks for Better Living* (www.mentalhealthhelp.com)
Luks, A. (1993). The healing power of doing good. New York: Ballantine Books.
Marlatt, G. & Kristeller, J. (1999). Mindfulness and meditation. In Miller, W. (ed.). Integrating spirituality in treatment. (pp. 67–84). Washington, D.C.: American Psychological Association.
Maslow, A. H. (1962). *Toward a psychology of being.* Princeton, NJ: Van Nostrand.
Maslow, A. (1968). *Toward a psychology of being. Second edition.* New York: Van Nostrand.
McCullough, M. E. (1999). Research on religion-accommodative counseling: Review and meta-analysis. *Journal of Counseling Psychology, 46*, 92–98.
McSherry, W., & Cash, K. (2004). The language of spirituality: An emerging taxonomy. *International Journal of Nursing Studies, 41*, 151–161.
Miller, W., & C'de Baca, J. (2001). *Quantum change: When epiphanies and sudden insights 'transform ordinary lives.* New York: Guilford.
Moon, G. W., & Benner, D. G. (2002). Psychotherapy and spiritual direction, Part I [Special Issues]. *Journal of Psychology and Theology, 30(4).*
Moon, G. W., & Benner, D. G. (2003). Psychotherapy and spiritual direction, Part II [Special Issue]. *Journal of Psychology and Theology, 31(1).*
Moon, G. W., & Benner, D. G. (2004). *Spiritual direction and the care of souls.* Downers Grove, IL: InterVarsity Press.
Moriarty, G. (2006). *Pastoral care of depression: Helping clients heal their relationship with God.* New York: Haworth Press.
Pargament, K. I. (1997). *The psychology of religion and coping: Theory, research, practice.* New York: The Guilford Press.
Pargament, K. (1999). The psychology of religion and spirituality? Yes and no. *International Journal of Psychology of Religion, 9*, 3–16.
Pargament, K. I., Smith, B. W., Koenig, H. G., & Perez, L. (1999). Patterns of positive and negative religious coping with major life stressors. *Journal for the Scientific Study of Religion, 37*, 710–724.
Pennington, B. (1998). *Lectio divina: Renewing the ancient practice of praying the scriptures.* New York: Crossroads.
Piedmont, R. (1999). Does spiritual represent the sixth factor of personality? Spiritual transcendence and the five-factor model. *Journal of Personality, 67*, 985–1013.
Poloma, M. & Pendleton, B. (1989). Exploring types of prayer and quality of life. A research note. *Review of Religious Research, 31,* 46–53
Propst, L. R. (1980). The comparative efficacy of religious and nonreligious imagery for the treatment of mild depression in religious individuals. *Cognitive Therapy and Research, 4*, 167–178.
Propst, L. R., Ostrom, R., Watkins, P., Dean, T., & Mashburn, D. (1992). Comparative efficacy of religious and nonreligious cognitive-behavioral therapy for the treatment of clinical depression in religious individuals. *Journal of Consulting and Clinical Psychology, 60*, 94–103.
Reed, P. (1991). Toward a nursing theory of self-transcendence: Deductive reformulation using developmental theories. *Advances in Nursing Science, 13(4)*, 64–77.
Richards, P., & Bergin, A. (1997) *A spiritual strategy for counseling and psychotherapy.* Washington, DC: American Psychological Association.
Rolheiser, R. (1999). *The holy longing: The search for a Christian spirituality.* New York: Doubleday.

Rye, M. S., Pargament, K. I., Ali, M. A., Beck, G. L., Dorff, E. N., Hallisey, C., Narayanan, V., & Williams, J. G. (2000). Religious perspectives on forgiveness. In M. E. McCullough, K., Pargament, & C. E. Thoresen (Eds.), *Forgiveness: Theory, research, and practice*. New York: Guilford Press.

Sperry, L. (2002). *Spirituality in clinical practice: Incorporating the spiritual dimension in psychotherapy and counseling*. New York: Brunner-Routledge.

Sperry, L. (2003). Integrating spiritual direction functions in the practice of psychotherapy. *Journal of Psychology and Theology, 31,* 3–13.

Sperry, L., & Shafranske, E. (2005), Introduction. In L. Sperry & E. P. Shafranske (Eds.), *Spiritually oriented psychotherapy* (pp. 3–8). Washington, DC: American Psychological Association.

Sperry, L. (2006). Is a consensus definition of spirituality possible? Theory construction in spiritually-oriented psychotherapy. *Research in the Social Scientific Study of Religion, 17*, 10–22.

Sawatzky, R, Ratner, P. A., & Chiu, L. (2005). A meta-analysis of the relationship between spirituality and quality of life. *Social Indicators Research, 72*, 153–188.

Stawaski, C. (2003). Definitions and hypotheses: William James, religion and spiritual transformation. *Cross Currents, 53(3)*, 424–437.

Tan, S.-Y. (1987). Cognitive-behavior therapy: A biblical approach and critique. *Journal of Psychology and Theology, 15*, 103–112.

Tan, S.-Y. (1994). Ethical considerations in religious psychotherapy: Potential pitfalls and unique resources. *Journal of Psychology and Theology, 22*, 389–394.

Tan, S.-Y., & Dong, N. J. (2001). Spiritual interventions in healing and wholeness. In T. G. Plante & A. C. Sherman (Eds.), *Faith and health: Psychological perspectives* (pp. 291–310). New York: The Guilford Press.

Tan, S.-Y., & Johnson, W. B. (2005). Spiritually oriented cognitive-behavioral therapy. In L. Sperry & E. P. Shafranske (Eds.), *Spiritually oriented psychotherapy* (pp. 77–103). Washington, DC: American Psychological Association.

Teasdale, J. D., Segal, Z., & Williams, J. M. G. (1995). How does cognitive therapy prevent depressive relapse and why should attentional control (mindfulness) training help? *Behavior Research and Therapy, 33*, 25–39.

Tloczynski, J., & Fritzsch, S. (2002). Intercessory prayer in psychological well-being: using a multiple-baseline, across-subjects design. *Psychological Reports, 91*, 731–741. [Abstract] Retrieved November 17, 2005, from PsycINFO database.

Tisdale, T. C., Key, T. L., Edwards, K. J., Brokaw, B. F., Kemperman, S. R., Cloud, H., Townsend, J., & Okamoto, T. (1997). Impact of treatment of God image and personal adjustment, and correlations of God image to personal adjustment and object relations development. *Journal of Psychology and Theology, 25*, 227–239.

Walsh, R. (1999). *Essential spirituality: The seven central practices to awaken heart and mind*. New York: Wiley.

Section VI

Tertiary Multi-Personal Approaches

Admittedly, the dividing line between secondary and tertiary is artificial and arbitrary. One could use, for instance, survival versus enjoyment as a dividing line. However, that line already exists between Sections II and III. One cannot enjoy without surviving while surviving physically may occur without enjoyment, with a great deal of pain. At this point, the only line that can be drawn lies in the level of complexity involved in relational, multi-personal activities and alliances that include groups, or animal-human relationships directed toward a common, observable activity or goal. In the previous Section V, some chapters dealt with intrapsychic topics that were produced by dyadic relational experiences. For instance, intimacy, forgiveness, and spirituality might have been directly affected by close physical contact, extended touch, and affection. In this section, activities or interventions are directed toward relationships that may be dyadic, as in animal companions, but that could be extended to groups of intimates, as in the animal-family connection, groups of friends, and support groups.

23

Friendship, Social Support, and Health

Patricia M. Sias and Heidi Bartoo

Both researchers and popular press writers have contributed to the recent media buzz linking friendship to physical and mental health. *Psychology Today* (1999) touts research that indicates individuals in general, and women in particular, underutilize friendship as a powerful healing force for physical and mental illness. According to the article, a group of chronically depressed women experienced substantial improvement in mental health when they were prescribed personal "befrienders" who visited, went on outings with, and became confidants of the participants over a 12-month period. The findings after the first year of befriending yielded the same success rate as traditional medical and psychological interventions (i.e. antidepressants or cognitive therapies). Further, the most successful women in the study group experienced a feeling of renewal in their personal and social lives that enabled them to move forward in more healthy ways (Raymond, 1999).

Having friends can apparently also lead to differences in an individual's physical and biochemical reactions to environmental stressors (Taylor, Klein, Lewis, Gruenewald, Gurung, & Updegraff, 2000). Specifically, studies conducted at UCLA revealed that some individuals (women, in particular) have the tendency to "tend and befriend," rather than resort to the more common "fight or flight" response as a first line of defense against environmental and social stressors. Tending and befriending deals specifically with the act of self-disclosure between trusted companions to talk or work through the stresses in one's life. Because friendships are grounded in communication, functional friendships provide a strong sense of personal support. Individuals who feel supported by their close friends tend to live longer, stay healthier, and have a more positive outlook when faced with adversity (Taylor et al., 2000).

Understanding the health benefits of friendships can provide individuals with a sense of safety, security, and support against life's unknowns. These feelings are similar to the sense of security we feel when we receive medical vaccines for proactive prevention of diseases. Friends are also an outward reflection of parts of our self and this provides us the opportunity to more deeply understand our own place and behavior. This chapter addresses the link between friendship and overall health by conceptualizing friendship as a behavioral vaccine.

Friendship as "Behavioral Vaccine"

As Duck and Pittman (1994) note, relationships are mental creations constituted by interaction. Our relationships with others are defined by how we communicate with those others and exist in our perceptions of that interaction. Across many interpersonal interactions, we develop cognitive maps of our friendships as they are interconnected within our social network (Duck and Pittman, 1994). In many ways, this cognitive map is similar to keeping an updated medical immunization record. Maintaining the "optimal dosage" of friendship requires constant monitoring and negotiation, because our relationship needs vary along with our personal and emotional needs (Duck and Pittman, 1994). In our view, the friendships fostered and developed at different points in our lives are a snapshot of our personal and communication needs at particular points in the lifespan.

Just as there are recommended doses for over-the-counter medications, prescriptions, and medical vaccines depending upon one's age, gender, illness, and risk factors, personal relationships should be a "match" to the individual enacting them. While we cannot offer a "one-size-fits-all" friendship vaccine to meet everyone's relational needs, we believe that understanding how friendship is associated with health is an effective starting point toward proactive physical and mental health.

We maintain that friendship functions as a behavioral vaccine primarily through its social support functions. In the following sections, we develop a model outlining the links between friendship, social support, and health. We conclude by providing practical advice regarding the initiation and maintenance of friendship networks with the goal of improved physical and mental health.

Health and Social Support

The goal of behavioral vaccines is the proactive promotion of positive physical and mental health by way of behavioral, rather than medical, means. Fundamental to the concept of a behavioral vaccine is the notion that an individual's physical and mental health is framed by his/her social environment. Humans are social beings who interact with others to make sense of their social experience (Weick, 1979). Social interaction enables individuals not only to understand their personal and social experiences, but also to develop, learn, and ultimately survive across their lifespan. Social support is a crucial form of such interaction.

Social support is conceptually defined as verbal and nonverbal communication between receiver and provider that reduces uncertainty about a situation, one's self, another, or a relationship, and enhances the perception of control over one's life (Albrecht & Adelman, 1987). Thus, social support is, by definition, a communicative phenomenon.

Individuals obtain three primary types of social support in the context of interpersonal relationships: emotional, informational, and tangible (Schaefer, Coyne, & Lazarus, 1981). *Emotional support* is characterized by direct empathetic and compassionate behaviors (e.g., being a "shoulder to cry on"). *Informational support* involves sharing knowledge to help others make sense of specific social experiences. *Tangible support* involves the provision of tangible resources such as money and help with tasks. In other words, emotional support is "feeling", informational support is "telling," and tangible support is "doing" (Schaefer et al., 1981). All three types of social support share an important quality in that they are all enacted through human communication.

In their extensive review, Albrecht, Burleson, & Goldsmith (1994) discuss two widely cited explanations of the relationship between social support and mental health. The first explanation suggests that social support leads to positive mental health in a direct and linear fashion. According to this perspective, positive mental health is a product of healthy interpersonal interaction within one's social support networks. The quality of one's mental health is proportional to the actual support given or received, in addition to the perceived availability of support within one's network. An underlying assumption of this position is that a "supported individual" has more opportunities to develop and adopt healthy behaviors and attitudes as a result of modeling and the demonstration of desirable characteristics from within one's social support network (Hammer, 1983; Seeman & Sayles, 1985). For example, receiving information or encouragement from others regarding healthy lifestyle choices in the form of informational or emotional social support will enhance the likelihood that the "supported" individual will make healthy life choices.

The second position suggests that social support influences health by buffering the negative physical and mental health effects caused by stress. This position conceptualizes social support networks as an important moderating link between stress and health (i.e. Cohen & McKay, 1984; DeLongis, Folkman, & Lazarus, 1988). This position offers a triangulated view of the relationship between social support, mental health, and stress. It provides the complexity necessary to account for differences (i.e., specific events) in individuals' social experiences.

Although these positions are often presented as conflicting, we maintain that they actually reflect two different, but complementary, forms of social support – *general social support* and *targeted social support*. General social support, reflected by the first position, refers to ongoing, supportive behavior that occurs under normal circumstances. Targeted social support, reflected by the second position, refers to supportive behavior that is targeted toward, and reactive to, specific events that induce a stress response and threaten an individual's mental health. These are explained in greater detail below.

General Social Support

Social support functions generally as individuals share feelings, information, and activities during their everyday lives. Fortunately, most individuals' lives are not rife with stressful events such as illness, marital problems, and the like. Day-to-day functioning is typically routine, stable, and predictable. Despite the lack of critical stressful events, however, individuals still require and rely upon social support from others. Social support is enacted in several ways during "everyday conversation (Barnes & Duck, 1994)." For example, "everyday" social support communication performs a *ventilation* function through which individuals vent about routine stressors in order to prevent them from escalating (e.g., complaining to, and seeking advice from, a friend about your consistently annoying boss). Everyday social support communication also performs a *perpetuation* function by helping individuals maintain "continuity in relationships which increases support availability and greater ease in mobilization of support." Relatedly, they argue, through the *regulation* function, that everyday social support communication "provides regulation of face needs within relationships by reducing the severity of potentially embarrassing requests for help." Thus, "everyday" communication performs a general social support function by helping individuals deal with routine, recurring events, and by helping individuals maintain balance and stability in their interpersonal relationships. Returning to our "inoculation" metaphor, this position conceptualizes social support as akin to a "daily vitamin" that provides the body with the nutrients required for overall health. Figure 23.1 illustrates the general social support model.

It is important to note that general social support is related to, and in fact, enables, targeted social support, which is discussed in the next section.

Targeted Social Support

Although not typically a constant feature of everyday life, stress-inducing events such as illness, marital problems, or workplace trauma, do occur. During such times, social support performs a buffering function, reducing the extent to which stress harms the individual's mental health (Helgeson & Lepore, 1997). In contrast to general social support, this type of social support is explicitly *targeted* toward helping individuals cope with a specific stressful event (Hoybye, Johansen & Tjornhoj-Thomsen, 2005). Metaphorically speaking, in contrast to the "daily vitamin" provided by general social support, we suggest that targeted social support is akin to a vaccine targeted toward a specific disease or health threat. Imagine, for example, a situation in which a woman has been diagnosed with breast cancer. Once that information is shared with others in her social support network, targeted social support is triggered. Friends may provide informational social support by sharing information regarding similar experiences they, or others they know, have gone through. Toward this end, they may share information regarding particular health care providers, support groups, or suggestions for managing treatment effects (e.g., where to purchase wigs and scarves to deal with chemo-induced hair loss). Support network members will likely provide instrumental support such as driving the individual to doctor's appointments, providing meals when the individual is feeling sick, taking care of the patient's children, and the like. And, of course, friends will likely offer much emotional support targeted toward providing empathy and sympathy to the patient as she processes her new role as cancer patient. Figure 23.2 illustrates our targeted social support model.

Although targeted social support cannot inoculate the target individual against the cancer, it can help "minimize" the psychological damage of the disease by buffering its stressful effects on the patient's mental health. Just as an inoculated child may nonetheless develop a very mild case of chicken

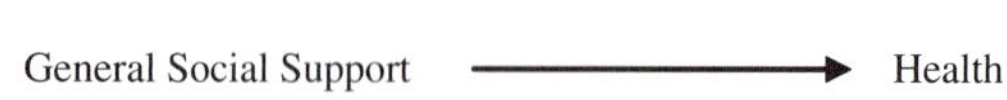

Figure 23.1. General Social Support Model.

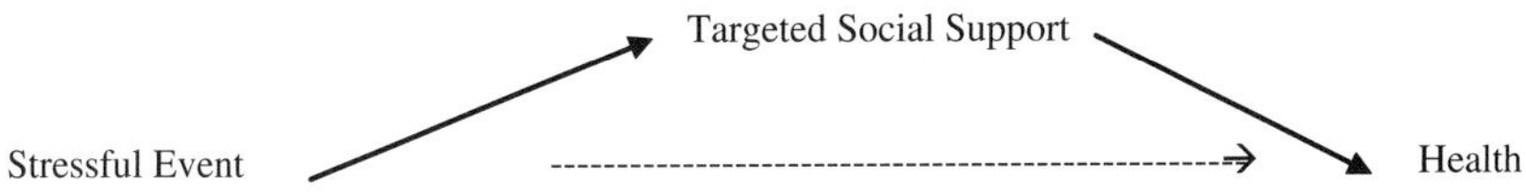

Figure 23.2. Target Social Support Model.

pox, the targeted social support "vaccine" minimizes the mental and physical health effects the cancer patient would have experienced without the vaccine (Helgeson & Lepore, 1997; Lepore & Helgeson, 1998).

Social Support Reciprocity

We have focused thus far on explaining the link between social support and health from the perspective of *receiving* social support. Research indicates, however, that individuals can also reap mental health benefits by *providing* social support to others (i.e. Schroeder, Penner, Dovidio, & Piliavin, 1995). This likely results from two dynamics. First, again returning to our "vaccine" metaphor, reciprocal social support among the various members of a social support network enhances the overall health of those members. For example, if an individual quits smoking cigarettes (a behavioral vaccine against physical diseases like cancer and heart disease), they may or may not talk to others about their decision. If they don't share that information with others, their choice to quit smoking will, technically, only "vaccinate" that nonsmoking individual. If, however, they talk about their choice with others (through informational social support), the behavioral vaccine can function at both the individual and network levels by encouraging others to make the positive choice to quit smoking. In essence, the most potent behavioral vaccine not only vaccinates an individual, but also opens the door for others to engage in similar health behavior, via the provision of social support. This is demonstrated in the findings of the British study where many of the befriended companions became more likely to befriend others after the 12-month study time frame.

Second, and relatedly, effective targeted social support depends largely on effective general social support. Maintaining a network of general social support providers increases the likelihood that you will receive targeted social support when you need it. If an individual has not developed a general social support network, when faced with a traumatic event, such as illness, it will be more difficult to obtain the targeted social support so important for buffering that trauma. As mentioned earlier, for example, providing "regulative" general social support is crucial for maintaining social relationships and, as a consequence, reducing the potential embarrassment that accompanies requests for help which one might need during times of crisis (Barnes & Duck, 1994). Thus, providing general social support over time increases the likelihood that you will receive targeted social support when needed. This explanation highlights the reciprocal relationship between general and targeted social supported, illustrated in Figure 23.3.

Having established the link between social support and health, the following section discusses friends – important members of social support networks.

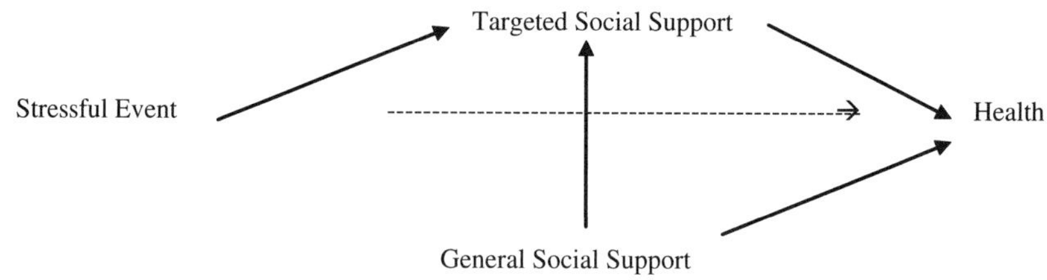

Figure 23.3. Relationship between General and Targeted Social Support.

Social Support and Friendship

Social support networks are essentially systems of social relationships. Just as social support is a communicative phenomenon, we conceptualize relationships as social categories that are created, maintained and altered through communication (Sigman, 1995). Relationships do not exist outside the partners involved but are social phenomena constituted in partners' interaction (Duck & Pittman, 1994). At the same time, partners' perceptions of their relationship influence their communication with one another. Thus, communication between relationship partners is influenced by their past interaction and informs their future interaction. As a consequence, relationships are defined by *patterned* interaction that occurs over *time*. Such a conceptualization emphasizes the dynamic nature of relationships, yet recognizes stability (patterned behavior over time) within that dynamism (Sias, Krone, & Jablin, 2002). Such a conceptualization also acknowledges both the general and targeted social support functions discussed above.

A long line of research has identified the important role a particular type of relationship – friendship – plays in social support. Friends are typically the people to whom we turn first, and most frequently, when dealing with life crises (Pennebaker & O'Heeron, 1984; Lowenthal & Haven, 1968). A discussion of the characteristics and qualities of friendship explains why.

What is Friendship?

Friendship is a unique, and uniquely important, type of relationship, distinguished by two primary characteristics. First, friendships are *voluntary*. Unlike family or work relationships which are typically imposed upon an individual, we choose our friends and voluntarily spend time with them. Second, friendships have a *personalistic focus* in which we come to know and view our friends as "whole persons" rather than simply occupants of particular roles (e.g., our boss or next-door neighbor).

Friendship's foundation rests on two important qualities – liking and trust. Friends like each other and share an affinity for one another (Hill & Stull, 1981). The affinity found in friendship, while not romantic (this is what makes friendship unique from a romantic relationship), is nonetheless strong and, in close friendships, intimate. Friends also trust one another and, therefore, share information with one another that they would not share with mere acquaintances (Davidson & Duberman, 1982). Accordingly, self-disclosure is an important dynamic in friendship initiation, development, and maintenance (Altman & Taylor, 1973).

These characteristics and qualities make friendships particularly useful sites of social support. As many researchers note, seeking social support can be "face-threatening" (Goldsmith, 1992). Asking others for help or sympathy threatens the individual's image as an independent, capable, and strong person (all highly valued qualities in the U.S. culture). The characteristics and qualities of friendship described above minimize such threats. For example, because friends interact with one another as "whole persons," they are more likely than others (workplace acquaintances, for example); to be aware that their friend is experiencing stress or trauma and, therefore, are well-placed to provide *unsolicited* social support, so that the target individual does not need to ask for it. As information about our imaginary individual's breast cancer diagnosis makes its way through the network, for example, friends are likely to phone the individual, send cards, drop by with gifts, food, and information, often without the patient requesting such help.

Sharing your troubles and concerns with others requires that you like and trust them. Toward this end, outside of family, it is our friends upon whom we rely for trusted information and supportive dialogue. The realization that one is supported by and trusted to support another is an empowering idea that may direct and define the strength and reliability of social support behavior and the perception of social support availability within one's social network.

It is important to note, however, the reciprocal relationship between friendship and social support. While friends are key sources of both general and targeted social support, acts of social support often lead to the initiation, and development of, friendship. As the befrienders study indicates, even professional friends who are, in essence, "prescribed" to provide social support often end up maintaining/further developing the friendships at the interpersonal level (Raymond, 1999).

Social support interaction is characterized by self-disclosure (Barnes & Duck, 1994), which is a key factor in friendship initiation and development (Altman & Taylor, 1973). Friendships often begin when one individual discloses information to another that demonstrates similarity (with respect to values, attitudes, or social status) or an attractive personality trait (Sias & Cahill, 1998). This disclosure, and its positive reception, encourages further, reciprocal disclosure, between the partners (Davis & Perkowitz, 1979). As the self-disclosure escalates, the relationship develops the personalistic focus characteristic of friendship. In addition, as the disclosure process continues, trust between the members grows. Thus, stressful events, and the social support communication that accompanies them, often provide the seeds of friendship. As Wills (1985) noted, "Under normal circumstances, most people probably have the information necessary for effective functioning. It is only when environmental stresses exceed the person's available knowledge and problem-solving ability that (additional resources and support) become necessary" (p. 70). In such cases, a stressful experience leads to seeking, and receiving, social support from individuals who are not friends, but the act of social support leads them to become friends.

Consider, again, our imaginary breast cancer patient. If none of her friends has experienced breast cancer themselves, the social support they provide will be limited and likely will not fulfill all of her support needs. Instead, the patient will likely turn to others for support, particularly informational and instrumental support. Cancer "support" groups are so called because their

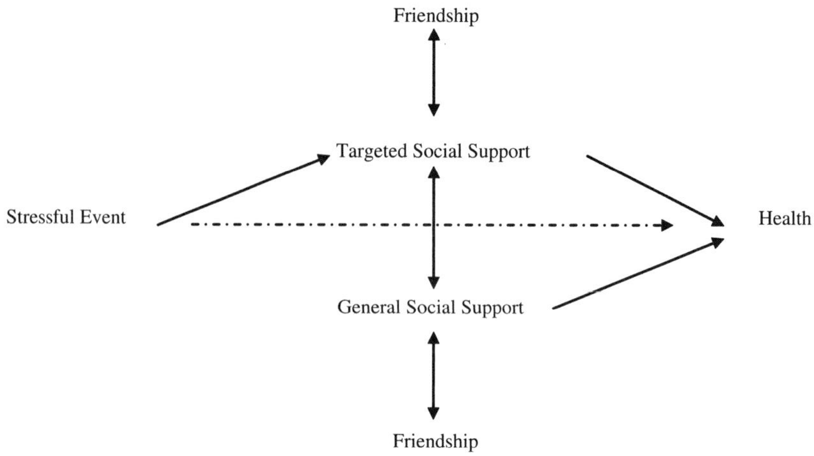

Figure 23.4. Stress, Friendship, Social Support and Health.

members (all cancer participants or survivors) provide social support to one another that the participants' friends and family cannot. It is not uncommon for relationships developed in support groups to continue and grow even closer once the cancer treatments end and the patient is no longer involved in the "official" support group (Ornish, 1998). Similar dynamics occur with support groups that address other types of stressful events such as divorce (Oygard, 2003) and spousal abuse (Brandl, Hebert, Rozwadowski & Spangler, 2003). In sum, friendships developed and maintained by way of general social support become important sources of targeted social support when stressful events occur. At the same time, individuals experiencing stressful events develop new friendships as they seek targeted social support they cannot obtain through their existing social support network. These new friends, in turn, eventually become important sources of general social support. Figure 23.4 illustrates the complete reciprocal model of friendship, social support, and health.

Understanding Friendship Development

Clearly, friendship is an important site for social support. Given its voluntary nature, the use of friendship as a behavioral vaccine to promote mental health is difficult to manipulate and monitor. You cannot force people to like and trust one another. You cannot force them to spend time with one another. It is possible, however, to influence the social environment in ways that provide individuals with opportunities to develop supportive friendships if they so desire. Such "interventions" require a solid understanding of friendship initiation and development processes (Blieszner & Adams, 1992).

Friendship Developmental Influences

As mentioned earlier, human relationships are socially constructed. They exist in, and are constituted by, the communication of the relationship partners. Accordingly, as communication changes, so does the relationship. And the extent to which the communication is stable reflects the stability of the relationship. This notion is empowering because it emphasizes that individuals have more control over their relationships than they think. It is also critical for understanding friendship initiation and development processes, and, therefore, developing effective ways of "prescribing" friendships to promote health.

Friendship researchers have identified several factors that influence friendship initiation, development, and deterioration. These factors fall into two main categories – *individual* and *contextual/environmental* (Fehr, 1996; Sias & Cahill, 1998). Individual factors are those that derive from the relationship partners themselves, such as personality and perceived similarity. Contextual factors derive from the context in which the friendship exists, such as important events in the friends' lives (e.g., marital problems, health concerns) and proximity (e.g., neighbors) (Sias, Smith & Avdeyeva, 2003).

We note that all of these developmental factors result from, or are enabled by, communication. Thus, opportunities to develop friendships require opportunities for interaction. We address individual factors first. *Perceived similarity* and *personality/liking* are the two primary individual factors that influence friendship initiation and development. Self-disclosure enables these dynamics. By communicatively disclosing information about yourself, others are able to gauge the extent to which they share your values, experiences, and beliefs. The more similar they perceive themselves to you, the more likely a friendship will begin (Sias & Cahill, 1998). Similarly, it is only through communication that our personalities become apparent to others. The more other individuals like our personality traits, the more likely a friendship will begin (Rodin, 1978).

Contextual factors influence friendship initiation and development primarily by way of the opportunities they provide for interaction. Along these lines, much research indicates the importance of *proximity* (also referred to as "propinquity") to friendship development (Newcomb, 1961). We tend to become friends with people with whom we have physical contact such as neighbors (Newcomb, 1961) or coworkers whose desks or workstations are near ours (Sias & Cahill, 1998). This is largely due to the opportunities for interaction provided by their proximity. We talk to people we come into contact with. These discussions provide opportunities for self-disclosure and, consequently, friendship development.

Relatedly, although they may not live or work near one another, individuals may become friends through *shared activities*. This may derive from club membership (e.g., PTA, Kiwanis, etc.) or shared work projects (Sias & Cahill, 1998). The common activity or task, again, provides opportunities for interaction that lead to friendship development. This is an important developmental influence in that individuals do not necessarily need to be in physical proximity to develop a friendship. They simply must interact with one another on a particular project or task. Thus, researchers note the possibility of "virtual friendships" that develop absent physical proximity (Sias & Cahill, 1998; Wright, 2004).

Life events, another important contextual factor, influence friendship development (Sias & Cahill, 1998; Sias et al., 2001). Life events are important events that occur in individuals' personal lives, including marriage, divorce, illness, childbirth, workplace problems, and the like. This contextual factor is particularly relevant to this chapter because life events impact friendship development explicitly through the context they provide for social support. The breast cancer diagnosis and ensuing treatment discussed above would be considered a life event and, as explained in the previous section, provides opportunities for the individual experiencing that event to seek out and receive social support. In doing so, the social support network becomes dynamic and elaborate. It provides valuable friendship resources when necessary and encourages others to turn to or seek out support from the cancer patient and from within his/her network as the friendships develop.

Friendship Phases

Friendships develop through a series of phases or transitions and the developmental factors discussed above become more or less important as the relationship evolves. Researchers have labeled the phases of friendship in various ways (Fehr, 1996). Sias & Cahill (1998) provide a phase model that includes three main transitions in friendship development: Acquaintance-to-Friend, Friend-to-Close Friend, and Close friend-to-Best Friend. Although this research was conducted with respect to workplace friendships, these transitions are consistent with interpersonal research conducted with nonworkplace samples (Davis & Todd, 1985).

Friendship initiation occurs during the "acquaintance-to-friend" transition. In this early stage, friendships begin as individuals perceive they are similar to one another in a variety of ways (e.g., values, opinions, background, etc.) and as they develop an appreciation of one another's personality and an affinity for one another. Shared activities or tasks also are important during this early transition, as they provide multiple opportunities for the interaction necessary for individuals to learn about each other. In essence, the communication that occurs during the "acquaintance-to-friend" transition helps the relationship develop the "personalistic focus" necessary for friendship.

The first transition sets the stage for the next two: friend-to-close friend and close friend-to-best friend. As the relationship takes on a personalistic focus, and as the partners communicate more frequently, more openly, and more broadly, trust develops and the friendship grows closer. At these latter stages, life events become more important. Again, this is due to the opportunity such events provide for social support communication (Sias & Cahill, 1998). Thus, as friendships within one's social network become more stable and developed, they rely less on the common predictors and indicators of friendship as an entity and take on a unique identity in one's social network through communication interaction between friendship partners.

With this understanding of friendship development, we turn in the next section to advice for "prescribing" friendship.[1]

---

[1] Much research has examined the extent to which men and women differ with respect to friendship development. Results have generally been mixed. A review of this research led Fehr (1996) to conclude that while men and women differ in some ways (e.g., women talk more frequently to their friends, have more sources of emotional support, communicate somewhat more intimately with their friends than do men), they are also quite similar – both men and women's relationships development via self-disclosure, proximity, shared activities, etc.

Prescribing Friendship

In their seminal chapter, Blieszner and Adams (1992) identified various levels appropriate for friendship intervention. Interventions targeted at the *individual level* focus on altering individuals' personalities, attitudes, and social skills. As the authors noted, interventions at the individual level are extremely difficult, if not unrealistic, because, "First, it is difficult to change basic personality attributes and second, individual-level interventions that conflict with the values and norms of the person's network will be neutralized or discredited by network members" (Blieszner & Adams, 1992, p. 113).

Network level interventions are founded on the notion that social support is a primary function of friendship – a notion fundamental to this chapter. Such intervention involves developing enriched and effective social support networks, important elements of which are friendships. In a way, this chapter is a network-level intervention. It is designed to help individuals, through their mental health practitioners, understand the importance of friendship for mental health, and to develop effective and supportive friendship networks.

Toward this end, the following sections provide suggestions for interventions that both broaden and strengthen individuals' friendship networks, and consequently, social support, networks. Given space limitations, we do not provide an exhaustive list of interventions, but instead offer a few to illustrate how our understanding of the links between friendship and health, and our understanding of friendship developmental processes can inform the design of friendship interventions.

These interventions are grounded in the understanding that friendship initiation requires multiple opportunities for interaction. Accordingly, we suggest a variety of ways in which social environments (i.e., the immediate environment and communities) may be altered to encourage and better enable the formation of friendships by way of opportunities for interaction, thus laying the foundation for effective social support. We offer recommendations for "prescribing" friendship for individuals particularly "at risk" for stress and health problems. Again, due to space limitations, we do not address all such types of individuals, but instead focus on two particular populations to illustrate specific types of "friendship behavioral vaccine interventions": the elderly (as they illustrate general social support) and the seriously ill (as they illustrate targeted social support).

Interventions for the Elderly

A primary mental health threat to the elderly is loneliness (Lopata, 1970). Loneliness is an ongoing feature of everyday life for many seniors and the mental health effects of loneliness include stress, depression, and anxiety (Tweedy, Morrison, & DeMichele, 2002). Research has consistently demonstrated the ways in which friendship helps alleviate loneliness for the elderly and, consequently, mitigates the potential negative effects of the mental health of these individuals (Angel, Angel, & Henderson, 1997). This is due to the general social support provided by friends. Friends are key to combating loneliness and its negative impact on mental health and, according to some, are even more important in this area than are family members (Russell, 1981; Wister, 1990).

As mentioned earlier, friendship initiation is made more likely when individuals have physical/geographical contact with one another. A variety of interventions are available for elderly populations, including adult neighborhoods such as retirement communities and adult-only housing developments. Recent research indicates the health benefits such communities have for seniors specifically through friendship. Buys (2001) examined the extent to which living in a retirement village influenced the friendship networks of residents. Her results indicate that living in close proximity to other seniors increased the amount of interaction residents had with other elderly residents. Recall that perceived similarity is important to the initiation of friendship. Accordingly, the contact afforded by living in close proximity enables the initiation of friendships among these similar retirement village residents. In addition, the longer individuals live in such communities, the closer and stronger their friendships become (Perkinson & Rockemann, 1996). This logically results from the opportunities available to reciprocally engage the three types of social support that would likely be abundant in this type of living community between residents.

An important finding from the Buys (2001) study was that elderly individuals living in retirement villages actually reduced the amount of interaction, and friendships, with individuals living outside the village and in the broader community. This result demonstrates the importance of *close* and *consistent* proximity – the closer individuals live to one another, the more likely they will become friends. This is likely especially true for the elderly who may have less access to transportation that would enable them to travel farther to visit friends (e.g., they may lack a driver's license or their own automobile).

Of course, not all individuals have the opportunity, or desire, to move to a retirement village. For such individuals, other interventions can afford opportunities for friendship. Recall that shared activities or tasks are important triggers for friendship initiation. Senior centers or city recreation departments can offer a variety of activities and outings specifically for the elderly. These might include outings to a variety of nearby events, parks, or shopping malls. Particularly effective are programs that encourage seniors to work together on a specific task such as an arts and crafts class, a volunteer project to benefit the City, and the like. Again, these activities provide opportunities for interaction with similar individuals that lay the foundation for friendship.

To the extent that these activities or programs are ongoing (rather than a one-time event), they can provide the context for an ongoing, and increasingly close, friendship. Thus, senior centers should emphasize activities that require ongoing contact between participants such as luncheon groups and community action groups.

While our discussion about the elderly illustrates the importance of ongoing general social support from friends, the seriously ill demonstrate the importance of targeted social support.

Interventions for the Seriously Ill

Chronic or critical illness is a life event that creates a great deal of stress for the afflicted individual. Mental health problems associated with this stress include anxiety, depression, fear, and anger (Mutran, Danis, Bratton, Sudha, & Hanson, 1997). Illnesses such as these trigger targeted social support.

This support (emotional, informational, and instrumental) is targeted toward helping the patient deal specifically with the stress created by the illness.

As discussed earlier, a well-established general social support network is crucial for effective targeted social support. Once an individual is diagnosed with a serious illness, his/her friends will begin to provide targeted emotional, instrumental, and informational social support. "Life events" such as these often function as a developmental factor in transforming existing friendships into closer friendships (Sias & Cahill, 1998). The opportunities for self-disclosure, empathy, and the provision of targeted social support from current friends increases the breadth and depth of the friendships, moving the relationships toward closer and more intimate levels (e.g., friend-to-close friend or best friend).

As we also noted, however, one's current group of friends is likely not able to fulfill all of a seriously ill individual's social support needs. Consequently, interventions are needed that enable the initiation and development of additional friendships.

Our understanding of friendship development processes suggests a number of friendship interventions for this population. Proximity, for example, is important. Toward this end, the effectiveness of illness-specific support groups (e.g., cancer support groups, HIV/Aids support groups, diabetes support groups) is well established. Participation in such support groups is effective in buffering the mental and the physical effects of these illnesses (e.g., Ciambrone, 2002; Dunn, Steginga, Rosoman, & Millichap, 2003; Hipkins, Whitworth, Tarrier, & Jayson, 2004). These groups provide important physical access to others undergoing a similar experience, which, in turn, provides opportunities for interaction specifically targeted toward the illness itself. Thus, illness-specific support groups enable the initiation of friendships through the developmental influences of proximity and perceived similarity. Participation in a support group is an important venue for a "friendship" behavioral vaccine.

Many individuals, however, lack access to face-to-face groups. participants living in rural or isolated locations, for example, may find it very difficult to travel a significant distance to attend a support group meeting. Others may simply lack the self-confidence or social skills necessary to be comfortable participating in a face-to-face interaction. Fortunately, new communication technologies have made participating in a "face to face" support group (e.g., groups that provide physical proximity) less necessary for initiating relationships that provide targeted social support. The past 5 years have seen a large increase in the number of participants participating in online support groups or chat rooms by way of internet communication. Recent studies indicate that online support groups provide mental health benefits similar to those of face-to-face groups, specifically through the opportunities such groups provide for interaction and relationship development (e.g., Houston, Cooper, & Ford, 2002; Hoybye et al., 2005).

Support groups are not the only avenue toward initiating and developing supportive relationships, however. Although research has focused primarily on psychological social support interventions such as the efficacy of support groups for helping individuals cope with serious illness, interventions in the medical treatment of the patient may also prove helpful in the development of targeted social support networks. Such interventions provide proximity and access to similar individuals in the treatment of the illness itself. Segmented hospital wards, for example, can enable individuals undergoing inpatient procedures to form supportive relationships with one another. Clinics specializing in a specific illness, such as comprehensive or integrated cancer care centers, enable participants with the same disease to interact with one another. Such centers foster the interaction of caregivers (e.g., surgical oncologist, chemical oncologists, radiologists, nurses, etc.). Improved interaction between specialists for a specific disease can lead to improvement in the overall treatment of the patient (Laliberte, Fennell, & Papandonatos, 2005; McMorrow, 1995). These specialized centers may also benefit participants *psychologically* by providing them opportunities to develop relationships with individuals suffering from a similar disease. Along these lines, for instance, many oncology care centers offer participants their chemotherapy treatments in large communal rooms with others also receiving chemotherapy at the same time. These group chemotherapy environments provide a social, at times, convivial, atmosphere that can help combat the loneliness and depression participants often experience during such treatments. For those uncomfortable with social interaction, of course, private therapy sessions are available. To the best of our knowledge, research has yet to examine the psychological benefits of medical treatments such as this and we encourage such studies in the future to develop more effective friendship and social support interventions to this population.

Friendship Variety

In the preceding sections, we discuss the elderly and the seriously ill to illustrate how an understanding of friendship development dynamics can inform and guide friendship interventions in the pursuit of mental health. Returning to our "vaccine" metaphor, we turn now to a discussion of friendship variety. While many believe, for instance, that old friends are the best friends, in fact, friends of all types are necessary for overall health. Just as a daily vitamin should provide a variety of nutrients, our friendship networks should comprise a variety of types of friends, for maximum efficacy.

The importance of complex and varied friendship networks is reinforced, somewhat ironically, by acknowledging that a common source of stress (and accompanying mental health problems) is the loss of a friend. The elderly, for example, are at high risk for losing friends who die as they grow older (Angel, et al., 1997). Similarly, if an individual has friends in only one sphere of his/her life (e.g., only workplace friends, or neighborhood friends), s/he will be unable to mitigate the anxiety and stress caused in the event s/he loses those friends (e.g., a coworker takes a job with a different organization and leaves the area, a neighbor moves to a different community). The larger and more varied a person's friendship network, the more likely s/he is to obtain social support necessary for coping with the loss of such friends and other stressors. Accordingly, interventions should be designed with friendship network multiplexity in mind. The better the nutrient formulation in the vitamin we take, the better prepared we are to deal with the potential stressors in our social environment.

Friendship behavioral vaccines also must be tailored toward the specific needs and characteristics of the individual. A great deal of research demonstrates that different types of people have different needs for, and approaches toward, friendship. For example, although men garner mental health benefits from social support and friendship (e.g., Helgeson & Lepore, 1997), women appear to profit more, or at least differently, from such relationships with respect to the extent to which friendship helps relieve stress (e.g., Taylor et al., 2000). Research also indicates individuals' friendships needs change over their lifespan (e.g., Angel, et al., 1997). In addition, researchers have identified cultural differences in reliance upon friends and social support (e.g., Angel, et al., 1997; Mutran et al., 1997). Finally, people's friendship and social support needs vary depending on the life events they experience such as serious illness, divorce, and abuse. Thus, just as a woman needs a vitamin higher in iron than does a man, people have differing "friendship" requirements based on their age, sex, health, culture, and the like. The key to effective use of friendship as a behavioral vaccine is understanding friendship dynamics and applying them appropriately to specific individuals (while recognizing their goals and motivation).

Conclusion

Our primary goal in writing this chapter was to provide a model of the links between friendship, social support, and health. This model helps us understand the health benefits of friendship, as well as guide interventions that can foster the use of friendship as a "behavioral vaccine" for improved physical and mental health.

Conceptualizing friendship as a behavioral vaccine highlights a variety of issues and concerns with respect to friendship and health. First, each individual's needs for friendship "vaccines" are unique because each individual's physical and social conditions and needs are unique. Friendship interventions must be designed specifically for individuals and/or specific populations (e.g., people who suffer social anxiety will likely not benefit from face-to-face support group interaction).

Perhaps most importantly such a conceptualization emphasizes that individuals can be proactive in maintaining physical and mental health through social relationships, while acknowledging that individuals do have some control over their mental and physical health. You don't need a physician's prescription to make a friend. You don't need money or health insurance to obtain the health benefits of friendship. You simply need to talk to people and offer social support to others in a reciprocal manner. Understanding friendship as a behavioral vaccine reveals that individuals are more empowered and in control of their health than they might realize. A behavioral vaccine is self-administered for the promotion of one's positive mental health. Consistent with this, we emphasize that friendship is an enacted communicative phenomenon. It is something that we engage in and do proactively, not something that happens to us passively.

References

Albrecht, T. L., & Adelman, M. B. (1987). *Communicating social support*. Newbury Park, CA: Sage.

Albrecht, T., Burleson, B., & Goldsmith, D. (1994). Supportive communication. In Knapp, M. L., & Miller, G. R. (Eds.), *Handbook of Interpersonal Communication* (pp. 419–449). Thousand Oaks: Sage.

Altman, I., & Taylor, D. A. (1973). *Social penetration: The development of interpersonal relationships*. New York: Holt, Rinehart & Winston.

Angel, J. L., Angel, R. J., & Henderson, K. J. (1997). Contextualizing social support and health in old age: Reconsidering culture and gender. *The International Journal of Sociology and Social Policy, 17*, 83–117.

Barnes, M. K., & Duck, S. (1994). Everyday communicative contexts for social support. In B. R. Burleson, T. L. Albrecht, & I. G. Sarason (Eds.), *Communication of social support: Messages, interactions, and community* (pp. 175–194). Thousand Oaks, CA: Sage.

Blieszner, R., & Adams, R. G. (1992). *Adult friendship*. Newbury Park, CA: Sage.

Brandl, B., Hebert, M., Rozwadowski, J., & Spangler, D. (2003). *Violence against women, 9*, 1490.

Buys, L. R. (2001). Life in a retirement village: Implications for contact with community and village friends. *Gerontology, 47*, 55–60.

Ciambrone, D. (2002). Social support networks among women with HIV/AIDS: Present support and future prospects. *Qualitative Health Research, 12*, 876–897.

Cohen, S., & McKay, G. (1984). Social Support, stress, and the buffering hypothesis: A theoretical analysis. In A. Baum, S. E Taylor, & J. E. Springer (Eds.), *Handbook of Psychology and Health, 4*, 253–267. Hillsdale, NY: Erlbaum.

Davidson, L., & Duberman, L. (1982). Friendship: Communication and interactional patterns in same-sex dyads. *Sex Roles, 8*, 809–822.

Davis, D., & Perkowitz, W. T. (1979). Consequences of responsiveness in dyadic interaction: Effects of probability of response and proportion of content-related responses on interpersonal attraction. *Journal of Personality and Social Psychology, 37*, 534–551.

Davis, K. E., & Todd, M. J. (1985). Assessing friendships: Prototypes, paradigm cases and relationship description. In S. Duck, & D. Perlman (Eds.), *Understanding personal relationships: An interdisciplinary approach* (pp. 17–38). London: Sage.

DeLongis, A., Folkman, S., & Lazarus, R. (1988). The impact of daily stress on health and mood: Psychological and social resources as mediators. *Journal of Personality and Social Psychology, 54*, 486–495.

Duck, S., & Pittman, G. (1994). Social and personal relationships. In. M. L. Knapp, & G. R. Miller (Eds.), *Handbook of interpersonal communication* (2nded.) (pp. 676–695). Thousand Oaks, CA: Sage.

Dunn, J., Steginga, S. K., Rosoman, N., & Millichap, D. (2003). A review of peer support in the context of cancer. *Journal of Psychosocial Oncology, 21*, 55.

Fehr, B. (1996). *Friendship processes*. Thousand Oaks, CA: Sage.

Goldsmith, D. J. (1992). Managing conflicting goals in supportive interaction: An integrative theoretical framework. *Communication Research, 19*, 264–286.

Hammer, M. (1983). "Core" and "extended" social networks in relation to health and illness. *Social Science and Medicine, 17*, 405–411.

Helgeson, V. S., & Lepore, S. J. (1997). Men's adjustment to prostate cancer: The role of agency and unmitigated agency. *Sex Roles, 37*, 251–268.

Hill, C. T., & Stull, D. E. (1981). Sex differences in effects of social and value similarity in same-sex friendship. *Journal of Personality and Social Psychology, 41*, 488–502.

Hipkins, J., Whitworth, M., Tarrier, N., & Jayson, G. (2004). Social support, anxiety and depression after chemotherapy for ovarian cancer: A prospective study. *British Journal of Health Psychology, 9*, 569–582.

Houston, T. K., Cooper, L. A., & Ford, D. E. (2002). Internet support groups for depression: A 1-year prospective cohort study. *The American Journal of Psychiatry, 12*, 2062–2069.

Hoybye, M. T., Johansen, C., & Tjornhoj-Thomsen, T. (2005). Online interaction: Effects of storytelling in an internet breast cancer support group. *Psycho-Oncology, 14*, 211.

Laliberte, L., Fennell, M. L., & Papandonatos, G. (2005). The relationship of membership in research networks to compliance with treatment guidelines for early-stage breast cancer. *Medical Care, 43*, 471.
Lepore, S. J., & Helgeson, V. S. (1998). Social constraints, intrusive thoughts, and mental health after prostate cancer. *Journal of Social and Clinical Psychology, 17*, 89–107.
Lopata, H. Z. (1970). The social involvement of American widows. In E. Shanas (Ed.) *Aging in Contemporary Society*. Beverly Hills, CA: Sage Publications.
Lowenthal, N. F., & Haven, L. (1968). Interaction and adaptation: Intimacy as a critical behavior. *American Sociological Review, 33*, 20–30.
McMorrow, E. (1995). Treating the big C. *Facilities Design & Management, 14*, 39.
Mutran, E. J., Danis, M., Bratton, K.A., Sudha, S., & Hanson, L. (1997). Attitudes of the critically ill toward prolonging life: The role of social support. *The Gerontologist, 37*, 192–200.
Newcomb, T. M. (1961). *The acquaintance process*. New York: Holt, Rinehart & Winston.
Ornish, D. (1998). *Love & survival: The scientific basis for the healing power of Intimacy*. New York: HarperCollins.
Oygard, L. (2003). Divorce support groups: What factors are of importance regarding friendship development in the groups? *Social Work with Groups, 26*, 59.
Pennebaker, J. W., & O'Heeron, R. C. (1984). Confiding in others and illness rate among spouses of suicide and accidental-death victims. *Journal of Abnormal Psychology, 93*, 473–476.
Perkinson, M. A., & Rockemann, D. D. (1996). Older women living in a continuing care retirement community: Marital status and friendship formation. In K. A. Roberto (Ed.). *Relationship between women in later life* (pp. 159–177). Binghamton: Harrington Park Press.
Raymond, N. (1999). Hug drug: Friendship heals. *Psychology Today*, p.1.
Rodin, M. J. (1978). Liking and disliking. *Personality and Social Psychology Bulletin, 4*, 473–478.
Russell, C. (1981). *The aging experience*. Sydney: Allen and Unwin.
Schaefer, C., Coyne, J. C., & Lazarus R. S. (1981). The health-related functions of social support. *Journal of Behavioral Medicine, 4*, 381–406.
Schroeder, D. A., Penner, L. A., Dovidio, J. F., & Piliavin, J. A. (1995). *The psychology of helping and altruism: Problems and puzzles*. New York: McGraw-Hill.
Seeman, T., & Sayles, M. (1985). Social networks and health status: A longitudinal analysis. *Social Psychology Quarterly, 48*, 237–248.
Sias, P. M. & Cahill, D. J. (1998). From coworkers to friends: The development of peer friendships in the workplace. *Western Journal of Communication, 62*, 273–299.
Sias, P. M., Krone, K. J., & Jablin, F. M. (2001). An ecological systems perspective on workplace relationships. In M. L. Knapp & J. Daly (Eds.), *Handbook of interpersonal communication* (3rded.). Newbury Park, CA: Sage.
Sias, P. M., Smith, G., & Avdeyeva, T. (2003). Sex and sex composition similarities and differences in workplace friendship development. *Communication Studies, 54*, 322–340.
Sigman, S. J. (1995). Order and continuity in human relationships: A social communication approach to defining 'relationship.' In W. Leeds-Hurwitz (Ed.), *Social approaches to communication* (pp. 188–200). New York: Guilford Press.
Taylor, S. E., Klein, L. C., Lewis, B. P., Gruenewald, T. L., Gurung, R. A. R., & Updegraff, J. A. (2000). Female responses to stress: Tend and befriend, not fight or flight. *Psychology Review, 107*, 41–429.
Tweedy, K., Morrison, M. F., & DeMichele, S. G. (2002). Depression in older women. *Psychiatric Annals, 32*, 417–433.
Weick, K. E. (1979). *The social psychology of organizing* (2nded.). New York: Random House.

Wills, T. (1985). Supportive functions of interpersonal relationships. In S. Cohen, & S. L. Syme, (Eds.), *Social Support and Health* (pp. 61–82). Orlando, FL: Academic Press.

Wister, A. (1990). Living arrangements and informal social support among the elderly. In P. A. Psatalan (Ed.), *Aging in Place: The role of housing and social support.* London: Haworth Press.

Wright, K. (2004) On-line relational maintenance strategies and perceptions of partners within exclusively internet-based and primarily internet-based relationships. *Communication Studies, 55*, 239–254.

24

Animal Companions

Luciano L'Abate

> Pets provide unconditional love and acceptance; they offer spontaneous affection and undying loyalty. (Cusak, 1998, p. 9).

The term human-animal bond was first used in Scotland, but this term was first articulated by Konrad Lorenz and Boris Levinson, respectively, in ethology and in therapy. The two major kinds of animal companions (AC) dogs and cats have different evolutionary ages in domestication. The dog was domesticated about 30,000 years ago, while cats might have been domesticated about 9,000 years ago (Catanzaro, 2003). Twenty year old estimates (Katcher, 1986) counted 63 million cats, 55 million dogs, 25 million birds, 250 million fish, and upward of 125 million assorted pets of various kinds. These figures can only be conservative when counting increases in populations and parallel increases in animal ACs. What functions or purposes do these companions perform for so many people? Why do so many people own ACs? Considering the sheer size of these figures, clearly ACs could provide physical and mental health benefits, acting as approaches according to our original definition of the term (see Chapter 1 this volume). Animal pets seem to work as "approaches" in the sense that they are purported to be relatively easy to manage and provide years of comfort and even joy to their owners.

Presently, the major focus of attention to ACs lies in the relationship between this bond and human health and well-being (Hines, 2003). There is no question that, at least in secondary references (Beck & Katcher, 1996; Crawford & Pomerinke, 2003; Fine, 2000; Gunter, 1999; Podberscek, Paul, & Serpell, 2000), pets may provide seemingly physical and mental health benefits (Cusack, 1988; Wilson & Turner, 1998b), in the home (Triebenbacher, 1998, 2000), in child development (Melson, 2000, 2003), for the elderly (Baun & McCabe, 2000), in Alzheimer's Type dementia (Baun & McCabe, 2003), for those with cancer (Johnson, Meadows, & Haubner, 2003), for people with AIDS and other chronic/terminal illnesses (Gorczyca, Fine, & Spain, 2000), for people with disabilities, for the blind (Steffens & Bergler, 1998), for grieving people (Toray, 2004), for workaholics (Santarpio-Damerjian, 2002), and for prison inmates (Strimple, 2003). ACs are even being used as aids in child psychotherapy (Levinson & Mallon, 1997) and in psychotherapy with adults (Fine, 2000).

Given such widespread beliefs about the positive influence of ACs, what are the scientific bases for so many claims about their beneficial effects on humans? The sheer number of millions of people who form attachments with their ACs should alert mental health professionals, and not only psychologists, to the significance of their loss in grieving owners (Sharkin & Knox, 2003). The flip side of so much anecdotal goodness in using pets is found in their being abused rather than cared for, where animals remain helpless targets of their owners psychopathology (Ascione, Kaufman, & Brooks, 2000).

The purpose of this chapter is to provide a review of the evidence of what appears to be the relatively inexpensive and apparently long-lasting effects of ACs, and to separate the facts from fiction. ACs can be viewed as "good companions," as "family," as "parts of the self." These parts of the self crave talking, touching, and intimacy, qualities apparently not present in one's life (Beck & Katcher, 1996). Since this Handbook is not concerned with psychotherapy for the few but with interventions with lasting effects for the masses, the topic of using pets as aids in psychotherapy, no matter how valid, widespread and validated (Cusack, 1998; Fine, 2000; Hines & Fredrickson, 1998; Levinson & Mallon, 1997) will not be reviewed in this chapter. Even though Wilson & Turner (1998a) extended the focus from health to "quality of life," we are still concerned with whether ACs, of whatever kind, show empirically-based physical and mental health benefits, and quality of life, also including "well being on humans."

Theory

Among the many theoretical viewpoints that abound in this field, one must distinguish among sociological and psychological explanations. For instance, socialization and symbolic interactionism are terms favored by sociologists (Flynn, 2000; Irvine, 2004; Odendall, 2002; Sanders, 2003). Among psychological explanations, Cusack offered a "naturalistic/psycho-analytic" approach, after decrying the lack of scientific interest in the "centuries-old" humans-animals bond (p. 25). First, animals serve as *symbols* of that part of ourselves that includes the "natural environment". Cusack quotes Bruno Bettelheim and Carl Jung to support the position that animals serve as "symbols." It remains to be seen whether human-animal relationships are derived from a "genetic template" or "cultural transmission" as Cusack contends. Second, animals serve as *surrogates* for taking the place of people, assuming projected human qualities that may be lacking in the owner's experience. Third, the presence and contact with animals may have therapeutic effects, as demonstrated by secondary references to that effect (Crawford & Pomerinke, 2003; Levinson & Mallon, 1997), including greater socialization effects in participants with Alzheimer's disease (Batson, McCabe, Baun, & Wilson, 1998).

In addition to the naturalistic/psychoanalytic approach, Cusack considered learning theory in terms of acquired social roles from childhood on. Classical and operant conditioning and observational learning, in the form of intrinsic reinforcements, may explain the relationship between animals and humans. Pets may serve as anxiety reduction and distraction from everyday stresses. Indeed, animals may reduce depression by allowing owners to focus outside of themselves. Initial research with caged birds, for instance, seemed to have positive effects on psychiatric participants, even though this evidence was anecdotal rather than experimental. Supposedly, even delinquents may profit by having to care for animals (Cusack, 1998). The contention that ACs fulfill roles as friends, family, and as part of the self was supported in part by the work of Hirschman (1994). Her work was based on in-depth interviews with a large sample of pet owners. Psychoanalytic aspects of pet ownership have been updated by Bennett's (2005) and by Serpell's (2000) contribution. The latter proposed that ACs may fulfill three roles as mediators: (1) as *social lubricants* by catalyzing social relationships; (2) as *ambassadors* of a link between themselves and other animal species; and (3) as *the animal within*, connecting and reuniting people with something that is fundamentally conscious within themselves.

Current major theoretical formulations for the use of ACs are found in the "social support paradigm" (Wilson & Turner, 1998a) versus Bowlby's attachment model (Collis & McNicholas, 1998). However, while the latter has been specifically validated in thousands of studies with humans around the world, the social support model, even though possibly valid, is theoretically weak and vague in its many forms. When both models are evaluated using cats, for instance, in 1,548 participants, a positive correlation was found between scores on two attachment scales and the number of significant others listed in two measures of social support. Attachment to the cat correlated negatively with the number of significant others and with both emotional and tangible human support. Apparently, neither model could be eliminated since there is relationship between them, i. e., positive correlations (Stammbach, & Turner, 1999).

When the attachment model is applied to measures of human-animal attachment bonds and two measures of loneliness and stress: "...animals could become supplementary attachment figures for older people (Keil, 1998, p. 123)." Whether this hypothesis needs to be validated further remains to be reviewed in the next section. For instance, the relationship between personality type and pet attachment was explored by administering Keirsey's Four Types Sorter and the Lexington Attachment to Pets Scale to 163 participants. Idealist personality types showed significantly higher attachment scores than Rationals and Artisans, but not Guardians. The longer the owner cared for the pet, the stronger was the attachment (Bagley & Gonsman, 2005).

Research: The Outcome of Pet Ownership

Research about human-animal interaction is still beset by many challenges, like design, control of extraneous variables, sample selection, intervention development, and outcome measurement (Wilson & Barker, 2003). Three possible ways to research relationships among ACs and health benefits are: (1) straightforward antecedents of pet ownership leading to health; (2) indirect results mediated by external variables, such as contact with people; and (3) antecedent factors that effect both health and the desire to own a pet (McNicholas & Collis, 1998). In their review of empirical evidence between the years from 1990 to 1995 to support the hypothesis that ACs may enhance "quality of life," for instance, Garrity and Stallones (1998) located 25 such studies. Using the social support paradigm introduced earlier as an overall theoretical framework, Garrity and Stallones (1998) concluded that:

> ...although research progress continues to be slow in this area, findings of quality of life benefits derived from AC contact are consistent with the research reported during the last two decades...These benefits are evident on the psychological, physical, social, and behavioral levels. The quality of life benefits of pet association, however, are apparent only in certain situations and under certain circumstances (p. 3).

An update of Garrity and Stallones' review of the literature can be found in Barker, Rogers, & Turner (2003). Since the present chapter cannot perform another review of the literature, certain selected research highlights will be reported to support a hypothesis that is somewhat more stringent than just "quality of life" or "well-being," and that is: "Do ACs improve physical and mental health, however defined, by controlled evidence?" "Under what situations and what circumstances are such benefits found?"

As a beginning answer to this question, Wilson (1998a) reviewed research that supports positive outcomes with ACs – lowering blood pressure, heart rates, anxiety, and, in addition, enhancing social environments, and decreasing depression. In an effort to measure "quality of life," Barofsky and Rowan (1998) reviewed the validity of measures for happiness and sources of satisfaction in everyday life, including cognitive and psychometric models as well as the positive relationship between psychosocial adjustment and quality of life. Most of the research reviewed above and below, unless noted otherwise, has been conducted with dogs (Johnson, Odentaal, & Meadows, 2002). If and when other kinds of ACs are used, this exception will be noted.

Child and Adolescent Development

More than three/fourths of all children in America live with pets and are now more likely to grow up with a pet than with both parents (Melson, 2001). Some consistent pattern about the effects of pets in child and adolescent development were culled from the empirical literature (Melson, 1998, 2003): (1) Families with children are more likely to own ACs than are families without children; (2) Families with either very young children or teenagers are less likely to own pets than are families with school-age children; (3) Multiple pet ownership is also common; and (4) Many child, family, and environmental factors influence pet ownership. "Quality of life" in children is "...defined as the subjective symptoms, feelings, and well-being relevant to the child's ability to meet developmental challenges" (Melson, 1998, pp. 222–224).

These challenges concern: (1) *basic trust*, where pets offer a secure base with attachments for both pets and humans, and support for parents to provide responsivity and inculcation of cultural values; (2) *autonomy* initiative, where pets become playmates in relation to human playmates, with neighborhood and community availability, and cultural values of animals as play partners; (3) *industry*, where pets are used as a learning aid in relation to other learning aids, the learning environment, i.e., school with cultural values; and (4) *identity*, where pets become a source of support in relation to other supports for identity exploration and achievement, as well as support for parents and peers (Melson (1998, 2001). Apparently, children from single-parent families do show significantly higher levels of attachment to dogs than children in two-parent families. This difference may be due to children in the early childhood stage of development in single-parent families showing significantly higher levels of bonding with dogs than children of two-parent families at the same childhood stage (Bodsworth & Coleman, 2001)

A sample of 752 Swiss adolescents between 12 and 16 years of age equally divided for gender, contained 405 adolescent pet owners. Pet owners reported a higher level of well-being and more family resources than nonowners. Apparently, pet ownership per se does not seem to serve as a buffer for adolescents reporting few familial resources (Bodmer, 1998). On the other hand, children with pets show no difference in empathy from nonowners. There is no correlation between empathy and attachment to pets, and higher empathy scores were not related to pet preference (Daly & Morton, 2003). Hence, at this point one cannot claim that there is a direct relationship between pet ownership and health. Additional sources of evidence will be necessary.

For instance, girls of middle-school age with pets other than a dog or cat showed the highest levels of Posttraumatic stress reactions (PTSR), while boys without pets and girls with a dog or a cat showed the lowest levels of PTSR. Apparently, owing a dog or cat has a stronger effect in reducing PSTR in girls than in boys. Additionally, children with a dog or cat, in comparison to children without a pet or children with other pets, were able to express more emotions, and seek social support and help with problem solving. (Asambasic, Kerestes, & Kuterovac-Jagodic, 2000). There is statistically significant less behavioral distress in children between 2 and 6 years of age during a physical examination when a dog is present (Hansen, Messinger, & Baun, 1999).

Cardiovascular Risk

Jennings et al. (1998) examined the relationship between animals and cardiovascular risk factors in 5,741 healthy participants. Pet owners showed significantly lower systolic blood pressure and plasma triglycerides than nonowners. These investigators further found significantly lower cholesterol values in men but not in women. However, pet owners exercised more regularly. These investigators quoted additional research from Australia that found dog owners to have 8% fewer doctor visits than non-dog owners. Cat owners had 12% fewer visits than non-cat owners. For instance, coronary prone Type A personalities may tend to desire an AC because their energies are directed toward externally immediate goals. By the same token, pet ownership may lower stress-related illnesses, and thus, be useful to Type A personalities. To evaluate the validity of this hypothesis, McNicholas and Collis (1998) administered a brief questionnaire to evaluate the level of Type A personality in 541 participants. Results proved their hypothesis to be inaccurate: pet owners showed higher Type A scores than nonowners! Perhaps these results suggest that pet owners may be more active and more involved in a variety of activities, including per ownership, than nonowners. Whether animal ownership lowers rates of medication for high blood pressure, cholesterol, sleeping difficulties, or heart problems remains to be seen by further evidence.

Social support and pet ownership apparently increase chances of coronary artery disease survival. However, other factors need to be considered, such as disease severity and socioeconomic status. After completing various psychosocial questionnaires, randomly assigned participants (N = 421) participating in Cardiac Arrthythmia Suppression Trials, were evaluated for one-year survival rates. From the resulting 369 participants (87%), 112 (30.4%) owned pets and 20 (5.4%) died. Among various variables affecting these results, high social support and owning a pet tended to predict survival rates independent from disease severity and other demographic and psychosocial factors. Dog owners seemed less likely to die within one year than nonowners. Amount of social support was also an independent predictor of survival (Friedman & Thomas, 1998).

Relative to people without pets, people with pets showed significantly smaller increases in cardiovascular reactivity from baseline levels during mental arithmetic and cold compressor tests, as well as faster recovery. Among pet owners, lowest reactivity and quickest recovery was observed when the pet was present during testing. Whether people perceive of their pets as important, supportive parts of their lives, and whether this importance translates into cardiovascular and behavioral benefits, remains to be seen and supported by additional evidence. For instance, the mere presence of an unknown, friendly pet, traditional or non-traditional can significantly reduce physiological arousal in normotensive adults, regardless of gender, general pet attitude, and subjective reports (DeMello, 1999).

Health

Mood factors are related to cat ownership, presence or absence of a partner, and a respondent's gender. Only the partner, but not the cat, enhanced positive moods. Cats, on the other hand, seem to alleviate negative moods, and that affect seemed comparable to the affect of a human partner. This compensatory effect of cat ownership on negative moods was not comparable to a similar effect of degree of attachment towards the cat on human mood (Turner, Rieger, & Gygax, 2003). Whether mood is related to physical and mental health remains to be seen. In a middle-age sample of 1,844 participants, compared to nonowners, pet owners were more likely to be working married women. Measures of physical and mental health, including information obtained by general practitioners, were not significantly affected by pet ownership and caring. Indeed, pet owners used pain-relief medication more frequently than nonowners. (Parslow & Jorm, 2003). These findings, of course, run counter to results from other studies which suggested health benefits for pet ownership. For instance, there were no significant differences between pet owners and nonowners in level of happiness or life satisfaction, or medical problems (Crowley-Robinson & Blackshaw, 1998).

For older people, there may not be health benefits from owning a pet. Using survey information, caring for a pet may be associated with more depressive symptoms, more negative health outcomes, and higher rates of pain-relief medication. Men pet owners, as a whole, showed higher extraversion scores than women. A major finding, however, was that pet owners and carers and those who care for them reported higher levels of psychoticism, as measured by the Revised Eysenck Personality Questionnaire (Parslow, Jorm, & Christensen, 2005). A different outcome was found for older women from the Australian database. Age, living arrangements, and housing all strongly related to both living with AC and health (Pachana, Ford, & Andrew, 2005).

When the social support system and psychological well-being of men with AIDS were evaluated by contrasting the contribution of cats versus dogs, their comfort from ACs was significantly associated with having cats but not dogs, closeness with friends, dissatisfaction with their practical support system, and listing pets as a source of support. Cats appeared to complement supportive relationships with friends and family as protection against loneliness (Castelli, Hart, & Zasloff, 2001).

Pet ownership seems related to two measures of well-being, self-esteem and locus of control, but only for men (Hecht, McMillin, & Silverman, 2001). As far as the age of pet owners is concerned, they are younger, married, or living with someone, and more physically active than nonpet-owners. The Activities in Daily Living score level of nonowners deteriorated more on average than the level of pet owners over a one-year period. Ownership significantly modified the relationship between social support and changes in psychological well-being over the one-year period (Raina, Waltner-Toews, & Bonnett, 1999).

Practice

Owning pets is a widespread responsibility that is usually fulfilled seriously by most owners, with few exceptions. On the other hand, training standards and policy issues to insure safety and safeguard the welfare of animals need to be implemented (Duncan, 1998) in both private and public settings (Hubrecht, 1998). Even though Catanzaro (2003) advocated the use of the human-animal bond in primary prevention, in a way that supports the use of this bond to promote physical and mental health. Results reported here are still too inconsistent to make a recommendation. The use of pets as ACs needs to be a responsible decision that may not necessarily lead to positive physical and mental health benefits. One needs to decide what kind of pet would be more appropriate to people, according to age, gender, and health status.

Conclusions

From this review it can be safely concluded that ACs can be helpful in some circumstances and hurtful in others. Their use still depends a great deal on how pets are conceived of and needed. The variability in outcomes of pet ownership is still too great to conclude with a vast recommendation. Whether pets should be used to promote physical and mental health is still a question open to further research.

References

Asambasic, L., Kerestes, G., & Kuterovac-Jagodic, G. (2000). The role of pet ownership as a possible variable in traumatic experiences. *Studia Psychologica, 42*, 135–146.

Ascione, F. R., Kaufman, M. E., & Brooks, S. M. (2000). Animal abuse and developmental psycho-pathology: Recent research, programmatic, and therapeutic issues and challenges for the future. In A. H. Fine (Ed.), *Handbook on animal-assisted therapy: Theoretical foundations and guidelines for practice* (pp. 325–354). San Diego, CA: Academic Press.

Bagley, D. K., & Gonsman, V. L. (2005). Pet attachment and personality type. *Anthrozoos, 18*, 28–42.

Barker, S. B., Rogers, C. S., & Turner, J. W. (2003). Benefits of interacting with companion animals: A bibliography of articles published in refereed journals during the past 5 years. *American Behavioral Scientist, 47*, 94–99.

Barofsky, I., & Rowan, A. (1998). Models for measuring quality of life: Implications for human-animal interaction research. In C. C. Wilson & D. C. Turner (Eds.), *Companion animals in human health* (pp. 91–101). Thousand Oaks, CA: Sage

Batson, K., McCabe, B., Baun, M. M., & Wilson, C. (1998). The effect of a therapy dog on socialization and physiological indicators of stress in persons diagnosed with Alzheimer's disease. In C. C. Wilson & D. C. Turner (Eds.), *Companion animals in human health* (pp. 203–215). Thousand Oaks, CA: Sage.

Baun, M. M., & McCabe, B. W. (2000). The role animals play in enhancing quality of life for the elderly. In A. H. Fine (Ed.), *Handbook on animal-assisted therapy: Theoretical foundations and guidelines for practice* (pp. 137–251). San Diego, CA: Academic Press.

Baun, M. M., & McCabe, B. W. (2003). Companion animals and persona with dementia of the Alzheimer's Type: Therapeutic possibilities. *American Behavioral Scientist, 47*, 42–51.

Beck, A., & Katcher, A. (1996). *Between pets and people: The importance of animal companions*. West Lafayette, IN: Purdue University Press.

Bennett, S. R. (2005). Pets and psychoanalysis: A clinical contribution. *Psychoanalytic Review, 92*, 453–467.

Bodmer, N. C. (1998). Impact of pet ownership on the well-being of adolescents with few family resources. In C. C. Wilson & D. C. Turner (Eds.), *Companion animals in human health* (pp. 237–247). Thousand Oaks, CA: Sage.

Bodsworth, W., & Coleman, G. J. (2001). Child-companion animal attachment bonds in single- and two-parent families. *Anthrozoos, 14*, 216–223.

Castelli, P., Hart, L. A., & Zasloff, R. L. (2001). Companion cats and social support system of men with AIDS. *Psychological Reports, 89*, 177–187.

Catanzaro, T. E. (2003). Human-animal bond and primary prevention. *American Behavioral Scientist, 47*, 29–30.

Collis, G. M., & McNicholas, J. (1998). Theoretical basis for health benefits of pet ownership: Attachment versus psychological support. In C. C. Wilson & D. C. Turner (Eds.), *Companion animals in human health* (pp. 105–122). Thousand Oaks, CA: Sage.

Crawford, J. J., & Pomerinke, K. A. (2003). *Therapy pets: The animal-human healing partnership*. Amherst, NY: Prometheus Books.

Crowley-Robinson, P. & Blackshaw, J. K. (1998). Pet ownership and health status of elderly in the community. *Anthrozoos, 11*, 168–171

Cusack, O. (1988). *Pets and mental health*. New York: Haworth.

Daly, B., & Morton, L. L. (2003). Children with pets do not show higher empathy. A challenge to current views. *Anthrozoos, 16*, 298–314.

DeMello, L. R. (1999). The effect of the presence of a companion-animal on physiological changes following the termination of a cognitive stressor. *Psychology & Health, 14*, 859–868.

Duncan, S. L. (1998). The importance of training standards and policy for service animals. In C. C. Wilson & D. C. Turner (Eds.), *Companion animals in human health* (pp. 251–254). Thousand Oaks, CA: Sage.

Fine, A. H. (2000). Animals and therapists: Incorporating animals in outpatient psychotherapy. In A. H. Fine (Ed.), *Handbook on animal-assisted therapy: Theoretical foundations and guidelines for practice* (pp. 179–211). San Diego, CA: Academic Press.

Flynn, C. P. (2000). Battered women and their animal companions: Symbolic interaction between human and nonhuman animals. *Science & Animals, 8*, 99–127.
Friedman, E., & Thomas, S. A. (1998). Pet ownership, social support, and one-year survival after acute myocardial infarction in the cardiac arrhythmia trial (CAST). In C. C. Wilson & D. C. Turner (Eds.), *Companion animals in human health* (pp. 187–201). Thousand Oaks, CA: Sage.
Garrity, T. F. & Stallones, L (1998). Effects of pet contact on human well being. In C. C. Wilson & D. C. Turner (Eds.), *Companion animals in human health* (pp. 3–22). Thousand Oaks, CA: Sage.
Gorczyca, K., Fine, A. H., & Spain, C. V. (2000). History, theory, and development of human-animal support services for people with AIDS and other chronic/terminal illnesses. In A. H. Fine (Ed.), *Handbook on animal-assisted therapy: Theoretical foundations and guidelines for practice* (pp. 254–302). San Diego, CA: Academic Press.
Gunter, B. (1999). *Pets and people: The psychology of pet ownership*. London, England: Whurr Publishers.
Hansen, K. M., Messinger, C. J., & Baun, M. M. (1999). Companion animals alleviating distress in children. *Anthrozoos, 12*, 142–148.
Hecht, L., McMillin, J. D., & Silverman, P. (2001). Pets, networks and well-being. *Anthrozoos, 14*, 95–108.
Hines, L. M. (2003). Historical perspectives on the human-animal bond. *American Behavioral Scientist, 47*, 7–15.
Hines, L., & Fredrickson, M. (1998). Perspectives on animal-assisted activities and therapy. In C. C. Wilson & D. C. Turner (Eds.), *Companion animals in human health* (pp. 23–40). Thousand Oaks, CA: Sage.
Hirschman, E. C. (1994). Consumers and their animal companions. *Journal of Consumer Research, 20*, 616–631.
Hubrecht, R. & Turner, D. C. (1998). Companion animal welfare in private and institutional settings. In C. C. Wilson & D. C. Turner (Eds.), *Companion animals in human health* (pp. 267–289). Thousand Oaks, CA: Sage.
Irvine, L. (2004). A model of animal selfhood: Expanding interactionist possibilities. *Symbolic Interaction, 27*, 3–21.
Jennings, G. L. R., Reid, C. M., Christy, I., Jennings, J., et al. (1998). Animals and cardiovascular health. In C. C. Wilson & D. C. Turner (Eds.), *Companion animals in human health* (pp. 161–171). Thousand Oaks, CA: Sage.
Johnson, R., Meadows, R. L., & Haubner, J. S. (2003). Human-animal interaction: A complementary/alternative medical (CAM) intervention for cancer patients. *American Behavioral Scientist, 47*, 55–69.
Johnson, R. A., Odentaal, J. S. J., & Meadows, R. I. (2002). Animal-assisted intervention research: Issues and answers. *Western Journal of Nursing Research, 24*, 422–440.
Katcher, A. H., (1986). Man and the living environment. In A. H. Katcher & A. M. Beck (Eds.). *New perspectives in our lives with companion animals* (pp. 519–531). Philadelphia, PA: University of Pennsylvania Press.
Keil, C. P. (1998). Loneliness, stress, and human-animal attachment among older adults. In C. C. Wilson & D. C. Turner (Eds.), *Companion animals in human health* (pp. 123–134). Thousand Oaks, CA: Sage.
Levinson, B. M., & Mallon, G. P. (1997). *Pet-oriented child psychotherapy*. Second Edition. Springfield, IL: C. C. Thomas.
McNicholas, J., & Collis, G. M. (1998). Could Type A (coronary prone) personality explain the association between pet ownership and health? In C. C. Wilson & D. C. Turner (Eds.), *Companion animals in human health* (pp. 173–185). Thousand Oaks, CA: Sage.
Melson, G. F. (1998). The role of companion animals in human development. In C. C. Wilson & D. C. Turner (Eds.), *Companion animals in human health* (pp. 219–236). Thousand Oaks, CA: Sage.

Melson, G. F. (2000). Companion animals and the development of children: Implications for the biophilia hypothesis. In A. H. Fine (Ed.), *Handbook on animal-assisted therapy: Theoretical foundations and guidelines for practice* (pp. 376–383). San Diego, CA: Academic Press.

Melson, G. F. (2001). *Why the wild things are: Animals in the lives of children.* Cambridge, MA: Harvard University Press.

Melson, G. F. (2003). Child development and the human-companion animal bond. *American Behavioral Scientist, 47*, 31–39.

Odendall, J. (2002). *Pets and our mental health: The why, the what, and the how.* New York: Vantage Press.

Pachana, N. A., Ford, J. H., & Andrew, B. (2005). Relations between companion animals and self-reported health in older women: Cause, effect or artifact? *International Journal of Behavioral Medicine, 12*, 103–110.

Parslow, R. A., & Jorm, A. F. (2003). The impact of pet ownership on health and health service use: Results from a community sample of Australians aged 40 to 44 years. *Anthrozoos, 16*, 43–56.

Parslow, R. A., Jorm, A. F., & Christensen, H. (2005). Pet ownership and health in older adults: Findings from a survey of 2,551 community-based Australians aged 60–64. *Gerontology, 51*, 40–47.

Podberscek, A. L., Paul, E. S., & Serpell, J. A. (2000). *Companion animals and us: Exploring the relationship between people and pets.* New York: Cambridge University Press.

Raina, P., Waltner-Toews, D., & Bonnett, B. (1999). Influence of companion animals on the physical and psychological health of older people: An analysis of a one-year longitudinal study. *Journal of the American Geriatrics Society, 47*, 323–329.

Sanders, C. R. (2003). Actions speak louder than words: Close relationships between humans and nonhuman animals. *Symbolic Interaction, 26*, 405–425.

Santarpio-Damerjian, M. A. (2002). Identifying and rescribing the roles of companion animals in the lives of workaholics: An exploratory study of workaholism, animal companionship, and intimacy. *Dissetation Abstracts International, 63*, 100.

Serpell, J. A. (2000). Creatures of the unconscious: Companion animals as mediators. In A. L. Podberscek & E. S. Paul (Eds.), *Companion animals and us: Exploring the relationship between people and pets* (pp. 198–121).

Sharkin, B. S., & Knox, D. (2003). Pet loss: Issues and implications for the psychologist. *Professional Psychology: Research & Practice, 34*, 414–421.

Stammbach, K. B., & Turner, D. C. (1999). Understanding the human-cat relationship: Human social support or attachment. *Anthozoos, 12*, 162–168.

Steffens, M. C., & Bergler, R. (1998). Blind people and their dogs: An empirical study on change in everyday life, in self-excperience, and in communication. In C. C. Wilson & D. C. Turner (Eds.), *Companion animals in human health* (pp. 149–157). Thousand Oaks, CA: Sage.

Strimple, E. O. (2003). A history of prison inmate animal interaction programs. *American Behavioral Scientist, 47*, 70–78.

Toray, T. (2004). The human-animal bond and loss: Providing support for grieving clients. *Journal of Mental Health Counseling, 26*, 244–259.

Triebenbacher, S. L. (1998). The relationship between attachment to companion animals and self-esteem: A developmental perspective. In C. C. Wilson & D. C. Turner (Eds.), *Companion animals in human health* (pp. 135–148). Thousand Oaks, CA: Sage.

Triebenbacher, S. L. (2000). The companion animal within the family system: The manner in which animals enhance life within the home. In A. H. Fine (Ed.), *Handbook on animal-assisted therapy: Theoretical foundations and guidelines for practice* (pp. 357–374). San Diego, CA: Academic Press.

Turner, D. C., Rieger, G., & Gygax, L. (2003). Spouses and cats and their effects on human mood. *Anthrozoos, 16*, 213–228.

Wilson, C. C. (1998). A conceptual framework for human-animal interaction research:The challenge revisited. In C. C. Wilson & D. C. Turner (Eds.), *Companion animals in human health* (pp. 61–90). Thousand Oaks, CA: Sage.

Wilson, C. C., & Barker, S. B. (2003). Challenges in designing human-animal interaction research. *Human-Animal Interaction & Wellness, 47*, 16–28.

Wilson, C. C., & Turner, D. C. (1998a). Beyond health: Extending the definition of health to quality of life. In C. C. Wilson & D. C. Turner (Eds.), *Companion animals in human health* (pp. 58–60). Thousand Oaks, CA: Sage.

Wilson, C. C., & Turner, D. C. (1998b). Quality of life outcomes: Psychosocial aspects of human-animal interaction. In C. C. Wilson & D. C. Turner (Eds.), *Companion animals in human health* (pp. 103–104). Thousand Oaks, CA: Sage.

Wilson, C. C., & Turner, D. C. (1998c). Quality of life outcomes: The relevance of animals to health and disease. In C. C. Wilson & D. C. Turner (Eds.), *Companion animals in human health* (pp. 159–160). Thousand Oaks, CA: Sage.

25

Applications of Emotional Intelligence to Schools and Workplace

David Ryback and Laura Sweeney

The first glimmer of what we now know as emotional intelligence (EI) seems to have come from the term "social intelligence," articulated by Thorndike (1920). Empathy along with active, reflective thinking as one anticipates events (Kelly, 1955) has long been the core value of effective communication. Understanding the perspective of the other—whether that be client, spouse, student or business associate—has been the backbone of healthy relationships. Add to this Gardner's (1983) theory of multiple intelligences, particularly interpersonal intelligence (empathy, social responsibility) and intrapersonal intelligence ("*access to one's feeling life*...as a means of understanding and guiding one's behavior" p. 239) and you witness the birth of EI.

Theory

EI is a term first coined by Salovey and Mayer who defined it as "the ability to monitor one's own and others' feelings and emotions...to use this information to guide one's thinking and actions." (1989/1990, p. 189) They eventually identified its four central components (1997) and later defined it simply as "a form of intelligence that combines emotions and thinking." (Mayer, Caruso, & Salovey, 2002, p. 338) Now we have the full-blown construct of EI, popularized by Goleman (1995) and based to a large extent on the research of Bar-On (1997) as he developed the basis for his Emotional Quotient Inventory (EQ-i).

Goleman (1995) originally classified emotional competencies to consist of five components: (1) self-awareness and accurate self-assessment, (2) self-regulation, impulse management and conscientious responsibility along with integrity, (3) motivation and higher achievement through optimistic thinking, (4) using empathy to help others to develop, and (5) managing relationships and building collaborative teams—influencing change through empathy.

A more pointed perspective of this same concept is offered by Zeidner, Matthews, and Roberts (2001) as culture-bound knowledge of emotion, such as how to act in specific social settings. Later, Matthews, Zeidner, and Roberts (2002) describe EI as focusing on "character and aspects of self-control, such as the ability to delay gratification, tolerate frustration, and regulate impulses (ego strength)...suggestive of a kinder, gentler intelligence" (pp. 6–7) and as "learned skills for handling emotional situations." (p. 267) Prati, Douglas, Ferris, Ammeter et al. (2003) see EI as "the ability to read and understand others in social contexts, and to utilize such knowledge to influence others through emotional regulation and control." (p. 21)

"Amygdala hijack," popularized in Goleman's book, refers to the part of the brain—the amygdala—where emotional decisions are made at an unconscious level as we lose our temper or engage in behaviors that that don't appear to be under our control. When we "lose it," the amygdala takes over and communication to the thinking part of the brain is blocked (LeDoux, 1996). Emotional intelligence helps us learn how to avoid this by anticipating and avoiding such thoughtless reactions to stress. Emotional intelligence is a concept that has had a strong influence on many spheres of our culture, education and business in particular.

The first concern is whether or not EI meets the traditional standards to be accepted as a construct of a type of intelligence. Three criteria must be met in order to fulfill this test: (1) Is it capable of being operationalized as a set of abilities? (2) Is it intercorrelated with preexisting forms of intelligence, while at the same time showing some unique variance? (3) Does it develop with age and experience? Based on a review of the literature and their own research, Mayer, Caruso, and Salovey (2000) concluded that EI meets these three criteria to a sufficient degree to declare, "Perhaps a general intelligence that includes emotional intelligence will be a more powerful predictor of important life outcomes than one that does not." (p. 295)

A second concern is the possibility of overstatement as to the utility of EI as a scientific construct. Popular claims as to the potency of EI may be overstated and unsupported by evidence (Mayer, Salovey, & Caruso, 2000). It is our intention, in this chapter, to provide reliable evidence of the effectiveness of the application of EI to enhance human welfare in the classroom and in the workplace.

The theory of emotional change, from the early glimmer of the precedents of EI to the best methods application technology, challenges us to look at what has been done so far. What is the research from which we can learn?

Research

Research on the Classroom

Beyond teaching the basic three Rs of " 'readin', 'ritin' and 'rithmetic,' " it is critical that schools also get involved in teaching a fourth R—reflection of self and social environment, i.e., social and emotional development or, as Henley and Long (1999) prefer, responsibility (Goleman, 1995; Mayer & Salovey, 1997; Scales & Leffert, 1999, among others).

"Securely attached children," writes Scharfe (2000) upon review of the literature, "tended to be emotionally expressive, have superior understanding of emotions, and have superior abilities to regulate emotions than insecure children." (p. 258) One important consideration is the age at which insecure children begin to be affected. One study revealing the developmental consistency of EI is the marshmallow test made popular by Goleman (1995). Shoda,

Mischel, and Peake (1990) tempted four-year-olds with a second marshmallow as a prize if they could delay their gratification by not eating a first marshmallow. Those who demonstrated their impulse management at age 4 were more confident, self-assured and trustworthy at age 16 and scored higher on their SATs at age 18. Interestingly, the marshmallow test was a better predictor of SAT success than was IQ—twice as good! Was this an indication that early training had long-lasting effects or that these same children had consistently good or bad caregivers throughout their childhoods?

A study of one-year-old infants and their mothers may be of particular help in understanding student deficiencies in skills relating to EI. Mothers of infants with an avoidant detachment style responded minimally to their children's expression of negative affect; mothers of resistant/ambivalent infants were responsive to negative affect but gave less attention to positive affect; and mothers of securely attached infants were responsive to positive, negative and neutral affect expressions (Goldberg, MacKay-Soroka, & Rochester, 1994). Apparently the caregiver's capacity for self-awareness and her/his ability to transmit this capacity to the child is of paramount importance. The more we can do at this early level of development to enhance emotional communication, the easier might be the job of "fixing" students later on.

Equally significant, for similar reasons, are the findings that children suffering early physical or sexual abuse show abnormal EEG readings indicating a higher prevalence of right-left hemispheric asymmetries (Teicher, Ito, Glod, Schiffer & Gelbard, 1996), reversed asymmetry (Ito, Teicher, Glod, & Ackerman, 1998) and abnormalities of the corpus callosum (van der Kolk, 1998). These findings point out even more dramatically the need for appropriate intervention at the earliest stages if we are to affect emotional considerations of development. They also suggest that this asymmetry can be corrected through various types of writing (L'Abate, 1992; 2002).

These results are confirmed by more current research that the early years of development are crucial to emotional development. Olds et al. (2004) had nurses drop in on 400 high-risk, low-income teenage girls during their first pregnancy to offer basic instruction and counseling on emotional communication skills and infant care. Not only did the children suffer less abuse; when they were followed up 15 years later, they were found to have 81% fewer criminal convictions than peers from similar backgrounds as well as fewer sex partners and less substance abuse (Kalb, Underwood, & Springen, 2005, p. 45).

The above-cited research is quite convincing about the efficacy of EI but the best research would involve pre- and posttests with experimental and control groups. One such project (Matthews, Zeidner, and Roberts, 2002, pp. 293–295) compared a control group with three stress groups, with all groups being tested for degree of stress before and after. Without going into the details, results supported Salovey, Bedell, Detweiler, and Mayer's (1999) hypothesis that EI is associated with less distress and worry.

The research on worry itself is complex and somewhat paradoxical. Worry, according to Matthews et al. (2002), "may serve some useful functions such as viewing a problem from different perspectives and exploring its various implicitations" (p. 276). Zeidner and Saklofske (1996) seem to agree that avoidant types of behavior, i.e., not worrying, act against mental health. Objective performance is impaired by such "avoidance." (Matthews & Campbell, 1998)

So do we want to inoculate against worry? Probably not. Some worry, especially when done effectively (see Ryback, 1995, pp. 117–118), is apparently good for mental well-being. However, the research on worrying and avoidance seems to be mixed (see L'Abate, 2005).

Ultimately, a review of the literature (Hardy, Power, & Jaedicke, 1993) suggests that there are three primary factors that affect a child's ability to cope with stress: (1) parental support which makes a child feel comfortable and facilitates a sense of self-efficacy, (2) parental control in setting boundaries and (3) structure providing a predictable environment.

To the extent that the classroom can harbor good influence, it can also help facilitate the qualities of EI that would follow. Successful social and emotional learning results in: (1) relationships becoming transformed, (2) problem-solving becoming commonplace, (3) diversity being respected and valued, (4) norms discouraging violence or bias, and (5) democracy and teamwork flourishing (Lantieri, 2003a, pp. 188–190).

The EI approach to education has been successfully utilized for different types of educational settings, such as special education (Cohen, Ettinger, & O'Donnell, 2003) and boarding schools (Wallace, 2003); across the country, including Alaska (Lantieri, 2003a); and even as far away as the mideast (Shadmi & Noy, 2003). Clearly, the research on applications of EI in the classroom is strongly encouraging.

Research on the Workplace

The psychological conditions of personal engagement and disengagement at work involve many interpersonal issues, all subsumed under the rubric of EI. Those individuals sensitive to paradigm shifts in the workplace cannot but see how the values expressed by EI have finally made an impact on the world of business (Thottam, 2005). But can this impact be scientifically validated and harnessed for the welfare of those involved? Can we create an approach that, once injected into a workplace, will continue to provide enhanced welfare for the inoculated? And, furthermore, inoculated against what?

The focus on the human-relations aspect of workers reaches back to the earlier part of the last century. The Hawthorne studies of the late 1920s gave birth to interest in the influence of research on human and emotional aspects of work style (Roethlisberger & Dickson, 1939). This research offered an early glimpse into the relative importance of employee satisfaction being a function of more than just monetary reward.

Introduction to the Workplace

The October 2, 1995 issue of *Time* magazine had "The EQ Factor" as its cover story, in which the success of EI in business was extolled. Since then, most business magazines have had at least one article explaining the concept of EI to their readers. As well, this has been a favorite topic for conferences and seminars.

The concept of EI is fairly new in industry, but it looks at a way of approaching teamwork in business organizations that is not too different from what took place in the encounter and t-group experiences so popular in the 1960s and 1970s. Personal feedback, the main vehicle in this modern team-building approach, is reminiscent of what took place in those encounter groups of decades past, albeit somewhat toned down in intensity now to keep the heat to a manageable level in this more politically correct climate.

The shift to this new paradigm in the workplace did not take place overnight. An overview of the history of job performance assessment reveals four stages: (1) The "efficiency expert" approach in which workers' movements were analyzed to uncover the most efficient use of labor by discovering and removing extraneous movements. (2) The reliance on IQ as a measure of employee selection. (3) The emergence of focus on personality traits, especially as revealed by the Minnesota Multi-Phasic Personality Inventory and Myers-Briggs. (Personality testing for purposes of hiring is now a $400 million industry [Handler, 2005].) (4) The current, contemporary emphasis on competencies in EI, in which empathy was introduced as a viable factor in the marketplace for the first time (Goleman, Boyatzis, & McKee, 2002).

Improved people skills, Goleman (1998) maintains, likely account for tens of millions of dollars worth of improved business. Emotionally competent managers ("stars" in the contemporary lingo) spend more time socializing with customers and collaborating helpfully with their peers. The skills used involve the five components described earlier, done well and often. In addition to empathy, such skills include political awareness of group dynamics and team leadership.

Those high only in IQ, as it turns out, seem to be less adept with such winning characteristics, pointing to a somewhat inverse relationship between heart and mind. "The value of self-awareness and management, relationship building, being intuitive, and factoring feelings into your life's work is unquestionable," declares Dearborn (2002, p. 529).

Leadership

Human relations-oriented training began entering the picture in the 1950s, followed by training groups (or t-groups) in the 1960s and 1970s. By the 1990s, there was a focus on "transformational leadership" (Barling, Weber, & Kelloway, 1996), which differentiated "following orders" from visionary empowerment. Barling, Slater, and Kelloway (2000) found that EI was associated with idealized influence, individualized focus and inspirational motivation, three attributes of transformational leadership. Leader charisma, a principal characteristic of the transformational leader, was primarily responsible for engendering a feeling of cooperation among team members (DeCremer & van Knippenberg, 2002).

A number of studies in the late 1970s and early 1980s shed light on the effectiveness of programs using a social-learning-modeling approach to leadership training (Burnaska, 1976; Byham, Adams, & Kiggins, 1976; Latham & Saari, 1979; Moses & Ritchie, 1976). In one study, for example, the trained supervisors were more successful than controls in terms of monthly productivity and lower absenteeism (Porras & Anderson, 1981). Results were sustained even after six months following the training.

Although executive skill learning has become quite popular over the past few years, there are few studies confirming its effectiveness. One exception is a program (Peterson, 1996) involving an assessment over one or two days, followed by monthly all-day intensive sessions, accumulating in about 50 hours of intense one-on-one work. Results of one published study (Peterson,

1993) revealed improvement on targeted behaviors with no change in nontargeted behaviors and changes persisted over time.

Moreover, the current climate of sensitivity to moral leadership among executives in this "post-Enron" period makes EI all the more important (Mussig, 2003). As one Australian executive put it, the integrity of a business could emerge as its greatest sustainable competitive advantage (Hornery, 2000). After all, transparency and achievement—subcomponents of the self-management component of EI leadership (Goleman et al., 2002, pp. 254–255)—involve authenticity and high personal standards.

The connection between EI competencies and effective leadership skills seems apparent at an intuitive level but statistical validation is always necessary and this has been demonstrated (Dulewicz & Higgs, 2000; 2004; Higgs & Rowland, 2000; 2001). Kobe, Reiter-Palmon, and Rickers (2001) found a significant correlation between leadership measures and the EQ-i ($r = .35$, $p < .01$). Higgs and Aitken (2003) provided further evidence by correlating success in leadership with scores on the EIQ-Managerial for 40 senior managers. In addition, according to Lewis (2000), the positive emotion of the leader elevates the team's emotional state and inspires members to perform with more enthusiasm. Conversely, a leader's lack of emotional control was related to leader ineffectiveness.

In order to test the effectiveness of EI training, Dulewicz, Higgs, and Slaski (2003) tested 59 middle managers with the EIQ before, and six months after, taking EI training one day a week for four weeks. They also used performance ratings pre and posttest. They found a statistically significant improvement with both measures at the.01 level of confidence and higher.

In a study using both pre and posttests as well as control groups, Dulewicz and Higgs (2004) tested team leaders (14 in experimental group and 13 in control) with the EIQ prior to EI training and 12 months after. They also measured job performance with "a composite of ratings by the bosses' boss, the HR director and the CEO" (p. 102). Paired sample t-tests showed significant improvement on conscientiousness in the experimental group but not in the control group.

Coping and Job Performance

The relationship between coping processes and adaptational outcomes has become a major concern for personality researchers (Zeidner, Matthews & Roberts, 2000). So no matter what aspect of human welfare in the workplace we explore, the common denominator involves individuals' abilities to cope effectively with stressful situations, be they personal or environmental, short-term or long-term, physical or psychological. In virtually all cases, effective coping is often seen as a critical skill of EI (Salovey, Bedell, Detweiler, & Mayer, 1999, p. 161).

Further empirical evidence reveals that high EI factors are associated with increased creativity (Moses & Stahelski, 1999) and that EI factors leading to high job satisfaction and sense of commitment result in less turnover and higher productivity (Tesluk, Vance, & Mathieu, 1999).

In Great Britain, call centers were established mostly by financial organizations to deliver services remotely over the phone, thus replacing the need for face-to-face interactions with customers (Richardson, 1994) and significantly reducing the cost of service delivery (Fernie & Metcalfe, 1997). A high correlation ($r = 0.217$, $p < .001$) was found between overall EI and the performance of agents at such centers as well as between a number of specific EI elements and performance (Higgs, 2004). Those with the highest correlations were conscientiousness ($r = 0.254$, $p < 0.001$), emotional resilience ($r = 0.186$, $p < 0.001$), motivation ($r = 0.183$, $p < 0.002$) and interpersonal sensitivity ($r = 0.170$, $p < 0.004$).

Douglas, Frink, and Ferris (2003) found that (1) of all EI factors, conscientiousness (primarily subcomponents initiative and achievement under self-management) is the most consistent predictor of job performance, (2) EI "moderated" the conscientiousness-job performance relationship, and (3) EI demonstrated a significant direct effect on job performance.

One of the most misunderstood aspects of EI training has to do with the intransigent nature of emotional change. Clearly, one-day workshops, no matter how experiential or intense, will not likely result in significant, lasting change. It takes months to make a dent in behaviors that emanate from the limbic system (Dempster, 1988; Howard, Kopta, Krause, & Orlinsky, 1986). One option for scheduling is a 2- or 3-day retreat followed by a half-day session on a monthly basis for at least six months. All this can be done with built-in support from either the group itself or from individual mentors or coaches or at least a buddy system (Kolb, Winter, & Berlew, 1968).

Physicians

One area for EI training is with physicians. Such training benefits not only the participants but, in a very critical way, the doctors themselves. Doctors who lack EI skills with their participants are much more likely to get sued for malpractice (e.g., Rice, 2000). "What comes up again and again in malpractice cases," writes Gladwell (2005), "is that participants say they were rushed or ignored or treated poorly." (p. 40) Levinson et al. (1997) recorded hundreds of conversations between surgeons and their participants to discover why half the doctors were sued. Those that weren't sued spent more time (18.3 minutes versus 15 minutes) with their participants and were much more likely to be empathetic. Both groups gave equal amounts of medical information so the difference was the EI in their communications.

To explore even further the fascinating details of this research, Ambady et al., (2002) selected two ten-second clips from each surgeon for analysis. She "content-filtered" the slices to remove the high-frequency sounds making the tapes unintelligible. The remaining garble was analyzed for such qualities as warmth, hostility, dominance and anxiousness.

Using a blind procedure, the sued doctors could be separated from their unsued peers merely by the degree of sounding dominant, a quality surely missing qualities of EI. Gladwell, who interviewed Ambady, writes "Malpractice sounds like one of those infinitely complicated and multidimensional problems. But in the end it comes down to a matter of respect ... through tone of voice." (2005, pp. 42–43) If these "dominant" surgeons had invested some time and energy in learning EI skills, their return on investment would have been stupendous!

There has been good evidence in the past decade for effective programs training doctors in social competence skills (Evans, Stanley, Mestrovic, & Rose, 1991; Greco, Francis, Buckley, Brownlea, & McGovern, 1998; Roter et al., 1998).

Police Officers

Klinger (2004) describes police officers inadvertently making a scene more violent than it need be by drawing their guns and sometimes killing victims in error. The lack of training in EI skills here involves a much greater issue than money or career status. It involves lost lives because of poor social judgment. To reduce stress in police officers and to reduce the chance that they might react violently rather than professionally because of such stress is a job for EI training. Officers high in EI skills are least prone to violence escalation (Brondolo et al., 1996).

Practice

The most thorough guidelines for effective EI training are offered by Cherniss (2000, pp. 450–452). Here follows an abridged version:
The Best Practice Guidelines

Phase 1: Preparation for Change

1. *Assess the organization's needs.* Determine critical needs and make sure they're congruent with culture and overall strategy.
2. *Assess each person's strengths and limits on the key competencies and deliver the results with care.* Deliver the results in a safe and supportive environment.
3. *Gauge readiness of the learners before starting the development process.* Don't begin until learners are ready.
4. *Set clear goals, link them to personal values, and break them into manageable steps.* Make sure goals are clear, specific and meaningful.
5. *Make learning self-directed.* Allow people to set the goals themselves. Let them continue to be in charge.
6. *Help learners build positive expectations for the training.*

Phase 2: Training

1. *Foster a positive relationship between the trainer and the learner.* Give trainers ongoing evaluation and feedback.
2. *Use "live" models to teach the competencies.* High status models inspire change.
3. *Rely on experiential methods.* Less lecture, more demonstration and practice.
4. *Provide opportunities for practice and give frequent feedback on practice efforts*, over a period of months.
5. *Inoculate against setbacks so that they are not seen as signals of defeat.* Anticipate and prepare for lapses.

Phase 3: Encouraging, Maintaining and Evaluating Change

1. *Build in social support.* Encourage formation of groups (or buddy or coach) to offer support throughout the change effort.
2. *Create an encouraging environment.* Integrate new learning into existing culture with support from above.

3. *Conduct ongoing evaluation research.* Find unobtrusive measures before and after training and after follow-up.

Whether in the classroom or in the workplace, solid and supportive social networks appear to help the high EI individual in coping with and adapting to stress (Salovey et al., 1999). The first two steps of Phase 3 above clearly involve a network of support. It would seem that a supportive network would be essential for the success of the entire program, though this is not spelled out clearly. Changes in behavior, one would expect, would come about more comfortably with a supportive network for encouragement. Virtually none of the changes in behavior are accomplished in isolation.

Consequently, it would be wise to consider forming tightly knit, trust-building groups as the context in which vaccinations for better life would be "injected." Such groups could be formed on the basis of mutual sharing of past or current problems to be worked on. According to Salovey et al. (1999), high EI individuals possess the skills involved in disclosing their past personal traumas. So these individuals within a group could model such disclosure. The process of subsequent disclosure by those lower in EI could help them improve their psychological well-being. According to Pennebaker (1997), such disclosure in writing improves mental health, including decreased depression and improved grades.

Such groups could then go on to create other groups for which these original groups could act as models and mentors. At a point of "maturity," when the group is reaching a plateau of EI growth, it could assign different tasks to its own members so that, for example, one third of the group could take on the task of inviting other of their peers to consider joining a similar group; one third could take on the task of logistics for the new group setting; and the remaining third could take on the task of "teaching" the principles and guidelines that make for effective learning.

When lectures are used for teaching EI principles, it should be remembered that the most effective schedule of presentation consists of 20 minutes of lecture, followed by 10 minutes of "downtime" to practice what's been learned, followed by 10 minutes "to further elaborate, reinforce, and summarize".

Classroom Applications

To advance such goals as responsible decision-making in school-age children, as prescribed by a consortium of educators known as the Collaborative to Advance Social and Emotional Learning (Graczyk et al., 2000), Cowen (1998) proposed the following strategies: (1) encouraging the development of positive bonding between a child and a primary caregiver; (2) helping children attain effective communication and friend-making skills; (3) teaching children how to deal with stressors; (4) helping children gain a sense of control of their destinies; and (5) providing them with wellness-enhancing school environments.

Accordingly, a differentiation can be made between social and emotional learning (SEL) (gaining emotional intelligence about decision-making and establishing positive relationships) and social and emotional education (SEE) (the teaching of such skills to children) (Elias et al., 1997). The five categories of SEL are: (1) awareness of self and others, (2) positive attitudes and values, (3) responsible decision-making, (4) communication skills, and (5) social skills. Despite crowded school schedules and the perennial competing approaches to school reform, SEL has been accomplished "in a growing number of schools" (Elias & Weissberg, 2000, p. 186).

In terms of (1), (4) and (5) above, it should be pointed out that empathy begets empathy. Children who have experienced empathic caretakers are more able to be empathic to others (Taylor, Parker, & Bagby, 1999). Whatever the mechanism, the outcome is clear. Conversely, the more maltreatment by caregivers of elementary school-aged children, the lower the EI and all the characteristic shortfalls (Brenner & Salovey, 1997).

One of the most impactful principles for using EI as a approach in educational settings is the principle of cooperative goal setting, or cocreation of goals. This refers to the process of allowing the students to share meaningfully in the process of goal setting along with the more responsible individuals involved.

The sharing groups mentioned in the above paragraph can function in highly responsible fashion when all individuals feel mutually involved in the process of determining the goals and rules of the groups (see Brownlee & Yerkes, 2003).

There is a literature available (e.g., Rogers, 1980; Rogers & Freiberg, 1983) with many of the finer points and details for which there is insufficient space here. Suffice it to say that this is not a new technology. Its proper use can make EI available at very little cost once the philosophy of cocreation of goals is understood and applied. Students can use class meetings "to set class goals, norms, and ground rules; to make plans and decisions; and to discuss and resolve issues and problems" and work in pairs or small groups "to deepen both their understanding of subject matter and their capacity to work together effectively and respectfully" (Lewis, Watson, & Schaps, 2003, p. 102).

Specific instructions for structuring such EI-oriented classrooms can be acquired quite inexpensively in books (Child Development Project, 1996; Dalton & Watson, 1997). Evaluations of such programs, compared to matched comparison schools as controls, resulted in enhanced social development (Schaps, Watson, & Lewis, 1996; Watson, Battistich, & Solomon, 1997).

One of the bigger challenges in today's school systems is characterized by the Columbine tragedy and the many tragedies that followed. In response to this culture of violence, the Resolving Conflict Creatively Program was developed in which there is one model for kindergarten through 8th Grade and another for high schools. An evaluation of this program, involving over 5,000 children and 300 teachers from 15 public elementary schools over a 2-year period, revealed that nonviolent attitudes replaced those of violence (Aber, Brown, & Henrich, 1999). The benefits accrued to "all children, regardless of gender, grade level, or risk status" (Lantieri, 2003b, p. 84).

Workplace Applications

Why EI in the workplace? If for no other reason, because it works! Four out of five of the 50 leading-edge companies looked at by the American Society for Training and Development (1997) were already teaching it to their employees. As for-profit entities, they wouldn't be doing it if it weren't effective for them. As Bar-On & Parker point out, "One can find effective programs for improving emotional intelligence in a number of different areas associated with training and development. These include management training programs, communication and empathy training programs for physicians, programs to teach police how to handle conflict, stress management training, self-management training, and training for unemployed workers." (2000, p. 436)

Leadership

Fortunately, there is a clear history of successful practice of leadership training. A meta-analysis of management training programs based on self-analysis and other EI factors by Burke and Day (1986) reveals that such programs, as measured by objective criteria such as performance measures and absenteeism, were highly effective.

Often, the key to success was an ongoing program that integrated various modes of training. For example, one study (Hand & Slocum, 1972) involved 28 weekly, 90-minute sessions involving discussion of leadership styles and experiential exercises involving listening, decision-making and interviewing. Compared to a control group, managers who completed the training became more self-aware, empathic and more trustworthy when rated by subordinates and superiors. An 18-month follow-up revealed the changes to be persistent.

In order to have a clear perspective of the nature of EI competencies as they relate to leadership, the 18 emotional intelligence leadership competencies abridged from Goleman, Boyatzis, and McKee (2002, pp. 253–256) are presented here:

Self-Awareness

- Emotional self-awareness: Candid and authentic. Able to speak openly about their emotions. Able to express conviction about guiding vision.
- Accurate self-assessment: Know their limitations and strengths. Welcome constructive criticism.
- Self-confidence: Play to their strengths. Sense of presence, self-assurance.

Self-Management

- Self-control: Channel disturbing emotions in useful ways. Remain clear-headed during a crisis.
- Transparency: Authentic openness about their feelings and beliefs. Admit mistakes and faults.
- Adaptability: Comfortable with ambiguities. Flexible in adapting to new challenges.
- Achievement: High personal standards. Pragmatic. Continually learning.
- Initiative: Control their own destiny. Create opportunities rather than wait.
- Optimism: Roll with the punches. See others positively. "Glass half-full."

Social Awareness

- Empathy: Feel unspoken emotions. Listen attentively to grasp others' perspectives.
- Organizational awareness: Can read power relationships. Can understand unspoken rules.
- Service: Monitor customer or client satisfaction. Make themselves available.

Relationship management

- Inspiration: Create resonance. Inspire others to follow.
- Influence: Know how to build buy-in from key people. Persuasive and engaging.
- Developing others: Genuine interest in others' development. Natural mentors.
- Change catalyst: Challenge the status quo. Overcome barriers to change.
- Conflict management: Can understand different perspectives and find a common ideal.
- Teamwork and collaboration: Models of respect and helpfulness. Draw others into commitment.

A leader with many of the above characteristics (very few have all) would be expected to have a positive effect on associates in terms of productivity and loyalty. Such an approachable team leader would also be expected to encourage mutual trust and influence the group toward feelings of team empowerment. This is exactly what Koberg, Boss, Senjem, and Goodman (1999) found to be possible. They also found that empowerment of team members was tied to increased job satisfaction and increased team effectiveness and performance.

One important question is: "Do one-day training sessions have effects that last over time or, as is becoming increasingly apparent, are they merely entertainment to raise morale?" Those well versed in EI realize that lasting behavioral changes hardly occur as a result of singe-day training sessions. In-depth follow-up sessions weeks and months later are necessary to lock in any incipient changes that might come about. Furthermore, objective criteria are necessary to enable proper measurement.

It was to answer such concerns that Dearborn (2002) proposed a multi-rater assessment tool to help leaders obtain objective feedback from others as they attempt to grow toward their ideal selves. With such objective feedback regarding their EI, they might be more willing to extend themselves to personal growth than they would be with more traditional 360-degree feedback that is less objective.

Coping and Job Performance

Similarly, team identity has also been shown to increase effectiveness and performance (Worchel, Rothgerber, Day, Hart, & Butemeyer, 1998). Finally, Isen, Daubman, and Nowicki, (1987) and Amason (1996) found that the cooperative environment of emotionally intelligent teams fosters increased creative thought and innovative problem solving.

So, with all this evidence, why don't business schools focus on EI? Well, at least one does so, and successfully enough to offer a model for other schools. At Case Western Reserve University's Weatherhood School of Management, all beginning students go through an in-depth assessment for a two-week period. The next seven weeks are devoted to analyzing the results and planning the next two years of schooling. According to Boyatzis (1996), when compared with their more traditional peers, such students show superior EI skills across the board.

Physicians

The normal curriculum of medical studies typically involves some degree of skill in doctor-patient interaction (Fadem, 1994, pp. 165–172; Wiener, 1990, pp. 193–202). Since this is such a small part of conventional medical training, there is much benefit to learning EI skills once the licensed physician is practicing. As mentioned above, if for no other reason than to avoid costly malpractice suits, EI training is clearly worthwhile from the physicians' point of view.

One program in Israel (Kramer, Ber, & Moore, 1989) trained fifth-year medical students in ten 90-minute meetings over a 5-week period. Their training involved role-playing and observing live interviews. All students were then evaluated by independent observers. When compared with a control group, the trained medical students showed a significant and lasting increase in EI-related behaviors with actual participants while the students in the control group showed a significant decrease in these behaviors.

It is important to emphasize that the Israeli model mentioned above involves training over a 5-week period and includes role-playing and observing live interviews. Again, using the Cherniss (2000) guidelines above, EI training can be done with tight-knit groups cocreating their own goals and learning fairly independently within the groups.

Police Officers

Based on Zacker and Bard's (1973) original model, police officers can be trained through a number of modalities, including lectures, group discussions, real-life simulations and role-playing. Lectures and discussions on EI and its ramifications can be complemented by using the Best Practice Guidelines offered by Cherniss (2000) above to inculcate the officers with the EI values of self-management, empathy and successfully managing others.

If only one life were to be saved by such training, the return on investment from an EI program would be inestimable. The inoculation factor here is the opportunity to share stressful incidents on the job with peers thereby diffusing the buildup of stress if such incidents were withheld. The cost of such training is minimal given the availability of literature on these procedures. The groups involved can invite other groups to similar experience as mentioned above.

Conclusions

The large body of research on the application of EI to classroom settings, to the workplace, to physicians, and to police officers makes it clear that the principles involved are highly effective when done with integrity, perseverance and careful attention to the human factor.

Some may argue that many of the components are not new. What is new is the comprehensiveness of the entirety of the research and the conceptual consolidation that make further research and experimentation more meaningful. Consequently, vaccinations of EI for enhanced welfare in the sectors mentioned above can be continually examined over time, making it possible to judge the results within the integrated framework we call EI.

References

Aber, J. L., Brown, J. L., & Henrich, C. C. (1999). *Teaching conflict resolution.* NewYork: Columbia University, Joseph J. Mailman School of Public Health, National Center for Children in Poverty.

Amason, A. C. (1996). Distinguishing the effects of functional and dysfunctional conflict on strategic decision making. *Academy of Management Journal, 39*, 123–148.

Ambady, N., LaPlante, D., Nguyen, T., Rosenthal, R., et al. (2002). Surgeons' tone of voice. *Surgery, 132*, 5–9.

American Society for Training and Development. (1997). *Benchmarking forum member-to-member survey results.* Alexandria, VA.

Bar-On, R. & Parker, J. D. A. (2000). *Handbook of Emotional Intelligence.* San Francisco: Jossey-Bass.

Barling, J., Slater, F., & Kelloway, E. K. (2000). Transformational leadership and emotional intelligence. *Leadership and Organizational Development Journal, 21*, 157–161.

Barling, J., Weber, T., & Kelloway, E. K. (1996). Effects of transformational leadership training on attitudinal and financial outcomes. *Journal of Applied Psychology, 81*, 827–832.

Boyatzis, R. E. (1996). Competencies can be developed, but not in the way we thought. *Capability, 2*, 25–41.

Brenner, E. M. & Salovey, P. (1997). Emotion regulation during childhood. In P. Salovey & D. J. Sluyter (Eds.), *Emotional development and emotional intelligence.* NY: Basic Books.

Brondolo, E., Jellife, T., Quinn, C., Tunick, W. et al. (1996). Correlates of risk for conflict among New York City traffic agents. In G. R. VandenBos & E. Q. Bulatao (Eds.), *Violence on the job* (pp. 217–238). Washington, DC: American Psychological Association

Brownlee, M & Yerkes, R. (2003). Co-creating staff to facilitate adventure activities. *The Camping Magazine, 76*, 38–42.

Burke, M. & Day, R. (1986). A cumulative study of the effectiveness of managerial training. *Journal of Applied Psychology, 71*, 232–245.

Burnaska, R. F. (1976). The effects of behavior modeling training upon managers' behaviors and employees' perceptions. *Personnel Psychology*, 29, 329–335.

Byham, W. C., Adams, D. & Kiggins, A. (1976). Transfer of modeling training to the job. *Personnel Psychology, 29*, 345–349.

Cherniss, C. (2000). Social and emotional competence in the workplace. In R. Bar-On & J. D. A. Parker (Eds.), *The Handbook of Emotional Intelligence* (pp. 433–458). San Francisco, CA: Jossey-Bass.

Child Development Project, (1996). *Ways we want our class to be.* Oakland, CA: Developmental Studies Center.

Cohen, M., Ettinger, B., & O'Donnell, T. (2003). The children's institute model for building the social-emotional skills of students in special education. In M. J. Elias, H. Arnold, & C. S. Hussey (Eds.), *EQ + IQ = best leadership practices for caring and successful schools* (pp. 124–141). Thousand Oaks, CA: Corwin Press.

Cowen, E. L. (1998). Changing concepts of prevention in mental health. *Journal of Mental Health, 7*, 451–461.

Dalton, J. & Watson, M. S. (1997). *Among friends.* Oakland, CA: Developmental Studies Center.

Dearborn, K. (2002). Studies in emotional intelligence redefine our approach to leadership development. *Public Personnel Management, 31*, 523–530.

DeCremer, D. & van Knippenberg, D. (2002). How do leaders promote cooperation? *Journal of Applied Psychology, 87*, 858–866.

Dempster, F. N. (1988). The spacing effect. *American Psychologist, 43*, 627–634.

Douglas, C., Frink, D. D., & Ferris, G. R. (2003). Emotional intelligence as a moderator of the conscientiousness-performance relationship. Paper presented at the 18th Annual Conference of the Society for Industrial and Organizational Psychology, Orlando, FL.
Dulewicz, V. & Higgs, M. J. (2000). Emotional intelligence. *Journal of Managerial Psychology, 15*, 341–368.
Dulewicz, V. & Higgs, M. J. (2004). Can emotional intelligence be developed? *International Journal of Human Resource Management*, 15, 95–111.
Dulewicz, V., Higgs, M. J., & Slaski, M. (2003). Emotional intelligence. *Journal of Management Psychology, 18*, 405–420.
Elias, M. J. & Weissberg, R. P. (2000). Primary prevention. *The Journal of School Health, 70*, 186–190.
Elias, M. J., Zins, J. E., Weissberg, R. P., Frey, K. S., et al. (1997). *Promoting social and emotional learning*. Alexandria, VA: Association for Supervision and Curriculum Development.
Evans, B. J., Stanley, R. O., Mestrovic, R., & Rose, L. (1991). Effects of communication skills training on students' diagnostic efficiency. *Medical Education, 25*, 517–526.
Fadem, B. (1994). *Behavioral science* (2nd edition). Philadelphia, PA: Harwal.
Fernie, S. & Metcalf, D. (1997). *(Not) hanging on the telephone: Payment systems in the 'New Sweatshops'*. Working paper, Centre for Economic Performance, London School of Economics, London, England.
Gardner, H. (1983). *Frames of mind*. NY: Basic Books.
Gladwell, M. (2005). *Blink*. NY: Little, Brown
Goldberg, S., MacKay-Soroka, S., & Rochester, M. (1994). Affect, attachment, and maternal responsiveness. *Infant Behavior and Development, 17*, 335–339.
Goleman, D. (1995). *Emotional intelligence*. NY: Bantam
Goleman, D. (1998). *Working with emotional intelligence*. NY: Bantam
Goleman, D., Boyatzis, R., & McKee, A. (2002). *Primal leadership*. Boston: HBS Press.
Graczyk, P. A., Weissberg, R. P., Payton, J. W., Elias, M. J., et.al. (2000). Criteria for evaluating the quality of school-based social and emotional learning programs. In Reuven Bar-On & James D. A. Parker (Eds.), *The handbook of emotional intelligence* (pp. 391–410). San Francisco, CA: Jossey-Bass.
Greco, M., Francis, W., Buckley, J., Brownlea, A., & McGovern, J. (1998). Real-patient evaluation of communication skills teaching for GP registrars. *Family Practice, 15*, 51–57.
Hand, H. H. & Slocum, J. W. (1972). A longitudinal study of the effects of a human relations training program on managerial effectiveness. *Journal of Applied Psychology, 56*, 412–417.
Handler, R. (2005). The new phrenology: A critical look at the $400 million a year personality-testing industry. *Psychotherapy Networker, 29*, May/June, 77–81.
Hardy, D. F., Power, T. G., & Jaedicke, S. (1993). Examining the relation of parenting to children's coping with everyday stress. *Child Development, 64*, 1829–1841.
Henley, M. & Long, N. J. (1999). Teaching emotional intelligence to impulsive-aggressive youth. *Reclaiming Children and Youth, 7*, 224–229.
Higgs, M. (2004). A study of the relationship between emotional intelligence and performance in UK call centres. *Journal of Managerial Psychology, 19*, 442–454.
Higgs, M. & Aitken, P. (2003). An exploration of the relationship between emotional intelligence and leadership potential. *Journal of Managerial Psychology, 18*, 814–823.
Higgs, M. J. & Rowland, D. (2000). Building change leadership capability. *Journal of Change Management, 1*, 116–131.
Higgs, M. J. & Rowland, D. (2001). Developing change leadership capability. *Henley Working Paper Series*, HWP 01/21.

Hornery, S. (2000). Lend Lease's 2000 Annual Report, Lend Lease Corp. Ltd., Sydney, Australia.

Howard, K., Kopta, S. M., Krause, M. S., & Orlinsky, D. E. (1986). The dose-effect relationship in psychotherapy. *American Psychologist, 41*, 159–164.

Hunt, N. & Evans, D. (2004). Predicting traumatic stress using emotional intelligence. *Behavior Research and Therapy, 42*, 791–798.

Isen, A. M., Daubman, K. A., & Nowicki, G. P. (1987). Positive affect facilitates creative problem solving. *Journal of Personality and Social Psychology, 52*, 1122–1131.

Ito, Y., Teicher, M. H., Glod, C. A., & Ackerman, E. (1998). Preliminary evidence for aberrant cortical development in abused children. *Journal of Neuropsychiatry and Clinical Neuroscience, 10*, 298–307.

Kalb, C., Underwood, A., & Springen, K. (2005). Family matters. *Newsweek, CXLV*, April 25, 39–45.

Kelly, G. A. (1955). *A theory of personality*. NY: Norton.

Klinger, D. (2004). *Into the kill zone*. San Francisco: Jossey-Bass.

Kobe, L. M., Reiter-Palmon, R., & Rickers, J. D. (2001). Self-reported leadership experiences in relation to inventoried social and emotional intelligence. *Current Psychology, 20*, 154–163.

Koberg, C. S., Boss, R. W., Senjem, J. C., & Goodman, E. A. (1999). Antecedents and outcomes of empowerment. *Group and Organizational Management, 24*, 71–91.

Kolb, D. A., Winter, S. K., & Berlew, D. E. (1968). Self-directed change. *Journal of Applied Behavioral Science, 4*, 453–471.

Kramer, D., Ber, R., & Moore, M. (1989). Increasing empathy among medical students. *Medical Education, 23*, 168–173.

L'Abate, L. (1992). *Programmed writing: Self-administered interventions for individuals, couples, and families*. Pacific Grove, CA: Brooks-Cole.

L'Abate, L. (2002). *Beyond psychotherapy: Programmed writing and structured computer-assisted interventions*. Westport, CT: Ablex.

L'Abate, L. (2005). *Personality in intimate relationships: Socialization and psychopathology*. NY: Springer.

Lantieri, L. (2003a). A vision of schools with heart and spirit. In M. J. Elias, H. Arnold, & C. S. Hussey (Eds.), *EQ + IQ = best leadership practices for caring and successful schools* (pp. 184–198). Thousand Oaks, CA: Corwin Press

Lantieri, L. (2003b). Waging peace in our schools. In M. J. Elias, H. Arnold, & C. S. Hussey (Eds.), *EQ + IQ = best leadership practices for caring and successful schools* (pp. 76–88). Thousand Oaks, CA: Corwin Press

Latham, G. P. & Saari, L. M. (1979). Application of social-learning theory to training supervisors through behavioral modeling. *Journal of Applied Psychology, 64*, 239–246.

LeDoux, J. E. (1996). *The emotional brain*. NY: Simon & Schuster.

Levinson, W., Roter, D. L., Mullooly, J. P., Dull, V. T., et al. (1997). Physician-patient communication. *Journal of the American Medical Association, 277*, 553–559.

Lewis, K. M. (2000). When leaders display emotion. *Journal of Organizational Behavior, 21*, 221–234.

Lewis, C., Watson, M., & Schaps, E. (2003). Building community in school. In M. J. Elias, H. Arnold, & C. S. Hussey (Eds.), *EQ + IQ = best leadership practices for caring and successful schools* (pp. 100–108). Thousand Oaks, CA: Corwin Press

Matthews, G. & Campbell, S. E. (1998). Task-induced stress and individual differences in coping. *Proceedings of the 42nd Annual Meeting of the Human Factors and Ergnomics Society* (pp. 821–825). Santa Monica, CA: Human Factors and Ergnomics Society.

Matthews, G., Zeidner, M., & Roberts, D. R. (2002). *Emotional intelligence*. Cambridge, MA: MIT Press.

Mayer, J. D., Caruso, D. R., & Salovey, P. (2000). Emotional intelligence meets traditional standards for an intelligence. *Intelligence, 27*, 267–298.

Mayer, J. D., Caruso, D. R., & Salovey, P. (2002). Selecting a measure of emotional intelligence. In R. Bar-On & J. D. A. Parker (Eds.), *The handbook of emotional intelligence* (pp. 320–342). San Francisco, CA: Jossey-Bass.

Mayer, J. D. & Salovey, P. (1997). What is emotional intelligence? In P. Salovey & D. J. Sluyter (Eds.), *Emotional development and emotional intelligence* (pp.3–34). NY: Basic Books.

Mayer, J. D., Salovey, P., & Caruso, D. R. (2000). Emotional intelligence. In R. J. Steinberg, (Ed.), *Handbook of intelligence* (pp. 117–137). NY: Cambridge University Press.

Moses, J. L. & Ritchie, R. J. (1976). Supervisory relationships training. *Personnel Psychology, 29*, 337–343.

Moses, T. P. & Stahelski, A.J. (1999). A productivity evaluation of teamwork at an aluminum manufacturing plant. *Group and Organizational Management, 24*, 391–412.

Mussig, D. J. (2003). A research and skills training framework for values-driven leadership. *Journal of European Industrial Training, 27*, 73–79.

Olds, D. L., Robinson, J., Pettit, L. Luckey, D. W. et al. (2004). Effects of home visits by paraprofessionals and by nurses. *Pediatrics, 114*, 1560–1568.

Pennebaker, J. W. (1997). Writing about emotional experiences as a therapeutic process. *Psychological Science, 8*, 162–166.

Peterson, D. B. (1993). *Skill learning and behavior change in an individually tailored management coaching program.* Paper presented at the Annual Conference of the Society for Industrial and Organizational Psychology, San Francisco, April.

Peterson, D. B. (1996). Executive coaching at work. *Consulting Psychology Journal, 48*, 78–86.

Porras, J. L. & Anderson, B. (1981). Improving managerial effectiveness through modeling-based training. *Organizational Dynamics, 9*, 60–77.

Prati, L. M., Douglas, C., Ferris, G. R., Ammeter, A. P., et al. (2003). Emotional intelligence, leadership effectiveness, and team outcomes. *The International Journal of Organizational Analysis, 11*, 21–40.

Rice, B. (2000). How plaintiffs' lawyers pick their targets. *Medical Economics, 8*, 94.

Richardson, R. (1994). Back-officing front office functions—organizational and locational implications of new telemediated services. In R. Munsell (Ed.), *Management of information and communication technologies, emerging patterns of control* (pp. 309–335). London, England: ASLIB.

Roethlisberger, F. J. & Dickson, W. J. (1939). *Management and the worker.* Cambridge, MA: Harvard University Press.

Rogers, C. R. (1980). *A way of being*. Boston: Houghton Mifflin.

Rogers, C. R. & Freiberg, H. J. (1983). *Freedom to learn.* (3rd edition). New York: Merrill.

Roter, D., Rosenbaum, J., de Negri, B., Renaud, D., et al. (1998). The effects of continuing medical education programme in interpersonal communication skills on doctor practice and patient satisfaction in Trinidad and Tobago. *Medical Education, 32*, 181–189.

Ryback, D. (1995). *Look 10 years younger/live 10 years longer*. Englewood Cliffs, NJ: Prentice Hall.

Salovey, P., Bedell, B. T., Detweiler, J. B., & Mayer, J. D. (1999). Coping intelligently. In C. R. Snyder (Ed.), *Coping: The psychology of what works* (pp. 141–164). NY: Oxford University Press.

Salovey, P. & Mayer, J. D. (1989/1990). Emotional intelligence. *Imagination, Cognition, and Personality, 9*, 185–211.

Scales, P. C. & Leffert, N. (1999). Developmental assets. Minneapolis, MN: Search Institute.

Schaps, E., Watson, M., & Lewis, C. (1996). A sense of community is key to effectiveness in fostering character education. *Journal of Staff Development, 17*, 42–47.

Scharfe, E. (2000). Development of emotional expression, understanding, and regulation in infants and young children. In R. Bar-On & J. D. A. Parker (Eds.), *Handbook of emotional intelligence* (pp. 244–262). San Francisco: Jossey-Bass.

Shadmi, C. & Noy, B. (2003). Promoting students' social-emotional and intellectual well-being and the school as ecosystem. In M. J. Elias, H. Arnold, & C. S. Hussey (Eds.), *EQ + IQ = best leadership practices for caring and successful schools* (pp. 154–173). Thousand Oaks, CA: Corwin Press

Shoda, Y., Mischel, W., & Peake, P. K. (1990). Predicting adolescent cognitive and self-regulatory competencies from preschool delay of gratification. *Developmental Psychology, 26*, 978–986.

Taylor, G. J., Parker, J. D. A., & Bagby, R. M. (1999). Emotional intelligence and the emotional brain. *Journal of the American Academy of Psychoanalysis, 27*, 339–354.

Teicher, M. H., Ito, Y., Glod, C. A., Schiffer, F., & Gelbard, H. A. (1996). Neurophysiological mechanisms of stress response in children. In C. R. Pfeffer (Ed.), *Severe stress and mental disturbance in children* (pp. 59–84). Washington, DC: American Psychiatric Press.

Tesluk, P. E., Vance, R. J., & Mathieu, J. E. (1999). Examining employee involvement in the context of participative work environments. *Group and Organizational Management, 24*, 271–299.

Thorndike, E. L. (1920). Intelligence and its uses. *Harper's Magazine, 140*, 227–235.

Thottam, J. (2005). Thank God It's Monday! *Time, 165*, January 17, A58–A61.

van der Kolk, B. A. (1998). *The psychobiology of developmental trauma.* Paper presented at the 151st Annual Meeting of the American Psychiatric Association, Toronto, Canada, May.

Wallace, F. (2003). Social-emotional learning at North Country School. In M. J. Elias, H. Arnold, & C. S. Hussey (Eds.), *EQ + IQ = best leadership practices for caring and successful schools* (pp. 142–153). Thousand Oaks, CA: Corwin Press.

Watson, M. S., Battistich, V., & Solomon, S. (1997). Enhancing students' social and ethical development in schools. *International Journal of Educational Research, 27*, 571–586.

Wiener, J. M. (1990). *Behavioral science* (2nd edition). Baltimore, MD: Williams & Wilkins.

Worchel, S., Rothgerber, H., Day, E. A., Hart, D., & Butemeyer, J. (1998). Social identity and individual productivity within groups. *British Journal of Social Psychology, 37*, 389–413.

Zacker, J. & Bard, M. (1973). Effects of conflict management training on police performance. *Journal of Applied Psychology, 58*, 202–208.

Zeidner, M., Matthews, G., & Roberts, R. D. (2001). Slow down, you move too fast. *Emotion, 1*, 265–275.

Zeidner, M. & Saklofske, D. S. (1996). Adaptive and maladaptive coping. In M. Zeidner & N. S. Endler (Eds.), *Handbook of coping* (pp. 505–531). NY: John Wiley & Sons.

Section VII

Conclusion

We have come full circle from complete internality, as in the digestive process involved in nutrition, to activities involving some kind of external, individual action, as in exercise, or in some seemingly internal inaction, as in meditation. From there, levels of complexity, externality, and probably costs, increase, going from individualized writing to computers and the Internet. Chances of survival and enjoyment increase with the larger complexity of activities and interventions, going ultimately to groups and classrooms. Finally, we enter the community level, which could not be included because it constitutes deservedly a tier of its own, with its own organizations and methodologies that increase the complexity of interventions. Nonetheless, Cornelius Hogan offers a glimpse of what can be achieved even at the State policy level, when one can use sensitivity, ingenuity, and creativity to solve difficult social problems. Chapter 26 shows how it is possible to change potentially expensive behavior through relatively inexpensive interventions.

26

Implications of Prescriptive Approaches for Policy, Health Promotion, Epidemiology, and Public Health

Cornelius Hogan

The purpose of this chapter is to offer a practical overview of this writer's first-hand experience with low-cost interventions in the field of public health promotion. Hence, no references will be cited because they are no substitutes for the actual experience shown with real data.

General Theory

There are several important constructs that can serve as important elements of theory that can serve as a grounding for low-cost promotional strategies in a world where we are spending ever more resources to fix serious problems of the human condition after the odds of positive change become long. The three theories of low-cost change on which I will focus are the power of human relationships in human change, the power of common purpose across people and organizations to effect change, and the power of community to mold change. These are very related ideas but will be considered separately here for the sake of clarity and presentation.

The Power of Human Relationships

The power of human relationships is at the center of most human change. We can all relate to the power that our favorite and early teacher or had on our lives. We know the impact of that great coach that we had early on. We know the power of transference in the therapist client relationship. And we know the incredible power of the attachment of a mother to her newborn. And now considerable literature is emerging that speaks to the positive impact of intact families over time. The chapter which shows us the impact that confidants, family, friends, and companions play in our leading healthy lives gives us important examples of the possibilities (Chapter 23 this volume).

Efficient and effective systems, as important as they are, cannot create the kind of lasting and deep change in people that human relationships can. This is being ever more recognized in new ways to reach our youth, many of who are suffering from an anomie born of fragile and broken human relationships. This is recognized with the large and increasing concentration of mentorship programs, which aim to develop strong and positive human relationships among many of our disaffected youth and successful and strong adults. And, the new knowledge coming our way regarding the impact of small animals on nursing home residents, and the role that horses play in the rehabilitation of inmates in Texas and other places shows us that the idea of companionship and human relationships go well beyond what we have previously accepted and known.

In the Trondheim region of Norway, the many and excellent child serving organizations have adopted a common purpose of "All children have a human relationship they can depend upon." The Norwegians know and act on the power of human relationships. There are some deeply worrisome trends in the data we follow in this country that are working strongly against strong relationships among family members. The birth rate to single parents is now over 50%. The percent of children living in single parent homes parallels this trend. And there are many other trends, which are connected to these realities, which serve to lessen the quality of relationships among people. The steady and inexorable trend toward ever more individualization of our entertainment, and particularly the entertainment of our children are a case in point. The average number of hours that individuals, and particularly children, watch television is now over an astounding 8 hours per day. Individualized computer games where young people play in isolation are another case in point. And studies associated with the level of violence that children experience on television in their early years of life and the impact that this depersonalization of human life has on later behavior and attitudes, have been well studied and documented.

These realities in our lives by and large are not a question of money. They are questions of common sense and culture. In the simplest sense it has been said that one of the most low-cost steps that parents can take is to simply unplug the television set. And in our rapidly moving world common sense is often in short supply in the context of a culture where time needed to build the kind of relationships we need to have with other human beings, has been generally set aside for our more material side of life.

Having two jobs to survive economically works against human relationships as does the over scheduling and the lack of free time and free play time for our children. These are not alone questions of money, but are more a function of our speeding lives. Having a meal as a family together is less and less the norm. Can we think of a lower cost and more effective way of leading our lives other than making sure our families share a meal together so that important family relationships can be cemented in a systematic way over time?

The Power of Common Purpose

The 'power of common purpose' is also well-known and well-documented. And common purpose can occur at every level of our lives. It can occur on the largest stage at the national level and beyond. It can occur with the smallest units of life in and with our friends and family. The powerful common purpose of 'putting a man on the moon and bringing him back safely' was an utterance by President Kennedy in the early 1960s that galvanized a nation, the machinery of government, and the imagination of our people. And, that common purpose brought together the talent, resources, and energy of government, the private sector, the military, and others and resulted in the first moon landing in the late 1960s, which captured the interest of most of the people on Earth.

From that lofty example of common purpose, comes the work and energy of a family who gets behind one of their children to be the first of any generation to achieve success in college. Individuals in the family sacrifice, encourage, support, and find many ways to make sure this common purpose is achieved. A strong common purpose is intangible. It can bring forth and summon tangible resources, such as the resources appropriated by Congress to properly support the moon landing, but that common purpose also served to set a tone and climate, within which adequate resources were focused, and where those in the project simply knew that they had the spirit of the country behind them.

The Power of Community

A major power for change is the collective power of the people in a community. By definition a community is a collection of people who live in a place and share the general values of that place. Most of the people in a community contribute resources and energy to the infrastructure of the community and in a sense have invested in that place through their taxes and employment. Communities develop powerful cultures over time that help shape the lives of the people who live there. Those cultures can be positive or negative. In the positive community culture people take pride in the appearance, the educational system, its recreational opportunities, and in the history and traditions of the community. Often the mobility rates of people moving in and out of the community are relatively low.

In a more negative culture, there is a sense of disconnect and anomie where people tend to shy away from working on behalf of the community, and the indicators of community problems and dysfunction are noticeable and real. Classic indicators of child abuse, school dropouts, teen pregnancies, and crime rates, among other indicators are significantly higher in troubled communities, and become self fulfilling particularly when these communities have high mobility rates with many people, in effect, just passing through.

Understanding the dynamics of a community in terms of the imbedded assets and liabilities associated with a community leads us to powerful low-cost strategies on behalf of positive change. Many communities now systematically measure their positive assets as a way to begin determining how to employ those assets on behalf of the people who live in the community. The quality of the schools, and other educational centers, the viability of the housing stock, the strength of neighborhoods, are all functions in one way or another of the quality and power of the understanding of how communities function.

In sum, we also need to constantly remind ourselves that the best governance, and the potential for the most and best change, lies in our communities. That there is more power for positive change locked up in our communities that all of the money in government programs. Strong common purpose, backed up with adequate resources, is a powerful and effective combination for change.

Practice

The power of human relationships, common purpose, and community, together, serve as a lens through which other more specific capacities for low cost-intervention and change can be considered. There are great resources beyond money that are available to help contribute to change. Most are straightforward common sense ways of doing business but which fall into disuse because of our inability to break out of our day to day way of doing business, and to put technique into the larger context of human relationships, common purpose and community, but which, if applied hold great promise for strong, low-cost, and effective results. There are a variety of low-cost, high value techniques that are available to us to improve the overall well-being of our people.

The Power of the Internet

The Internet is the most recent form of community that has emerged, as discussed in greater and more relevant detail in Chapter 15 (this volume). New communities of interest are constantly being developed on the Internet. The Internet is providing a new form of market where ideas, values, goods and materials are all bought, sold, and otherwise exchanged. One can take university level courses, find medical information, do almost unlimited research, 'talk' to people around the world, and serve as social network, all of this 24 hours a day.

The Internet is changing how we buy and sell things, how we elect our presidents and other public officials, how we trade humor, and how we learn about the world. It is increasingly becoming lower in cost, so that it is within the means of most of us. There are even current efforts to build a "100 dollar computer," which will bring the cost of the hardware to lows where a computer is within the means of virtually all of us.

The internet has become a low-cost venue for opportunities for individuals to know more about more in less and less time. The Internet may be having a negative impact on traditional community life, and it is certainly a different form and way of forming human relationships, and it is too soon to know what the longer-term impact on communities and individuals will be. But there is no doubt that the interest can serve as a low-cost, high-leverage medium for change. The speed of the development of the Internet has been breathtaking, as has the increasing numbers of people using the Internet for their many purposes. It has added a complete new range of words to our language, and it seems that the speed of Internet development is accelerating.

The Internet burst upon the scene 20 years ago, and is rapidly changing our traditional definition of community. There are now 'virtual' communities of people from different places who have common interest, regardless of where they live. We have seen both positive and negative consequences from this development.

There is much more personalized time on the Internet, in place of traditional group and community based activity. Many people now create and participate in their own communities of interest on the Internet at the expense of their traditional participation in group activities in their own communities. There is also a related lowering of personal accountability on the Internet. Any thing goes it seems. People can say anything and not be held accountable. About one half of all of the news now consumed by the general public is obtained through Internet "blogging" sites. The traditional news over the air outlets have come under much greater pressure to report the news sooner and earlier as a result of blogger pressure, with the result that the traditional news outlets are losing considerable market share.

We've seen the Internet greatly change how political campaigns are conducted. The Dean for President phenomenon was in large measure, Internet driven. Over half the households in the United States now have direct Internet access. We now do much of our business over the Internet. On the other hand, people now get their news from many sources, rather than just one or two. And the Internet has contributed to a kind of democracy where everyone's voice is just as important as anyone else's. And using Tom Friedman's analogy of a flattening of the earth, Internet users are simply several clicks away from almost all of the knowledge known to man. As a result, we are now in direct economic competition with people in China, India, and Brazil, where what you know, how we learn, and how quickly we can know it, is at the center of huge personal change, opportunity, danger, and knowledge accumulation.

All in all, the Internet has been an explosion of a relatively low-cost technology, which is changing our lives in ways that we easily recognize, and in ways that cannot yet be contemplated. It is truly a low cost-strategy available for future change.

The Power of Volunteerism

The power of volunteerism, which speaks to community, common purpose, and human relationships, is quite remarkable. Volunteerism is one of the very low-cost strategies at our disposal that can make big differences in outcomes and results. A current and effective version of volunteerism is the current mentoring movement. Mentoring combines the idea of volunteerism with building fundamental human relationships upon which human change can occur.

Even though we have seen a significant decline in the volunteerism of formal church attendance, which was the basis for strong volunteerism for many years, we have seen a resurgence in the power of other organizations to bring volunteered improvements to their communities, such as the volunteer roles that service organizations such as Rotary, Lions, Kiwanis, and other community service groups bring to the table. Further, volunteers are the backbone of many of our youth sports groups and teams. Every week the newspapers are filled with notices about the need for volunteers to take on one project or another in a community.

These opportunities fill a large need by the people who volunteer, in addition to the benefits to those who are the recipient of the volunteer time and energy. Volunteerism meets an innate need of human beings to contribute to the common good. And it is a way to contribute without getting caught up into long-term rigid arrangements and where there is much flexibility in the way that the volunteerism is applied. Guardians Ad Litem, for example, combine well the elements of providing an important human relationship to a young person in difficulty, but also melds in the aspect of community support for the individual through volunteerism.

A strong and vital ethic of volunteerism in a community is a low-cost way to contribute to positive change in a community. And, the well is much deeper than we have experienced to date. The current wave of volunteer mentors is only now grabbing hold in our communities and has the potential to change many lives for the better in the process.

The Use of Multi-Year Operational Budgets

Using a longer time frame in government budgeting processes is an example of away to promote low cost interventions. The current reality of government budgeting is that it is by and large a single year focused exercise. This makes it difficult for longer-term investments to be made in operating systems. The pressure to balance current year budgets makes serious investment in prevention problematical. One only needs to think about the general fund spending for corrections, the most remedial program in government, which now represents over 6% on average of general fund spending in the states, and continues to grow. Spending for corrections also exceeds the spending for higher education in most states. This is a most visible expression of the imbalance between remedial efforts and the much lower spending on prevention. This imbalance is due in large measure to the inability to fashion investment oriented multi-year budgets.

Finding ways to connect some portion of current year spending to longer term multi-year budgeting would go a long way to improving the prospects for meaningful prevention spending. Using corrections as an example, a budgeting process that would take the equivalent of 10% of the corrections budget for multi-year investments in prevention activities and programs, would unleash a new energy around the idea of calculating longer term cost benefit of investments in prevention.

Understanding the Power of Mid- to Longer-Term Cost Benefit

One of the ideas that naturally flows from multi-year operating budgets is a better understanding of the power of mid to longer term cost benefit thinking. Multi-year budgets allow us to think in more investment terms. Investing early in the lives of our people will provide bigger benefits at a later date. In the year-to year maelstrom of year to year budgets, this way of thinking and benefiting is not possible, unless there is a surplus of resources beyond what is needed for this year's governmental operational requirements. This is rarely the case.

One of the implications of longer term budgetary and operational planning is the opportunity to move beyond the requirements of the traditional domains of government – health, safety, environment, culture, sports, and education – toward a more developmental view of important well-being outcomes such as: All Pregnant Women and Young Children Thrive; All Children Are Ready for School; and All Children Succeed in School, and so on up the developmental ladder. This kind of construction of outcomes, and their related indicators, along with budgetary resources connected to these points on the life cycle, present the opportunity for us to think about our operational budgetary investments over a longer period. The natural effect of this way of thinking is to consider operating investments to be applied earlier in the life cycle than investments in the traditional budgetary and program domains. This results in earlier consideration of the overall well-being of the people and has social and budgetary effects throughout the remaining life cycle.

The Potential of Health Promotion

Longer term budgeting allows new models for thinking about investment. Multi-year investment models then unlock the idea of promotion to become a primary budgeting technique, rather than being the recipient of budget leftovers. The power lies in the basic idea that a relatively small investment can result in relatively large benefits. The algorithms regarding the economic power of investing in immunizations early in life that can preempt later costly and debilitating diseases makes the point. Investing in promotion to prevent young teen pregnancies, which can reduce the number of teen pregnancies over time, has been shown to avoid considerable direct cost of intervention connected to a young teen pregnancy. The budgetary implications of this example are clear. These budgetary implications do not include the social benefits of avoiding unwanted children, and the difficult long-term economic circumstances often associated with teen pregnancies for the mother and child.

Once again, we talk a lot about this kind of promotion, but we don't fund it very well, as we continue to fund well the back end more tertiary realities that can largely exist as a result of our not funding promotion strongly enough, particularly promotion that benefits those early in their life cycle. This is an example of a low-cost intervention, which can have significant benefit down the road.

An Example of Promotion: Universal Visits to all Families with Newborns

In Vermont in the early 1990s, a simple and low-cost strategy was employed to improve the well-being of the children of Vermont. Simply put, an effort to offer visits to the families of all newborns, conducted by people in local communities, was begun. Following is a graphic, which shows how that strategy unfolded over the years.

There are about 6,000 births per year in Vermont. The visits were conducted by a variety of local organizations and entities, and ranged from public health nurses in several areas of Vermont, to the school nurse in other places, to trained neighborly volunteers in other places. The cost of the intervention was low, by most standards, and has been calculated at the level of several hundred dollars per visit. Being careful about claiming cause and effect, following are some of the indicators of children's well-being that changed for the better over the years.

The 'story behind the story' of lowered lead levels was the informal conversation between family and visitor. "How old is the house? Is it older than 1974? If so, can we look to see if there are any paint chips around the window? It looks like there is some ground paint dust around the windows, which undoubtedly has some lead in it. Can we arrange for a lead screen for your toddler?" Those were the low cost neighborly conversations that contributed to the above result.

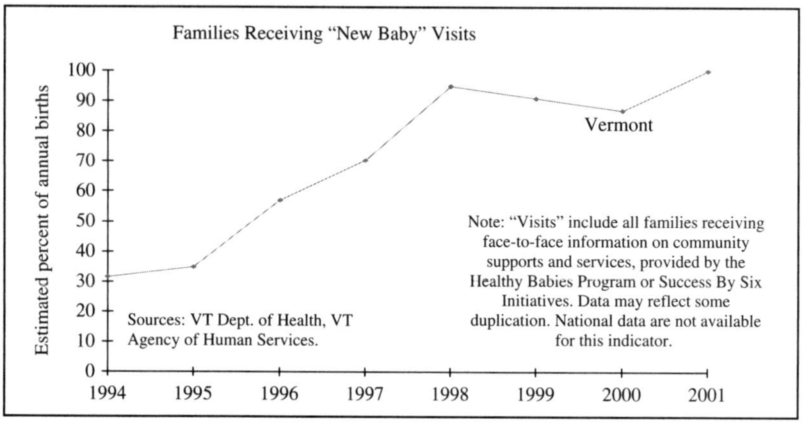

Figure 26.1. Families Receiving "New Baby" Visits.

This steadily declining child death rate, was a function of many interventions, but the key insight is that when preventable deaths versus non preventable deaths are tracked, it is clear that the preventable death rate declined greatly. Again, quiet, educational conversations with families who describe what shaking a baby can do to the brain stem, or what is the best way to have a baby sleep in a crib, along with the sharing of literature and current information, is a low-cost strategic way that can contribute to measurable positive change.

Declines in child abuse can be clearly shown over the period. And declines in young baby child sexual abuse were remarkable with declines of over 50% over the period. Again, the neighborly sense of caring and communication with families of newborns were contributors to this phenomenon.

The visits also allowed stronger connections to school systems. Educational and friendly conversations in the home between the family and the home visitor made it easier for young children who were entering school or who were already in school to take advantage of school breakfast and lunch programs, and ensured that they did. Again, there are many reasons for

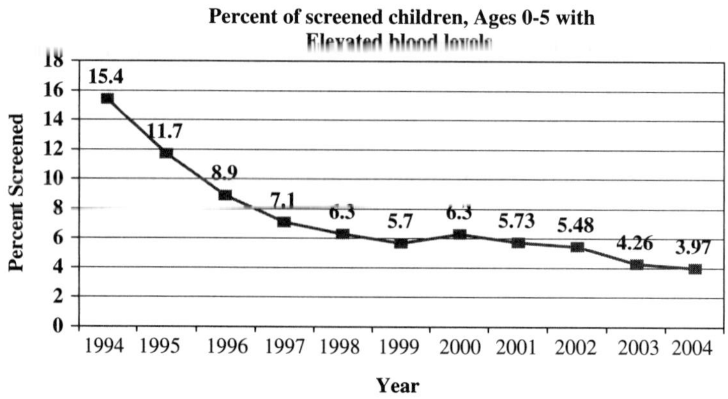

Figure 26.2. Percent of Screened Children, Ages 0–5 with Elevated Blood Levels.

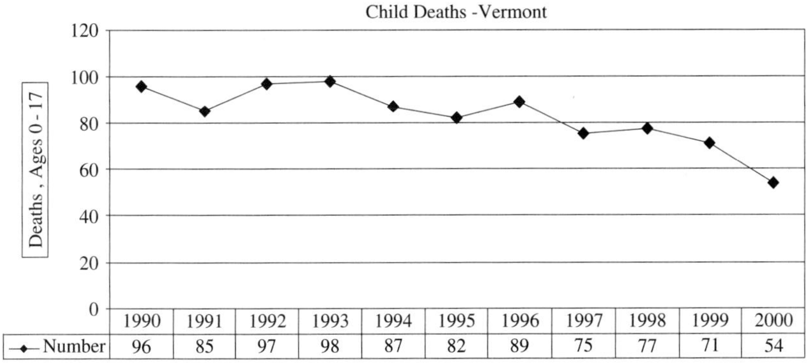

Figure 26.3. Child Deaths-Vermont.

this indicator improvement, but the early referrals and education certainly contributed to this result.

Knowing who the father of a newborn is can contribute greatly to the longer term well-being of a child. And there is a moment when a child is born, that everyone rallies around the mother. And the feelings that a father may have for a child can be stronger at this point, and often they are visible in the family in those early months. That is the time when fathers are asked to accept paternity responsibility for the child. In many cases, this can have long-term positive economic consequences for the child and family. This is certainly a low-cost intervention that has positive results. This can also be seen in the next graph, which tracks the rising value of child support over the period. The opportunity to have families sign their children up for state-sponsored health insurance in these visits also contributed significantly to the virtual universal coverage of children for health insurance in Vermont, as shown by the following graph.

The impact of this low cost intervention can also be seen in the rate of immunizations.

In sum, Vermont saw consistent and long-term improvements in indicators of child-well being over the course of the 1990s, which have continued during the course of the first half of the current decade. The low-cost intervention of

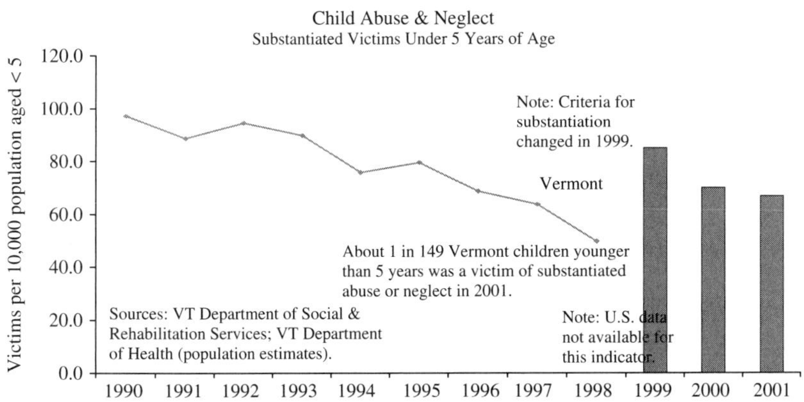

Figure 26.4. Child Abuse and Neglect.

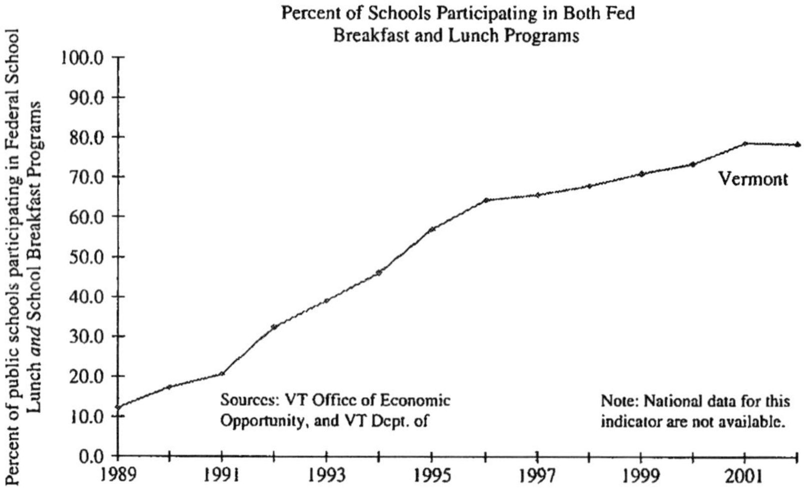

Figure 26.5. Percent of Schools Participating in Both Federal Breakfast and Lunch Programs.

offering visits to the families of newborns over that course of time translated into the contribution of noticeable and measurable improvement in important indicators of well-being.

Arranging for Dividends

We can build "dividends" into budgetary transactions where it can clearly be shown that the benefit of an investment is greater than the investment itself. To obtain the benefit is a technique that is well within our knowledge and capacity, but which is rarely used in a governmental setting.

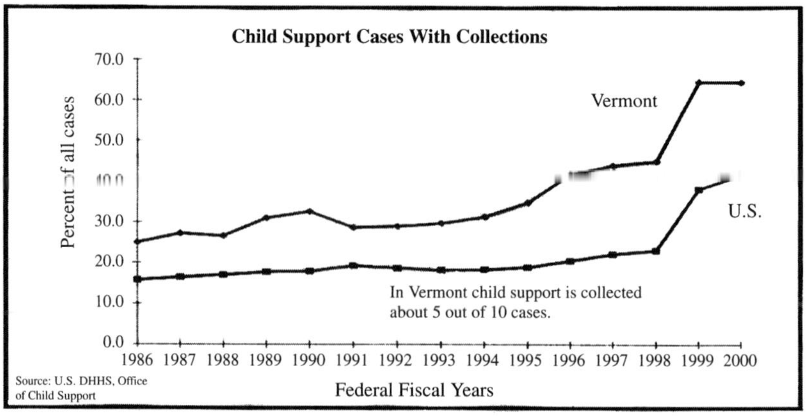

	1986	1987	1988	1989	1990	1991	1992	1993	1994	1995	1996	1997	1998	1999	2000
Vermont	25.0	27.0	26.6	31.0	32.6	28.7	29.0	29.7	31.3	34.8	41.7	43.9	44.9	64.5	64.4
U.S.	15.7	16.4	17.0	17.7	17.9	19.3	18.7	18.2	18.3	18.9	20.5	22.1	23.0	38.1	41.6
VT Rank	12	9	8	3	1	1	1	1	8	6	1	1	1	3	7

("1" is highest)

Figure 26.6. Child Support Cases with Collections.

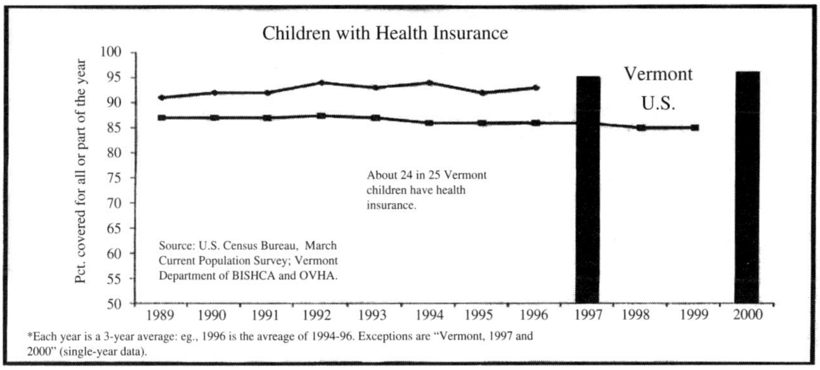

	1989	1990	1991	1992	1993	1994	1995	1996	1997	1998	1999	2000
Vermont	91	92	92	94	93	94	92	93	95	n/a	n/a	96
U.S.	87	87	87	87	87	86	86	86	86	85	85	86
VT Rank	n/a	12	14	9	3	1	2	1	n/a	n/a	n/a	n/a

("1" is highest)

Figure 26.7. Children with Health Insurance.ections.

One example that readily comes to mind was an experiment in one of the local regions of Vermont human services in the late 1990s. The opportunity came as a result of localized data which was showing that one particular region of the state was showing considerably higher rates of out of area placements for children in the custody of the child protective services unit of government. That realization caused a calculation of the direct cost of serving a child in the region, versus the cost of serving the same child outside the region, often in a very costly out-of-area facility. Those calculations produced no surprise – namely that it is much more costly to serve a child out of the area than it would be to keep the child in the region and in the process purchase high quality services.

With this comparative data in hand, the child protection division proposed to the local community partnership that if the number of children from that region served out of the region could be reduced, it would result in net lower

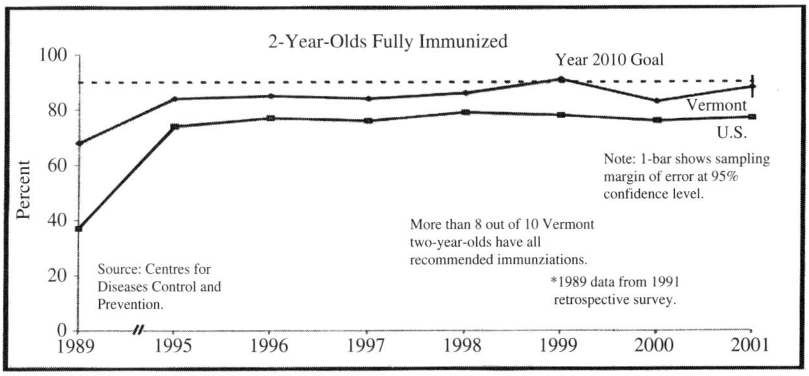

	1989	1995	1996	1997	1998	1999	2000	2001
Vermont	68	84	85	84	86	91	83	88
U.S.	37	74	77	76	79	78	76	77
VT Rank	2	3	3	4	6	1	8	1

("1" is highest)

Figure 26.8. Two-year-Olds Fully Immunized.

aggregate costs of serving all children from the region. Further, the proposition was made that the "savings" as a result of serving more children in their home region be split between the local children's services partnership and the state's budget. It was to be a clear demonstration of a win/win scenario if fewer children were served out of the region.

As time unfolded, fewer children were indeed served out of the home area, and were served well inside their home region, and the savings were divided as planned between the local and state budgets. And, the only condition placed on the use of the money sent back to the district was that it be used for further intervention work, thus priming the pump for even further and future savings as a result of handling even more children in their home district.

This is but one example as to how arranging for intervention dividends can not only save important resources, but can result in a more healthy set of local interventions that have a greater chance of making the lives of children better.

Having Formal Outcomes and Indicators

A system of formal outcomes of well-being and their regular and visible measurement is virtually a no-cost way to engage the energy of wide-ranging people and organizations around commonly held desired results. Powerful outcomes and their indicators that are clear and declarative, positive in a world of negative indicators, that are big enough to engage a range of people toward a common outcome. The indicators are presented over enough time to determine whether or not there is progress toward a widely held outcome. This approach can pull the energy and resources of government, nonprofits, the private sector, churches, communities, families and others toward the strongly stated common purpose.

A strong system of outcomes and indicators, wisely managed, can tell us where we've been, where we are, and where we are going. Managed well, it can help build critical mass for change, build public confidence that positive change is possible, and generally motivate us to improve. This approach to contributing to desired change is another tool that is at our disposal, that does not require large sums of money to implement, but over time can accumulate results that improve the overall well-being of our people, and help us to use our resources more wisely.

Having Knowledgeable and Committed Leaders

There are also things that we can do that don't cost a lot of money. These things will have a major impact on the results we seek, and, if not done, will and do cause us considerable agony and great cost. I'm referring to one of the major and visible lessons of Hurricane Katrina, where it became painfully clear that appointing people to key positions because of their political contributions instead of their professional experience and expertise had terrible, costly, and even deadly consequences.

There has been a long-standing trend by the two political parties to place partisans in as many places in the government as possible, toward the end of enhancing the ability to enact the policies of the party in power. This system wasn't a problem, as long as the partisans had the kind of professional backgrounds needed to do a good job. However, that standard appears to be slipping, with the result that more and more people are appointed to key positions with little regard for professional experience or credentials. The American public got a taste of the impact of this trend as we all watched with horror the mega failure, arrogance, and ineptitude of the leader of FEMA, which contributed to the loss of life, limb, and property in the aftermath of Katrina. There could not have been a stronger and clearer expression of this danger. Simply put, poor leadership in key governmental functions can result in unnecessary and large cost. A little applied common sense could upright this problem.

More Attention and Training in the Use of Science Based Decision Making

The body of knowledge that science is providing us regarding the human condition has continued to develop and enlarge. However, the application of what we are learning is lagging far behind our understanding about what is possible. Much of the reason for this is that people who become public servants at any level receive little training or education about the possibilities that science provides. One significant exception to this would be in the public health world, where a constant stream of scientific findings regarding issues such as the use of tobacco, the role that obesity plays in our overall health, and the ability of seat belts to help us avoid death and injury, are but a few examples. Current attention by the American public to diet and nutrition show us clearly the mass potential of the application of the expanding body of knowledge. New findings regarding the combined role of exercise and diet in the lives of diabetics are occurring rapidly.

However, in other important and expensive areas of our lives, science or data- based decisions give way to emotionalism and value-based decisions. In this instance I find myself thinking about policies and practices regarding criminal justice, and particularly those connected to corrections. Very few programs and interventions connected to corrections work are based on data and science. We know much about the relationship of diet to behavior for example. We also know that generally, the longer sentences of incarceration are the less likely successful behavior will occur after release, yet, we continue to incarcerate numbers and rates of people seen only at levels in the Soviet Union and South Africa. We almost ignore the results of other systems and policies of incarceration such as those in the Scandinavian countries. For instance, we know how to supervise nonviolent people in community settings, using the rapidly emerging technology and science of globally positioned satellites, yet we continue to use bricks and mortar, and pay in the neighborhood of $30,000 for each nonviolent person we incarcerate. We continue to increase the numbers of people incarcerated even though crime rates have dropped significantly over the last decade. And there is no rational basis for the over incarceration of black people verses white people. On this subject we seem to have abandoned even the pretense of using data based and science based decision-making. And yet, it is one of most rapidly growing costs in our society.

In a more general view, we could benefit from requiring science-based assessments of the possibilities similar to required environmental assessments that we use regularly and effectively in the world of construction development.

The earlier discussion (Chapter 2 this volume) regarding the biological foundations for behavioral and psychological approaches are a demonstration of how the boundaries of what we know are rapidly expanding.

Ways to Influence the Behavior of People Beyond Money

Earlier in this chapter there was a display of graphs, which showed a set of substantial indicator improvements as they related to a common purpose outcome of "All Children Are Ready for School." One of the key elements of the outcomes work is that virtually everyone can contribute to an improving outcome. And in that situation, it then follows that everyone can receive approbation and credit for the improvement. This set of dynamics fosters change about how people think about their work, and can improve the overall satisfaction that people have in their work. And a sense of satisfaction and achievement is an important reward for people, beyond money.

Toward the end of a sustained effort to improve fundamental outcomes for people by the agency and its departments of human services in Vermont, in 1999 an effort was made to measure the overall impact that the work had on the 2,700 people who worked in the agency. A survey was constructed and sent out to every employee, along with their paycheck. Basically the survey asked a brief set of questions that would help us determine whether the outcomes work over the previous eight years was influencing the employees' views of the importance of their jobs.

Four hundred and thirty employees responded. Of those that responded, 94% indicated that their work clearly contributed to the improving outcomes. The responses came from every department, and from every level of the organization. We also left room on the survey for people to write a short narrative if they so wished regarding their view of their contribution. The richness of the narrative responses was telling. Employees truly saw their work as contributing in specific ways to the improving outcomes. Seeing the bigger picture was a strong and important motivator and source of satisfaction as people now had a better sense of what the overall purpose of their work was, and how they could contribute to a much broader outcome beyond the confines of their specific work role or job description.

This intangible, in the form of energy, focus, and attention to broader purpose, helped each employee contribute to a larger and more universal outcome. It is an example of a low-cost preventative strategy which can help achieve results in a broad based manner.

Policy Implications of Low-Cost Interventions

None of the interventions discussed in this book are beyond our technical ability to implement them. Singly or accumulatively, implementation would result in measurable and long-term improvement in the well-being of the people we serve. And yet, we don't do these things, or if we do attempt some of them we merely nibble at the edges.

Our working lives have become so complex, and the speed of our working lives has increased to breathtaking levels. We simply, as organizations and individuals, do not take the time to determine thoughtfully what we want to achieve, and how to go about it.

The policy implications of not taking the time to put in place known interventions are costly both in fiscal and human terms. The cost of bad results can be calculated and they are impressively depressing. In a world where there are major forces increasingly competing for our relatively fixed resources, we have a duty and responsibility to use our resources in ways we know can work the best way possible.

The interventions discussed in this book can have impact, for example, on the unacceptable rising cost of healthcare, which is already under pressure from our rapidly aging population. Some of the interventions could have impact on the hyper costly toll in the rapidly expanding numbers of people incarcerated in the country, which has recently passed the two million-person mark.

But these changes will require disciplined changes in the way we construct important policy. We need to shift from short-range policy making to a longer term view. And longer term policy views need to apply the discipline of longer term cost benefit thinking. And longer term cost benefit decisions then need to result in freeing up some proportion of avoided costs to apply to a higher and more liberal application of resources for more interventions that work.

In summary, we need to, in effect, create a new kind of machine, a prevention machine, fueled by the existing knowledge about what can and could work, if we only applied what we now know to the human condition.

Some Conclusive Thoughts

Most of the above thoughts are about broad ideas that if implemented don't cost a lot of money. But, if implemented they have the potential, applying the rules of cost benefit, to improve substantially the well-being of the people we all serve in one way or another, and at the same time to avoid the spending of considerable sums of money that we now spend unnecessarily. The strategies enumerated here, along with strategies and interventions not noted here are large enough to have an impact of considerable scale.

Few of the strategies discussed would require new laws. But all would require more formal administrative policy to implement. And all of the enumerated strategies could be implemented over a relatively short period of time.

In a world where the need for better performance and investment is greater than our readily available resources to meet those needs, the wise spending of taxpayer dollars becomes even more important. These low-cost ideas of earlier and more effective intervention can contribute strongly to effective public policy strategies and have long reaching and lasting effects.

Subject Index

Printed in the United States of America.